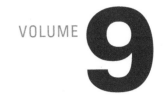

DISEASE CONTROL PRIORITIES • THIRD EDITION

Disease Control Priorities: Improving Health and Reducing Poverty

DISEASE CONTROL PRIORITIES • THIRD EDITION

Disease Control Priorities: Improving Health and Reducing Poverty

EDITORS

Dean T. Jamison
Hellen Gelband
Susan Horton
Prabhat Jha
Ramanan Laxminarayan
Charles N. Mock
Rachel Nugent

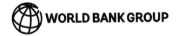 **WORLD BANK GROUP**

ISBNs and DOIs:

Softcover:
ISBN (paper): 978-1-4648-0527-1
ISBN (electronic): 978-1-4648-0528-8
DOI: 10.1596/978-1-4648-0527-1

Hardcover:
ISBN (paper): 978-1-4648-0529-5

DOI: 10.1596/978-1-4648-0529-5

Cover photo: © World Bank. Further permission required for reuse.

Chapter opener photo: © Frank Spangler/Worldview Images. Used with the permission of Worldview Images. Further permission required for reuse.

Library of Congress Cataloging-in-Publication Data has been requested.

Contents

PART 1   OBJECTIVES AND CONCLUSION OF *DISEASE CONTROL PRIORITIES,*
THIRD EDITION

1. Universal Health Coverage and Intersectoral Action for Health   3

*Dean T. Jamison, Ala Alwan, Charles N. Mock, Rachel Nugent, David A. Watkins, Olusoji Adeyi,
Shuchi Anand, Rifat Atun, Stefano Bertozzi, Zulfiqar Bhutta, Agnes Binagwaho, Robert Black,
Mark Blecher, Barry R. Bloom, Elizabeth Brouwer, Donald A. P. Bundy, Dan Chisholm,
Alarcos Cieza, Mark Cullen, Kristen Danforth, Nilanthi de Silva, Haile T. Debas, Peter Donkor,
Tarun Dua, Kenneth A. Fleming, Mark Gallivan, Patricia Garcia, Atul Gawande, Thomas Gaziano,
Hellen Gelband, Roger Glass, Amanda Glassman, Glenda Gray, Demissie Habte, King K. Holmes,
Susan Horton, Guy Hutton, Prabhat Jha, Felicia Knaul, Olive Kobusingye, Eric Krakauer,
Margaret E. Kruk, Peter Lachmann, Ramanan Laxminarayan, Carol Levin, Lai Meng Looi,
Nita Madhav, Adel Mahmoud, Jean-Claude Mbanya, Anthony R. Measham, María Elena Medina-Mora,
Carol Medlin, Anne Mills, Jody-Anne Mills, Jaime Montoya, Ole Norheim, Zachary Olson,
Folashade Omokhodion, Ben Oppenheim, Toby Ord, Vikram Patel, George C. Patton, John Peabody,
Dorairaj Prabhakaran, Jinyuan Qi, Teri Reynolds, Sevket Ruacan, Rengaswamy Sankaranarayanan,
Jaime Sepúlveda, Richard Skolnik, Kirk R. Smith, Marleen Temmerman, Stephen Tollman,
Stéphane Verguet, Damian Walker, Neff Walker, Yangfeng Wu, and Kun Zhao*

2. Intersectoral Policy Priorities for Health   23

*David A. Watkins, Rachel Nugent, Helen Saxenian, Gavin Yamey, Kristen Danforth,
Eduardo González-Pier, Charles N. Mock, Prabhat Jha, Ala Alwan, and Dean T. Jamison*

3. Universal Health Coverage and Essential Packages of Care   43

*David A. Watkins, Dean T. Jamison, Anne Mills, Rifat Atun, Kristen Danforth,
Amanda Glassman, Susan Horton, Prabhat Jha, Margaret E. Kruk, Ole F. Norheim,
Jinyuan Qi, Agnes Soucat, Stéphane Verguet, David Wilson, and Ala Alwan*

Foreword

Bill and Melinda Gates
Gates Foundation, Seattle, Washington, United States

During the past 25 years, many countries have achieved significant improvements in human health and well-being. Huge problems persist, and terrible inequities must still be addressed to ease the suffering of the world's poorest and most vulnerable. But that does not diminish several remarkable accomplishments: Since the early 1990s, the world has seen substantial reductions in extreme poverty; child and maternal mortality; and the incidence of deadly and debilitating diseases, such as tuberculosis, malaria, and HIV/AIDS. The incidence of polio has decreased by 99 percent, bringing the world to the verge of eradicating a major infectious disease for only the second time in history.

Credit for these and other advances in global health belongs to many institutions, governments, and individuals, including the scholars who organized and contributed to the first and second editions of *Disease Control Priorities*. We hope and expect this third edition also will have a large, salutary impact.

The first edition, *DCP1*, was published by the World Bank in 1993. It was the first comprehensive effort to systematically assess the effectiveness of interventions against the major diseases of low-income and middle-income countries. *DCP1* also analyzed the relative costs of interventions, enabling policy makers and aid donors to make smarter decisions about how to allocate scarce health dollars for the greatest impact. *DCP1* helped bring about dramatic shifts in how countries and the global community invest in health.

Indirectly, *DCP1* also influenced our personal decision to devote much of our philanthropy to improving the health of people in poor countries. This came about because data from *DCP1* was a basis for the World Bank's 1993 *World Development Report*, which focused on investing in health and catalyzed our thinking about how and where we could make a difference. We were

stunned to read that 11 million young children were dying every year from preventable causes such as pneumonia, diarrhea, malaria, and other infections that are rare or rarely fatal in the developed world. We were shocked by the disparities in health outcomes between rich countries and poorer ones. Every page screamed out that human life was not being valued as it should be.

In addition, our eyes were opened to the fact that most preventable deaths and disability in lower-income countries were caused not by hundreds of diseases but by relatively few, and that the costs of preventing and treating them were often low, relative to the benefits. Our shock turned to excitement. Here were points of leverage where we could work to reduce inequity and help realize a world where every person has the opportunity to live a healthy, productive life.

DCP2, published in 2006, again advanced the conversation on global health. Where *DCP1* focused on the benefits and costs of interventions against individual diseases, contributors to *DCP2* also considered how countries might gain greater traction by organizing their efforts around multi-purpose health platforms, ranging from village clinics and school-based health programs to district hospitals with emergency services and surgical units. *DCP2* showed how investments in health platforms, especially for community-based primary care, could magnify impact despite limited budgets. Several countries, particularly India and Ethiopia, have pursued this approach with good results.

In important and useful ways, this third edition of *Disease Control Priorities* further widens the frame for discussion of health policies and priorities, innovatively addressing the different needs of countries at different stages in the development of their health systems. This edition maps out pathways—essential packages of related, cost-effective interventions—that countries can consider to speed their progress toward universal health coverage. *DCP3* also draws attention to the catastrophically impoverishing effects that many medical procedures can have on poor families. This analysis, combined with data on the lost productivity caused by various diseases, provides insights into how investing in health, particularly in expanded access to health insurance and prepaid care, can not only save lives but also help alleviate poverty and bolster financial security.

Across the three editions, some conclusions remain constant. Childhood vaccinations, nutrition programs, access to treatment for common infections—these pay enormous returns in lives saved and suffering avoided. Family planning, maternal health programs, and gender equity benefit communities and society as a whole. Major infectious diseases can be beaten through collaborative, international efforts, as the past 25 years have shown. Overall, improving the health of the world's most vulnerable people remains one of the best investments the global community can continue to make toward realizing a better, safer world.

Introduction

Lawrence H. Summers
Harvard University, Boston, Massachusetts, United States

Most economists pride themselves on combining social concern with hard analysis. This trait they share with an important strand of the human rights community working on global health. The late Jonathan Mann, to take a leading example, both argued for an idealistic vision of health as a human right for all and created, from almost nothing, the World Health Organization's (WHO) effective and pragmatic Global Programme against AIDS. Paul Farmer continues to provide global leadership in advocating health as a human right, but he rightly emphasizes that advocacy alone remains insufficient. In Partners in Health, an organization Farmer cofounded with Jim Kim (now president of the World Bank), Farmer created a vehicle to go beyond advocacy and develop the practical dimensions of the aspiration to provide the highest quality of health care in rural Haiti, Rwanda, and elsewhere. In his essay "Rethinking Health and Human Rights," Farmer points to the importance of research in this agenda: "The purpose of this research should be to do a better job of bringing the fruits of science and public health to the poorest communities" (2010, p. 456). Farmer and I may well have a different take on the contributions that have been made over time by the World Bank and other international financial institutions. But I think it fair to say that the pragmatic task of bringing technical knowledge to bear on the needs of the poor is a shared goal—and a goal that the *Disease Control Priorities* series has sought to advance for over two decades.

Each year the World Bank's flagship publication, the *World Development Report (WDR)*, attempts to assemble knowledge and to inspire action that serves the world's poorest communities. These reports develop and take stock of research and other evidence on a specific topic to inform the World Bank's own policies and to stimulate discourse among member countries, other development agencies, civil society, and the academic community. The *WDR*s are probably the world's most widely distributed economic publication. They are prepared by the World Bank's research arm, under the direction of its Chief Economist, a position I had the good fortune to hold in the period 1991–93. I selected health as the topic for *WDR 1993*.

Why health? First, health and poverty intertwine closely, and having a *WDR* on health provided an opportunity to provide insight into the World Bank's central goal of reducing poverty. Second, health represents an area where governments can play a necessary and constructive role. And third, I believed that the potential gains from getting health policy right were enormous. Thus, the *WDR 1993: Investing in Health*, was published in June of 1993 (World Bank 1993).

Several features dominated the global health landscape at the time of *the WDR 1993*. First, and most visibly, the HIV/AIDS epidemic had emerged from nowhere to grow into a major problem in Africa and globally. Second, but much less visibly, government policies to control undernutrition, excess fertility, and infection had begun to bear fruit. Consolidating and expanding the scope of these successes promised enormous gains. As a consequence of success, however, China and other countries with early progress were already experiencing substantial relative growth in their older populations—and concomitant growth in the incidence of cancer, heart disease, and stroke. Intervention against these diseases is less decisive and often far more costly than intervention against infection. Policy makers thus experienced strong pressures to divert resources from high payoff infection control to responding to noncommunicable diseases.

In response to these features of the health landscape, the World Bank's policy staff had initiated a review of priorities for disease control. Its purpose was to identify effective yet affordable responses to the epidemics of HIV/AIDS and noncommunicable disease while expanding successes in control of childhood infection. Work began on the *WDR 1993* while the priorities review was drawing to a close. The detailed analyses of value for money in that review provided strong intellectual underpinnings for the *WDR 1993*. Oxford University Press published the *WDR 1993* and the first edition of *Disease Control Priorities in Developing Countries* at about the same time (Jamison, Mosley, Measham, and Bobadilla 1993; World Bank 1993).

On the occasion of the 20th anniversary of publication of the *WDR 1993*, *The Lancet* invited me to chair a commission to reassess health policies in light of two decades of remarkable change (mostly for the good) in health and related institutions around the world. *Global Health 2035*, the report of the *Lancet* Commission on Investing in Health (Jamison, Summers, and others 2013) took stock of those changes and drew policy implications for coming decades. Perhaps the most important message from Global Health 2035 is that our generation, uniquely in history, has the resources and knowledge to close most of the enormous health gap between rich and poor within a generation. The work of the *Lancet* Commission provided a policy framework for this concluding volume of the third edition of *Disease Control Priorities* (*DCP3*). For evidence-oriented decision makers in ministries and in development agencies, and for a broader community, the *DCP* series has provided (as it did for *Global Health 2035*) a wealth of information relevant to informing policies for improving health and reducing health-related poverty.

Let me close by placing *DCP3* into a context not just of health policy formulation but also of macroeconomic policy formulation. Macroeconomic policy encompasses three major components:

- Establishing and enforcing an environment for secure and inclusive economic growth. Creating this environment includes finance of domestic and international security, enforcement of contracts and property rights, regulation of cross border flows (goods and services, capital, persons), and establishing the broad structure and regulation of the financial system. Global warming and the risk of severe pandemics pose particular challenges to long-term economic growth. In chapter 18 of this volume, I report work undertaken with several colleagues that assesses the magnitude of pandemic influenza risk (Fan, Jamison, and Summers 2018). Suffice it to say that low probability but potentially devastating pandemics pose a global risk—but particularly a risk to lower-income countries—that warrants inclusion on the macroeconomic policy agenda.

- Establishing mechanisms for social insurance—insurance that enables income security in old age; that provides a financial safety net against permanent disability, against transitory job loss, and against inadequate earning power; and that provides financial protection against medical expenses. *DCP3*'s extended cost-effectiveness analysis introduces an approach to efficient purchase of financial protection against medical expenses.

- Allocation of resources within and across those sectors where efficient levels of investment require substantial public finance. These sectors include much of physical infrastructure, research, education, environmental protection and population health.

DCP3's methods and conclusions provide critical guidance on resource allocation to and within the health sector. Spending the resources available for health investments on the wrong interventions is worse than inefficient: it costs lives. As *DCP3*'s findings make clear, huge variation remains in how many lives can be saved from a million dollars spent on different interventions. Transferring resources from low- to high-yield health interventions is, therefore, a moral imperative. Nor should resources available to the health sector be taken as given. Careful consideration of the social returns to increasing the health sector's share of national budgets and of national income suggests that, in many countries, macroeconomic policy makers underinvest in health.

My own career has centered on macroeconomic policy and on research to improve macroeconomic policy. Over the years I have increasingly come to feel that getting health policy right contributes importantly to improving the social insurance and public sector investment dimensions of macroeconomic policy. For this reason, I have closely followed the 20-year evolution of the disease control priorities agenda. This new edition continues *DCP*'s tradition of informing the efficient selection of health interventions. And it extends that agenda to informing choices where health policy can contribute to poverty reduction as well as health improvement.

REFERENCES

Fan, V. Y, D. T. Jamison, and L. H. Summers. 2018. "The Loss from Pandemic Influenza Risk." In *Disease Control Priorities* (third edition): Volume 9, *Disease Control Priorities: Improving Health and Reducing Poverty*, edited by D. T. Jamison, H. Gelband, S. Horton, P. Jha, R. Laxminarayan, C. N. Mock, and R. Nugent. Washington, DC: World Bank.

Farmer, P. 2010. "Rethinking Health and Human Rights: Time for a Paradigm Shift." In *Partner to the Poor: A Paul Farmer Reader*, chapter 21, 435–70, edited by H. Saussy. Berkley, Los Angeles, and London: University of California Press.

Jamison, D. T., W. H. Mosley, A. R. Measham, and J. L. Bobadilla, eds. 1993. *Disease Control Priorities in Developing Countries*. New York: Oxford University Press for the World Bank.

Jamison, D. T., L. H. Summers, G. Alleyne, K. J. Arrow, S. Berkley, and others. 2013. "Global Health 2035: A World Converging within a Generation." *The Lancet* 382 (9908): 1898–1955.

World Bank. 1993. *World Development Report: Investing in Health*. New York: Oxford University Press for the World Bank.

Preface

Budgets constrain choices. Policy analysis helps decision makers achieve the greatest value from limited available resources. In 1993, the World Bank published *Disease Control Priorities in Developing Countries* (DCP1), an attempt to systematically assess the cost-effectiveness (value for money) of interventions that would address the major sources of disease burden in low- and middle-income countries (LMICs). The World Bank's 1993 *World Development Report* on health drew heavily on *DCP1*'s findings to conclude that specific interventions against noncommunicable diseases were cost-effective, even in environments where high burdens of infection and undernutrition remained top priorities.

DCP2, published in 2006, updated and extended *DCP1* in several aspects, including explicit consideration of the implications for health systems of expanded intervention coverage. One way health systems expand coverage is through selected *platforms* that deliver interventions that require similar logistics but address heterogeneous health problems. Platforms often provide a more natural unit for investment than do individual interventions. Analysis of the costs of providing platforms—and of the health improvements they can generate in given epidemiological environments—can help to guide health system investments and development.

DCP3 differs importantly from *DCP1* and *DCP2* by extending and consolidating the concepts of platforms and by offering explicit consideration of the financial risk protection objective of health systems. In populations lacking access to health insurance or prepaid care, medical expenses that are high relative to income can be impoverishing. Where incomes are low, seemingly inexpensive medical procedures can have catastrophic financial effects. *DCP3* offers an approach (extended cost-effectiveness analysis, or ECEA) to explicitly include financial protection as well as the distribution across income groups of financial and health outcomes resulting from policies (for example, public finance) to increase intervention uptake. *DCP3* provides interested policymakers with evidenced-based findings on financial as well as health interventions to assist with resource allocation.

This volume of *DCP3*, volume 9, places the findings from the first eight volumes into a framework identifying an efficient pathway toward essential universal health coverage (EUHC) through the identification of 21 essential *packages* that include health interventions, and fiscal and intersectoral policies. The intervention packages are defined by groups with common professional interests (for example, child health or surgery) and include interventions delivered across a range of platforms. The volume also provides an up-to-date summary of levels and trends in deaths by cause and an early attempt to assess which elements of disease burden most contribute to impoverishment. While most of *DCP3*'s 21 packages of interventions are developed in the first eight volumes, several of the packages are presented here, including discussion of pandemic preparedness. Along with these new elements, *DCP3* updates the efforts of *DCP1* and *DCP2* to synthesize cost-effectiveness analysis of health interventions.

The overall convergence of many countries and international development partners around the UN Global Goals for 2030 has raised in particular the need for careful analytic work that informs priorities and choices. DCP3 stands unique in taking on this challenge, providing analyses of the contributions of 218 health system interventions and 71 intersectoral policies grouped into 21 essential packages.

DCP3 is a large-scale enterprise involving an international community of authors, editors, peer reviewers, and research and staff assistants who contributed their time and expertise to the preparation and completion of this series. We convey our acknowledgements elsewhere in this volume. Here we express our particular gratitude to the Bill & Melinda Gates Foundation for its sustained financial support, to the University of Washington's Department of Global Health for hosting *DCP3*'s Secretariat, and to the World Bank, the original home for the *DCP* series and accomplished publisher of its products.

Dean T. Jamison
Hellen Gelband
Sue Horton
Prabhat Jha
Ramanan Laxminarayan
Charles N. Mock
Rachel Nugent

Abbreviations

ACE	Advisory Committee to the Editors
AIDS	acquired immune deficiency virus
ANM	auxiliary nurse midwifery
ARI	acute respiratory illness
ART	antiretroviral therapy
BCA	benefit-cost analysis
BMI	body mass index
CCT	conditional cash transfer
CEA	cost-effectiveness analysis
CEPI	Coalition for Epidemic Preparedness Innovations
CHE	catastrophic health expenditure
CHWs	community health workers
CLAS	local health administration communities
COPD	chronic obstructive pulmonary disease
CPD	continuing professional development
CRS	Creditor Reporting System
CVD	cardiovascular disease
DAC	Development Assistance Committee
DALY	disability-adjusted life year
DCP2	*Disease Control Priorities in Developing Countries* (second edition)
DCP3	*Disease Control Priorities* (third edition)
DOTs	directly observed treatment, short course
ECEA	extended cost-effectiveness analysis
EP	essential package
EPHF	Essential Public Health Functions
EQA	external quality assurance
EUHC	essential universal health coverage
FRP	financial risk protection
FTE	full-time equivalent
Gavi	Gavi, the Vaccine Alliance
GBD	global burden of disease
GBHS	global burden of health-related suffering
GDP	gross domestic product

GHE	Global Health Estimates
GST	goods and services tax
HICs	high-income countries
HIV	human immunodeficiency virus
HIV/AIDS	human immunodeficiency virus/acquired immune deficiency syndrome
HPP	highest-priority package
IAMP	Interacademy Medical Panel
ICD	International Classification of Diseases
ICER	incremental cost-effectiveness ratio
ICU	intensive care unit
IHD	ischemic heart disease
IHME	Institute of Health Metrics and Evaluation
IHR	International Health Regulations
INEGI	National Institute of Statistics and Geography (Mexico)
IPCC	Intergovernmental Panel on Climate Change
LC-GAPCPC	*The Lancet* Commission on Global Access to Palliative Care and Pain Control
LICs	low-income countries
LIS	laboratory information systems
LMICs	low- and middle-income countries
LPG	liquefied petroleum gas
MDGs	Millennium Development Goals
MERS	Middle East respiratory syndrome
MICs	middle-income countries
MTB/RIF	mycobacterium tuberculosis/rifampicin
NAM	National Academy of Medicine
NCDs	noncommunicable diseases
NCEF	National Clean Energy Fund
NGO	nongovernmental organization
NTCP	National Tobacco Control Programme
NTDs	neglected tropical diseases
ODA	official development assistance
OECD	Organisation for Economic Co-operation and Development
OOP	out of pocket
P4P	pay for performance
PDS	public distribution system
PEF	Pandemic Emergency Financing Facility
PEPFAR	U.S. President's Emergency Plan for AIDS Relief
POCT	point-of-care testing
PPA	public-private alliance
PPP	purchasing power parity
PT	proficiency testing
QALYs	quality-adjusted life years
QIDS	Quality Improvement Demonstration Study
RBF	results-based financing
R&D	research and development
RNTCP	Revised National Tuberculosis Control Program
SARA	Service Availability and Readiness Assessment
SARS	severe acute respiratory syndrome

SDGs	Sustainable Development Goals
SMU	standard mortality unit
SRS	Sample Registration System
SSB	sugar-sweetened beverage
SSRI	selective serotonin reuptake inhibitor
STIs	sexually transmitted diseases
TB	tuberculosis
UHC	universal health coverage
UMICs	upper-middle-income countries
UN	United Nations
UNAIDS	Joint United Nations Programme on HIV/AIDS
UNPD	United Nations Population Division
UPF	universal public finance
USAID	U.S. Agency for International Development
VPD	vaccine preventable disease
VSL	value per statistical life
VSLr	VSL-to-income ratio
VSMU	value of a standard mortality unit
WHO	World Health Organization
WHO-CHOICE	Choosing Interventions That Are Cost-Effective
YLGs	years of life gained

Objectives and Conclusion of
Disease Control Priorities, Third Edition

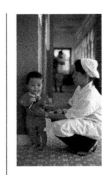

Universal Health Coverage and Intersectoral Action for Health

Dean T. Jamison, Ala Alwan, Charles N. Mock, Rachel Nugent, David A. Watkins, Olusoji Adeyi, Shuchi Anand, Rifat Atun, Stefano Bertozzi, Zulfiqar Bhutta, Agnes Binagwaho, Robert Black, Mark Blecher, Barry R. Bloom, Elizabeth Brouwer, Donald A. P. Bundy, Dan Chisholm, Alarcos Cieza, Mark Cullen, Kristen Danforth, Nilanthi de Silva, Haile T. Debas, Peter Donkor, Tarun Dua, Kenneth A. Fleming, Mark Gallivan, Patricia Garcia, Atul Gawande, Thomas Gaziano, Hellen Gelband, Roger Glass, Amanda Glassman, Glenda Gray, Demissie Habte, King K. Holmes, Susan Horton, Guy Hutton, Prabhat Jha, Felicia Knaul, Olive Kobusingye, Eric Krakauer, Margaret E. Kruk, Peter Lachmann, Ramanan Laxminarayan, Carol Levin, Lai Meng Looi, Nita Madhav, Adel Mahmoud, Jean-Claude Mbanya, Anthony R. Measham, María Elena Medina-Mora, Carol Medlin, Anne Mills, Jody-Anne Mills, Jaime Montoya, Ole Norheim, Zachary Olson, Folashade Omokhodion, Ben Oppenheim, Toby Ord, Vikram Patel, George C. Patton, John Peabody, Dorairaj Prabhakaran, Jinyuan Qi, Teri Reynolds, Sevket Ruacan, Rengaswamy Sankaranarayanan, Jaime Sepúlveda, Richard Skolnik, Kirk R. Smith, Marleen Temmerman, Stephen Tollman, Stéphane Verguet, Damian Walker, Neff Walker, Yangfeng Wu, and Kun Zhao

INTRODUCING *DISEASE CONTROL PRIORITIES*, THIRD EDITION

In 1993, the World Bank published *Disease Control Priorities in Developing Countries (DCP1)*, an attempt to systematically assess value for money (cost-effectiveness) of interventions that would address the major sources of disease burden in low- and middle-income countries (LMICs) (Jamison and others 1993). A major motivation for *DCP1* was to identify reasonable responses in highly resource-constrained environments to the growing burden of noncommunicable diseases (NCDs) and of human immunodeficiency virus/acquired immune deficiency syndrome (HIV/AIDS) in LMICs. The World Bank had highlighted the already substantial NCD problem in country studies for Malaysia (Harlan, Harlan, and

Oii 1984), for China (Jamison and others 1984), and in a *New England Journal of Medicine* Shattuck Lecture (Evans, Hall, and Warford 1981). Mexican scholars (Bobadilla and others 1993; Frenk and others 1989) pointed to the rapid growth of NCDs in Mexico and introduced the concept of a protracted epidemiological transition involving a dual burden of NCDs combined with significant lingering problems of infectious disease. The dual burden paradigm remains valid to this day. The World Bank's first (and so far only) *World Development Report* (1993) dealing with health drew heavily on findings from *DCP1* to conclude that a number of specific interventions against NCDs (including tobacco control and multidrug secondary prevention of vascular disease) were attractive even in environments where substantial

Corresponding author: Dean T. Jamison, University of California, San Francisco, California, United States; djamison@uw.edu.

burdens of infection and insufficient dietary intake remained policy priorities (World Bank 1993).

Disease Control Priorities, second edition (*DCP2*), published in 2006, updated and extended *DCP1* most notably by explicit consideration of implications for health systems of expanded coverage of high-priority interventions (Jamison and others 2006). One important link to health systems was through examination of selected *platforms* for delivering logistically related interventions that might address quite heterogeneous sets of problems. Platforms examined included the district hospital as a whole, the surgical and emergency room platforms within the district hospital, and school-based platforms for delivering a range of services. Platforms often provide a more natural unit for investment—and for estimating costs—than do individual interventions. Analysis of the costs of providing platforms—and of the health improvements they can generate in a given epidemiological environment—can thus help guide health system investments and development. Both *Disease Control Priorities,* third edition (*DCP3*), and the World Health Organization's (WHO)

major investment case for health (Stenberg and others 2017) continue to utilize platforms and their costs as important organizing concepts.

This chapter conveys the main findings of *DCP3*, and in particular its conclusions concerning intersectoral policy priorities and essential universal health coverage (EUHC). Like its two predecessors, *DCP3*'s broad aim is to assist decision makers in allocating often tightly constrained budgets so that health system objectives are maximally achieved. Beyond informing policy discourse, the granularity of analysis reported in *DCP3*'s nine volumes is intended to serve officials within ministries at the implementation level. Beginning with *DCP3* volume 1 on *Essential Surgery*, *DCP3*'s first eight volumes (and related overviews of six of them in *The Lancet*) appeared between 2015 and 2017. This final volume contains cross-cutting and synthesizing chapters. Box 1.1 lists *DCP3*'s nine volumes and their editors.

DCP3 differs importantly from *DCP1* and *DCP2* in terms of its multivolume format, in terms of extending

---

Box 1.1

DCP3's Nine Volumes

The World Bank has published *DCP3* in 2015–2018. In contrast to the single (very large) volume formats of *DCP1* and *DCP2*, *DCP3* appeared in nine smaller topical volumes, each with its own set of editors. Coordination across volumes is provided by seven series editors: Dean T. Jamison, Rachel Nugent, Hellen Gelband, Susan Horton, Prabhat Jha, Ramanan Laxminarayan, and Charles N. Mock. The topics and editors of the individual volumes are as follows:

Volume 1: *Essential Surgery,* edited by Haile T. Debas, Charles N. Mock, Atul Gawande, Dean T. Jamison, Margaret E. Kruk, and Peter Donkor, with a foreword by Paul Farmer

Volume 2: *Reproductive, Maternal, Newborn, and Child Health,* edited by Robert E. Black, Ramanan Laxminarayan, Marleen Temmerman, and Neff Walker, with a foreword by Flavia Bustreo

Volume 3: *Cancer,* edited by Hellen Gelband, Prabhat Jha, Rengaswamy Sankaranarayanan, and Susan Horton, with a foreword by Amartya Sen

Volume 4: *Mental, Neurological, and Substance Use Disorders,* edited by Vikram Patel, Dan Chisholm, Tarun Dua, Ramanan Laxminarayan, and María Elena Medina-Mora, with a foreword by Agnes Binagwaho

Volume 5: *Cardiovascular, Respiratory, and Related Disorders,* edited by Dorairaj Prabhakaran, Shuchi Anand, Thomas Gaziano, Jean-Claude Mbanya, Yangfeng Wu, and Rachel Nugent, with a foreword by K. Srinath Reddy

Volume 6: *Major Infectious Diseases,* edited by King K. Holmes, Stefano Bertozzi, Barry R. Bloom, and Prabhat Jha, with a foreword by Peter Piot

Volume 7: *Injury Prevention and Environmental Health,* edited by Charles N. Mock, Rachel Nugent,

box continues next page

Olive Kobusingye, and Kirk R. Smith, with a foreword by Ala Alwan

Volume 8: *Child and Adolescent Health and Development,* edited by Donald A. P. Bundy, Nilanthi de Silva, Susan Horton, Dean T. Jamison, and George C. Patton, with a foreword by Gordon Brown

Volume 9: *Disease Control Priorities: Improving Health and Reducing Poverty,* edited by Dean T. Jamison, Hellen Gelband, Susan Horton, Prabhat Jha, Ramanan Laxminarayan, Charles N. Mock, and Rachel Nugent, with a foreword by Bill and Melinda Gates and an introduction by Lawrence H. Summers.

Figure 1.1 Policies for Health

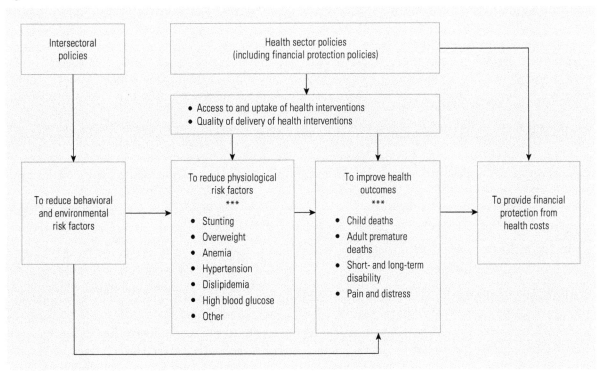

and consolidating the concept of platforms, and in terms of explicit consideration of a broad range of intersectoral and fiscal policies for health. Figure 1.1 illustrates the division of *DCP3*'s analyses between intersectoral policies and health sector policies and shows examples of the risk factors and conditions that the policies address. Importantly, the *DCP3* structure views the role of intersectoral action to be reduction of behavioral and environmental risks, which themselves affect the level of physiological risks and health outcomes directly. The health sector's role in reducing behavioral and environmental risk is viewed as modest—rather the health sector's main role is in reducing (some of) the physiological risk factors and reducing the duration and severity of health conditions and their sequelae. Appropriate health sector policies also offer the potential for reducing health-related financial risks in a population.

DCP3 has four major objectives that go beyond previous editions. The first is to address explicitly the financial risk protection and poverty reduction objective of health systems, as well as other objectives such as provision of contraception, reduction in stillbirths, and palliative care or enhancement of the physical and cognitive development of children. Standard health metrics such as the quality-adjusted life year (QALY) and disability-adjusted life year (DALY) fail to encompass these other objectives of health systems, and *DCP3* has endeavored to be explicit about them and their importance. The second extension lies in systematic attention to the intersectoral determinants of health.

The third major way that *DCP3* goes beyond previous editions lies in organizing interventions into 21 essential packages reflecting professional communities. Table 1.1 lists *DCP3*'s 21 packages. *DCP3* defines a concept of EUHC in the health systems components of the essential 21 packages. *DCP3* further identifies a subset of EUHC, the highest-priority package (HPP), that can potentially be afforded by low-income countries (LICs) and that offers the most potential achievement (given limited resources) of health, financial protection, and other objectives. Finally, *DCP3* provides estimates for low- and lower-middle-income countries of incremental and total costs in 2030 for both EUHC and HPP and of the magnitude of their impact on mortality. In addition to these new elements, *DCP3* updates the efforts of *DCP1* and *DCP2* to assemble and interpret the literature on economic evaluation of health interventions.

This chapter introduces the substantive topics addressed by *DCP3* and relays our main conclusions. Before turning to that, we briefly describe the context in which *DCP3*'s analyses have been undertaken.

CONTEXT

Five considerations set the context for *DCP3*: (a) the 20th-century revolution in human health, (b) the scientific underpinnings of that revolution, (c) the high estimated returns to (carefully chosen) health investments, and (d) the increasing implementation of universal health coverage (UHC) as a practical goal for domestic finance of health systems. Skolnik (2016) provides further discussion of these four issues. A fifth consideration concerns evolution in the thinking about the international dimension of health finance—development assistance for health broadly defined.

Chile exemplifies the two key elements of the 20th-century revolution in human health. One is the

sheer magnitude of improvement. As recently as 1910, Chilean life expectancy fell below 32 years. By 2012, life expectancy exceeded 78 years. Second, time has narrowed cross-country differences. In 1910, world leaders (such as Australia and New Zealand) achieved life expectancies almost 30 years greater than Chile, but by 2010 that gap had narrowed to around 4 years. The magnitude of Chile's success has been unusual, but the broad story it conveys is not. That said, Sub-Saharan Africa now lags 20 years behind global life expectancy of 72 years, and countries in other regions (and regions within large countries) remain similarly disadvantaged. *DCP3*'s main purpose is to provide information to help close those gaps.

Income growth in the past century and past decades has contributed to increased life expectancy as has, to a somewhat greater extent, improvements in education levels (Pradhan and others 2017). Most improvements, however, have resulted from an ever-expanding menu of drugs, diagnostics, vaccines, and knowledge (Jamison, Jha, and others 2013). Nurturing continuation of the scientific investment therefore remains a policy priority, as was extensively discussed in *DCP2* (Bloom and others 2006; Mahmoud and others 2006; Meltzer 2006; Weatherall and others 2006). *DCP3* has devoted less attention to research and development (R&D) than did *DCP2*—in part because of the coverage there. While R&D is discussed in several places (for example, Bundy and others 2017; Trimble and others 2015), a careful mining of *DCP3* for its implications for R&D remains to be done.

Valuation of mortality decline (or health change more generally) is excluded from the global system of national income and product accounts. Economists have nonetheless expended substantial effort tracing the effect of health improvements on household and national income and in assessing the value of the small reductions in mortality risk that have occurred year by year. *Global Health 2035* (GH2035), the report of the *Lancet* Commission on Investing in Health (Jamison, Summers, and others 2013), reviewed and extended the literature on the value of health improvements. That literature points to high returns indeed. The Copenhagen Consensus, a project that comparatively assesses returns across all major development sectors, has likewise found high returns: its 2012 assessment found that 9 of the 15 highest return investments were health-related, including all of the top 5 (Kydland and others 2013).

As national incomes rise, countries typically increase the percentage of national income devoted to health.

Equally significantly, they increase the proportion of health expenditures that are prepaid, usually through public or publicly mandated finance. WHO's leadership in advancing a global UHC agenda has accelerated this underlying movement of political systems toward UHC. Dr. Tedros Ghebreyesus, WHO's new Director-General, has reaffirmed the WHO commitment to UHC and to the use of evidence and data in support of achieving that goal (Ghebreyesus 2017). *GH2035* advocated variants on a pathway toward UHC, "progressive universalism," that emphasized two initial priorities for action: (a) universal coverage of publicly financed interventions and (b) reductions of user payments at the point of service to very low levels (Jamison, Summers, and others 2013). With inevitable constraints on public budgets, these two priorities point to the need for initial selectivity in the range of interventions to be publicly financed, the so-called benefits package. Many considerations will influence national choices of how benefits packages will evolve over time and on the appropriate pathways to universalism. Hence, the importance of maintaining the focus on the highest priority health investments as *DCP3* is intended to facilitate.

With substantial income growth in most LMICs and an increasing number of countries committed to public finance of UHC, the role of development assistance is being reexamined (Bendavid and others 2018; Jamison, Summers, and others 2013). As the World Bank and others have long argued, finance ministers will often reduce domestic allocations to sectors receiving substantial foreign aid. The challenge to those concerned with aid effectiveness thus becomes one of identifying and supporting important activities that national finance ministries are likely to underfinance (such as R&D, pandemic preparedness, and control of antimicrobial resistance). A recent assessment found that support for these international functions already constitutes more than 20 percent of development assistance broadly defined; the authors make the case that percentage should steadily increase over time (Schäferhoff and others 2015). This view of development assistance has clear implications for the construction of model benefits packages for domestic finance; other things being equal, domestic finance needs to emphasize services having minimal *international* externalities.

PACKAGES, PLATFORMS, AND POLICIES

DCP3 defines *packages* of interventions as conceptually related interventions—for example, those dealing with cardiovascular disease or reproductive health or surgery.

An objective of each *DCP3* volume was to define one or more essential packages and the interventions in that package that might be acquired at an early stage on the pathway to UHC. The essential packages comprise interventions that provide value for money, are implementable, and address substantial needs.

Platforms are defined as logistically related delivery channels. *DCP3* groups EUHC interventions within packages that can be delivered on different types of platforms. The temporal character of interventions is critical for health system development. Patients requiring nonurgent but substantial intervention—repair of cleft lips and palates is an example—can be accumulated over space and time, enabling efficiencies of high volume in service delivery. Urgent interventions, which include a large fraction of essential surgical interventions, are ideally available 24/7 close to where patients live—with important implications for dispersal of relevant platforms and integration of different services. Nonurgent but continuing interventions to address chronic conditions (for example, secondary prevention of vascular disease or antiretroviral therapy for HIV–positive individuals) provide a major and quite distinct challenge. One new product of *DCP3* has been to explicitly categorize all essential interventions into one of these three temporal categories and to draw relevant lessons, including concerning cost, for health systems.

In total, 71 distinct and important intersectoral policies for reducing behavioral and environmental risk were identified, and 29 of those were identified as candidates for early implementation. In addition to intersectoral policies, *DCP3* reviews policies that affect the uptake of health sector interventions (such as conditional cash transfers) and the quality with which they are delivered (Peabody and others 2018).

METHODS

DCP3's authors have thoroughly updated findings from *DCP2* on costs, effectiveness, and cost-effectiveness. The literature provides much of specific interest, but formulation of policy, when informed by evidence at all, requires expert judgment to fill extensive gaps in the literature. The first subsection of this section discusses *DCP3*'s approach. The second and third subsections discuss methods of economic evaluation and *DCP3*'s extension of standard methods to include analysis of the financial protection objectives of health systems. The final subsection discusses the process of formulation of *DCP3*'s packages.

Table 1.1 *DCP3*'s Clusters of Essential Packages

	Packages
Age-related cluster	1. Maternal and newborn health; 2. Child health; 3. School-age health and development; 4. Adolescent health and development; 5. Reproductive health and contraception
Infectious diseases cluster	6. HIV and STIs[a]; 7. Tuberculosis; 8. Malaria and adult febrile illness[b]; 9. Neglected tropical diseases; 10. Pandemic and emergency preparedness
Noncommunicable disease and injury cluster	11. Cardiovascular, respiratory, and related disorders; 12. Cancer; 13. Mental, neurological, and substance use disorders; 14. Musculoskeletal disorders; 15. Congenital and genetic disorders; 16. Injury prevention; 17. Environmental improvement[c]
Health services cluster	18. Surgery; 19. Rehabilitation; 20. Palliative care and pain control; 21. Pathology

Note: HIV = human immunodeficiency virus; STIs = sexually transmitted infections.

a. Most forms of hepatitis are in part sexually transmitted and hence control of hepatitis is included in this package.

b. Dengue is included among adult febrile illnesses.

c. Environmental improvements affect the incidence of risk factors both for infectious and for noncommunicable disease. We include them under the noncommunicable disease and injury cluster because the more significant consequences lie there.

Use of Evidence

Using research (or other) evidence to guide policy is most simply done when randomized controlled trials of the relevant intervention (or mix of interventions) have been undertaken on the population of interest in the appropriate ecological setting. Even in high-income countries, such strong evidence is rarely available. In lower-income environments, the problem of the quality of evidence is compounded. As always, evidence must be used to help decision makers (a) avoid adopting interventions that don't work in a given context and (b) avoid rejecting those that do. Box 1.2 discusses the *DCP3* thinking on this issue.

Economic Evaluation

The methods and findings of *DCP3*'s approaches to economic evaluation appear in three separate chapters of this volume: one on cost-effectiveness, one on benefit-cost analysis, and one on extended cost-effectiveness analysis (Horton 2018; Chang, Horton, and Jamison 2018; Verguet and Jamison 2018). Table 1.2 provides a high-level overview. Several of the entries in that table—covering value for money, dashboards, and extended cost-effectiveness analysis—point to the desirability of multicriteria decision analysis of the sort explored by Youngkong (2012) and others.

The bottom row of table 1.2 takes the multioutcome extended cost-effectiveness analysis (ECEA) approach one step further to discussion of the "dashboard" *DCP3* uses to help inform and structure setting priories. This health dashboard concept is a natural extension of the dashboard approach that Stigliz, Sen, and Fitoussi (2010) propose to go beyond gross domestic product

(GDP) as a macroeconomic indicator. The health dashboard is likewise a natural step beyond use of cost-effectiveness league tables in constructing health benefit packages, an approach consistent with that of Glassman, Giedion, and Smith (2017).

Protecting against Financial Risk

In populations lacking access to health insurance or prepaid care, medical expenses that are high relative to income can be impoverishing (figure 1.2 illustrates mechanisms). Where incomes are low, seemingly inexpensive medical procedures can be catastrophic. WHO's *World Health Report 2010* documented the (very substantial) magnitude of medical impoverishment globally and pointed to the value of universal health coverage for addressing both the health and the financial protection needs of populations (WHO 2010). Most of the literature on medical impoverishment fails to identify the medical conditions responsible. Essue and others (2018) point to where specific causes of medical impoverishment information are known, an obviously central point for construction of benefits packages.

Although multiple studies document the overall magnitude of medical impoverishment, most economic evaluations of health interventions and their finance (including those in *DCP1* and *DCP2*) have failed to address the important question of *efficiency* in the purchase of financial protection. In work undertaken for *DCP3*, an approach was developed—ECEA—to explicitly include financial protection and equity in economic evaluation of health interventions. Smith (2013) has developed an approach that addresses the same concern from

Box 1.2

Evidence for Policy: From Research Findings to Policy Parameters

Analysis in *DCP3* proceeds by attempting to make the best use of the evidence available for informing important decisions rather than exclusively using what ideally generated evidence has to say (Jamison 2015). The distinction is important. An example illustrates. Quite good evidence is available on the effect of vector control on malaria mortality in specific environments. Likewise there is strong evidence concerning treatment efficacy. Very little evidence, however, exists on how different mixes of vector control and treatment affect mortality, but this is the important question for policy.

Inevitably imperfectly, our task in the *Disease Control Priorities* series, beginning with the first edition, has been to combine the (sometimes) good science about unidimensional intervention in very specific locales with informed judgment to reach reasonable conclusions about the effect of intervention mixes in diverse environments. To put this in a slightly different way: the parameters required for assessing policy differ, often substantially, from what has been addressed (so far) in the research literature. The transition from research findings to policy parameters requires judgment to complement the research and, often, a consideration of underlying mechanisms (for example, use of incentives) that might suggest generalizability (Bates and Glennerster 2017).

In particular, four types of judgments were often needed in the course of *DCP3* to make the transition from research findings to evidence for policy. Examples illustrate:

1. *Similar interventions.* Assume we have evidence that intervention A is effective, and we believe intervention B is quite similar. (Think of two lipid-lowering agents.) We use judgment to infer that intervention B is (or perhaps is not) also effective.

2. *Combined interventions.* As in the malaria example, assume that evidence shows interventions A and B are both effective. What about A + B? Is the combination's effect the sum of the separate effects? Or are the two substitutes? Hard evidence on combinations is far more rare than evidence on individual interventions.

3. *Changed settings.* Assume we have strong evidence that intervention A works in environment Y, for example, that antimalarial bednets reduce all causes of child mortality when mosquitos bite indoors at night, at moderate intensity. Good evidence concludes that bednets were effective where evaluated, but other, biological considerations suggest that that evidence be rejected in an environment with very high-biting intensity. Economists have discussed this point in the context of "external validity." Ozler (2013) provides a clear overview.

4. *Trait-treatment interactions.* Finally, patient characteristics may differ. Measles immunization in healthy child populations may have been shown to have no effect on mortality rates. Generalizing that finding to a population with different traits (for example, undernourished or sickly children) might and in this case would generate an unfortunate false negative.

***

Evidence can be weak. Or, as in the examples above, evidence can be strong but only partially relevant. Often weak evidence for effectiveness, or partially relevant evidence for effectiveness, is likewise weak evidence concerning lack of effectiveness. Interpreting weak evidence as grounds for rejecting an intervention could generate false negatives that cost lives. The attempt in *DCP3* has been to unashamedly combine evidence with informed judgment in order to judiciously balance false positives and false negatives.

a different perspective. ECEA is the approach that *DCP3* used to address issues of both reduction in financial risk and distribution across income groups of financial as well as health outcomes resulting from policies, such as public finance, to increase intervention uptake. ECEA has been used to evaluate tobacco taxation and regulatory policies (Verguet and Jamison 2018). An important implication of the ECEA evaluations of tobacco taxation in China and in Lebanon was that such taxation, when the full range of consequences is considered, is progressive in

Table 1.2 Economic Evaluation Methods

Economic method	Costs	Consequences
1.1 *Cost-effectiveness analysis (CEA)* Horton (2018) overviews *DCP3*'s findings on CEA. Wilkinson and others (2016) and Sanders and others (2016) provide recent guidelines for health CEA. Jamison (2009) provided earlier guidelines that pointed to inclusion of financial protection outcomes and nonfinancial constraints in CEA.	• Social costs[a]	• Changes in specific outcomes (child deaths, new HIV infections) • Changes in aggregated measures (YLL, QALY, DALY)
1.2 *Value-for-money assessment* Value-for-money assessment of health sector interventions includes CEA but acknowledges the CEA is irrelevant for some health sector outcomes.	• Social costs[a]	Important outcomes of health sector intervention are not measurable in mortality or DALY terms (and are therefore excluded from CEA) include the following: • Contraception provided • Stillbirths averted • Palliative care • IQ or stature enhanced.
1.3. *Extended cost-effectivess analysis (ECEA)* Verguet and Jamison (2018) overview of *DCP3*'s findings on ECEA.	• Costs are viewed separately from perspectives of provider, patient, and society.	• Consequences are reported from a distributional perspective (for example, by gender, income, or membership in a disadvantaged group). See, for example, Asaria, Griffin, Cookson, and others (2015). • Valuation of financial risk protection is included.
1.4. *Benefit-cost analysis (BCA)* Chang, Horton, and Jamison (2018) overview of *DCP3*'s findings on BCA.	• Social costs[a]	• Changes in income or gross domestic product • Changes in income plus the monetary value of change in mortality (or health)
1.5. Economic dashboard *DCP3*'s judgments about interventions to include in ECEA and in the HPP involved combining multiple strands of evidence. While intervention cost-effectiveness was typically most important, in the end judgments involved considering a dashboard of information including disease burden, value for money assessment, ECEA, and BCA. Stiglitz, Sen, and Fitoussi (2010) propose making this dashboard explicit and the primary guide to decision making in the macroeconomic context.	• As with ECEA	• Poverty reduction consequences or insurance value are explicitly considered. • Distribution of costs and consequences across income quintiles are explicitly considered. • Dashboard contains a fuller and more disaggregated list of consequences than ECEA, which is itself much more comprehensive than CEA.

Note: DALY = disability-adjusted life year; *DCP3 = Disease Control Priorities* third edition; HIV = human immunodeficiency virus; HPP = highest-priority package; IQ = intelligence quotient; QALY = quality-adjusted life year; YLL = years of life lost.

a. Social costs refer to the value of real resources used to implement an intervention. For example, if a health ministry needs to pay import taxes on pharmaceuticals, the social cost is the pretax cost not the posttax cost, as the tax simply represents a transfer (from the health to the finance ministry). Taxation itself is often considered by economists to involve a real cost (the so-called deadweight loss from taxation) arising from distortion of prices and hence decisions of actors in the economy. *DCP3* follows standard practice in health-related CEA in not considering deadweight losses from taxation. Inclusion of deadweight losses as currently assessed would typically increase the cost per unit of outcome by 50 to 70 percent.

terms of health outcomes and unlikely to be regressive in terms of financial outcomes (Salti, Brouwer, and Verguet 2016; Verguet and others 2015). A 13-country ECEA of tobacco taxation found results similar to those from China and Lebanon (Jha and Global Tobacco Economics Consortium 2017).

The tobacco ECEAs suggest a more general point about government policies to provide populations with protection against financial risk. Policy can operate either upstream or downstream. Upstream provision of financial risk protection (FRP) attenuates the need for costly medical intervention. Upstream measures include

Figure 1.2 Financial Risk Protection

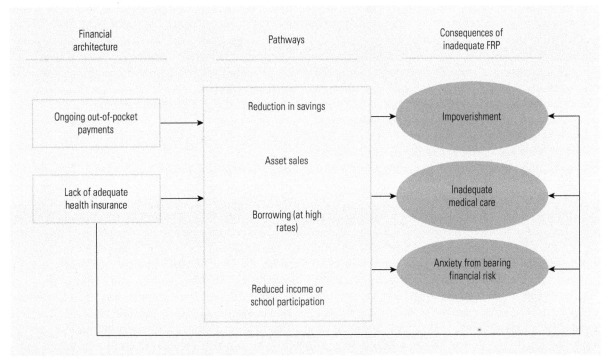

Note: FRP = financial risk protection.

prevention, early treatment, and investment in improved medical technologies (see Lakdawalla, Malani, and Reif 2017). Most health systems emphasize downstream measures through payment for expensive procedures in the hospital. Downstream measures will always be needed. That said, resource constraints will sharply limit public finance of downstream financial protection; provision only of downstream measures perverts incentives in the obvious way and in many (but not all) cases upstream measures more efficiently purchase FRP given budget constraints.

Construction of Packages

Editors of *DCP3* volumes and authors of specific chapters in volume 9—on rehabilitation (Mills and others 2018), on pathology (Fleming and others 2018), on palliative care (Krakauer and others 2018) and on pandemic preparedness (Madhav and others 2018)—constructed the 21 essential packages listed in table 1.1. The series editors and authors of this paper then consolidated those policies and formats into a common level of aggregation and a common structure (for example, screening was not considered an intervention by itself but only in conjunction with the indicated response). This generated a set of harmonized essential packages. The originals

appear as an annex to this chapter, and chapters 2 and 3 provide a full discussion of methods. Several interventions appear in more than one package as the final lists of 71 intersectoral policies, and 218 EUHC interventions remove this duplication. A consequence is that the cost of EUHC is less than the sum of the costs of the packages within it.

INTERSECTORAL POLICIES FOR HEALTH

Eleven of *DCP3*'s 21 packages contain a total of 71 intersectoral policies. These policies fall into four broad categories: taxes and subsidies (15 of 71), regulations and related enforcement mechanisms (38 of 71), built environment (11 of 71), and information (7 of 71). These policies are designed to reduce the population level of behavioral and environmental risk factors—tobacco and alcohol use, air pollution, micronutrient deficiencies in the diet, unsafe sexual behavior, excessive sugar consumption, and others (figure 1.1). Watkins, Nugent, and others (2018) provide a thorough overview of *DCP3*'s findings on intersectoral policy. Here we highlight several of *DCP3*'s points:

First, at initially low levels of income, the levels of many risk factors rise with income, creating headwinds against which health sector policy must proceed. These rises are at least potentially countered by sound policy. We identify 29 of 71 intersectoral policies to be well worth considering for early adoption.

Second, for important categories of risk, such as pollution and transport risks, there are multiple sources of the risk, each of which is addressed through different modalities. Rather than a clear set of "first priorities," there are multiple country- or site-specific actions to be taken. Perhaps the single most important point to note is that the success of many high-income countries in reducing these risks to very low levels points to the great potential that these multiple policies can have for dealing, in particular, with air pollution and road traffic injuries.

A third point of importance is that fiscal policies—finance ministry policies—are likely of key significance. Discussion of these policies has most prominently involved taxes on tobacco, alcohol, and sugar-sweetened beverages. But the possibilities for taxation are broader: sugar production and imports, fossil fuels (or carbon), and industrial or vehicle emissions. Also of importance is reducing expensive subsidies that now exist on fossil fuels and often on unhealthy food production or unhealthy child dietary supplements. While health improvement may be only one of several objectives for lowering subsidies, it is an important one. The literature

on the health potential for removing subsidies remains limited. But the sheer magnitude of some of these subsidies, as the International Monetary Fund has stressed, points to the value of careful further analysis. In all likelihood, a country's finance ministry is the most important ministry (after health) for improving population health. And many—not all—of the measures it can take can enhance public sector revenue.

ESSENTIAL UNIVERSAL HEALTH COVERAGE

The heart of *DCP3* consisted of reviewing available evidence on health sector interventions' costs, effectiveness, ability to be implemented, and capacity to deliver significant outcomes. *DCP3*'s nine volumes provide granular overviews of this evidence, overviews directed to the implementation community as well as to the policy community. Chapter 3 of volume 9 provides an integrative overview (Watkins, Jamison, and others 2018).

Figure 1.3 provides a schema of how *DCP3* defines EUHC. Beyond EUHC is the full range of available, efficacious health sector interventions, or UHC. While no country publicly finances all interventions, many high-income countries come close and can reasonably be described as having achieved UHC. Short of EUHC is what *DCP3* labels the HPP. Individual countries' highest priorities will differ from our model list for multiple reasons. That said, the HPP is intended to provide a useful starting point for national or subnational assessments. As with EUHC, *DCP3* provides estimates for the cost and effects of EUHC. *GH2035* (Jamison, Summers, and others 2013) pointed to the possibility of a "grand convergence," across most countries, in our lifetimes, in levels of under-age-five mortality and major infections. Figure 1.3 illustrates grand convergence in the *DCP3* structure. The two following subsections provide our estimates of the costs and mortality-reducing consequences of EUHC.

Costs

We generated two estimates of costs for the health system component of each of *DCP3*'s 21 packages. The first was an estimate of how much additional funding it would take—in the 2015 cost and demographic environment—to implement each package to the extent judged feasible. The packages were designed so that for most cases, "full" implementation, defined as 80 percent effective coverage, was judged feasible by 2030. The second estimate of cost was of total cost for the package, defined as incremental cost plus the amount already (in 2015) being spent on the intervention. These costs were estimated both for LICs and for lower-middle-income

Figure 1.3 Essential Universal Health Coverage and Highest-Priority Packages

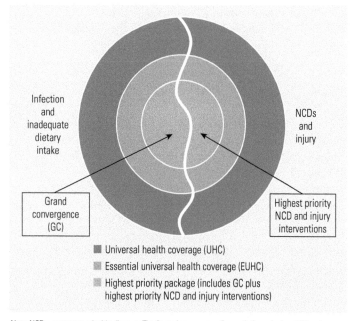

■ Universal health coverage (UHC)

■ Essential universal health coverage (EUHC)

■ Highest priority package (includes GC plus highest priority NCD and injury interventions)

Note: NCD = noncommunicable disease. The "grand convergence" agenda for reducing child and infectious disease mortality was advanced by the *Lancet* Commission on Investing in Health (Jamison, Summers, and others 2013).

countries. Some interventions were included in several packages, which was a natural outcome of a package formulation process that delineated packages as areas of concern to specific professional communities, such as surgeons or reproductive health specialists. Eliminating this duplication resulted in 218 distinct EUHC interventions. This implies that the sum of the package costs will exceed the cost of providing all packages. The subset of EUHC that was judged by explicit criteria to be highest priority (the HPP) was costed in the same way as for EUHC. All these costs are the estimated costs associated with expanding coverage in the 2015 environment, an environment for which we have substantial, if incomplete, information without making assumptions about the evolution of costs and epidemiology over time. Costs should be interpreted as long-term steady state costs, that is, costs that include (a) training of staff to replace retirements and (b) investment to counter depreciation of equipment and facilities.

Table 1.3 reports the calculated expenditure increases required above baseline and expresses those numbers as a percentage of gross national income (GNI). (Chapter 3, volume 9, of *DCP3* reports costs by package.) We consider it reasonable to think of the costs in 2030 of EUHC and the HPP in these percentage terms (as well as in numbers of dollars). Only a small fraction of reasonably anticipated economic growth in most countries would cover the incremental costs of EUHC, although achieving the increased percentage of gross national income

required would require substantial reallocation of public sector priorities (Jamison, Summers, and others 2013). In principle, projections could be made of changes in both the tradable and nontradable components of cost, of the responsiveness of costs to demography (and in particular to fertility decline), and on whether improved transport and other infrastructure might reduce our estimates of the cost of expanding coverage to ever-more difficult-to-reach parts of the population. In a country-specific context, this might well be worthwhile. But for purposes of reasonable overall cost estimates we judge that adding these layers of assumption would add little or nothing to the information content of table 1.3.

Table 1.4 presents our cost assessments divided along two other relevant dimensions. Panel a provides estimates of the costs associated with each platform, and about half of our calculated costs occur at the health center level. For EUHC, another 15 to 25 percent each of incremental expenditures would go to the first-level hospital and to the community level. Panel b reports intervention cost estimates by degree of urgency. The health systems implications for increasing intervention coverage differ markedly by urgency. Continuing interventions require appropriate community capacity for delivery. Examples include antiretroviral therapy or antihypertensive therapy. A full half of incremental costs are needed to finance continuing, very long-term intervention. Urgent interventions—for example, for trauma or obstructed labor—require that first-level hospitals be

Table 1.3 Total and Incremental Annual Costs of Essential UHC and the Highest Priority Package, 2015 (in 2012 US$)

	Low-income countries[a]		Lower-middle-income countries[a]	
	HPP	EUHC	HPP	EUHC
1. Incremental annual cost (in billions, 2012 US$)	$23	$48	$82	$160
2. Incremental annual cost per person[b] (in US$)	$26	$53	$31	$61
3. Total annual cost (in billions, US$)	$38	$68	$160	$280
4. Total annual cost per person[c] (in US$)	$42	$76	$58	$110
5. Incremental annual cost as a share of current GNI per person[b]	3.1%	6.4%	1.5%	2.9%
6. Total annual cost (as percentage of current GNI per person)[d]	5.1	9.1	2.8	5.2

Source: Watkins, Jamison, and others 2018.
Note: EUHC = essential universal health coverage; GNI = gross national income; HPP = highest-priority package.
a. This paper uses the World Bank's 2014 income classification of countries. As a country's income changes, its classification can also change; for example, both Bangladesh and Kenya moved from low- to lower-middle income after 2014.
b. Incremental annual cost is the estimated cost of going from current to full (80%) coverage of the EUHC and HPP interventions. The *total* annual cost is the incremental cost plus the cost of the current level of coverage assuming the same cost structure for current as for incremental coverage. Estimated costs are inclusive of estimates for (large) health system strengthening costs and are steady state (or long-term average) costs in that investments to achieve higher levels of coverage and to cover depreciation are included.
c. The 2015 population of low-income countries was 0.90 billion. For lower-middle-income countries, it was 2.7 billion.
d. The 2015 GNI of low-income countries was $0.75 trillion. For lower-middle-income countries, it was $5.6 trillion.

Table 1.4 Incremental Costs of the HPP and EUHC by Platform and by Intervention Urgency, Percent

	Low-income countries		Lower-middle-income countries	
	HPP (percent)	EUHC (percent)	HPP (percent)	EUHC (percent)
(a) Incremental costs by platform, percentage of total				
Population based	0.57	2.3	0.6	2.0
Community	18	16	12	14
Health center	50	52	57	52
First-level hospital	25	25	22	25
Referral and specialty hospitals	6.4	5.2	9.1	6.1
	100	**100**	**100**	**100**
(b) Incremental costs by intervention urgency, percentage of total				
Urgent	35	28	27	24
Continuing	41	48	50	52
Nonurgent	24	24	23	24
	100	**100**	**100**	**100**

Source: Watkins, Jamison, and others 2018.
Note: EUHC = essential universal health coverage; HPP = highest-priority package.

accessible quickly (Reynolds and others 2018). About one-quarter to one-third of incremental costs are required to provide this capacity. Nonurgent (but potentially important) interventions (for example, cataract extraction) allow patients to be accumulated over space and time with concomitant potential for efficiency and quality resulting from high volume.

Mortality Reduction from Essential UHC

DCP3 generated estimates of mortality in 2015, as well as estimates for a "counterfactual 2015" and of how many fewer deaths would have occurred following implementation of EUHC and the HPP. This analysis thus provides a reasoned estimate of the costs and consequences of using—in the 2015 demographic context—today's medical and public health technology as fully as reasonably possible (as well as associated cost-effectiveness estimates). This subsection discusses estimates of mortality reduction.

Norheim and others (2015) developed a structure—40x30—for thinking about mortality reduction goals for the Sustainable Development Goal (SDG) period. Their starting point was the United Nations Population Division's (UNPD) projected age distribution of population in 2030 and an age distribution of deaths generated from that age distribution of population and age-specific mortality rates from 2010. The overall 40x30 goal was, then, to reduce the calculated

number of premature deaths by 40 percent, where *premature* is defined as under age 70 years. Subgoals were to reduce under-age-five and major infectious disease deaths by two-thirds and NCD and injury deaths by one-third.

Our approach in *DCP3* followed the approach of Norheim and others (2015) in broad terms but inserts into it our "counterfactual 2015" analysis. We start with a baseline age distribution of deaths by age and (broad) cause generated from the UNPD's projected 2030 age distribution of population and age combined with cause-specific death rates from 2015 (Mathers and others 2018). We then estimate the effect of EUHC (and HPP) on mortality by assuming that the underlying intervention packages are implemented over the 15 years from 2015 to 2030. (The packages were designed to make this assumption reasonable.) The age- and cause-specific mortality rates from counterfactual 2015 were then applied to the UNPD 2030 age distributions to give the age distributions of death by cause estimated to result from implementation of EUHC.

These calculations enable comparison of the EUHC mortality profile to an explicit counterfactual baseline. Table 1.5 shows these comparisons for EUHC and for the HPP. What we can see from this comparison is that full implementation of the HPP could achieve about half of the 40x30 goal. Full implementation of EUHC could achieve about two-thirds of the

Table 1.5 Implementation of *DCP3's* Essential Packages: Estimated Reduction in Premature Deaths in 2030[a] (in Millions)

Age group or condition	Low-income countries[b]				Lower-middle-income countries[b]			
	Projected number of premature deaths, 2030	40x30 reducton target[c]	Expected reduction in premature deaths from		Projected number of premature deaths, 2030	40x30 reducton target[c]	Expected reduction in premature deaths from	
			HPP	EUHC			HPP	EUHC
By age group								
0–4	2.2	1.5	0.62	0.77	3.3	2.2	1.1	1.3
5–69	5.2	1.5	0.99	1.2	14	4.8	2.2	2.9
0–69	**7.4**	**3.0**	**1.6**	**2.0**	**17**	**7.0**	**3.2**	**4.2**
By cause (age 5+)[d]								
Group I	**1.9**	**0.76**	**0.59**	**0.65**	**3.2**	**1.5**	**0.85**	**0.94**
Tuberculosis	0.34	0.22	0.11	0.13	0.90	0.60	0.29	0.35
HIV/AIDS	0.44	0.29	0.18	0.20	0.48	0.32	0.23	0.26
Malaria	0.087	0.058	0.051	0.051	0.055	0.037	0.026	0.026
Maternal conditions	0.17	0.11	0.075	0.086	0.20	0.13	0.079	0.026
Other diseases	0.90	0.074	0.18	0.18	1.6	0.40	0.22	0.22
Group II	**2.5**	**0.60**	**0.36**	**0.53**	**8.9**	**2.7**	**1.3**	**1.9**
Neoplasms	0.65	0.22	0.010	0.039	1.8	0.60	0.10	0.16
Cardiovascular diseases	0.93	0.31	0.24	0.36	4.0	1.3	0.89	1.4
Other diseases	0.93	0.076	0.11	0.13	3.2	0.80	0.28	0.35
Group III	**0.77**	**0.13**	**0.043**	**0.060**	**2.0**	**0.54**	**0.070**	**0.10**
Road injuries	0.25	0.085	0.032	0.046	0.57	0.19	0.048	0.069
Other injuries	0.52	0.042	0.010	0.014	1.4	0.36	0.022	0.032

Sources: Watkins, Norheim, and others 2017; Watkins, Qi, and others 2017; Watkins, Jamison, and others 2018.

Note: EUHC = essential universal health coverage; HIV/AIDS = human immunodeficiency virus/acquired immune deficiency syndrome; HPP = highest-priority package. All estimates are in millions of deaths. The 40x30 reduction target includes a 40 percent reduction in deaths ages 0–69 overall; a two-thirds reduction in under-age-five deaths and adult deaths from tuberculosis, HIV/AIDS, malaria, and maternal conditions; and a one-third reduction in deaths from major noncommunicable diseases. The quantitative targets above reflect these goals; however, targets for the residual categories ("other diseases" and "other injuries") have been calculated in light of the targets for specific causes of death so that the total number of target deaths for ages 5–69 is sufficient to meet the 40x30 target.

a. A death under age 70 is defined as premature.

b. This paper uses the World Bank's income classification of countries.

c. A reduction target of 40x30 is defined as a 40 percent reduction in premature deaths by 2030, relative to the number that would have occurred had 2015 death rates persisted to 2030. The *United Nations Population* Prospects (UN 2017) median population projection for 2030 was used to provide the population totals for calculating deaths by age and sex.

d. World Health Organization's Global Health Estimates provided the 2015 cause distributions of deaths for these calculations (Mathers and others 2018).

40x30 goal. In a sensitivity analysis, Watkins, Norheim, and others (2018) demonstrate that higher levels of coverage (on the order of 95 percent) and more optimistic assumptions about the quality and efficiency of intervention delivery could acheive the 40x30 goal in lower-middle-income countries and exceed it by about 20 percent in low-income countries. If we were to assume that both tools and implementation capacity improve over the period to 2030—*Global Health 2035* (Jamison, Summers, and others 2013) made an assumption of a 2 percent rate of technical progress in one of their scenarios—then the reduction in deaths from EUHC could be more substantial than shown in this table. Such progress is certainly possible, but may be unlikely. Likewise there could be more than anticipated reduction in behavioral and environmental risk. Our model is estimating what is technically and economically feasible given today's tools. The results are indeed substantial—and are viable options for decision makers. But required resources are substantial, and at realistic (that is, 80 percent) coverage levels the goals are incompletely met. The actual decision to commit resources remains, of course, in the hands of national authorities.

CONCLUSIONS

DCP3 has been a large-scale enterprise involving multiple authors, editors, and institutions. The first volume appeared in 2015 and the last of the nine volumes is being published at the beginning of 2018. The volumes appear as serious discussion continues about quantifying and achieving SDGs, including SDG 3 for health.

DCP3's analyses complement those of *GH2035* and WHO's recent assessments of the cost of attaining SDG 3 (Jamison, Summers, and others 2013; Stenberg and others 2017). Each of these analyses addresses somewhat different questions (table 1.6), but the broad results they convey are mutually supportive.

DCP3 reached six broad conclusions:

1. *DCP3* has found it useful to organize interventions into 21 essential packages that group the interventions relevant to particular professional communities. Each package can contain both intersectoral interventions and health system interventions. Specific findings from packages point to the attractiveness of widely available surgical capacity, the value of meeting unmet demand for contraception, the potential of a multipronged approach to air pollution and the importance of maintaining investment in child health and development far beyond the first 1000 days.
2. Interventions were selected for packages by a systematic process using criteria of value for money, burden addressed, and implementation feasibility. Collectively, the selected interventions are defined to constitute "essential" universal health coverage

Table 1.6 Comparison of *Global Health 2035, DCP3*, and WHO 2017 Resource Estimates for Costs and Consequences of Large Scale Investment in Health Systems

	Global Health 2035	DCP3	WHO 2017
1. *Countries included*	34 low-income and 3 (large) lower-middle-income countries. Separate estimates for the low- and lower-middle-income countries groups are provided.	34 low-income and 49 lower-middle income countries. Separate estimates for the low- and lower-middle-income countries groups are provided.	67 low-, lower-middle, and upper-middle-income countries individually estimated and then aggregated. Reported results are for all included countries combined.
2. *Key definitions and intervention range covered*	Grand convergence (GC) interventions are defined as ones leading to very substantial crosscountry convergence in under age 5, maternal, tuberculosis, malaria, and HIV/AIDS mortality and in the prevalence of neglected tropical diseases (NTDs).	• 21 packages of care (table 1.1) are identified in terms that include intersectoral and health sector interventions (71 distinct intersectoral interventions and 218 distinct health sector interventions). • Essential universal health coverage (EUHC) is defined as health sector interventions in the 21 packages (covered in national health accounts and potentially included in benefits packages). • A highest priority subset of EUHC. The highest-priority package (HPP) includes the GC interventions but goes beyond it, including a limited range of interventions against noncommunicable diseases (NCDs) and injuries, and cross-cutting areas such as rehabilitation and palliative care.	• Investments were modeled for 16 SDGs, including 187 health interventions and a range of health system strengthening strategies (the latter of which included investments required to achieve target levels of health workforce, facilities, and other health system building blocks). • Two scenarios were modeled, a *progress scenario* (in which coverage is limited by the absorptive capacity of current systems to incorporate new interventions) and an *ambitious scenario* (in which most countries achieve high levels of intervention coverage and hence SDG targets).

table continues next page

Table 1.6 Comparison of *Global Health 2035, DCP3,* and WHO 2017 Resource Estimates for Costs and Consequences of Large Scale Investment in Health Systems **(continued)**

	Global Health 2035	DCP3	WHO 2017
3. *Intersectoral action for health*	Extensive discussion of intersectoral actions for health but not included in modeling grand convergence.	Intersectoral interventions defined as those typically managed and financed outside the health sector. Each of the 21 packages contains the intersectoral interventions deemed relevant. The costs and effects of intersectoral action on mortality reduction not explicitly modelled.	WHO 2017 scenarios include some finance of intersectoral interventions, from the health sector perspective, as well as their effects on mortality.
4. *Intervention coverage*	Full coverage defined as 85%; rates of scale-up defined using historical data on "best performers" among similar groups of countries.	Full coverage defined as 80%. The HPP differs from EUHC not in coverage rate but in the scope of interventions included.	Full coverage defined as 95% for most interventions in the ambitious scenario, with a range from 53–99% depending on the intervention.
5. *Estimated additional costs (including requisite investment in health system capacity), in US$*	For low-income countries in 2035: US$30 billion annually between 2016 and 2030. For lower-middle-income countries in 2035: US$61 billion per year.	Low-income countries, 2030: HPP—US$23 billion/year EUHC—US$48 billion/year Lower middle-income countries, 2030: HPP—US$82 billion/year EUHC—US$160 billion per year. (Costs presented in 2012 US$)	Low-income countries: $64 billion in 2030. Lower-middle-income countries: $185 billion in 2030. (Costs presented in 2014 US$)
6. *Estimated deaths averted*[a, b, c]	For low-income countries: 4.5 million deaths averted per year between 2016 and 2030. For lower-middle-income countries: 5.8 million deaths averted per year between 2016 and 2030.	Low-income countries: 2.0 million premature deaths averted in 2030. Lower-middle-income countries: 4.2 million premature deaths averted in 2030.	Low-income countries: 2.9 million deaths averted in 2030. Lower-middle-income countries: 6.1 million deaths averted in 2030.

Sources: Global Health 2035: Jamison, Summers, and others 2013; Boyle and others 2015. *DCP3:* Watkins, Qi, and others 2017; Watkins, Norheim, and others 2017. Stenberg and others 2017.

Note: HIV/AIDS = human immunodeficiency virus/acquired immune deficiency syndrome; SDGs = Sustainable Development Goals.

a. *DCP3* reports the number of *premature* deaths averted, that is, deaths under age 70.

b. Averted deaths included stillbirths averted in *GH2035* and WHO 2017, but not in *DCP3.*

c. For *GH2035* and *DCP3* the reported deaths averted included only deaths averted among children actually born. Family planning averts unwanted pregnancies and hence potential deaths of children from those pregnancies who were never born. The difference is major. For low-income countries, a *GH2035* sensitivity analysis estimated that the more comprehensive figure was 7.5 million deaths averted rather than the 4.5 million shown in the table. The WHO 2017 headline numbers do include deaths averted from pregnancies averted but sensitivity analyses were undertaken. Ambitious scale-up of family planning services accounted for 50 percent of averted child and maternal deaths and over 65 percent of averted stillbirths in the WHO analysis (K. Stenberg 2017, personal communication).

or EUHC. A subset of 97 of these interventions, selected using more stringent criteria, are suggested as the highest-priority package or HPP, constituting an important first step on the path to EUHC. Five platforms—from population-based through the referral hospital—provide the delivery base for 218 health sector interventions. The specific interventions selected for the HPP and for EUHC and the definitions of platforms and packages are necessarily quite generic. Every country's definitions and selections will differ from these and from each other's. Nonetheless, we view *DCP3*'s selections as a potentially useful model—as a starting point for what are appropriately country-specific assessments.

3. The costs estimated for the HPP and EUHC are substantial. The HPP is, however, affordable for LICs prepared to commit to rapid improvement in population health, and the EUHC is affordable for lower-middle-income countries. Many upper-middle-income countries have yet to achieve EUHC and they, too, might find that the EUHC interventions are a useful starting point for discussion.

4. The goal of a 40 percent reduction in premature deaths by 2030 (Norheim and others 2015), 40x30, represents a goal for mortality reduction closely mirroring the quantitative content of SDG 3. Our calculations suggest that implementing EUHC or the HPP by 2030 will make substantial progress

toward 40x30. Higher levels of coverage than we have assumed here would be required to reach 40x30, but this might be a realistic target for some early-adopter UHC countries.

5. *DCP3* has shown that it is possible to identify the main sources of health-related financial risk and impoverishment to estimate the value of risk reduction and to use ECEA to help achieve efficiency in purchase of risk reduction. Although *DCP3* has made a beginning in applying these methods, much remains to be done.

6. In addition to the aggregate conclusions of *DCP3* just summarized, each volume provides rich detail on policy options and priorities. This granularity in the volumes makes them of use to the implementation level of government ministries as well as the policy level.

ACKNOWLEDGMENTS

We wish to acknowledge three institutions that have played key roles in *DCP3*. One is the World Bank, original home for the *DCP* series and accomplished publisher of its products. In the World Bank, Carlos Rossel and Mary Fisk oversaw the editing and publication of the series and served as critical champions for *DCP3*. The second is the Interacademy Medical Panel (IAMP) and its U.S. affiliate, the National Academy of Medicine (NAM). IAMP/NAM have organized a peer review process to cover chapters in the nine volumes; they established an Advisory Committee to the Editors (ACE), chaired by Anne Mills, that has been of enormous value. The Department of Global Health of the University of Washington has provided a congenial home for *DCP* for the past five years. We wish in particular to acknowledge the intellectual and practical support of the department's two chairs during that period: King Homes and Judith Wasserheit. We also wish to acknowledge Brianne Adderley, Shamelle Richards, and Nazila Dabestani for their management, administrative, and research support to the production of *DCP3*.

ANNEX

The following annex to this chapter is available at http://www.dcp-3.org/DCP.

- Annex 1A: Essential Packages as They Appear in *DCP3* Volumes 1 through 9

NOTE

World Bank Income Classifications as of July 2014 are as follows, based on estimates of gross national income (GNI) per capita for 2013:

- Low-income countries (LICs) = US$1,045 or less
- Middle-income countries (MICs) are subdivided:
  (a) lower-middle-income = US$1,046 to US$4,125.
  (b) upper-middle-income (UMICs) = US$4,126 to US$12,745.
- High-income countries (HICs) = US$12,746 or more.

REFERENCES

Asaria, M., S. Griffin, R. Cookson, S. Whyte, and P. Tappenden. 2015. "Distributional Cost-Effectiveness Analysis of Health Care Programmes: A Methodological Case Study of the UK Bowel Cancer Screening Programme." *Health Economics* 24: 742–54.

Bates, M. A, and R. Glennerster. 2017. "The Generalizability Puzzle." *Stanford Social Innovation Review* (summer). https://ssir.org/articles/entry/the_generalizability_puzzle.

Bendavid E., T. Ottersen, P. Liu, R. Nugent, N. Padian, and others. 2018. "Development Assistance for Health." In *Disease Control Priorities* (third edition): Volume 9, *Improving Health and Reducing Poverty*, edited by D. T. Jamison, H. Gelband, S. Horton, P. Jha, R. Laxminarayan, C. N. Mock, and R. Nugent. Washington, DC: World Bank.

Bloom, B. R., C. M. Michaud, J. R. La Montagne, and L. Simonsen. 2006. "Priorities for Global Research and Development of Interventions." In *Disease Control Priorities in Developing Countries*, second edition, edited by D. T. Jamison, J. G. Breman, A. R. Measham, G. Alleyne, M. Claeson, D. B. Evans, P. Jha, A. Mills, and P. Musgrove. Washington, DC: World Bank and Oxford University Press.

Bobadilla, J. L., J. Frenk, R. Lozano, T. Frejka, C. Stern, and others. 1993. "The Epidemiologic Transition and Health Priorities." In *Disease Control Priorities in Developing Countries*, first edition, edited by D. T. Jamison, W. H. Mosley, A. R. Measham, and J. L. Bobadilla. New York: Oxford University Press.

Boyle, C. F., C. Levin, A. Hatefi, S. Madriz, and N. Santos. 2015. "Achieving a 'Grand Convergence' in Global Health: Modeling the Technical Inputs, Costs, and Impacts from 2016 to 2030." *PLOS ONE* 10 (10).

Bundy, D. A. P., N. de Silva, S. Horton, D. T. Jamison, and G. C. Patton, eds. 2017. *Child and Adolescent Health and Development*. Volume 8, *Disease Control Priorities* (third edition), edited by D. T. Jamison, R. Nugent, H. Gelband, S. Horton, P. Jha, R. Laxminaryan, and C. N. Mock. Washington, DC: World Bank.

Chang, A., S. Horton, and D. T. Jamison. 2018. "Benefit-Cost Analysis in *Disease Control Priorities*, Third Edition." In *Disease Control Priorities* (third edition): Volume 9, *Improving Health and Reducing Poverty*, edited by D. T. Jamison, H. Gelband, S. Horton, P. Jha, R. Laxminarayan, C. N. Mock, and R. Nugent. Washington, DC: World Bank.

Essue, B. M., T.-L. Laba, F. M. Knaul, A. Chu, H. V. Minh, and others. 2018. "Economic Burden of Chronic Ill Health and Injuries for Households in Low- and

Middle-Income Countries." In *Disease Control Priorities* (third edition): Volume 9, *Improving Health and Reducing Poverty*, edited by D. T. Jamison, H. Gelband, S. Horton, P. Jha, R. Laxminarayan, C. N. Mock, and R. Nugent. Washington, DC: World Bank.

Evans, J. R., K. L. Hall, and J. Warford. 1981. "Shattuck Lecture; Health Care in the Developing World: Problems of Scarcity and Choice." *New England Journal of Medicine* 305: 1117–27.

Fleming, K., M. Naidoo, M. Wilson, J. Flanigan, S. Horton, and others. 2018. "High Quality Diagnosis: An Essential Pathology Package." In *Disease Control Priorities* (third edition): Volume 9, *Improving Health and Reducing Poverty*, edited by D. T. Jamison, H. Gelband, S. Horton, P. Jha, R. Laxminarayan, C. N. Mock, and R. Nugent. Washington, DC: World Bank.

Frenk, J., J. L. Bobadilla, J. Sepúlveda, and M. Lopez-Cervantes. 1989. "Health Transition in Middle-Income Countries: New Challenges for Health Care." *Health Policy and Planning* 4 (1): 29–39.

Glassman, A., U. Giedion, and P. C. Smith. 2017. *What's In, What's Out: Designing Benefits for Universal Health Coverage.* Washington, DC: Center for Global Development.

Ghebreyesus, T. A. 2017. "All Roads Lead to Universal Health Coverage." Commentary. *The Lancet*, July 17.

Harlan, W. R., L. C. Harlan, and W. L. Oii. 1984. "Changing Disease Patterns in Developing Countries: The Case of Malaysia." In *Health Information Systems*, edited by P. Leaverton and L. Massi. New York: Praeger Scientific.

Horton, S. E. 2018. "Cost-Effectiveness in *Disease Control Priorities*, Third Edition." In *Disease Control Priorities* (third edition): Volume 9, *Improving Health and Reducing Poverty*, edited by D. T. Jamison, H. Gelband, S. Horton, P. Jha, R. Laxminarayan, C. N. Mock, and R. Nugent. Washington, DC: World Bank.

Jamison, D. T. 2009. "Cost-Effectiveness Analysis: Concepts and Applications." In *Oxford Textbook of Public Health* (fifth edition). Volume 2, *The Methods of Public Health*, edited by R. Detels, J. McEwen, R. Beaglehole, and H. Tanaka, 767–82. Oxford, UK: Oxford University Press.

———. 2015. "Disease Control Priorities: Improving Health and Reducing Poverty." *The Lancet.* Comment. doi: 10.1016/S0140-6736(15)60097-6.

Jamison, D. T., A. Alwan, C. N. Mock, R. Nugent, D. A. Watkins, and others. 2018. "Universal Health Coverage and Intersectoral Action for Health." In *Disease Control Priorities* (third edition): Volume 9, *Improving Health and Reducing Poverty*, edited by D. T. Jamison, H. Gelband, S. Horton, P. Jha, R. Laxminarayan, C. N. Mock, and R. Nugent. Washington, DC: World Bank.

Jamison, D. T., J. G. Breman, A. R. Measham, G. Alleyne, M. Claeson, D. B. Evans, P. Jha, A. Mills, and P. Musgrove, eds. 2006. *Disease Control Priorities in Developing Countries*, second edition. Washington, DC: Oxford University Press and World Bank.

Jamison, D. T., J. R. Evans, T. King, I. Porter, N. Prescott, and others. 1984. "China: The Health Sector." Country Study. World Bank, Washington, DC.

Jamison, D. T., W. H. Mosley, A. R. Measham, J. L. Bobadilla, eds. 1993. *Disease Control Priorities in Developing Countries*, first edition. New York: Oxford University Press.

Jamison, D. T., P. Jha, V. Malhotra, and St. Verguet. 2013. "Human Health: The Twentieth-Century Transformation of Human Health—Its Magnitude and Value." In *How Much Have Global Problems Cost the World?: A Scorecard from 1900 to 2050*, edited by B. Lomborg. New York: Cambridge University Press.

Jamison, D. T., L. H. Summers, G. Alleyne, K. J. Arrow, S. Berkley, and others. 2013. "Global Health 2035: A World Converging within a Generation." *The Lancet* 382 (9908): 1898–955.

Jha, P., and Global Tobacco Economics Consortium. 2017. *The Health, Poverty and Financial Consequences of a Large Tobacco Price Increase among 0.5 Billion Male Smokers in 13 Low- and Middle-Income Countries.* Toronto: Centre for Global Health Research.

Krakauer, E., Z. Ali, H. Arreola, A. Bhadelia, S. Connor, and others. 2018. "Palliative Care." In *Disease Control Priorities* (third edition): Volume 9, *Improving Health and Reducing Poverty*, edited by D. T. Jamison, H. Gelband, S. Horton, P. Jha, R. Laxminarayan, C. N. Mock, and R. Nugent. Washington, DC: World Bank.

Kydland, F. E., R. Mundell, T. Schelling, V. Smith, and N. Stokey. 2013. "Expert Panel Ranking" In *Global Problems, Smart Solutions: Costs and Benefits*, edited by B. Lomborg, 701–16. Cambridge, UK: Cambridge University Press.

Lakdawalla, D., A. Malani, and J. Reif. 2017. "The Insurance Value of Medical Innovation." *Journal of Public Economics* 145: 94–102.

Madhav, N., B. Oppenheim, M. Gallivan, P. Mulembakani, E. Rubin, and others. 2018. "Pandemics: Risks, Mitigation, and Costs." In *Disease Control Priorities* (third edition): Volume 9, *Improving Health and Reducing Poverty*, edited by D. T. Jamison, H. Gelband, S. Horton, P. Jha, R. Laxminarayan, C. N. Mock, and R. Nugent. Washington, DC: World Bank.

Mahmoud, A., P. M. Danzon, J. H. Barton, and R. D. Mugerwa. 2006. "Product Development Priorities." In *Disease Control Priorities in Developing Countries*, second edition, edited by D. T. Jamison, J. G. Breman, A. R. Measham, G. Alleyne, M. Claeson, D. B. Evans, P. Jha, A. Mills, and P. Musgrove. Washington, DC: Oxford University Press and World Bank.

Mathers, C., G. Stevens, D. Hogan, A. Mahanani, and J. Ho. 2018. "Global and Regional Causes of Death: Patterns and Trends, 2000–15." In *Disease Control Priorities* (third edition): Volume 9, *Improving Health and Reducing Poverty*, edited by D. T. Jamison, H. Gelband, S. Horton, P. Jha, R. Laxminarayan, C. N. Mock, and R. Nugent. Washington, DC: World Bank.

Meltzer, D. 2006. "Economic Approaches to Valuing Global Health Research." In *Disease Control Priorities in Developing Countries*, second edition, edited by D. T. Jamison, J. G. Breman, A. R. Measham, G. Alleyne, M. Claeson, D. B. Evans, P. Jha, A. Mills, and P. Musgrove. Washington, DC: World Bank and Oxford University Press.

Mills, J. A., E. Marks, T. Reynolds, and A. Cieza. 2018. "Rehabilitation: Essential Along the Continuum of Care." In *Disease Control Priorities* (third edition): Volume 9, *Improving Health and Reducing Poverty*, edited by D. T. Jamison, H. Gelband, S. Horton, P. Jha, R. Laxminarayan, C. N. Mock, and R. Nugent. Washington, DC: World Bank.

Norheim, O. F., P. Jha, K. Admasu, T. Godal, R. H. Hum, and others. 2015. "Avoiding 40% of the Premature Deaths in Each Country, 2010–30: Review of National Mortality Trends to Help Quantify the UN Sustainable Development Goal for Health." *The Lancet* 385 (9964): 239–52.

Ozler, B. 2013. "Learn to Live without External Validity." *Development Impact* (blog). World Bank, Washington, DC. https://blogs.worldbank.org/impactevaluations/learn-live-without-external-validity.

Peabody, J., R. Shimkhada, O. Adeyi, H. Wang, E. Broughton, and others. 2018. "Quality of Care." In *Disease Control Priorities* (third edition): Volume 9, *Improving Health and Reducing Poverty*, edited by D. T. Jamison, H. Gelband, S. Horton, P. Jha, R. Laxminarayan, C. N. Mock, and R. Nugent. Washington, DC: World Bank.

Pradhan, E., E. M. Suzuki, S. Martínez, M. Schäferhoff, and others. 2017. "The Effects of Education Quantity and Quality on Child and Adult Mortality: Their Magnitude and Their Value." In *Disease Control Priorities* (third edition): Volume 8, *Child and Adolescent Health and Development,*" edited by D. A. P. Bundy, N. de Silva, S. E. Horton, D. T. Jamison, and G. C. Patton. Washington, D.C.: World Bank.

Reynolds, T., H. Sawe, A. M. Rubiano, S. D. Shin, and others. 2018. "Strengthening Health Systems to Provide Emergency Care." In *Disease Control Priorities* (third edition): Volume 9, *Improving Health and Reducing Poverty*, edited by D. T. Jamison, H. Gelband, S. Horton, P. Jha, R. Laxminarayan, C. N. Mock, and R. Nugent. Washington, DC: World Bank.

Salti, N., E. D. Brouwer, and S. Verguet. 2016. "The Health, Financial, and Distributional Consequences of Increases in the Tobacco Excise Tax among Smokers in Lebanon." *Social Science and Medicine* 170 (December): 161–69.

Sanders, G. D., P. J. Neumann, A. Basu, D. W. Brock, and others. 2016. "Recommendations for Conduct, Methodological Practices, and Reporting of Cost-Effectiveness Analyses: Second Panel on Cost-Effectiveness in Health and Medicine." *Journal of the American Medical Association* 316 (10): 1093–103.

Schäferhoff, M., S. Fewer, J. Kraus, E. Richter, L. H. Summers, and others. 2015. "How Much Donor Financing for Health Is Channelled to Global Versus Country-Specific Aid Functions?" *The Lancet* 386 (10011): 2436–41.

Skolnik, R. 2016. *Global Health 101* (third edition). Burlington, MA: Jones & Bartlett Learning.

Smith, P. C. 2013. "Incorporating Financial Protection into Decision Rules for Publicly Financed Healthcare Treatments." *Health Economics* 22 (2): 180–93.

Stenberg, K., O. Hanssen, T. Tan-Torres Edejer, M. Bertram, and others. 2017. "Financing Transformative Health Systems Towards Achievement of the Health Sustainable Development Goals: A Model for Projected Resource Needs in 67 Low-Income and Middle-Income Countries." *The Lancet Global Health.* doi:http://dx.doi.org/10.1016/S2214-109X(17)30263-2.

Stigliz, J., A. Sen, and J. P. Fitoussi. 2010. *Mis-Measuring Our Lives: Why GDP Doesn't Add Up*. New York and London: The New Press.

Trimble, E. L., P. Rajaraman, A. Chao, T. Gross, and others. 2015. "Need for National Commitments to Cancer Research to Guide Public Health Investment and Practice." In *Disease Control Priorities* (third edition): Volume 3, *Cancer*, edited by H. Gelband, P. Jha, R. Sankaranarayanan, and S. Horton. Washington, D.C.: World Bank.

UN (United Nations). 2017. *World Population Prospects: The 2017 Revision*. New York: Population Division, United Nations Department of Economic and Social Affairs.

Verguet, S., C. L. Gauvreau, S. Mishra, M. MacLennan, and others. 2015. "The Consequences of Tobacco Tax on Household Health and Finances in Rich and Poor Smokers in China: An Extended Cost-Effectiveness Analysis." *The Lancet Global Health* 3 (4): e206–e216.

Verguet, S., and D. T. Jamison. 2018. "Health Policy Analysis: Applications of Extended Cost-Effectiveness Analysis Methodology in *Disease Control Priorities*: (third edition)." In *Disease Control Priorities* (third edition): Volume 9, *Improving Health and Reducing Poverty*, edited by D. T. Jamison, H. Gelband, S. Horton, P. Jha, R. Laxminarayan, C. N. Mock, and R. Nugent. Washington, DC: World Bank.

Verguet, S., R. Laxminarayan, and D. T. Jamison. 2015. "Universal Public Finance of Tuberculosis Treatment in India: An Extended Cost-Effectiveness Analysis." *Health Economics* 24 (3): 318–32.

Watkins, D. A., D. T. Jamison, A. Mills, R. Atun, K. Danforth, and others. 2018. "Universal Health Coverage and Essential Packages of Care." In *Disease Control Priorities* (third edition): Volume 9, *Improving Health and Reducing Poverty*, edited by D. T. Jamison, H. Gelband, S. Horton, P. Jha, R. Laxminarayan, C. N. Mock, and R. Nugent. Washington, DC: World Bank.

Watkins, D. A., O. F. Norheim, P. Jha, and D. T. Jamison. 2017. "Mortality Impact of Acheiving Essential Universal Health Coverage in Low- and Lower Middle-Income Countries." *DCP3 Working Paper* no. 21. World Bank, Washington, DC.

Watkins, D. A., R. A. Nugent, H. Saxenian, G. Yamey, and others. 2018. "Intersectoral Policy Priorties for Health." In *Disease Control Priorities* (third edition): Volume 9, *Improving Health and Reducing Poverty*, edited by D. T. Jamison, H. Gelband, S. Horton, P. Jha, R. Laxminarayan, C. N. Mock, and R. Nugent. Washington, DC: World Bank.

Watkins, D. A., J. Qi, S. E. Horton, E. Brouwer, and others. 2017. "Costs and Affordability of Essential Universal Health Coverage in Low- and Middle-Income Countries." *DCP3 Working Paper* no. 20. World Bank, Washington, DC.

Weatherall, D., B. Greenwood, H. L. Chee, and P. Wasi. 2006. "Science and Technology for Disease Control: Past, Present, and Future." In *Disease Control Priorities in Developing*

Countries, second edition, edited by D. T. Jamison, J. G. Breman, A. R. Measham, G. Alleyne, M. Claeson, D. B. Evans, P. Jha, A. Mills, and P. Musgrove. Washington, DC: World Bank and Oxford University Press.

WHO (World Health Organization). 2010. *The World Health Report 2010: Health Systems Financing: The Path to Universal Coverage.* Geneva: WHO.

Wilkinson, T., M. J. Sculpher, K. Claxton, P. Revill, and others. 2016. "The International Decision Support Initiative Reference Case for Economic Evaluation: An Aid to Thought." *Value Health* 19 (8): 921–28.

World Bank. 1993. *World Development Report 1993: Investing in Health.* New York: Oxford University Press. https://open knowledge.worldbank.org/handle/10986/5976.

Youngkong, S. 2012. "Multi-Criteria Decision Analysis for Including Health Interventions in the Universal Health Coverage Benefit Package in Thailand." PhD dissertation, Radboud University, Nijmegen, the Netherlands.

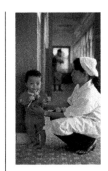

Chapter 2

Intersectoral Policy Priorities for Health

David A. Watkins, Rachel Nugent, Helen Saxenian, Gavin Yamey,
Kristen Danforth, Eduardo González-Pier, Charles N. Mock,
Prabhat Jha, Ala Alwan, and Dean T. Jamison

INTRODUCTION

Many aspects of population health can be addressed solely by services delivered through the health sector. These services include health promotion and prevention efforts as well as treatment and rehabilitation for specific diseases or injuries. At the same time, policies initiated by or in collaboration with other sectors, such as agriculture, energy, and transportation, can also reduce the incidence of disease and injury, often to great effect. These policies can make use of several types of instruments, including fiscal measures (taxes, subsidies, and transfer payments); laws and regulations; changes in the built environment (roads, parks, and buildings); and information, education, and communication campaigns (see chapter 1 of this volume, Jamison and others 2018). In addition, a range of non–health sector social services can mitigate the consequences of ill health and provide financial protection. These intersectoral policies that promote or protect health, when implemented as part of a coherent plan, can constitute a whole-of-government approach to health (UN 2012).

Ideally, a whole-of-government approach to health would involve the systematic integration of health considerations into the policy processes of all ministries. This collaborative approach is often termed *Health in All Policies* (Khayatzadeh-Mahani and others 2016). Some governments have achieved such collaboration by employing ministerial commissions or other mechanisms comprising top-level policy makers to enable health-related decisions to be made across government sectors (Buss and others 2016). The goal is to create benefits across sectors by taking actions to support population health and beyond that, to ensure that even "nonhealth" policy decisions and implementation have beneficial, or at least neutral, effects on determinants of health. Intersectoral involvement increases the arsenal of available tools to improve health, helps ensure that government policies are not at cross-purposes to each other, and can generate sizable revenue (as in the case of tobacco and alcohol taxes).

Many countries do not practice a Health in All Policies approach, and doing so is especially challenging when there are extreme resource constraints, low capacity, and weak governance and communication structures (Khayatzadeh-Mahani and others 2016), as in many low- and middle-income countries (LMICs). As an alternative in these settings, a ministry of health could engage other sectors opportunistically and strategically on specific issues that are likely to produce quick successes and have substantial health effects (WHO 2011a). Thus, a concrete menu of policy options that are highly effective, feasible, and relevant in low-resource environments is needed. This need is particularly relevant in light of the ambitious targets specified in the United Nations Sustainable Development Goals (SDGs) for 2030 (UN 2015).

Rachel Nugent, Helen Saxenian, and Gavin Yamey are co-second authors for this chapter.

Corresponding author: David A. Watkins, University of Washington, Seattle, Washington, United States; davidaw@uw.edu.

The *Disease Control Priorities* series has consistently stressed the importance of intersectoral action for health and the feasibility of intersectoral action in LMICs. *Disease Control Priorities in Developing Countries*, second edition (*DCP2*) (Jamison and others 2006), included chapters that emphasized intersectoral policies for specific diseases, injuries, and risk factors, and it also included a chapter devoted to fiscal policy (Nugent and Knaul 2006). *Disease Control Priorities*, third edition (*DCP3*), has reinforced many of these messages—usually with newer and stronger evidence—and has also explored some emerging topics and new paradigms, particularly for control of noncommunicable disease risk factors. Volume 7 of *DCP3* is especially noteworthy in this respect: it provides a list of 111 policy recommendations for prevention of injuries and reduction of environmental and occupational hazards, 109 of which are almost entirely outside the purview of health ministers to implement (Mock and others 2017).

Despite the political barriers to developing an intersectoral agenda for health, this chapter contends that not only is intersectoral action a good idea for health—it is a must. Much of the reduction in health loss globally over the past few decades can be attributed to reductions in risk factors such as tobacco consumption and unsafe water that have been implemented almost exclusively by actors outside the health sector (Hutton and Chase 2017; Jha and others 2015). An environment that increases health risks at early stages of industrial and urban growth often, although not always, gives way to a cleaner natural environment at higher levels of per capita income. Yet these risks can be associated with dramatic health losses along the way (Mock and others 2017). Furthermore, the health risks produced by advanced industrialization—such as unhealthy diet and physical inactivity—require policy interventions across multiple sectors if they are not to worsen substantially with economic development.

This chapter is based on a close look at the intersectoral policies recommended across the *DCP3* volumes, and it proposes 29 concrete early steps that countries with highly constrained resources can take to address the major risks that can be modified. The chapter also touches on broader social policies that address the consequences of ill health and stresses that the need for such policies will increasingly place demands on public finance. This chapter can be viewed as a complement to chapter 3 of this volume (Watkins and others 2018) concerning health sector interventions in the context of universal health coverage. It also provides illustrative examples of successful health risk reduction through intersectoral policy and discusses various aspects of policy implementation. By synthesizing non–health sector policies separately and in greater depth

in this chapter, *DCP3* seeks to reinforce the importance of these policy instruments and provide a template for action for ministers of health when engaging other sectors and heads of state.

HEALTH CONDITIONS AND RISK FACTORS AMENABLE TO INTERSECTORAL ACTION

Most of this chapter discusses policies that influence the distribution of selected risk factors for diseases and injuries across the population (Jamison and others 2018). Risk factors fall into three broad categories:

1. *Individual personal characteristics.* Important characteristics include an individual's genetics (including epigenetic factors arising very early), age, height, body mass index, blood lipid profile, blood pressure, and many others. Although age and genetics cannot be modified, they may provide information to guide medical treatment and behavior.
2. *Diseases.* Some diseases increase the risk of other diseases or increase their severity. Important examples include diabetes, hepatitis, severe mood disorders, and malaria. In some cases, the burden from diseases as risk factors well exceeds their intrinsic burden. Diabetes is one of the most prominent examples in this regard (Alegre-Díaz and others 2016).
3. *Behavior and environment.* Important examples of behavioral risk factors include diets that contribute to adiposity and vascular risk; diets that contribute to undernutrition; lack of exercise; unsafe sex; and abuse of addictive substances such as tobacco, alcohol, and narcotics. Important environmental risk factors include air and water pollution and unsafe occupational and transport conditions.

This chapter's main focus is on instruments of policy intended to change the third category of risk factors: behavior and environment. Changes in behavior and environment can influence disease incidence or severity either directly or by modifying other risk factors. Interventions that address both individual personal characteristics and diseases as risk factors are covered in chapter 3 of this volume (Watkins and others 2018).

Conceptual Model for Interactions among Health Risks

Behavioral and environmental risk factors can be disaggregated into multiple specific risks, illustrating sources and pathways of risk exposure. The more disaggregated set of risk factors outlined in figure 2.1 has two

Figure 2.1 Conceptual Model of Interactions among Key Risk Factors and Diseases That Can Be Modified

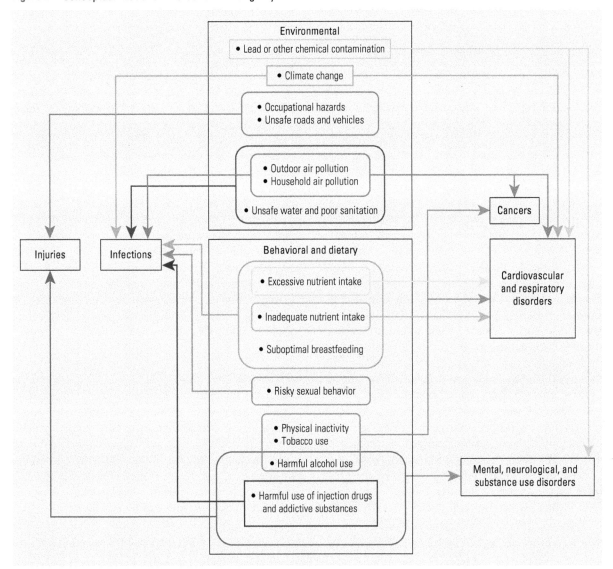

striking features. First, multiple risk factors can overlap and interact to influence the incidence of specific diseases or injuries; for example, smoking, dietary risks, and physical inactivity can all contribute to the development of ischemic heart disease (Ajay, Watkins, and Prabhakaran 2017). Second, single risk factors can be responsible for a substantial fraction of cases of multiple diseases or injuries; for example, air pollution from outdoor sources can lead to chronic obstructive pulmonary disease and asthma, among other conditions (Smith and Pillarisetti 2017). One implication of these interactions is that aggressive targeting of a few major risk factors, such as tobacco smoke and air pollution, can greatly improve population health.

Magnitude of Health Loss from Specific Risk Factors

There are theoretical and practical challenges to quantifying the effect of specific risk factors on fatal and nonfatal outcomes. Comparative risk assessment is the most commonly used approach for this purpose, and its limitations have been reviewed elsewhere (Hoorn and others 2004). Whereas expanded direct measurement of deaths by cause has led to greater precision in mortality estimates in recent years, especially in LMICs (Jha 2014), methods and data sources that can be used to quantify risk factor–attributable mortality are much less developed and subject to greater uncertainty. Nonetheless, for priority setting, information on mortality patterns by broad cause group and the relative proportion of cases that can be attributed to modifiable risk factors, the latter of which is taken from comparative risk assessment studies, is useful. The data shown in table 2.1 suggest that perhaps one-fourth or more of the 57 million deaths globally in 2015 can be attributed to one or more behavioral or environmental risk factors.

In addition, several environmental and behavioral risk factors have been studied for their effects on life expectancy. Air pollution studies have estimated life expectancy losses of 3.3 years in India (Sudarshan and others 2015) and 5.5 years in northern China (Chen and others 2013). (It is important to note that the methodological challenges to estimating the relative risks from air pollution appear to be considerable in settings where there is widespread exposure [Lipfert and Wyzga 1995]). The losses from unsafe water and sanitation appear to be somewhat smaller—ranging from one month in more-developed areas of Mexico to one year or more in the least-developed areas (Stevens, Dias, and Ezzati 2008). In the behavioral risk factor cluster, tobacco studies have estimated that smokers in India, Japan, the United Kingdom, and the United States have about 10 years' lower life expectancy than their nonsmoking peers (Jha and Peto 2014). A U.S. study estimated that physical inactivity, defined as sitting for more than three hours a day, decreases life expectancy by three years (Katzmarzyk and Lee 2012).

Yet another way of appreciating the importance of various risk factors is simply to compare estimates of the proportion of the population exposed to specific risks. The World Health Organization (WHO) Global Health Observatory database contains estimates of the prevalence of a number of important risk factors (WHO 2016b). In the environmental cluster, 95–99 percent of cities across low- and lower-middle-income countries exceed WHO-recommended limits on ambient particulate matter. Further, 91 percent and 56 percent of households in these two income groups, respectively, still used solid fuels for cooking in homes in 2013. Water, sanitation, and hygiene indicators appear to be more favorable: 34 percent and 11 percent, respectively, lack access to improved water sources; and 71 percent and 48 percent, respectively, lack access to improved sanitation. These proportions have declined significantly over the past decade (Hutton and Chase 2017).

As for the behavioral cluster of risk factors, insufficient physical inactivity appears to be the most prevalent risk, particularly among adolescents, with estimates ranging from 78 to 85 percent across World Bank income groups in 2010. The prevalence of risky sexual behavior among reproductive-age individuals in low-income and lower-middle-income countries was an estimated 74 percent and 30 percent, respectively, over 2007–13. The prevalence of tobacco smoking—likely the most hazardous behavior of all—was about 17–18 percent among adults in low- and lower-middle-income countries in 2012 (WHO 2016b).

Distal Determinants of Health

Inadequate individual or household income constrains access to clean water, adequate sanitation, safe shelter, medical services, and other goods and services potentially important for health. Inadequate education results in less likelihood that individuals will acquire information relevant to their health-related behaviors or use that information well. For these reasons, income, education, and other social (or socioeconomic) determinants of health have received much attention for many years.

Table 2.1 Magnitude of Effect of Top Environmental and Behavioral Risk Factors on Major Causes of Death, 2015

Risk category	Number of deaths globally in 2015 (millions)	Share of deaths attributable to one or more behavioral or environmental risks (%)	Top risk factors
Communicable, maternal, perinatal, and nutritional conditions[a]	12	30	Unsafe water, sanitation, and handwashing; maternal and child nutritional risks; unsafe sex; air pollution; tobacco smoke
Noncommunicable diseases	40	24	Dietary risks; tobacco smoke; air pollution; alcohol and drug use; low physical activity; occupational hazards
Injuries[b]	5	20	Alcohol and drug use

Sources: GBD Risk Factors Collaborators (Forouzanfar and others 2016).
Note: Mortality data are taken from World Health Organization (WHO) Global Health Estimates database (Mathers and others 2018, chapter 4 of this volume). Risk factor proportions are taken from the Global Burden of Disease (GBD) 2015 Study (Forouzanfar and others 2016) because similar data were not available from Mathers and others (2018). The table includes risk factors that were estimated to be responsible for 1 percent or more of total deaths globally.
a. For alternative estimates of the attributable burden of maternal and child nutritional risks, see the 2013 *Lancet* series on "Maternal and Child Nutrition" (*Lancet* 2013).
b. Unsafe roads are not included as a risk factor in the GBD 2015 project (Forouzanfar and others 2016); however, the WHO estimates that about 1.3 million road injury deaths occurred in 2015, comprising about 2 percent of all deaths in 2015 (Mathers and others 2018).

Two recent studies extend cross-country time-series studies dealing with income and education (Jamison, Murphy, and Sandbu 2016; Pradhan and others 2017). Three broad conclusions emerge from this literature:

1. *Countries' income levels* are highly statistically significant but quantitatively small factors in terms of influencing reductions in both adult and child mortality.
2. *Level and quality of education* are both statistically significant and quantitatively important. Pradhan and others (2017) concluded that about 14 percent of the decline in under-five mortality between 1970 and 2010 resulted from improvements in education levels. Likewise, about 30 percent of the decline in adult mortality resulted from improvement in education.
3. *Female education* is far more important than male education for reducing both adult and child mortality.

Aside from income and education, social norms and attitudes can greatly affect health. For example, discrimination and stigma have been shown to increase the risks of acquiring sexually transmitted infections, suffering from mental disorders, and incurring injuries from interpersonal violence (Drew and others 2011; Piot and others 2015). In some countries, legalized discrimination persists against vulnerable groups such as men who have sex with men and transgender people. Even in countries without harsh legal arrangements, pervasive discrimination—for example, against indigenous groups—can greatly limit access to needed health and other social services (Davy and others 2016).

Emerging evidence suggests that providing legal and human rights protections to vulnerable and stigmatized groups can reduce health risks or improve health outcomes. Conversely, the lack of such protections can increase health risks and worsen outcomes. For example, criminalization of sex work and same-sex relations is associated with increased risk of human immunodeficiency virus (HIV) among commercial sex workers and men who have sex with men, through mechanisms such as increased risk of sexual violence and decreased provision and uptake of HIV prevention services (Beyrer and others 2012; Shannon and others 2015). At the same time, decriminalization can "avert incident infections through combined effects on violence, police harassment, safer work environments, and HIV transmission pathways" (Piot and others 2015). In general, criminalization of same-sex relations and certain health conditions—such as drug addiction and abortion—often leads to worse health outcomes and cannot be supported on health grounds (Godlee and Hurley 2016; Sedgh and others 2016).

A review of the full range of potential social determinants or the health outcomes they affect is beyond the scope of this chapter. However, these findings are highlighted to note two implications for intersectoral action on health. First, the level of female education appears to be a quantitatively important social determinant of mortality reduction, so discussions of intersectoral policies for health need to stress the importance of female education. Second, discrimination and violation of human rights lead to worse health outcomes and need to be considered in conversations with ministers of justice and law enforcement.

INTERSECTORAL POLICY PACKAGES

Essential Intersectoral Policies

Chapter 1 of this volume (Jamison and others 2018) describes the 21 packages of disease interventions presented throughout the nine *DCP3* volumes that contain 327 interventions in total. Of these, 218 are health sector specific and are covered in chapter 3 of this volume (Watkins and others 2018). The remaining 119 intersectoral interventions are discussed in this chapter.

Annex 2A presents the contents of the intersectoral component of *DCP3*'s essential packages of interventions. These policy interventions varied across packages in terms of their level of specificity, and in a number of cases (such as tobacco taxation) they were duplicated across packages. The authors of this chapter critically reviewed this list of policies and consolidated and harmonized them. This process led to a list of 71 harmonized intersectoral interventions that were grouped by risk factor and type of policy instrument (annex 2B).

Annex 2C provides a few important additional characteristics of the interventions contained in the harmonized list. These include

- The risk factor(s) or cause(s) of death or disability addressed
- The ministry primarily responsible for implementation of the policy
- Whether there are health sector interventions that are equally or more effective (that is, to serve as so-called substitutes—in which cases a health sector approach may be more feasible than an intersectoral approach in limited resource settings)
- Where relevant, notable costs and benefits of the intervention to other sectors
- SDG target(s) addressed.

The vast majority of interventions in annexes 2A and 2B were featured in volume 7 of *DCP3*. Major areas of focus in this volume were air pollution, road injuries, and a number of individually small but collectively important environmental toxins such as lead, mercury, arsenic, and asbestos. This volume also included a number of interventions focused on occupational health, primarily by reducing occupational injury. Volumes 3, 4, and 5 of *DCP3* contained a number of interventions focused on noncommunicable disease risk, particular from addictive substances and excessive nutrient intake. The most common types of policy instruments recommended were legal and regulatory instruments (38 of 71), followed by fiscal instruments (15 of 71).

An Early Intersectoral Package

The 71 interventions listed in annex 2B constitute a demanding menu for policy makers, especially in low-resource settings. Even in well-resourced settings, an incremental approach to implementation of the essential intersectoral package may be politically or economically more tractable than a comprehensive approach. Further, epidemiological and economic conditions will dictate that some intersectoral interventions can await a more urgent need for their implementation. Nonetheless, initiating a subset of intersectoral interventions as soon as possible to achieve significant progress during the 2015–30 SDG period is important. The focus could be on those policies that are likely to provide the best value for money and to be feasible in a wide range of settings.

Table 2.2 outlines the authors' distillation of the contents of annex 2B into an *early* intersectoral package. This package draws on policy interventions that the authors have reviewed and determined to have the strongest evidence and the highest likely magnitude of health effect. (The specific interventions are shown in boldface in annex 2B.) In some cases, the policies have quickly and directly resulted in a measurable decline in mortality, with notable examples being in the area of household air pollution (box 2.1) and suicide prevention (box 2.2).

Table 2.2 Components of an Early Intersectoral Package of Policy Instruments

Key health risk	Policy	Instrument
Air pollution	1. Indoor air pollution: subsidize other clean household energy sources, including liquid propane gas (LPG), for the poor and other key populations.	Fiscal
	2. Indoor air pollution: halt the use of unprocessed coal and kerosene as a household fuel.	Regulatory
	3. Indoor air pollution: promote the use of low-emission household devices.	Information and education
	4. Emissions: tax emissions and/or auction off transferable emission permits.	Fiscal
	5. Emissions: regulate transport, industrial, and power generation emissions.	Regulatory
	6. Fossil fuel subsidies: dismantle subsidies for and increase taxation of fossil fuels (except LPG).	Fiscal
	7. Public transportation: build and strengthen affordable public transportation systems in urban areas.	Built environment
Addictive substance use	8. Substance use: impose large excise taxes on tobacco, alcohol, and other addictive substances.	Fiscal
	9. Substance use: impose strict regulation of advertising, promotion, packaging, and availability of tobacco, alcohol, and other addictive substances, with enforcement.	Regulatory
	10. Smoking in public places: ban smoking in public places.	Regulatory
Inadequate nutrient intake	11. School feeding: finance school feeding for all schools and students in selected geographical areas.	Fiscal
	12. Food quality: ensure that subsidized foods and school feeding programs have adequate nutritional quality.	Regulatory
	13. Iron and folic acid: fortify food.	Regulatory
	14. Iodine: fortify salt.	Regulatory

table continues next page

Table 2.2 Components of an Early Intersectoral Package of Policy Instruments **(continued)**

Key health risk	Policy	Instrument
Excessive nutrient intake	15. Trans fats: ban and replace with polyunsaturated fats.	Regulatory
	16. Salt: impose regulations to reduce salt in manufactured food products.	Regulatory
	17. Sugar sweetened beverages: tax to discourage use.	Fiscal
	18. Salt and sugar: provide consumer education against excess use, including product labeling.	Information and education
Road traffic injuries	19. Vehicle safety: enact legislation and enforcement of personal transport safety measures, including seatbelts in vehicles and helmets for motorcycle users.	Regulatory
	20. Traffic safety: set and enforce speed limits on roads.	Regulatory
	21. Traffic safety: include traffic calming mechanisms into road construction.	Built environment
Other risks	22. Pesticides: enact strict control and move to selective bans on highly hazardous pesticides.	Regulatory
	23. Water and sanitation: enact national standards for safe drinking water, sanitation, and hygenic behavior within and outside households and institutions.	Regulatory
	24. Hazardous waste: enact legislation and enforcement of standards for hazardous waste disposal.	Regulatory
	25. Lead exposure: take actions to reduce human exposure to lead, including bans on leaded fuels and on lead in paint, cookware, water pipes, cosmetics, drugs, and food supplements.	Regulatory
	26. Agricultural antibiotic use: reduce and eventually phase out subtherapeutic antibiotic use in agriculture.	Regulatory
	27. Emergency response: create and exercise multisectoral responses and supply stockpiles to respond to pandemics and other emergencies.	Regulatory
	28. Safe sex: remove duties and taxes on condoms, then introduce subsidies in brothels and for key at-risk populations.	Fiscal
	29. Exercise: take initial steps to develop infrastructure enabling safe walking and cycling.	Built environment

Box 2.1

Bans on Household Coal Use

Coal has been used for household cooking and heating for around 1,000 years, especially in places such as China and the United Kingdom where coal is easy to mine. The famous 1952 "London smog" (smoke and fog) episode, which killed 12,000 people, was mostly the result of indoor burning of coal for heating (Bell, Davis, and Fletcher 2004).

Household coal use has diminished in high-income countries. Today, it is mostly confined to LMICs, especially China and other countries in the Western Pacific region, where it constitutes around 20 percent of all household fuel use (Duan and others 2010). Indoor burning of coal and other solid fuels is a risk factor for cancer and cardiac and respiratory diseases in adults and children.

Bans on coal use, and successful enforcement of these bans have been followed by a reduction in premature deaths from these conditions. For example, during the six years after the Irish government banned the sale of coal in 1990, the age-standardized cardiovascular death rate fell by 10.3 percent and the age-standardized respiratory death rate by 15.5 percent (Clancy and others 2002). These reductions suggest that Dublin experienced about 243 fewer cardiovascular deaths and 116 fewer respiratory deaths per year after the coal ban.

Preventing Suicide in Sri Lanka by Regulating Pesticides

From 1950 to 1995, suicide rates in Sri Lanka increased eightfold to a peak of 47 per 100,000 in 1995, the highest rate in the world (Gunnell and others 2007). Around two-thirds of the suicide deaths during this period were due to self-poisoning with pesticides (Abeyasinghe 2002). Consensus is lacking on the chief contributors to the changing rates of suicide in Sri Lanka, but these are likely to include periods of civil war and economic recession, changes in the rates of mental illness and its treatment, and the easy availability of hazardous agrochemicals (Abeyasinghe 2002; Gunnell and others 2007).

In the 1980s and 1990s, a series of legislative activities led to the stepwise banning of the most toxic of the pesticides being used for self-poisoning. This legislation included (a) the 1984 ban on methyl parathion and parathion, (b) the 1995 ban on the remaining WHO Class I ("extremely" or "highly" toxic) organophosphate pesticides, and (c) the 1998 ban on endosulfan, a Class II ("moderately hazardous") pesticide that farmers had been using in place of Class I pesticides (figure B2.1.1, panel a).

An ecological analysis of time trends in suicide and suicide risk factors in Sri Lanka from 1975 to 2005 found that these bans coincided with marked declines in the suicide rates of both men and women (figure B2.1.1, panel a). Time trends in the data on suicide method showed that the large reduction in suicide was mostly due to a reduction in self-poisoning (figure B2.1.1, panel b). Further support for this interpretation came from in-hospital mortality data, which showed a halving in death rates from pesticide self-poisoning—from 12.0 per 100,000 population in 1998 to 6.5 per 100,000 population in 2005.

Figure B2.1.1 Suicide Rates in Relation to Selected Events in Sri Lanka, by Gender and Method, 1975–2005

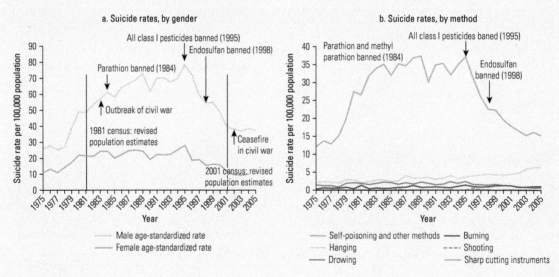

Source: Gunnell and others 2007.

A few general themes emerge from table 2.2:

- *Nearly all of the policies address risks that produce large negative externalities* such as polluted air (including from tobacco), unsafe driving, and environmental toxins, to name a few. The presence of such externalities justifies the use of aggressive fiscal and regulatory measures to correct the economic inefficiencies that result from the failure of households or firms to take negative externalities into account in their decision making.
- *Many of the policies attempt to regulate or alter markets for unhealthy and often addictive substances* such as tobacco, alcohol, and processed foods. These might be seen as important first steps toward a more comprehensive approach to reduce disease risks that would eventually include greater incentives for healthy eating and physical activity. Greater incentives for healthy eating and physical activity are likely to be much more disruptive and potentially expensive to fully incorporate into a whole-of-government policy but could lead to greater and more sustained gains in healthy life years as incomes grow.
- *These policies require cross-cutting engagement with a few key ministries*, including finance, justice, environment, agriculture, and trade. Ministers of health could seek to develop productive relationships across these key sectors early in the process.

POLICIES TO ADDRESS THE CONSEQUENCES OF ILLNESS OR INJURY

Globally, estimates of overall life expectancy have exceeded estimates of healthy life expectancy by several years on average over the past few decades, suggesting that nonfatal health losses are a significant—and in many countries, growing—concern for global health (WHO 2016b). One group has estimated that at the same time that global mortality has declined in absolute terms, absolute levels of disability have increased over time, particularly in regions that have experienced significant social and economic development (Kassebaum and others 2016). Thus, the general conclusion is that although rapid declines in child and adult mortality have facilitated population growth and aging, these changes have not been matched by improvements in overall rates of disability. In part, this phenomenon can be attributed to unchanged or increased levels of noncommunicable disease and injury risk factors that could potentially be addressed using intersectoral measures, as described previously. At the same time, an equally important question is the role of health and nonhealth

sectors in mitigating the consequences of illness and injury for the fraction of cases that are not effectively preventable by addressing the major risk factors.

Projection studies from high-income and selected middle-income countries raise concerns that, even in countries with high-performing health systems, spending on long-term care for individuals with chronic physical or mental disability is significant and likely to continue increasing (de la Maisonneuve and Oliveira Martins 2013). A recent study from the Netherlands found that health expenditure increases dramatically with age and nearness to death, with about 10 percent of aggregate expenditure devoted to individuals in their last year of life (Bakx, O'Donnell, and van Doorslaer 2016). Studies from other settings such as the United States validate these findings (Bekelman and others 2016). Yet another concerning result of the Dutch study is that about one-third of total health expenditure in recent years was on long-term care, and the distribution of this share of expenditure was skewed toward a relatively small number of individuals with severe disability (Bakx, O'Donnell, and van Doorslaer 2016). These expenditures were also persistent over time, highlighting the chronic, often lifelong, nature of ill health.

Several sources of long-term disabilities have been observed to accompany economic growth and population aging, including vision and hearing loss, dementias, disability from cerebrovascular disease, and injuries related to advanced age. These conditions are no longer limited to high-income countries; most LMICs are now experiencing substantial health burden related to population aging (WHO 2011b). In many cases, these trends are superimposed on continued high levels of disability at younger ages—for example, disabilities resulting from severe injuries (which can result from interpersonal violence, falls, or transport injury), severe psychiatric disorders, and intellectual disability (Kassebaum and others 2016). The growing population, elderly and nonelderly, needing long-term care in LMICs will inevitably require a greater response from government in the form of broad-based social support measures.

Support for those individuals with long-term disability will need to include health sector–based interventions such as home health services, institutional care (for example, in skilled nursing facilities), and palliative care, but it will need more than the health sector can provide to care adequately for the whole person. Intersectoral policies can be developed to provide these individuals with assistance in obtaining affordable food, housing, and transportation, all of which are instrumental to preventing further health loss. These policies usually fall under the category of transfer payments and may be delivered directly as grants (nonwage income) or through more targeted efforts such as subsidized housing or nutrition programs.

These transfer payments provide an important opportunity for ministries of health to work with ministries of social development and others to care for the whole individual. In some settings, intersectoral collaboration has led to large-scale anti-poverty, social welfare, and cash-transfer programs that integrate key social support measures and enable effective uptake of health interventions (Watkins and others 2018). There are examples of successful social support programs that effectively integrate health interventions, including support for older adults. One of these is Mexico´s Prospera program, which has been in operation since the late 1990s and covers the majority of the population living in poverty (Knaul and others 2017).

As a result, *DCP3* recommends that, as resources permit, countries consider income and in-kind social support for individuals living with long-term disability or severe, life-limiting illness (Krakauer and others 2018). Unfortunately, there is a limited evidence base on which to design and implement social support measures in LMICs. Further, the feasibility and sustainability of broad-based social support programs in low-income and lower-middle-income countries, in particular, are unknown. For example, Krakauer and others (2018) produce preliminary estimates of social support costs for individuals in need of palliative care. These costs could vary widely

by country and would depend on the proportion of the population in extreme poverty and the sorts of benefits (such as income, food, and transportation) included in the social support package. In low-income countries, such a comprehensive program would probably be unaffordable at current levels of government spending.

The following three general points can be emphasized for all countries, even those that are not currently able to implement fiscal policies that address long-term care:

1. The need for long-term care is increasing in nearly all countries because of population aging and high rates of nonfatal health loss.
2. Long-term care accounts for a significant fraction of government expenditure in high-income settings, and LMICs need to start preparing for this transition.
3. To address the needs of disabled persons adequately, non–health sectors will need to be engaged and willing to assume a large part of the fiscal responsibility.

This last point suggests that countries could begin to develop a more inclusive notion of national health accounts. Mexico's experience in developing inclusive national health accounts can be instructive for other LMICs (box 2.3). In light of the critical gaps in current evidence and the rapid shifts in disease burden in

---

Box 2.3

Inclusive National Health Accounts: The Case of Mexico

National health accounts (NHAs) show that Mexico spent 5.7 percent of its gross domestic product (GDP) on health in 2015. This share is low compared with an average of 9.3 percent among Organisation for Economic Co-operation and Development countries and an average of 8.2 percent for the Latin American region. However, the real figure is probably much larger because a significant part of health-related economic activities, in particular those related to long-term illness and injuries, goes unreported or unaccounted for by official NHA figures.

The National Institute of Statistics and Geography (INEGI) acknowledged this concern by producing

satellite accounts to estimate the value at market prices of informal health activities generated by economic agents. These satellite accounts are sizable: the value of unpaid work related to health care performed by households alone can add an extra 18.6 percent to the traditional GDP estimates for the health sector. An even more inclusive figure of the costs of ill health would add income transfers of voluntary and legally mandated sick leave and disability insurance. Figures from the main social security institutions would add another 9.2 percent, bringing total health spending estimates closer to 7.3 percent of GDP.

box continues next page

Box 2.3 (continued)

Conservative estimates from the satellite accounts of the combined value of (a) unpaid household members' activities aimed at preventing ill health and caring for and maintaining health both within and outside the household and (b) the volunteer work for nonprofit organizations averages 1 percent of GDP over the past 10 years (INEGI 2017). According to INEGI, the value of 69 percent of total hours and 82 percent of unpaid work comes from household members undertaking mostly specialty care of chronic ailments. Moreover, 70 percent of unremunerated caregivers are women (INEGI 2017).

A more inclusive approach toward NHA also helps estimate the economic consequences of ill health that are increasingly being borne outside of institutional settings. In 2015, approximately half of the burden of disease in Mexico was related to years lived with disability, out of which mental and substance abuse and musculoskeletal disorders accounted for 40 percent (Kassebaum and others 2016), and an estimated 16 percent of the adult population had diabetes (OECD 2016). This burden has not only increased pressure in an already overwhelmed and underfunded public health care system but also created significant pressure on social security institutions. Not surprisingly, about half of total health spending is from private sources, most of it paid out of pocket. Moreover, figures on the value of cash benefits for temporary disability (resulting from illness or accident, whether work or nonwork related, and maternity leave) paid through the main social security schemes—the Mexican Social Security Institute and the Institute of Social Security and Services for State Workers—amount to at least 9.2 percent of total health spending. Adding pensions for permanent disability would include this value. None of these figures are currently being accounted for as health-related spending neither in the NHA nor in the satellite accounts.

Naturally, families also face increased pressure as they seek ways to care for these patients, whether by reorganizing household members' roles and timetables, investing to adapt their homes to better suit their needs, hiring nonfamily caregivers, or sometimes even quitting their own jobs or reducing work hours. Because long-term care for the elderly or the chronically ill is not reimbursed by social or public health insurance schemes, families must step in and find ways to provide care, sometimes for long periods of time. The institutional response from the health system has been slow regarding long-term care. Elderly or chronically ill patients receive hospital care for acute events, but the supply of publicly funded long-term care or nursing homes to care for them over longer periods is very limited, and services provided by existing private nursing homes need to be paid for out of pocket.

Although social security institutions and other social assistance programs run day centers, which can include meals, families are by far the main provider of long-term care for the elderly (OECD 2007). Mexico's omission in reporting expenditure on long-term care only reflects this institutional void. Part of the value of the informal long-term care provided by families is included in the satellite health accounts, but a significant amount of nursing home services paid for out of pocket by families possibly still goes unregistered.

As health needs become more complex and require care that goes beyond the traditional clinical and acute care settings, a broader perspective is needed to tease apart the economic and organizational implications. Mexico's satellite accounts illustrate one step in this direction, highlighting the need to broaden the range of types of care and providers considered when estimating the production value of the health sector's share of GDP is necessary. Informal care undertaken by families and by nursing homes and other types of long-term care facilities needs to be accounted for, even if this means considering a mix of medical and other services (such as psychological and nutrition services). Yet the indirect costs of illness are also important, as confirmed by the large value of income transfers for temporary disability. These should also be considered for a more inclusive NHA. More comprehensive estimates of the production value of the health sector would increase awareness and inform policy formulation to better prepare for the long-term care transition.

LMICs, the issue of long-term care could be regarded as one of the most important priorities for policy research over the coming years.

IMPLEMENTATION OF AN INTERSECTORAL AGENDA FOR HEALTH

Translation of the Intersectoral Package into Action

The *DCP3* intersectoral package, including the early-priority actions outlined in table 2.2, is intended to provide a list of policy actions outside the health sector that could substantially improve population health through a whole-of-government approach. Of course, the application of this intersectoral package will vary according to epidemiological and demographic considerations. For instance, low- and lower-middle-income countries might place a higher priority on controlling indoor sources of air pollution, improving maternal and child nutrition through food fortification, and scaling up water and sanitation measures. Upper-middle-income and high-income countries would probably devote more efforts toward reductions in dietary risks. Most LMICs could consider implementing stronger road safety and tobacco control measures. All countries could work collectively to address climate change, antimicrobial resistance, and other global threats.

The WHO (2011b) has produced a practical guide to intersectoral engagement that includes a 10-step process for building and sustaining cross-sectoral collaboration. The guide—"Intersectoral Action on Health: A Path for Policy-Makers to Implement Effective and Sustainable Action on Health"—highlights three cross-cutting themes relevant to implementation:

- Careful consideration of the social, cultural, economic, and political context
- Emphasis on generating political will and commitment from all relevant sectors at the national and subnational levels
- Design and reinforcement of accountability mechanisms, which also integrate into the monitoring and evaluation process.

In addition, it stresses that historically major policy change has tended to occur at times of political or economic transition or crisis and that ministries of health should take advantage of these times to put their priorities on the agenda (WHO 2011b).

A number of countries have overcome barriers to implementation by mainstreaming intersectoral approaches to health. A common theme in these successes is that the government, including the health sector, recognized the legitimacy of intersectoral action for health, as the following examples show:

- *Iran* has established several national mechanisms for bringing sectors together to improve health, including the National Coordination Council for Healthy Cities and Healthy Villages (Sheikh and others 2012). The council oversees community-based health improvement initiatives based on strategies such as expanding access to financial credit, social services, and sanitation.
- *Vietnam* has established a national intersectoral coordination mechanism, the National Traffic Safety Committee, with representatives from 15 ministries and agencies, to advise the prime minister on improving road safety. The committee played a key role in the passage of Vietnam's national mandatory helmet law (box 2.4).

Box 2.4

Reducing Road Traffic Deaths in Vietnam through Helmet Laws

Nearly half of all road deaths worldwide are among groups of individuals who are the least protected—pedestrians, cyclists, and motorcyclists (WHO 2015). The risk to these different groups shows large regional variations. For example, in Sub-Saharan Africa pedestrians and cyclists are at highest risk, whereas in Southeast Asia motorcyclists are at greatest risk.

Head injuries from motorcycle crashes are a common cause of morbidity and mortality. A Cochrane systematic review of 61 observational studies concluded that motorcycle helmets reduce the risk of head injury by around 69 percent and death by around 42 percent (Liu and others 2008). Several countries in Southeast Asia have seen significant reductions in the rate of head injuries and deaths

box continues next page

Box 2.4 (continued)

Figure B2.4.1 Share of Motorcycle Drivers and Passengers Wearing Helmets in Vietnam, 2007 and 2008

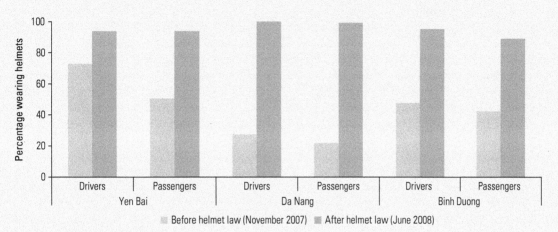

Before helmet law (November 2007)   After helmet law (June 2008)

Source: Passmore, Nguyen, and others 2010.
Note: Figure shows extent of motorcycle helmet wearing in three provinces of Vietnam before and after the introduction of mandatory helmet-wearing legislation.

among motorcyclists after the introduction of laws that made motorcycle helmet use mandatory (Hyder and others 2007). For example, after Vietnam's mandatory motorcycle helmet law went into effect in December 2007, an observational time-series study using data from a random selection of the road network in three provinces (Yen Bai, Da Nang, and Binh Duong) found significant increases in helmet wearing among both motorcycle riders and their passengers (Passmore, Nguyen, and others 2010), as shown in figure B2.4.1. Surveillance data from 20 rural and urban hospitals found that the risk of road traffic head injuries and deaths decreased by 16 percent and 18 percent, respectively (Passmore, Tu, and others 2010).

An extended cost-effectiveness analysis of the 2007 helmet policy suggests that it prevented about 2,200 deaths and 29,000 head injuries in the year following its introduction (Olson and others 2016). The analysis found that the wealthy owned the greatest number of motorcycles, so they accrued a larger share of the absolute health and financial benefits from the law. However, the policy probably prevented a larger number of cases of poverty among the poor and middle class as well.

- *Thailand* has vigorously promoted nationwide intersectoral action on health, including the use of health impact assessments. Such assessments are important tools for the health sector to engage other sectors by identifying the possible positive and negative health consequences of other sectoral policies (Kang, Park, and Kim 2011). They have been conducted for a wide range of policies or plans, including biomass power plant projects, patents on medicines, coal mining, and industrial estate development (Phoolcharoen, Sukkumnoed, and Kessomboon 2003).

A Key Role for Ministries of Finance

As shown in table 2.2 and annexes 2A and 2B, many of the essential intersectoral policies in *DCP3* are fiscal in nature. Even the nonfiscal instruments proposed have implications for non–health sector budgets and thus involve ministries of finance to a degree. By tracking the anticipated effects of interventions on government and private revenues and expenditures outside the health sector, annex 2C provides ministries of health with some sense of where opportunity and opposition may arise on fiscal grounds.

Estimating the costs and consequences of intersectoral intervention can be challenging for a variety of reasons, and evaluation of all-of-society costs and benefits of health-related policies is outside the scope of *DCP3*. Health economic evaluations usually implement cost-effectiveness and cost-utility analyses from a health sector perspective on costs. In some cases, cost-effectiveness analysis has been used to evaluate intersectoral interventions. However, this perspective is quite limited because many of the important economic costs and benefits of these interventions lie outside the health sector. Fortunately, interest in benefit-cost analysis has grown within health economics of late, and this approach is ideal for evaluating intersectoral policies (see chapter 9 of this volume, Chang, Horton, and Jamison 2018).

In volume 7 of *DCP3*, Watkins and others (2017) summarize benefit-cost studies, including program costs, of interventions focusing on injury prevention and environmental hazards, which are among the health topics with a significant benefit-cost literature. Although the costs reviewed in volume 7 are neither totally representative nor exhaustive, they can provide a rough sense of the magnitude of intersectoral costs. These range from negative costs in the case of taxes to less than US$1 per capita per year for regulation and legislation to more than US$10 per capita per year for certain education interventions or built-environment modifications (Watkins and others 2017).

Taxation-Based Strategies

This chapter strongly recommends taxation-based strategies for addressing harmful substance use and selected environmental hazards because of their clear effect on behavioral change and the positive revenue implications for governments. Tobacco, alcohol, carbon emissions, and unhealthy food products may all be considered as candidates for taxation. Although tobacco and alcohol were originally taxed solely to generate revenue—perhaps as early as the 1300s (Crooks 1989)—the long history of these taxes can provide insights into how to implement a variety of taxes to improve health. The fundamental question to answer first is *what* to tax. For example, is it more effective to tax sugar as a nutrient per se, to tax specific products such as sugar-sweetened beverages, or to opt for a hybrid approach (for example, a tax based on the amount of added sugar in a particular class of products, such as sugar-sweetened beverages)? The pros and cons of any specific tax target need to be evaluated in terms of consumption habits, possible substitution effects (as discussed below), and the administrative costs and feasibility of tax implementation given a country's tax administration. Taxing the amount of added sugar in a product group would also require information on the nutrient content in those foods.

Closely tied to what to tax is the issue of *substitution* effects—that is, how demand for another product might change when the price of the newly taxed product changes (Fletcher, Frisvold, and Tefft 2013). For example, if sugar-sweetened beverages are taxed, the decrease in sugar intake from reduced consumption of sugar-sweetened beverages might be offset by increased consumption of fruit juice or confectionary products. At the same time, not all substitution effects are negative: recently implemented soda taxes in Mexico were associated with increased consumption of bottled water (Colchero and others 2016, Colchero and others 2017). In some cases, substitution effects might mutually reinforce public health goals ultimately. For example, tobacco taxes appear to decrease binge drinking, presumably because tobacco and alcohol use disorders co-occur in many individuals (Young-Wolff and others 2014). Hence, when designing taxes, policy makers need to consider substitution effects and balance these against implementation feasibility. For example, a broader nutrient tax on sugar or on added sugar in processed foods would decrease the substitution effects relative to a tax on sugar-sweetened beverages alone, but it may not be easily implemented in many settings given the high tax administration requirements.

Several other tax design considerations are worth noting briefly:

- *The type of tax* is important to determine, and experience suggests that excise taxes can be more effective than sales taxes (IARC 2011). Tobacco taxes provide an important example in this regard. Tax rates can be simplified and based on the quantity of cigarettes, not their price (the latter of which is easier for the tobacco industry to manipulate). A related goal is to preempt downward substitution, when smokers switch to cheaper cigarette brands in response to a tax-rate hike on the brands they had previously smoked. Specific excises, as opposed to *ad valorem* (value-based) excises or other taxes, are more effective at doing so. The second strategy is to merge the multiple tobacco tax tiers that are used in most LMICs. This way, tax hikes raise prices by the same large amount on all brands at once, pushing smokers to quit completely rather than switch (Marquez and Moreno-Dodson 2017).
- *The amount of tax* needs to be large enough to change behavior. For example, the WHO recommends that the cigarette excise tax make up at least 70 percent of the final consumer price and that it be designed

to keep up with inflation and overall affordability (WHO 2011c).

- *Tax evasion and avoidance* are common problems that can be mitigated by having effective tax administration measures and harmonized tax rates within a country and with neighboring countries (WHO 2011c.).
- *Tax effectiveness* may improve as part of a comprehensive approach that includes public education, regulations, and other types of policies that support behavior change (WHO 2016a).
- *Public and industry opposition to taxes* needs to be anticipated and countered. A traditional tactic of industry groups is to argue that taxes will hurt employment and have a regressive effect on the poor. Yet low-income groups are generally more responsive to these taxes and are likely receive more of the long-term health and economic benefits from the tax (Chaloupka and others 2012).

Subsidy-Related Strategies

Recognizing the role that subsidies can play in increasing or reducing health risks is also important. In many countries, fossil fuels are heavily subsidized, representing a major economic barrier to clean energy (Coady and others 2015). In some countries, broad food subsidies (such as on bread, milk, or other products) are entrenched, but these measures are ineffective in promoting a healthy diet and may actually incentivize over-consumption in environments, such as in the Arab Republic of Egypt, that are experiencing forms of malnutrition currently (IFPRI 2013). Similarly, agricultural subsidies in some countries greatly influence food consumption, both in the producing country and in its trading partners, sometimes to the detriment of health (Fields 2004; Russo and Smith 2013).

In light of anticipated revenue streams and country experiences, a potential expansion path can be conceived for the rollout of fiscal policies directed toward a given substance. A first step would be to remove subsidies—especially important in the case of fossil fuels and unhealthy foods—or, at the very least, to prevent subsidies from being added. The next step would be to add taxes on the substance. The final step would be to add subsidies for healthier substitutes. The first two steps would generate revenue and create fiscal space for subsidies, including those that preferentially affect vulnerable populations.

Intersectoral Action in the SDG Era

One method for increasing political will and accountability is to design policies explicitly linked to international agreements to which governments are already signatories. Annex 2C demonstrates wide-reaching connections between the *DCP3* intersectoral package and the SDG targets—especially the nonhealth-related SDGs, which are of particular interest to other sectors. These connections and other international agreements that have intersectoral implications (for example, the WHO Framework Convention on Tobacco Control and the United Nations Convention on the Rights of the Child) can be leveraged both to engage other sectors on health issues and to put into place good accountability and reporting mechanisms for specific policies. This approach suggests a strong relationship with ministries of foreign affairs that are accountable for the implementation of these agreements (WHO 2011b).

The SDGs contain strong language on poverty alleviation (for example, SDG 1) and equity (for example, SDGs 5 and 10).[1] One new scientific contribution of *DCP3* has been the development of extended cost-effectiveness analysis (ECEA), which considers not only the health outcomes but also the financial risk protection and distributional (equity-enhancing) effects of policies (as further discussed in chapter 8 of this volume, Verguet and Jamison 2018). Although ECEA most naturally serves as a tool to prioritize various health services for public finance (covered in chapter 3 of this volume, Watkins and others 2018), several ECEAs have also been conducted on intersectoral policies, including tobacco taxation (Verguet and others 2015), regulation of salt in processed foods (Watkins and others 2016), and mandatory helmet laws (Olson and others 2016). These ECEAs show that intersectoral policies can—by reducing disease risk and hence reducing an individual's need for health care—prevent medical impoverishment, and in some cases they can be pro-poor (meaning the poor benefit disproportionately to their population share from the combined health and financial benefits of such interventions). One area of future work would be to integrate the ECEA approach into health impact assessment or benefit-cost analysis to illustrate the disaggregated nonhealth benefits of intersectoral policies, particularly when those benefits speak to SDG targets or goals.

ANNEXES

The following annexes to this chapter are available at http://www.dcp-3.org/DCP.

- Annex 2A: Intersectoral Policies of *DCP3*'s 21 Essential Packages
- Annex 2B: Essential Intersectoral Policies Covered in This Chapter
- Annex 2C: Characteristics of Essential Intersectoral Policies Covered in This Chapter

NOTES

World Bank Income Classifications as of July 2014 are as follows, based on estimates of gross national income (GNI) per capita for 2013:

- Low-income countries (LICs) = US$1,045 or less
- Middle-income countries (MICs) are subdivided:
  (a) lower-middle-income = US$1,046 to US$4,125.
  (b) upper-middle-income (UMICs) = US$4,126 to US$12,745.
- High-income countries (HICs) = US$12,746 or more.

1. SDG 1: "End poverty in all its forms everywhere"; SDG 5: "Achieve gender equality and empower all women and girls"; and SDG 10: "Reduce inequality within and among countries."

REFERENCES

Abeyasinghe, R. "Psychiatric Aspects of Pesticide Poisoning." 2002. In *Pesticides: Health Impacts and Alternatives. Proceedings of a Workshop held in Colombo 24 January 2002*, edited by L. A. M. Smit, 11–15. Working Paper 45. Sri Lanka: International Water Management Institute.

Ajay, V. S., D. A. Watkins, and D. Prabhakaran. 2017. "Relationships among Major Risk Factors and the Burden of Cardiovascular Diseases, Diabetes, and Chronic Lung Disease." In *Disease Control Priorities* (third edition): Volume 5, *Cardiovascular, Respiratory, and Related Disorders*, edited by D. Prabhakaran, S. Anand, T. Gaziano, J.-C. Mbanya, Y. Wu, and R. Nugent. Washington, DC: World Bank.

Alegre-Díaz, J., W. Herrington, M. Lopez-Cervantes, L. Gnatiuc, R. Ramirez, and others. 2016. "Diabetes and Cause-Specific Mortality in Mexico City." *New England Journal of Medicine* 375 (20): 1961–71.

Bakx, P., O. O'Donnell, and E. van Doorslaer. 2016. "Spending on Health Care in the Netherlands: Not Going So Dutch." *Fiscal Studies* 37 (3–4): 593–625.

Bekelman, J. E., S. D. Halpern, C. R. Blankart, J. P. Bynum, J. Cohen, and others. 2016. "Comparison of Site of Death, Health Care Utilization, and Hospital Expenditures for Patients Dying with Cancer in 7 Developed Countries." *Journal of the American Medical Association* 315 (3): 272–83.

Bell, M. L., D. L. Davis, and T. Fletcher. 2004. "A Retrospective Assessment of Mortality from the London Smog Episode of 1952: The Role of Influenza and Pollution. Environmental Health Perspectives 112 (1): 6–8.

Beyrer, C., P. S. Sullivan, J. Sanchez, D. Dowdy, D. Altman, and others. 2012. "A Call to Action for Comprehensive HIV Services for Men Who Have Sex with Men." *The Lancet* 380 (9839): 424–38.

Buss, P. M., L. E. Fonseca, L. A. Galvao, K. Fortune, and C. Cook. 2016. "Health in All Policies in the Partnership for Sustainable Development." *Revista Panamericana de Salud Pública* 40 (3): 186–91.

Chaloupka, F. J., A. Yurekli, and G. T. Fong. 2012. "Tobacco Taxes as a Tobacco Control Strategy." *Tobacco Control* 21 (2): 172–80.

Chang, A., S. Horton, and D. Jamison. 2018. "Benefit-Cost Analysis in *Disease Control Priorities*, Third Edition." In *Disease Control Priorities* (third edition): Volume 9, *Disease Control Priorities: Improving Health and Reducing Poverty*, edited by D. T. Jamison, H. Gelband, S. Horton, P. Jha, R. Laxminarayan, C. N. Mock, and R. Nugent. Washington, DC: World Bank.

Chen, Y., A. Ebenstein, M. Greenstone, and H. Li. 2013. "Evidence on the Impact of Sustained Exposure to Air Pollution on Life Expectancy from China's Huai River Policy." *Proceedings of the National Academy of Sciences of the United States of America* 110 (32): 12936–41.

Clancy, L., P. Goodman, H. Sinclair, and D. W. Dockery. 2002. "Effect of Air-Pollution Control on Death Rates in Dublin, Ireland: An Intervention Study." *The Lancet* 360 (9341): 1210–14.

Coady, D., I. Parry, L. Sears, and B. Shang. 2015. "How Large Are Energy Subsidies?" IMF Working Paper WP/15/105, International Monetary Fund, Washington, DC..

Colchero, M. A., B. Popkin, J. Rivera, and S. W. Ng. 2016. "Beverage Purchases from Stores in Mexico under the Excise Tax on Sugar Sweetened Beverages: Observational Study." *BMJ* 352: h6704/

———. 2017. "In Mexico, Evidence of Sustained Consumer Response Two Years after Implementing a Sugar-Sweetened Beverage Tax." *Health Affairs*. doi:10.1377.

Crooks, E. 1989. *Alcohol Consumption and Taxation*. London: The Institute of Fiscal Studies.

Davy, C., S. Harfield, A. McArthur, Z. Munn, and A. Brown. 2016. "Access to Primary Health Care Services for Indigenous Peoples: A Framework Synthesis." *International Journal for Equity in Health* 15 (1): 163.

De la Maisonneuve, C., and J. Oliveira Martins. 2013. "Public Spending on Health and Long-Term Care: A New Set of Projections." OECD Economic Policy Papers 6, Organisation for Economic Co-operation and Development, Paris.

Drew, N., M. Funk, S. Tang, J. Lamichhane, E. Chavez, and others. 2011. "Human Rights Violations of People with Mental and Psychosocial Disabilities: An Unresolved Global Crisis." *The Lancet* 378 (9803): 1664–75.

Duan, X., J. Zhang, H. Adair-Rohani, N. Bruce, H. Solomon, and K. R. Smith. 2010. "WHO Guidelines for Indoor Air Quality: Household Fuel Combustion—Review 8: Household Coal Combustion: Unique Features of Exposure to Intrinsic Toxicants and Health Effects." World Health Organization, Geneva. http://www.who.int/indoorair/guidelines/hhfc/Review_8.pdf.

Fields, S. 2004. "The Fat of the Land: Do Agricultural Subsidies Foster Poor Health?" *Environmental Health Perspectives* 112 (14): A820–23.

Fletcher, J., D. Frisvold, and N. Tefft. 2013. "Substitution Patterns Can Limit the Effects of Sugar-Sweetened Beverage Taxes on Obesity." *Preventing Chronic Disease* 10 (February 7): 120–95.

Forouzanfar, M., and others. 2016. "Global, Regional, and National Comparative Risk Assessment of 79 Behavioural, Environmental and Occupational, and Metabollic Risks or Clusters of Risks, 1990–2015: A Systematic Analysis for the Global Burden of Disease Study 2015." *The Lancet* 388 (10053): 1659–724.

Godlee, F., and R. Hurley. 2016. "The War on Drugs Has Failed: Doctors Should Lead Calls for Drug Policy Reform." *Britsh Medical Journal* 355: i6067.

Gunnell, D., R. Fernando, M. Hewagama, W. D. Priyangika, F. Konradsen, and M. Eddleston. 2007. "The Impact of Pesticide Regulations on Suicide in Sri Lanka." *International Journal of Epidemiology* 36 (6): 1235–42

Hoorn, S. V., M. Ezzati, A. Rodgers, A. D. Lopez, and C. J. L. Murray. 2004. "Estimating Attributable Burden of Disease from Exposure and Hazard Data." In *Comparative Quantification of Health Risks: Global and Regional Burden of Diseases Attributable to Selected Major Risk Factors*, Volume 2, edited by M. Ezzati, A. D. Lopez, A. Rodgers, and C. J. L. Murray, 2129–40. Geneva: World Health Organization.

Hutton, G., and C. Chase. 2017. "Water Supply, Sanitation, and Hygiene." In *Disease Control Priorities* (third edition): Volume 7, *Injury Prevention and Environmental Health*, edited by C. N. Mock, O. Kobusingye, R. Nugent, and K. Smith. Washington, DC: World Bank.

Hyder, A.A., H. Waters, T. Phillips, and J. Rehwinkel. 2007. "Exploring the Economics of Motorcycle Helmet Laws—Implications for Low and Middle-Income Countries." *Asia-Pacific Journal of Public Health* 19 (2): 16–22.

IARC (International Agency for Research on Cancer). 2011. *Effectiveness of Tax and Price Policies for Tobacco Control.* Volume 14, IARC Handbooks. Lyon, France: IARC.

IFPRI (International Food Policy Research Institute). 2013. "Food Subsidies in Egypt: A Help or Hindrance?" IFPRI blog, June 24, http://www.ifpri.org/blog/food-subsidies-egypt-help-or-hindrance.

INEGI (National Institute of Statistics and Geography, Government of Mexico). 2017. "Cuenta Satélite del Sector Salud de México, 2015" [Health Sector Satellite of Mexico, 2015]. Press release, March 23.

Jamison, D. T., A. Alwan, C. N. Mock, R. Nugent, D. A. Watkins, and others. 2018. "Universal Health Coverage and Intersectoral Action for Health: Findings from *Disease Control Priorities, Third Edition*." In *Disease Control Priorities* (third edition): Volume 9, *Disease Control Priorities: Improving Health and Reducing Poverty*, edited by D. T. Jamison, H. Gelband, S. Horton, P. Jha, R. Laxminarayan, C. N. Mock, and R. Nugent. Washington, DC: World Bank.

Jamison, D. T., J. G. Breman, A. R. Measham, G. Alleyne, M. Claeson, D. B. Evans, P. Jha, A. Mills, and P. Musgrove, eds. 2006. *Disease Control Priorities in Developing Countries*, second edition. Washington, DC: Oxford University Press and World Bank.

Jamison, D. T., S. M. Murphy, and M. E. Sandbu. 2016. "Why Has Under-5 Mortality Decreased at Such Different Rates in Different Countries?" *Journal of Health Economics* 48: 16–25.

Jha, P. 2014. "Reliable Direct Measurement of Causes of Death in Low- and Middle-Income Countries." *BMC Medicine* 12: 19.

Jha, P., M. MacLennan, A. Yurekli, C. Ramasundarahettige, K. Palipudi, and others. 2015. "Global Hazards of Tobacco and the Benefits of Smoking Cessation and Tobacco Tax." In *Disease Control Priorities* (third edition): Volume 3, *Cancer*, edited by H. Gelband, P. Jha, R. Sankaranarayanan, and S. Horton, 175–94. Washington, DC: World Bank.

Jha, P., and R. Peto. 2014. "Global Effects of Smoking, of Quitting, and of Taxing Tobacco." *New England Journal of Medicine* 370 (1): 60. doi:10.1056/NEJMra308383.

Jha, P., C. Ramasundarahettige, V. Landsman, B. Rostron, M. Thun, and others. 2013. "21st-Century Hazards of Smoking and Benefits of Cessation in the United States." *New England Journal of Medicine* 368 (4): 341–50.

Kang, E., H. J. Park, and J. E. Kim. 2011. "Health Impact Assessment as a Strategy for Intersectoral Collaboration." *Journal of Preventive Medicine and Public Health* 44 (5): 20109.

Kassebaum, N. J., M. Arora, R. M. Barber, Z. A. Bhutta, J. Brown, and others. 2016. "Global, Regional, and National Disability-Adjusted Life Years (DALYs) for 315 Diseases and Injuries and Healthy Life Expectancy (HALE) for 195 Countries and Territories, 1990–2015: A Systematic Analysis for the Global Burden of Diseases, Injuries, and Risk Factors (GBD) 2015 Study." *The Lancet* 388 (10053): 1603–58.

Katzmarzyk, P. T., and I. M. Lee. 2012. "Sedentary Behaviour and Life Expectancy in the USA: A Cause-Deleted Life Table Analysis." *BMJ Open* 2 (4): e000828.

Khayatzadeh-Mahani, A., Z. Sedoghi, M. H. Mehrolhassani, and V. Yazdi-Feyzabadi. 2016. "How Health in All Policies Are Developed and Implemented in a Developing Country? A Case Study of a HiAP Initiative in Iran." *Health Promotion International* 31 (4): 769–81.

Knaul, F. M., P. E. Farmer, E. L. Krakauer, L. de Lima, A. Bhadelia, and others. 2017. "Alleviating the Access Abyss in Palliative Care and Pain Relief: An Imperative of Universal Health Coverage. Report of the *Lancet* Commission on Global Access to Palliative Care and Pain Control." *The Lancet*. doi:10.1016/S0140-6736(17)32513-8.

Krakauer, E., X. Kwete, H. Arreola-Ornelas, A. Bhadelia, O. Mendez, and others. 2018. "Palliative Care in Response to the Global Burden of Health-Related Suffering." In *Disease Control Priorities* (third edition): Volume 9, *Improving Health and Reducing Poverty*, edited by D. T. Jamison, H. Gelband, S. Horton, P. Jha, R. Laxminarayan, C. N. Mock, and R. Nugent. Washington, DC: World Bank.

Lancet. 2013. "Maternal and Child Nutrition." Executive Summary of *The Lancet* Maternal and Child Nutrition Series, *The Lancet*, London. http://www.thelancet.com/pb/assets/raw/Lancet/stories/series/nutrition-eng.pdf.

Lipfert, F. W., and R. E. Wyzga. 1995. "Air Pollution and Mortality: Issues and Uncertainties." *Journal of the Air & Waste Management Association* 45 (12): 949–966, DOI: 10.1080/10473289.1995.10467427.

Liu, B.C., R. Ivers, R. Norton, S. Boufous, S. Blows, and S.K. Lo. 2008. "Helmets for Preventing Injury in Motorcycle Riders." *Cochrane Database of Systematic Reviews* 23 (1): CD004333. doi:10.1002/14651858.CD004333.pub3.

Marquez, P., and B. Moreno-Dodson. 2017. "Tobacco Control Program." Brief, World Bank, Washington, DC, July 19. http://www.worldbank.org/en/topic/health/brief/tobacco.

Mathers, C., G. Stevens, D. Hogan, A. Mahanani, and J. Ho. 2018. "Global and Regional Causes of Death: Patterns and Trends, 2000–15." In *Disease Control Priorities* (third edition): Volume 9, *Improving Health and Reducing Poverty*, edited by D. T. Jamison, H. Gelband, S. Horton, P. Jha, R. Laxminarayan, C. N. Mock, and R. Nugent. Washington, DC: World Bank.

Mock, C. N., O. Kobusingye, R. Nugent, and K. R. Smith, eds. 2017. "Injury Prevention and Environmental Health: Key Messages from This Volume." In *Disease Control Priorities* (third edition): Volume 7, *Injury Prevention and Environmental Health*, edited by C. N. Mock, O. Kobusingye, R. Nugent, and K. Smith. Washington, DC: World Bank.

Nugent, R., and F. Knaul. 2006. "Fiscal Policies for Health Promotion and Disease Prevention." In *Disease Control Priorities in Developing Countries*, second edition, edited by D. T. Jamison, J. G. Breman, A. R. Measham, G. Alleyne, M. Claeson, D. B. Evans, P. Jha, A. Mills, and P. Musgrove, eds., 211–24. Washington, DC: World Bank and Oxford University Press.

OECD (Organisation for Economic Co-operation and Development). 2007. "Conceptual Framework and Methods for Analysis of Data Sources for Long-Term Care Expenditure." Final report, OECD, Paris.

———. 2016. "OECD Reviews of Health Systems: Mexico 2016." OECD Publishing, Paris. http://dx.doi.org/10.1787/9789264230491-en.

Olson, Z., J. A. Staples, C. Mock, N. P. Nguyen, A. M. Bachani, and others. 2016. "Helmet Regulation in Vietnam: Impact on Health, Equity and Medical Impoverishment." *Injury Prevention* 22 (4): 233–38.

Passmore, J. W., L. H. Nguyen, N. P. Nguyen, and J.-M. Olivé. 2010. "The Formulation and Implementation of a National Helmet Law: A Case Study from Viet Nam." *Bulletin of the World Health Organization* 88 (10): 783–87.

Passmore, J., N. T. H. Tu, M. A. Luong, N. D. Chinh, and N. P. Nam. 2010. "Impact of Mandatory Motorcycle Helmet Wearing Legislation on Head Injuries in Viet Nam: Results of a Preliminary Analysis. *Traffic Injury Prevention* 11: 202–6.

Phoolcharoen, W., D. Sukkumnoed, and P. Kessomboon. 2003. "Development of Health Impact Assessment in Thailand: Recent Experiences and Challenges." *Bulletin of the World Health Organization* 81 (6): 465–67.

Piot, P., S. S. Abdool Karim, R. Hecht, H. Legido-Quigley, K. Buse, and others. 2015. "Defeating AIDS—Advancing Global Health." *The Lancet* 386 (9989): 171–218.

Pradhan, E., E. Suzuki, S. Martinez, M. Schaferhoff, and D. Jamison. 2017. "The Effects of Education Quantity and Quality on Child and Adult Mortality: Their Magnitude and Their Value." In *Disease Control Priorities* (third edition):

Volume 8, *Child and Adolescent Health and Development*, edited by D. A. P. Bundy, N. de Silva, S. Horton, D. T. Jamison, and G. Patton. Washington, DC: World Bank.

Russo, M., and D. Smith. 2013. "Apples to Twinkies 2013: Comparing Taxpayer Subsidies for Fresh Produce and Junk Food." CALPIRG (California Public Interest Research Group), Sacramento, July.

Sedgh, G., J. Bearak, S. Singh, A. Bankole, A. Popinchalk, and others. 2016. "Abortion Incidence between 1990 and 2014: Global, Regional, and Subregional Levels and Trends." *The Lancet* 388 (10041): 258–67.

Shannon, K., S. A. Strathdee, S. M. Goldenberg, P. Duff, P. Mwangi, and others. 2015. "Global Epidemiology of HIV among Female Sex Workers: Influence of Structural Determinants." *The Lancet* 385 (9962): 55–71.

Sheikh, M. R., M. M. Afzal, S. Z. Ali, A. Hussain, and R. Shehzadi. 2012. "Multisectoral Development for Improved Health Outcomes: Evaluation of Community-Based Initiatives in the Islamic Republic of Iran." *Eastern Mediterranean Health Journal* 16 (12): 1231–36.

Smith, K. R., and A. Pillarisetti. 2017. "Household Air Pollution from Solid Cookfuels and Health." In *Disease Control Priorities* (third edition): Volume 7, *Injury Prevention and Environmental Health*, edited by C. N. Mock, O. Kobusingye, R. Nugent, and K. Smith. Washington, DC: World Bank.

Stevens, G. A., R. H. Dias, and M. Ezzati. 2008. "The Effects of 3 Environmental Risks on Mortality Disparities across Mexican Communities." *Proceedings of the National Academy of Sciences of the United States of America* 105 (44): 16860–65.

Sudarshan, A., A. Sugathan, J. Nilekani, M. Greenstone, N. Ryan, and R. Pande. 2015. "Lower Pollution, Longer Lives: Life Expectancy Gains if India Reduced Particulate Matter Pollution." *Economic and Political Weekly* 50 (8): 40–46.

UN (United Nations). 2012. "Political Declaration of the High-Level Meeting of the General Assembly on the Prevention and Control of Non-Communicable Diseases." A/Res/66/2, UN, New York.

———. 2015. "Sustainable Development Goals." Sustainable Development Knowledge Platform, UN, New York. http://sustainabledevelopment.un.org/?menu=1300.

Verguet, S., C. L. Gauvreau, S. Mishra, M. MacLennan, S. M. Murphy, and others. 2015. "The Consequences of Tobacco Tax on Household Health and Finances in Rich and Poor Smokers in China: An Extended Cost-Effectiveness Analysis." *The Lancet Global Health* 3 (4): e206–16.

Verguet, S., and D. T. Jamison. 2018. "Health Policy Assessment: Applications of Extended Cost-Effectiveness Analysis Methodology in Disease Control Priorities, Third Edition." In Disease Control Priorities (third edition): Volume 9, Disease Control Priorities: Improving Health and Reducing Poverty, edited by D. T. Jamison, H. Gelband, S. Horton, P. Jha, R. Laxminarayan, C. N. Mock, and R. Nugent. Washington, DC: World Bank.

Watkins, D. A., N. Dabestani, R. Nugent, and C. Levin. 2017. "Interventions to Prevent Injuries and Reduce Environmental and Occupational Hazards: A Review of

Economic Evaluations from Low- and Middle-Income Countries." In *Disease Control Priorities* (third edition): Volume 7, *Injury Prevention and Environmental Health*, edited by C. N. Mock, O. Kobusingye, R. Nugent, and K. Smith. Washington, DC: World Bank.

Watkins, D. A., D. Jamison, A. Mills, R. Atun, K. Danforth, and others. 2018. "Universal Health Coverage and Essential Packages of Care." In *Disease Control Priorities* (third edition): Volume 9, *Disease Control Priorities: Improving Health and Reducing Poverty*, edited by D. T. Jamison, H. Gelband, S. Horton, P. Jha, R. Laxminarayan, C. N. Mock, and R. Nugent. Washington, DC: World Bank.

Watkins, D. A., Z. D. Olson, S. Verguet, R. A. Nugent, and D. T. Jamison 2016. "Cardiovascular Disease and Impoverishment Averted Due to a Salt Reduction Policy in South Africa: An Extended Cost-Effectiveness Analysis." *Health Policy and Planning* 31 (1): 75–82.

WHO (World Health Organization). 2011a. "Global Health and Aging." WHO and U.S. National Institute of Aging, Geneva and Washington, DC.

———. 2011b. "Intersectoral Action on Health: A Path for Policy-Makers to Implement Effective and Sustainable Action on Health." Guidance booklet, WHO Centre for Health Development, Kobe, Japan.

———. 2011c. *WHO Technical Manual on Tobacco Tax Administration*. Geneva: World Health Organization.

———. 2015. *Global Status Report on Road Safety*. Geneva: WHO. http://www.who.int/violence_injury_prevention /road_safety_status/2015/en/.

———. 2016a. "Fiscal Policies for Diet and Prevention of Noncommunicable Diseases: Technical Meeting Report, 5–6 May 2015 Geneva, Switzerland." Geneva: World Health Organization.

———. 2016b. Global Health Observatory (GHO) database, WHO, Geneva. http://www.who.int/gho/en/.

Young-Wolff, K., K. Kasza, A. Hyland, and S. McKee. 2014. "Increased Cigarette Tax Is Associated with Reductions in Alcohol Consumption in a Longitudinal U.S. Sample." *Alcoholism: Clinical and Experimental Research* 38 (1): 241–48.

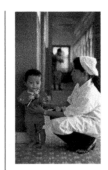

Chapter 3

Universal Health Coverage and Essential Packages of Care

David A. Watkins, Dean T. Jamison, Anne Mills, Rifat Atun,
Kristen Danforth, Amanda Glassman, Susan Horton,
Prabhat Jha, Margaret E. Kruk, Ole F. Norheim, Jinyuan Qi,
Agnes Soucat, Stéphane Verguet, David Wilson, and Ala Alwan

INTRODUCTION

Health systems have several key objectives; the most fundamental is to improve the health of the population. In addition, they are concerned with the distribution of health in the population—for example, with health equity—and they strive to be responsive to the needs of the population and to deliver services efficiently (WHO 2007). Notably, they also seek to provide protection against the financial risks that individuals face when accessing health services. Ideally, this financial risk protection (FRP) is accomplished through mechanisms such as risk pooling and group payment that ensure prepayment of most, if not all, health care costs (Jamison and others 2013).

An effective health system is one that meets these objectives by providing equitable access to affordable, high-quality health care—including treatment and curative services as well as health promotion, prevention, and rehabilitation services—to the entire population. Unfortunately, most countries lack health systems that meet this standard. Shortfalls in access, quality, efficiency, and equity have been documented extensively, both in low- and middle-income countries (LMICs) and in some high-income countries (HICs) (WHO 2010). In addition, in many countries, households routinely face catastrophic or impoverishing health expenditure when seeking acute or chronic disease care (Xu and others 2007). These financial risks can result in further health loss and reduced economic prosperity for households and populations (Kruk and others 2009; McIntyre and others 2006).

The current universal health coverage (UHC) movement emerged in response to a growing awareness of the worldwide problems of low access to health services, low quality of care, and high levels of financial risk (Ji and Chen 2016). UHC is now a core tenet of United Nations (UN) Sustainable Development Goal (SDG) 3.[1] UHC was preceded by the aspirational notion of a minimum standard of health for all, enshrined in the Universal Declaration of Human Rights (adopted by the UN General Assembly in 1948) and the declaration of Alma-Ata in 1978, and many HICs have provided universal coverage for decades. The World Health Assembly endorsed the modern concept of UHC as an aspiration for all countries in 2005. Subsequent *World Health Reports* by the World Health Organization (WHO) expanded on various technical aspects of UHC, and in 2015, UHC was adopted as a subgoal (target 3.8) of SDG 3 (UN 2016; WHO 2013b).

Corresponding author: David A. Watkins, University of Washington, Seattle, Washington, United States; davidaw@uw.edu.

Mechanisms and approaches, summarized elsewhere (WHO 2010; WHO 2013b), have been proposed or attempted as specific means of achieving UHC, but the objectives of UHC are the same in all settings, regardless of approach: improving access to health services (particularly for disadvantaged populations), improving the health of individuals covered, and providing FRP (Giedion, Alfonso, and Díaz 2013). There are three fundamental dimensions to UHC—proportion of population covered, proportion of expenditures prepaid, and proportion of health services included in UHC—that any given health care reform strategy seeks to achieve in some prioritized order (Busse, Schreyögg, and Gericke 2007). Recent reports, including the *Lancet* Commission on Investing in Health and the WHO *Making Fair Choices* consultation, have endorsed a "progressive universalist" approach to public finance of UHC (Jamison and others 2013; WHO 2014).[2] Progressive universalism makes the case, on the basis of efficiency and equity, for an expansion pathway through the three UHC dimensions that prioritizes full population coverage and prepayment, albeit for a narrower scope of services than could be achieved at lower coverage levels or through cost-sharing arrangements. (It has been argued that full population coverage and full prepayment are necessary conditions to ensure that UHC leaves no one behind [WHO 2014].)

If progressive universalism is the preferred approach to UHC, then a critical question for health planners is which health interventions should be included. HICs are able to provide a wide array of health services, but LMICs have the resources to deliver a smaller set of services, necessitating a more explicit and systematic approach to priority setting (Glassman and others 2016). In this spirit, the *Making Fair Choices* report recommended that UHC focus on interventions that are the most cost-effective, improve the health of the worst off, and provide FRP (WHO 2014). The extended cost-effectiveness analysis (ECEA) approach developed for this third edition of *Disease Control Priorities* (*DCP3*) assesses policies in these dimensions and can help identify efficient, fair pathways to UHC. Chapter 8 of this volume provides an overview of ECEA methods and results of ECEAs undertaken in conjunction with *DCP3* (Verguet and Jamison 2018).

The set of prioritized health services publicly financed through a UHC scheme has been termed a *health benefits package* (Glassman and others 2016). The limited experience of LMICs with benefits packages suggests that such packages can be part of a coherent and efficient approach to health system strengthening, but many countries lack the technical capacity to review a broad range of candidate interventions and

summarize the evidence for their effectiveness or cost-effectiveness. In this regard, *DCP3* provides guidance on priority health interventions for UHC in LMICs in the form of a model health benefits package that is based on *DCP3*'s 21 essential packages (see chapter 1 of this volume, Jamison and others 2018).

This chapter proposes a concrete set of priorities for UHC that is grounded in economic reality and is intended to be appropriate to the health needs and constraints of LMICs, particularly low-income countries and lower-middle-income countries. It develops a model benefits package referred to as essential UHC (EUHC) and identifies a subset of interventions termed the highest-priority package (HPP). The chapter presents a case that all countries, including low-income countries, could strive to fully implement the HPP interventions by the end of the SDG period (2030), and many middle-income countries could strive to achieve full implementation of EUHC. The chapter also presents estimates of the EUHC and HPP costs and mortality consequences. It concludes with a discussion of measures that improve the uptake and quality of health services and with some remarks on the implications of EUHC and the HPP for health systems.

The chapter does not, however, prescribe one correct approach to UHC, nor does it attempt to review the wide array of delivery mechanisms, policy instruments, and financial arrangements that support the transition to UHC; these have been covered in detail elsewhere (WHO 2010; World Bank 2016). Rather, this chapter stresses that the UHC priority-setting process is contextual, depending on political economy as well as local costs, budgets, and demographic and epidemiological factors—all of which influence the value for money of specific interventions.

Because the development and refinement of a benefits package is an incremental and iterative process, many ministries of health probably will not use *DCP3*'s recommendations as a template for their packages but rather as an aid in reviewing existing services, identifying outliers, and considering services that are not currently provided. The *DCP3* model benefits package can thus serve as a starting point for deliberation on a new health benefits package or refinement of an existing package. However, as construed here, it would not be a perfect package for a particular country. To translate the *DCP3* findings into an actionable UHC agenda at the national or subnational level will require context-specific technical analyses and public consultation, ideally as part of a clearly articulated political agenda and an institutionalized priority-setting process that can govern public and donor resource allocation in the health sector.

FROM ESSENTIAL PACKAGES TO ESSENTIAL UNIVERSAL HEALTH COVERAGE

Development of an Essential UHC Package

Identification of interventions for the HPP and EUHC began by compiling all of the interventions described in *DCP3*'s essential packages. As described in chapter 1 of this volume (Jamison and others 2018), the essential packages of volumes 1 through 9 of *DCP3* contain 327 interventions that have been deemed to accomplish the following:

- Provide good value for money in multiple settings.
- Address a significant disease burden.
- Be feasible to implement in a range of LMICs.

(Note that 119 of the interventions in these essential packages are intersectoral in nature, as discussed in chapter 2 of this volume, Watkins and others [2018]. Some interventions in *DCP3* are not easily classified as health sector or intersectoral; these were generally included in the present chapter as health sector interventions by default. Examples of such interventions include maternal and infant nutrition [that is, food as medicine] and vector control.)

The interventions recommended in these essential packages reflect the synthesis of a wide range of epidemiological and economic evidence instilled with the expert judgment required to extrapolate these findings to settings and policy questions for which data are very limited. Most of the economic evidence takes a health sector perspective on costs and draws on estimates of incremental value for money in settings where the number and scale of current health services are limited. Still, as summarized in chapter 7 of this volume (Horton 2018), the quality and applicability of economic evidence in these studies vary widely, requiring additional deliberation and judgment as described later in this chapter.

Notably, this chapter includes essential packages for two additional groups of conditions: congenital and genetic disorders (annex 3A) and musculoskeletal disorders (annex 3B). These conditions had been treated extensively in *Disease Control Priorities in Developing Countries,* second edition (*DCP2*) (Jamison and others 2006) and were touched upon in various volumes of *DCP3,* but they were deemed not to require dedicated chapters. The essential packages for these two groups of conditions reflect the key messages of the relevant sections of *DCP2,* with updated information on burden of disease and economic evidence in LMICs, particularly over the past decade.

After compiling the contents of *DCP3*'s 21 essential packages, the authors of this chapter took several additional steps to arrive at a final list of EUHC interventions:

- First, instances of duplicate or redundant interventions were removed. Although duplicate interventions were removed in the construction of the EUHC list, each essential package retained all of its interventions.
- Second, the authors worked with the editors responsible for each of these packages to revise intervention descriptions, when needed, to add specificity or clarity for a nonspecialist audience. On the advice of the editors of *DCP3* volumes 4 (Patel and others 2015) and 6 (Holmes and others 2017), only a subset of best-practice interventions from these two volumes was included in the EUHC package. This chapter also aggregated a number of specific health services into single interventions that would always be delivered together in practice, such as screening of at-risk individuals for a given disease plus treatment of individuals who have screened positive for that disease.
- The authors deemed some interventions not to be specific health services but rather measures to increase intervention uptake or quality. These interventions were removed from the EUHC list and are discussed as a group later in this chapter.
- Finally, the authors mapped all interventions to a standard typology of health system platforms that reflects the consensus of editors and members of the *DCP3* Advisory Committee (box 3.1). The grouping of interventions into platforms is intended to illustrate how they could be integrated with each other and within existing health systems.

Annex 3C presents the final contents of the EUHC package, by platform. The EUHC package includes 218 unique interventions, including 13 interventions at the population level, 59 at the community level, 68 at health centers, 58 at first-level hospitals, and 20 at referral and specialized hospitals. Annex 3D, which accompanies annex 3C, examines issues related to specific EUHC interventions. These issues include prices and their impact on cost-effectiveness in cases where prices are rapidly changing, health system requirements such as integration of urgent intervention across delivery platforms, and considerations of feasibility in certain settings.

Identifying a Highest-Priority UHC Package

The EUHC list of 218 unique interventions still constitutes an ambitious agenda for many countries, and achieving full coverage of EUHC by 2030, the end of the

Defining Delivery Platforms for Essential UHC in *DCP3*: A Standardized Typology

DCP3 volumes 1–9 present interventions in 21 packages tailored to various "platforms," defined as logistically related delivery channels. Thus, a platform is the level of a health system at which interventions can be appropriately, effectively, and efficiently delivered. These platforms, and the interventions that are delivered through them, were determined by the editors of the individual volumes. To compile a single list of unique interventions in Essential Universal Health Coverage and group them by platform, the authors of this chapter harmonized the definitions of the platforms and, in some cases, reallocated interventions to platforms different from those that appeared elsewhere in the *DCP3* volumes.

This platform model is a pragmatic typology rather than a comprehensive description of the myriad health facilities currently serving clients in low- and middle-income countries. Contextual factors, including local culture, disease burden, resources, and geography, will influence both the types of services provided at each level and the way in which patients interact with a health care system. With changes in technology and delivery know-how, it is likely and desirable that existing modalities of health care delivery will evolve and adapt over time. A platform's definition will also evolve as a country's health system becomes more advanced and offers a wider array of health services, particularly at lower levels of the system.

The five platforms of a health system as defined in this chapter are as follows:

Population-based health interventions: This platform captures all nonpersonal or population-based health services, such as mass media and social marketing of educational messages, as typically delivered by public health agencies. (Note that nonhealth-system platforms related to fiscal and intersectoral policies—for example, taxes, subsidies, regulatory policies, and changes in the built environment—are discussed in chapter 2 of this volume [Watkins and others 2018].)

Community services: The community platform encompasses efforts to bring health care services to clients, meeting people where they live. It includes a wide variety of delivery mechanisms. Specific subplatforms include the following:

- Health outreach and campaigns (such as vaccination campaigns, mass deworming, and face-to-face health information, education, and communication)
- Schools (including school health days)
- Community health workers, who may be based primarily in the community but also connected to first-level care providers, with ties to the rest of the system.

Health centers: The health center level captures two types of facility. The first is a higher-capacity health facility staffed by a physician or clinical officer and often a midwife to provide basic medical care, minor surgery, family planning and pregnancy services, and safe childbirth for uncomplicated deliveries. (In annexes 3C and 3F, this sort of health center is denoted with an asterisk.) The second is a lower-capacity facility (for example, health clinics, pharmacies, dental offices, and so on) staffed primarily by a nurse or mid-level health care provider, providing services in less-resourced and often more remote settings.

First-level hospitals: A first-level hospital is a facility with the capacity to perform surgery and provide inpatient care. This platform also includes outpatient specialist care and routine pathology services that cannot be feasibly delivered at lower levels, such as newborn screening. *DCP3* contends that a primary goal for all countries to achieve during the Sustainable Development Goals era could be to ensure most patients have access to fully resourced, high-quality, first-level hospitals—a goal that, although aspirational, could be feasible by 2030.

Referral and specialized (second- and third-level) hospitals: This platform includes general and specialist hospitals that provide secondary and tertiary services.

SDG period, would be challenging for most low-income countries. Further, as has been highlighted throughout *DCP3*, there is great heterogeneity in the strength of evidence and the magnitude of the health impact of these essential interventions.

Some helpful guidance comes from the WHO *Making Fair Choices* consultation, which outlined the principle of priority classes—namely, that health services could be grouped into three classes (high, medium, or low priority) based on their relative merits in the dimensions of cost-effectiveness, priority given to the worse off, and FRP (Chan 2016; WHO 2014). In this spirit, this chapter develops an illustrative HPP that parallels the high-priority class described in *Making Fair Choices*. It looks at the HPP through the lens of low-income countries, taking into consideration their aggregate epidemiological and demographic patterns as well as typical resource constraints.

Identifying the Highest-Priority UHC Interventions: Three Key Dimensions

To identify the subset of EUHC interventions that could be included in the HPP, the authors appraised each EUHC intervention in three dimensions: value for money, priority given to the worse off, and FRP afforded. Annex 3E provides details on the methods and data used in this appraisal process, and annex 3F displays the authors' assessments of each EUHC intervention in these dimensions.

Value for money. To assess value for money, the authors considered cost-effectiveness estimates where cost-effectiveness was a relevant metric of value for money. In these cases, the geometric mean of incremental cost-effectiveness ratios was calculated from the economic evaluation literature in LMICs (see chapter 7 of this volume, Horton 2018). In the cases of EUHC interventions not covered in chapter 7, other databases of cost-effectiveness studies were searched for relevant estimates. The authors also noted the major drivers of cost-effectiveness in cases where interventions would not be uniformly cost-effective in LMICs. These drivers include epidemiological context (such as high- versus moderate-transmission areas for malaria), price variations in key technologies (such as vaccines for which certain countries may be eligible for subsidies), and the quality and generalizability of the cost-effectiveness data. These factors were then synthesized into a summary assessment of cost-effectiveness that placed interventions into one of five categories. Where cost-effectiveness was not a relevant metric of value for money, the appropriate outcome and the efficiency of the intervention in achieving the outcome were

noted separately. These issues are noted where pertinent in annexes 3D and 3F.

A few additional remarks should be made on *DCP3*'s shift from the criterion of cost-effectiveness to the broader criterion of value for money. In general, *DCP3* has drawn upon cost-effectiveness or cost-utility analyses to assess interventions that primarily affect health outcomes, including disability and premature mortality. In these cases, referring to the cost-effectiveness of an intervention, measured by cost per adult or child death averted or cost per disability-adjusted life year (DALY) averted, is appropriate. At the same time, several important types of health sector interventions predominantly produce outcomes that are not easily measured in deaths, DALYs, or quality-adjusted life-years (QALYs); these include met need for family planning, reductions in stillbirth rates, palliative care and relief of suffering, and remediation of intellectual losses associated with illness or poor nutritional status. In these cases, metrics such as cost per death or DALY averted do not apply. As a result, the more general term *value for money* is used here to refer to the relative attractiveness of interventions in terms of relevant outcomes. Outside of a benefit-cost analysis framework, the commensurability of different value for money indicators (for example, cost per death averted versus cost per case of met need for contraception) is a matter of judgment and may require further empirical study (see chapter 9 of this volume, Chang, Horton, and Jamison [2018]).

Another limitation of the use of cost-effectiveness and value-for-money criteria is the potential disconnect between modeled estimates and real-world impact. If the quality of care in practice lags what is captured in effectiveness studies, cost-effectiveness ratios will be higher than reported in the literature. Variations in observed clinical practice suggest that differential benefits from health care are likely within and between populations. Unfortunately, the quality of health services in LMICs is an understudied topic and is generally not considered in economic evaluations (Akachi and Kruk 2017; Kruk and others 2017). In the assessments presented in annex 3F, the authors have attempted to account for potential real-world reductions in value-for-money caused by low quality of care, particularly for complex and longitudinal services in low-income countries. (Measures that can ensure the quality of EUHC interventions are discussed later in this chapter.)

Despite all the important limitations discussed above, the *DCP3* perspective is that estimates of cost-effectiveness and value-for-money are critical inputs to the priority-setting process.

Priority given to the worse off. To assess whether an intervention gave priority to the worse off, the authors identified the principal health condition addressed by each intervention. An indicator for the "worse off" was developed that attempted to identify individuals who, by virtue of having a particular disease or injury, would have a much lower level of lifetime health. This indicator was termed "health-adjusted average age of death" (annex 3E). In brief, this measure estimated the additional fatal and nonfatal health loss experienced by an individual affected by a specific cause of death or disability or both, as compared to the average levels of health in the population. In essence, the measure identified causes that would be very severe or result in extremely premature mortality or both. Because the focus of the illustrative HPP is low-income settings, aggregate epidemiological estimates for low-income countries as a group were used as the reference population for constructing this indicator. Estimates of health-adjusted average age of death by cause were assigned to ordinal groups using cutoffs described in annex 3E and then mapped to specific interventions that addressed each cause.

The criterion of priority to the worse off is one variant on the more general notion of "pro-poor" UHC. There is broad agreement that UHC schemes in LMICs should strive first and foremost to serve the needs of marginalized and low-income groups (Bump and others 2016). To accomplish this, some UHC reforms have focused on expanding all health services to the poorest areas, while others have identified interventions against a set of "diseases of poverty" (such as tuberculosis or neglected tropical diseases) as priorities for public finance. Whereas this chapter's approach shares more in common with the latter than the former, it takes a lifecourse perspective on ill health and gives greater weight, for example, to selected noncommunicable diseases (such as schizophrenia, congenital disorders, or childhood cancers) and injuries than might be given within a "diseases of poverty" framework that is oriented to communicable diseases.

Financial risk protection. A qualitative approach was taken to assess FRP. The authors used a composite indicator for FRP derived from expert judgments in three dimensions: (a) likelihood of medical impoverishment in the absence of public finance of the intervention, based on unit cost data; (b) urgency of need for the intervention with unpredictable, severe, acute events generally conferring higher financial risk; and (c) average age of death and level of disability, with more FRP provided by interventions that improve the health of wage earners or address diseases that cause high levels of disability, all else being equal (WHO 2014).

Criteria for Inclusion in the Illustrative Highest-Priority UHC Package

A working concept of the HPP can be defined as the sum of all interventions that meet the following criteria, balanced against each other:

- *Very good value for money in low-income countries.* In cost-effectiveness terms, this is on the order of less than US$5,000–US$7,500 per death averted, depending on average age of death (with a higher willingness to pay for child and adolescent deaths averted), or less than US$200–$300 per DALY averted (or QALY gained). This range of cost-effectiveness values draws from the growing literature on health care opportunity costs, which suggests that a figure approximating half of gross domestic product (GDP) per capita per DALY averted is a realistic level of willingness-to-pay for health care interventions in LMICs (Ochalek, Lomas, and Claxton 2015). (*DCP3* does not explicitly endorse this particular threshold—or the health care opportunity cost approach in general—as a normative one but rather uses it in this chapter as an example of a typical threshold that might be implemented in a highly resource-constrained country.) For interventions where cost-effectiveness is not a relevant metric of value for money, an assessment was made by the authors as to whether the intervention would be likely to efficiently lead to health outcomes important in low-income countries that are not captured in DALYs (for example, averted stillbirths, averted unwanted pregnancies, and provision of palliative care). As a matter of both value for money and ethical obligation, full coverage of basic palliative care services was included in the HPP by default.
- *Priority given to the worst off.* This criterion is met by an intervention being directed against a cause of disease or injury that has a low health-adjusted average age of death.
- *Likely to provide a high degree of FRP.* This criterion is met by an intervention receiving a high score on the composite indicator for FRP.
- *Part of the "grand convergence" agenda proposed by the* Lancet *Commission on Investing in Health.* These interventions—in the domains of reproductive, maternal or neonatal, and child health; human immunodeficiency virus and acquired immune deficiency syndrome (HIV/AIDS); tuberculosis; and malaria—underwent careful scrutiny for this report. They largely overlap with the essential packages of *DCP3* volumes 2 and 6: *Reproductive, Maternal, Newborn, and Child Health* (Black and others 2016) and *Major Infectious Diseases* (Holmes and others 2017), respectively, although they are more selective.

Three additional remarks can be made on the criteria above. First, the exact thresholds for including an intervention in a country's HPP are context specific and should be weighed against social preferences. For instance, how to compare cases of poverty averted to deaths averted is not obvious; UHC priority setting exercises will reasonably differ as to how they weigh health and nonhealth outcomes. A scheme that seeks to prioritize the needs of the poor but is relatively resource-constrained may include more interventions that score high on priority given to the worse off and fall below a strict willingness-to-pay threshold—reflecting high health care opportunity costs. Thus, policy makers may be somewhat less likely to include interventions that provide significant FRP but not much health for money. At the same time, different levels of willingness to pay may be defined for different health outcomes (Cairns 2016); for example, a country that is committed to tackling HIV/AIDS (especially with aid from foreign donors) may decide to include HIV-related interventions despite their being somewhat less cost-effective than interventions for other conditions. *DCP3* does not take a position on the ethics of a choice like this but simply advocates for transparency and public accountability in the priority-setting process (that is, for explicit statements about trade-offs) as well as for consideration of health care opportunity costs (inefficiencies) and the possibility of failure in achieving stated levels of coverage because of budget constraints.

Second, the last criterion listed above is predicated on the analytic work conducted for the *Lancet* Commission on Investing in Health. Before the commission issued its 2013 report, "Global Health 2035: A World Converging within a Generation" (Jamison and others 2013), not all of the interventions included in its "grand convergence" package had the same rigorous evidence of value for money. However, the commission's original analysis deemed them to be effective and important to implement as a package, and their costs and benefits were estimated for the commission as such. Hence, the commission's finding that the grand convergence package was affordable and cost-beneficial influenced this chapter's judgment of the individual interventions' value for money when implemented as part of a package, especially regarding interventions for which other economic evidence was not available.

Finally, it is acknowledged that the design and implementation of the criteria in this chapter required a considerable amount of judgment and de-emphasized quantitative precision and comparability of criteria. To some extent this is an artifact of the *DCP3* process, which is intended to be illustrative rather than prescriptive for a wide range of local contexts. Applying these criteria to specific real-world policy questions would involve (a) gathering more local information on demographics, disease burden, and costs which would influence local estimates of value for money and of who are the "worst off," and (b) conducting local or regional studies that could quantify tradeoffs across each of these criteria, such as the comparability of a child death averted and a case of poverty averted. Empirical advances in these areas could facilitate their incorporation into multi-criteria decision analysis as described by Youngkong (2012) and others.

Interventions that fulfill the criteria above are shown in boldface in annex 3C and also noted alongside the appraisals in annex 3F. In all, 97 of 218 interventions could be classified as high priority according to the four criteria above. Although the proposed HPP includes a preponderance of maternal and child health interventions and interventions against HIV/AIDS and tuberculosis in adults, a significant number of interventions also primarily address noncommunicable diseases (NCDs) and injuries. In terms of the scope of health conditions addressed, these interventions go far beyond the high-priority interventions typically included in the global NCD discourse (WHO 2011).

COSTS OF ESSENTIAL UHC AND THE HPP

Estimating the potential costs and health effects of packages of health interventions is technically challenging in the face of limitations of current data, uncertainty about future demographic and epidemiological patterns, and lack of established methods and tools that span disease groups. This chapter presents estimates of costs and consequences of EUHC and the HPP, treating low-income and lower-middle-income countries in the aggregate. These estimates are not intended to be normative or precise, but rather illustrative of the magnitude and balance of costs and health benefits that a given country might expect.

The authors took a comparative statics approach to estimating cost and health gains from EUHC and the HPP, estimating the change in costs and mortality patterns that would be expected following an instantaneous increase in the coverage of services in the EUHC and HPP lists and holding constant all other factors (for example, demographics, epidemiology, and local prices) that might influence costs. The perspective taken on costs was that of the ministry of health, which was assumed to be the payer for EUHC and the HPP.

For this analysis, "universal" coverage was defined as 80 percent coverage; other groups have chosen targets ranging from 80 percent to 100 percent depending on the costing perspective, intervention, and health condition (Black and others 2016; WHO 2013a). The rationale for our 80 percent target is that the authors determined it would be unrealistic and infeasible in nearly all cases to achieve greater than 80 percent intervention coverage during the SDG period.

Watkins, Qi, and others (2017) present in detail the methods, data, and assumptions behind this chapter's costing exercise. Costs were decomposed into the following three categories: *direct costs* of service delivery at the point of care—for example, personnel, drugs, and equipment; *costs of facility-level ancillary services* required to deliver these services—for example, rents, building maintenance, and laboratory and radiology services (sometimes referred to as overhead or indirect costs); and *program costs* that support health services but occur above and separate from facility-level costs and are not easily allocable to specific services—for example, administration, logistics, and surveillance activities. We refer to the first category of cost as "service delivery costs" and the second and third categories together as "health system costs."

For each intervention, representative datasets that contained relevant unit cost estimates were identified, and then costs were adjusted to "average" costs in low- and lower-middle-income countries using assumptions about the proportion of health care based on traded goods and, for the nontraded proportion, gradients in health care worker salaries across various countries and between low-income and lower-middle-income countries on average. Care was taken to extract unit cost estimates that reflected long-run average costs. Most unit cost studies included ample detail on service delivery costs but did not factor in health system costs, so these were added as markups on service delivery costs using supplementary datasets and assumptions (Boyle and others 2015, Seshadria and others 2015).

The next step was to identify the population in need of the intervention. Previously published estimates of incidence or prevalence of various causes of disease or injury were compiled and mapped against the EUHC interventions (Vos and others 2016; WHO 2016).[3] In some cases, additional adjustments were made to estimates of population in need; for example, the proportion of the population requiring screening for diabetes (based on risk level) was first estimated and then divided by three to reflect the recommendation for screening once every three years on average. The final step was to estimate current coverage of each intervention using coverage indicators from the WHO Global Health Observatory database or reasonable proxies for coverage (WHO 2016).

As described by Watkins, Qi, and Horton (2017), the authors attempted to quantify major sources of uncertainty in the cost estimates. Three scenarios were defined—base case, worst case, and best case. For a set of key parameters in the costing model, a base case, worst case, and best case value was identified. The overall best and worst case estimates of UHC costs were obtained by simultaneously varying the values of all the key parameters to their most optimistic and pessimistic values, respectively. The point estimates and uncertainty ranges presented subsequently reflect these three scenarios.

Table 3.1 presents potential annual EUHC costs by package, including per capita and total population estimates of current spending, incremental costs, and total costs (that is, the sum of current spending and incremental costs, where total costs reflect 80 percent coverage). The largest single cost component of EUHC is health system costs, comprising about 40 percent of total costs at full coverage. The second largest cost component is the service delivery costs related to the cardiovascular, respiratory, and related disorders package. In both country groups, the service delivery costs related to HIV/AIDS and STIs, malaria, and adult febrile illness were also very high. In lower-middle-income countries, the service delivery costs related to mental, neurological, and substance use disorders were relatively high. It is also noteworthy that the share of incremental costs attributed to NCDs is higher than the share of total costs attributed to NCDs. This finding reflects low levels of current spending on NCDs and suggests that, in order to achieve EUHC, all countries will need to pay particular attention to the incremental investments required to scale up NCD services.

Table 3.2 presents the potential total and incremental annual costs of EUHC and the HPP in low- and lower-middle-income countries, including uncertainty ranges derived from the best- and worst-case scenario analyses described previously. The total cost per person of sustaining the HPP and EUHC at full coverage would be US$42 and US$76, respectively, in low-income countries and US$58 and US$110, respectively, in lower-middle-income countries. Getting to full implementation of the HPP and EUHC would require, annually, an additional 3.1 percent and 6.4 percent, respectively, of current income in low-income countries and 1.5 percent and 2.9 percent, respectively, in lower-middle-income countries.

To put these cost estimates in context, combined annual per capita health expenditure by government and donors in low- and lower-middle-income countries is currently US$25 and US$31, respectively, with out-of-pocket spending by the population being about as large again (WHO 2016). Assuming that the objective of UHC is to successfully crowd out out-of-pocket spending at the point of care through prepayment mechanisms and

Table 3.1 Costs of Essential UHC in Low-Income and Lower-Middle-Income Countries, by *DCP3* Intervention Package

	Current annual spending, per capita	Current annual spending, population (US$ billions)	Incremental annual cost, per capita[a]	Incremental annual cost, population (US$ billions)[a]	Total annual cost, per capita[b]	Total annual cost, population (US$ billions)[c]	Share of total costs (%)[d]
Panel a. Low-income countries							
Age related							
1. Maternal and newborn health (MNH)	$1.3	$1.2	$1.8	$1.6	$3.1	$2.8	6.1
2. Child health (CHH)	$2.3	$2.1	$1.2	$1.0	$3.4	$3.1	6.7
3. School-age health and development (SAH)	$0.094	$0.085	$0.20	$0.18	$0.30	$0.27	0.58
4. Adolescent health and development (AHD)	$0.31	$0.28	$0.44	$0.40	$0.75	$0.68	1.5
5. Reproductive health and contraception (RHC)	$0.82	$0.74	$0.38	$0.34	$1.2	$1.1	2.3
Infectious diseases							
6. HIV and STIs (HIV)	$3.6	$3.2	$4.0	$3.6	$7.6	$6.8	15
7. Tuberculosis (TB)	$0.34	$0.31	$0.15	$0.13	$0.49	$0.44	0.95
8. Malaria and adult febrile illness (MAL)	$2.4	$2.1	$2.6	$2.4	$5.0	$4.5	9.7
9. Neglected tropical diseases (NTD)	$0.33	$0.30	$0.31	$0.28	$0.63	$0.57	1.2
10. Pandemic and emergency preparedness (PAN)	$0.016	$0.014	$0.71	$0.63	$0.75	$0.68	1.5
Noncommunicable disease and injury							
11. Cardiovascular, respiratory, and related disorders (CVD)	$0.67	$0.60	$13	$11	$13	$12	26
12. Cancer (CAN)	$0.21	$0.19	$2.5	$2.2	$2.7	$2.4	5.2
13. Mental, neurological, and substance use disorders (MNS)	$0.49	$0.44	$1.8	$1.6	$2.3	$2.1	4.5
14. Musculoskeletal disorders (MSK)	$0.75	$0.67	$1.2	$1.1	$1.5	$1.4	3.0

table continues next page

Table 3.1 Costs of Essential UHC in Low-Income and Lower-Middle-Income Countries, by *DCP3* Intervention Package (continued)

	Current annual spending. per capita	Current annual spending, population (US$ billions)	Incremental annual cost, per capita[a]	Incremental annual cost, population (US$ billions)[a]	Total annual cost, per capita[b]	Total annual cost, population (US$ billions)[c]	Share of total costs (%)[d]
15. Congenital and genetic disorders (CGD)	$0.59	$0.53	$1.2	$1.1	$1.8	$1.7	3.6
16. Injury prevention (IPR)	$0.0044	$0.0039	$0.039	$0.035	$0.044	$0.039	0.085
17. Environmental improvement (ENV)	$0.050	$0.045	$0.049	$0.044	$0.10	$0.089	0.19
Health services							
18. Surgery (SUR)	$1.6	$1.5	$1.3	$1.1	$2.9	$2.6	5.6
19. Rehabilitation (RHB)	$0.10	$0.089	$1.5	$1.3	$1.6	$1.4	3.1
20. Palliative care and pain control (PCP)	$0.11	$0.10	$1.6	$1.5	$1.7	$1.6	3.4
21. Pathology (PTH)	$0.71	$0.64	$1.8	$1.7	$2.6	$2.3	5.1
Totals							
Total service delivery costs (sum of costs by package)	$16	$14	$36	$32	$51	$46	60
De-duplicated service delivery costs	$12	$11	$31	$28	$43	$39	60
Total health system costs	$7.9	$7.1	$20	$18	$29	$26	40
Total cost (sum of service delivery and health systems)[c]	$20	$18	$51	$46	$72	$65	100

table continues next page

Table 3.1 Costs of Essential UHC in Low-Income and Lower-Middle-Income Countries, by *DCP3* Intervention Package **(continued)**

	Current annual spending, per capita	Current annual spending, population (US$ billions)	Incremental annual cost, per capita[a]	Incremental annual cost, population (US$ billions)[a]	Total annual cost, per capita[b]	Total annual cost, population (US$ billions)[b]	Package share of total costs
Panel b. Lower-middle-income countries							
Age related							
1. Maternal and newborn health (MNH)	$1.6	$4.4	$2.1	$5.5	$3.7	$9.9	5.3
2. Child health (CHH)	$3.0	$8.1	$0.99	$2.6	$4.0	$11	5.8
3. School-age health and development (SAH)	$0.083	$0.22	$0.21	$0.57	$0.29	$0.79	0.42
4. Adolescent health and development (AHD)	$0.37	$0.99	$0.53	$1.4	$0.90	$2.4	1.3
5. Reproductive health and contraception (RHC)	$1.6	$4.4	$0.45	$1.2	$2.1	$5.6	3.0
Infectious diseases							
6. HIV and STIs (HIV)	$2.6	$7.0	$4.1	$11	$6.7	$18	9.6
7. Tuberculosis (TB)	$0.34	$0.91	$0.19	$0.50	$0.53	$1.4	0.76
8. Malaria and adult febrile illness (MAL)	$4.1	$11	$2.3	$6.2	$6.4	$17	9.1
9. Neglected tropical diseases (NTD)	$0.37	$1.0	$0.39	$1.0	$0.74	$2.0	1.1
10. Pandemic and emergency preparedness (PAN)	0.094	0.25	$0.66	$1.8	$0.75	$2.0	1.1
Noncommunicable disease and injury							
11. Cardiovascular, respiratory, and related disorders (CVD)	$9.4	$25	$15	$40	$24	$65	35
12. Cancer (CAN)	$0.64	$1.7	$1.8	$4.7	$2.4	$6.4	3.5
13. Mental, neurological, and substance use disorders (MNS)	$1.8	$4.8	$3.7	$9.8	$5.47	$15	7.8
14. Musculoskeletal disorders (MSK)	$1.1	$3.0	$2.1	$5.6	$2.8	$7.5	4.0
15. Congenital and genetic disorders (CGD)	$0.74	$2.0	$1.3	$3.5	$2.0	$5.4	2.9
16. Injury prevention (IPR)	$0.021	$0.055	$0.11	$0.30	$0.13	$0.36	0.19
17. Environmental improvement (ENV)	$0.11	$0.30	$0.10	$0.26	$0.16	$0.42	0.23

table continues next page

Table 3.1 Costs of Essential UHC in Low-Income and Lower-Middle-Income Countries, by *DCP3* Intervention Package **(continued)**

	Current annual spending, per capita	Current annual spending, population (US$ billions)	Incremental annual cost, per capita[a]	Incremental annual cost, population (US$ billions)[a]	Total annual cost, per capita[b]	Total annual cost, population (US$ billions)[b]	Package share of total costs
Health services							
18. Surgery (SUR)	$1.6	$4.2	$0.97	$2.6	$2.6	$6.8	3.7
19. Rehabilitation (RHB)	$0.41	$1.1	$2.9	$7.6	$3.3	$8.7	4.7
20. Palliative care and pain control (PCP)	$0.071	$0.19	$0.50	$1.3	$0.57	$1.5	0.81
21. Pathology (PTH)	$1.0	$2.6	$2.1	$5.6	$3.6	$9.7	5.2
Totals							
Total service delivery costs (sum of costs by package)	$30	$81	$40	$110	$70	$190	
De-duplicated service delivery costs	$16	$44	$35	$93	$60	$160	60
Total health system costs	$11	$29	$23	$62	$40	$110	40
Total cost (sum of service delivery and health systems)[c]	$27	$73	$58	$160	$101	$270	100

Source: Watkins, Qi, and others 2017.

Note: All dollar amounts are in U.S. dollars. *DCP3 = Disease Control Priorities,* third edition; HIV = human immunodeficiency virus; STIs = sexually transmitted infections; UHC = universal health coverage.

a. Incremental cost of scaling is from current coverage to 80 percent coverage.

b. Cost is at 80 percent coverage.

c. Total costs are the sum of "de-duplicated service delivery costs" and "total health system costs." The de-duplicated service delivery costs are lower than the total service delivery costs because a number of interventions are included in more than one *DCP3* essential package.

d. Two types of shares are presented in this column. First, the shares of costs presented for each of the 21 essential packages use, as the denominator, the de-duplicated service delivery costs, so the sum of these shares exceeds 100 percent because of duplication; however the share of any given package can be interpreted as the remaining fraction of the total EUHC service delivery cost if the interventions in all other packages were removed. Second, the shares of costs presented in the totals section reflect the relative proportion of EUHC costs related to service delivery and to health system strengthening, with the sum of these two being the total cost of EUHC.

Table 3.2 Total and Incremental Annual Costs of Essential UHC and the Highest-Priority Package (HPP) in 2015

	Low-income countries		Lower-middle-income countries	
	HPP	EUHC	HPP	EUHC
1. Incremental annual cost (US$ billions)[a]	23 (9.2 to 51)	48 (20 to 100)	82 (32 to 180)	160 (66 to 350)
2. Incremental annual cost per person (US$)	26 (10 to 57)	53 (22 to 110)	31 (12 to 67)	61 (25 to 130)
3. Total annual cost (US$ billions)[a]	38 (19 to 71)	68 (34 to 130)	160 (81 to 280)	280 (150 to 500)
4. Total annual cost per person (US$)	42 (21 to 79)	76 (37 to 140)	58 (30 to 100)	110 (54 to 190)
5. Incremental annual cost as a share of current GNI (%)[b]	3.1 (1.2 to 6.9)	6.4 (2.6 to 13)	1.5 (0.57 to 3.2)	2.9 (1.2 to 6.2)
6. Total annual cost as a share of current GNI (%)[b]	5.1 (2.5 to 9.5)	9.1 (4.5 to 17)	2.8 (1.4 to 4.8)	5.2 (2.6 to 9.1)

Source: Watkins, Qi, and others 2017.

Note: EUHC = Essential Universal Health Coverage; GNI = gross national income; UHC = Universal Health Coverage. Incremental annual cost is the estimated cost of going from current to full implementation (80 percent population coverage) of the EUHC and HPP interventions. The total annual cost is the incremental cost plus current spending assuming the same cost structure for current and incremental investments. Estimated costs are inclusive of estimates for (large) health system strengthening cost and are steady-state (or long-run average) costs in that investments to achieve higher levels of coverage and to cover depreciation are included.

a. The 2015 population of low-income countries was 0.90 billion. For lower-middle-income countries, it was 2.7 billion. Population sizes were estimated using data from UN DESA 2017 according to the country classifications listed at the end of this chapter.

b. The 2015 GNI of low-income countries was $0.75 trillion and for lower-middle income countries it was $5.4 trillion. Aggregate GNI figures were estimated using data from the World Bank.[4]

pooled contributions, these cost estimates suggest that current government and donor spending will need approximately to double or triple to finance the HPP or EUHC packages. These implied shortfalls are comparable to a recent costing exercise in Ethiopia (Ethiopia, Ministry of Health 2015) that estimated that a 30–80 percent increase in available resources would be required to finance universal coverage of a very basic package of essential health services in Ethiopia.

The incremental cost of reaching full coverage is significant; probably feasible in lower-middle-income countries but unlikely to be feasible in low-income countries without additional external support. For comparison, the annual incremental cost of the *Lancet* Commission on Investing in Health's grand convergence package was about 1 percent of current per capita income overall as compared to 2–3 percent of current per capita income in this chapter's HPP (Jamison and others 2013). The higher cost of *DCP3*'s HPP results from the inclusion of a wider scope of interventions, including both the reproductive, maternal, neonatal, and child health interventions in the *Lancet* Commission on Investing in Health package and additional interventions for major infectious diseases in

adults and substantial investments in NCDs and injury care at health centers and first-level hospitals.

Finally, *DCP3*'s cost estimates are in line with those estimated by others. Earlier work based on the WHO Commission on Macroeconomics and Health and the High Level Taskforce for Innovative International Financing of Health Systems suggested that the minimum total annual public expenditure on UHC in LMICs would need to be about US$86 per capita or 5 percent of current GDP per capita, whichever is larger (McIntyre, Meheus, and Rottingen 2017). A more recent costing exercise by WHO has suggested that the incremental annual public expenditure on UHC in LMICs would need to be US$58 (ranging US$22–US$167) per capita (in 2014 U.S. dollars) across LMICs in order to achieve full implementation by 2030 (Stenberg and others 2017). (The WHO study only reported incremental costs, not total costs. Watkins, Qi, and others [2017] compare the contents of the WHO's package and *DCP3*'s EUHC and HPP.) Taken together, these figures also suggest that, if resources for UHC do not increase in low-income countries, even the HPP—however attractive on health and efficiency grounds—would need to be significantly reduced in scope.

HEALTH CONSEQUENCES OF ESSENTIAL UHC AND THE HPP

Watkins, Norheim, and others (2017) present in detail the data sources, methods, and assumptions that are used to estimate the mortality impact of EUHC and the HPP. In brief, the overall framework for the impact assessment was the supplementary SDG 3 target proposed by Norheim and others (2015) of a 40 percent reduction in deaths under age 70 years by 2030. This chapter projects total deaths in 2030—by age group, gender, and cause—using UN Population Division estimates of population size (UN DESA 2017) and cause-specific mortality rates (by age group and gender) using the WHO's most recent Global Health Estimates database (Mathers and others 2018)

Estimates of mortality reduction from specific HPP and EUHC interventions implemented a hybrid approach. For under-five years, maternal, HIV/AIDS, and tuberculosis deaths, the analysis drew on the impact modeling undertaken for the Commission on Investing in Health (Boyle and others 2015). For NCDs and injuries, as well as for selected causes of death from infectious disease in adults, the authors identified a subset of interventions for which there was strong evidence for a large relative effect on cause-specific mortality. These relative reductions in mortality were then applied to cause-specific mortality rates, focusing on deaths in the groups ages 5–69 years. The impact estimates were then adjusted to reflect the proportion of deaths that would be affected by an increase in intervention coverage. Effect sizes were also adjusted downward to account for suboptimal quality of delivery, including imperfect adherence. The adjusted effect sizes were then applied to projected 2030 estimates of deaths, by cause, in low-income and lower-middle-income countries.

Table 3.3 presents these estimates of the potential mortality consequences of the HPP and EUHC in 2030. They can be regarded as conservative estimates: other EUHC and HPP interventions can reduce mortality as well as disability (the latter of which is not the focus of this analysis). A subset of NCD interventions also reduces mortality over the age of 70 years, although these deaths are not counted toward the target. Finally, many EUHC and HPP interventions have well-known nonhealth benefits, such as increased productivity, educational attainment, economic benefits to women resulting from reduced fertility rates, and so on, that make the suite of societal benefits of UHC even larger.

The impact estimates in table 3.3 suggest that HPP and EUHC implementation will facilitate substantial progress toward the SDG 3 target in both low-income and lower-middle-income countries, with relatively more progress in low-income countries. However, at 80 percent coverage and usual levels of delivery quality, the HPP and EUHC would achieve roughly half and two-thirds, respectively, of the mortality reduction target.

There are two sets of factors that influence the shortfall in mortality reduction. First, 80 percent is a particularly modest target for some conditions, such as childhood illnesses and HIV/AIDS and tuberculosis among adults. Scaling up the child health and infectious diseases packages to 95% or higher coverage, with more optimistic assumptions about the quality of delivery, would facilitate countries reaching the mortality target at least for these conditions. Second, lower-middle-income countries face greater challenges in reaching the target because of the predominance of noncommunicable diseases and injuries. The HPP and EUHC interventions for these conditions, particularly for neoplasms, are relatively less effective even at high levels of coverage. In addition, these countries face demographic and epidemiologic headwinds, with greater increases in total deaths and in the share of projected deaths in 2030 due to noncommunicable diseases and injuries. The findings of this analysis suggest that, particularly in lower-middle-income countries, meeting the target will be feasible only if health sector interventions against NCDs and injuries are complemented by strong intersectoral policies such as tobacco taxation and control, reduction of air pollution, and road safety that can reduce the risk of incidence of fatal and nonfatal NCDs and injuries. These sorts of interventions are addressed in greater detail in chapter 2 of this volume (Watkins and others 2018).

IMPLEMENTING ESSENTIAL UHC

The primary focus of this chapter and of *DCP3* as a whole has been to develop detailed essential packages of care. At the same time, the interventions contained in EUHC and the HPP would translate to gains in population health only through expanded uptake and improved efficiency and quality of health care (figure 1.1 in chapter 1 of this volume, Jamison and others 2018). Further, EUHC and the HPP require health systems that have adequate human and material resources to deliver a wide range of services. This section of the chapter discusses some important considerations for implementing EUHC and the HPP. These include reducing barriers to the uptake of priority health services, improving the quality of services provided, strengthening the building blocks of health systems, and supporting the institutionalization of priority setting.

Table 3.3 Premature Deaths Averted in 2030, by Age Group and Cause, through Full Implementation of EUHC and the HPP, Low-Income and Lower-Middle-Income Countries

Age group or condition	Low-income countries[b]				Lower-middle-income countries[b]			
	Projected number of premature deaths, 2030[a]	40x30 reduction target[c]	Expected reduction in premature deaths from HPP	Expected reduction in premature deaths from EUHC	Projected number of premature deaths, 2030[a]	40x30 reduction target[c]	Expected reduction in premature deaths from HPP	Expected reduction in premature deaths from EUHC
By age group								
0–4	2.2	1.5	0.62	0.77	3.3	2.2	1.1	1.3
5–69	5.2	1.5	0.99	1.2	14	4.8	2.2	2.9
0–69	**7.4**	**3.0**	**1.6**	**2.0**	**17**	**7.0**	**3.2**	**4.2**
By cause (age 5+)[d]								
I. Group I	**1.9**	**0.76**	**0.59**	**0.65**	**3.2**	**1.5**	**0.85**	**0.94**
Tuberculosis	0.34	0.22	0.11	0.13	0.90	0.60	0.29	0.35
HIV/AIDS	0.44	0.29	0.18	0.20	0.48	0.32	0.23	0.26
Malaria	0.087	0.058	0.051	0.051	0.055	0.037	0.026	0.026
Maternal conditions	0.17	0.11	0.075	0.086	0.20	0.13	0.079	0.092
Other diseases	0.90	0.074	0.18	0.18	1.6	0.40	0.22	0.22
II. Group II	**2.5**	**0.60**	**0.36**	**0.53**	**8.9**	**2.7**	**1.3**	**1.9**
Neoplasms	0.65	0.22	0.010	0.039	1.8	0.60	0.10	0.16
Cardiovascular diseases	0.93	0.31	0.24	0.36	4.0	1.3	0.89	1.4
Other diseases	0.93	0.076	0.11	0.13	3.2	0.80	0.28	0.35
III. Group III	**0.77**	**0.13**	**0.043**	**0.060**	**2.0**	**0.54**	**0.070**	**0.10**
Road injuries	0.25	0.085	0.032	0.046	0.57	0.19	0.048	0.069
Other injuries	0.52	0.042	0.010	0.014	1.4	0.36	0.022	0.032

Source: Watkins, Norheim, and others 2017.

Note: All estimates are in millions of deaths. The 40x30 reduction target includes a 40 percent reduction in deaths 0–69 overall; a two-thirds reduction in under-five deaths and adult deaths from tuberculosis, HIV/AIDS, malaria, and maternal conditions; and a one-third reduction in deaths from major noncommunicable diseases. The quantitative targets above reflect these goals; however, targets for the residual categories ("other diseases" and "other injuries") have been calculated in light of the targets for specific causes of death so that the total number of target deaths 5–69 is sufficient to meet the 40 x 30 target.

a. A death under age 70 years is defined as premature.

b. See unnumbered endnote for World Bank classification of countries by income group. UN and WHO data were aggregated according to these groupings.

c. A reduction target of 40 x 30 is defined as a 40 percent reduction in premature deaths by 2030, relative to the number that would have occurred had 2015 death rates persisted to 2030. The *UN Population Prospects* (UN DESA 2017) median population projection for 2030 was used to provide the population totals for calculating deaths by age and sex.

d. WHO's Global Health Estimates (Mathers and others 2018) provided the 2015 cause distributions of deaths for these calculations.

Reducing Barriers to Intervention Uptake

Ng and others (2014) have proposed the concept of "effective coverage" as a quantitative indicator of the effect of UHC. The concept goes beyond the usual notion of coverage, which is often measured as the probability that specific health services are available at a given facility. Effective coverage, in contrast, incorporates measures of intervention uptake by those in need as well as measures of the quality of the care provided, and thus it considers the actual health gain that an intervention is likely to produce in the population. Although the use of quantitative indicators for UHC continues to stimulate international debate, the principle that the health impact of UHC is bounded by effective coverage—constraints on access to and quality of care—is intuitive. Hence, a UHC scheme and associated package can truly claim to be "universal" only once full *effective* coverage has been achieved.

Removing or reducing key barriers to intervention uptake is crucial to achieving full effective coverage. Barriers to intervention uptake fall into four broad types: economic, geographic, sociocultural, or legal.

Economic barriers feature prominently in the UHC discourse, and they can be partially remediated through public finance. Still, public finance usually addresses only the direct cost of care. Direct nonmedical costs such as transportation and food expenses that are borne by individuals are not easily remedied by prepayment, nor are the economic consequences of taking time off work or school to receive care. Despite currently limited evidence, these sorts of barriers may be more amenable to intersectoral action (for example, paid sick leave and subsidized public transportation for visits to health facilities) than to changes in the delivery or financing of health care. In addition, social development policies and other approaches complementary to public finance may be needed to improve access to marginalized groups, particularly in countries with high levels of political, economic, and social inequality. Ideally, health insurance should be integrated with broader social protection measures that are implemented outside the health sector. At a minimum, the spirit of the progressive universalist approach to UHC implies that user fees should be reduced as much as possible or eliminated entirely, and in some cases, additional steps—such as cash transfers or other financial incentives for the poor—could be considered.

Geographic barriers arise when the distribution of health facilities does not match the distribution of the population's health needs. The EUHC package's platform structure allows health planners to identify what sorts of health facilities are most needed and what sort of capacity is required at those facilities. In general,

longitudinal interventions (such as chronic management of HIV/AIDS) and acute care interventions (such as fracture reduction and fixation) need to be decentralized as much as possible because of the frequency or urgency of contact with the health system. Such services, which make up nearly 75 percent of the recommended EUHC interventions, require highly decentralized facilities at high density in communities, including in hard-to-reach populations, to reach universal coverage. The interventions on the community, health center, and first-level hospital platforms can build a foundation for efficient primary health care (annex 3C). At the same time, routine, one-off services (such as immunization programs or cataract surgery) can often be efficiently delivered through stand-alone, targeted programs appropriate to the epidemiology of the country or region (Atun and others 2010). Finally, complex, high-risk services (such as chemotherapy treatment of childhood leukemia) generally need to be centralized, with strong referral systems, to ensure sufficient quality.

Sociocultural and legal barriers, which may be intertwined in cause and effect, vary according to both the characteristics of the intervention and the country context. Disease stigma may influence individuals' willingness to seek care or—consciously or unconsciously—providers' attitudes toward these individuals. Low knowledge or health literacy can also impede intervention uptake, and this has been a major focus of information, education, and communication interventions. Finally, there may be legal barriers to care, or mandates to provide certain kinds of care, that have little to do with stigma or culture. For example, restrictions on prescribing by nurses or mid-level practitioners may reduce the opportunities for individuals with chronic illness to receive needed medications.

Table 3.4 provides examples from *DCP3* of measures that have been used to expand access to care, either by reducing access barriers or by inducing demand for health care.

Improving the Quality of Essential UHC

In addition to affordability and availability, the quality of services is also critical to the success of UHC schemes. If users do not perceive services as valuable, public support will falter, undermining the politics of implementing UHC (Savedoff and others 2012). Low quality of care can thus reduce the positive health impact of otherwise effective and cost-effective interventions. From an economic standpoint, low quality suggests that more money needs to be spent on a health service than the estimates of cost-effectiveness would imply. As discussed in

Table 3.4 Selected Examples of Measures to Address Barriers to Health Care Access, LMICs

Barrier type	Examples
Economic	Bus fares to support attendance at STI clinics
	Conditional cash transfers for antenatal care
Geographic	Decentralization of chronic disease care, for example, for HIV and diabetes
	Extension of antenatal care using community health workers
	Mobile units to provide screening and care for HIV and tuberculosis
Sociocultural	Information and education about cervical cancer and the benefits of screening
	Ensuring that health care providers of the same sex are available when requested
	Educational campaigns to reduce stigma concerning mental health
Legal	Easing legal restrictions on access to family planning measures
	Legal measures to ensure confidential reporting of and care following episodes of intimate partner violence

Sources: Black and others 2016; Gelband and others 2015; Patel and others 2015; Prabhakaran and others 2017; Holmes and others 2017.
Note: LMICs = low- and middle-income countries; STI = sexually transmitted infection.

chapter 10 of this volume (Peabody and others 2018), health planners can improve outcomes and reduce inefficiency in spending on the UHC intervention package by integrating into routine health care four types of measures that ensure high quality:

- Measuring activities and providing feedback
- Identifying relevant standards for these measures using scientific evidence, guidelines, and best practices
- Ensuring that providers are adequately trained to deliver the intervention with adequate management and oversight
- Motivating and aligning providers through incentives, which may be either financial (such as results-based financing) or nonfinancial (such as reputation enhancement among peers).

In some cases, investments in improving quality can translate to improvements in health over a shorter time frame than introducing a new health technology or policy. Costs related to quality improvement are covered in the EUHC and HPP cost estimates as part of health system costs (see table 3.1). The following are some examples from *DCP3* of measures that have been used to improve the quality of care for specific health conditions:

- Clinical checklists for complex tasks such as surgical procedures
- Hospital infection control policies and procedures
- Clinical guidelines for specific syndromes or diseases, including guidance on reducing unnecessary antibiotic use

- National essential medicines and diagnostics lists and formularies
- Use of community health workers and technologies (such as mHealth) to promote medication adherence
- Creation of high-volume, specialized centers to deal with complex but not urgent problems
- Adequate control of pain, including pain related to acute injuries or severe life-limiting illnesses.

Implications of EUHC for the Building Blocks of Health Systems

Once consensus has been reached on a health benefits package such as the HPP or EUHC, with political and public buy-in, the next step would be to implement this agenda within the context of the current health system. Using the WHO health systems framework (WHO 2007) as a point of reference, the most critical implications of the EUHC package for health systems can be identified, particularly leadership and governance challenges, UHC financing issues, health workforce constraints, gaps in medical product and technology availability, and limited information and research functions.

Leadership and Governance

A recent case series of early-adopter UHC countries highlighted the importance of leadership and governance as well as the strategic use of social and economic crises as opportunities for moving forward with UHC reforms (Reich and others 2016). National UHC plans and strategies would rely on strong regulatory measures and bureaucracy. As mentioned, well-considered management of private interests and agendas (such as donors, industries, and advocacy groups) can help ensure that an economically efficient and equitable form of UHC moves forward. At the same time, mechanisms for feedback and response can ensure that governments are accountable to constituents (Kieslich and others 2016).

In addition, management competence at a subnational level is incredibly important in ensuring that health services are delivered effectively. In particular, large clinics and first-level and referral hospitals require robust administrative capacity and health information management systems. A variety of studies have demonstrated that the quality of management is critical to the delivery of high-quality health services (Mills 2014).

UHC Financing

Issues around financing UHC have been reviewed by others and are not treated in detail here (WHO 2010; World Bank 2016). Nevertheless, it is important to recognize that all early-adopter countries, regardless of income level, have faced challenges in raising sufficient public revenues for UHC (Reich and others 2016). This chapter provides some general conclusions on the likely magnitude of UHC costs (table 3.2), which in most countries suggests a need for increases in both total health expenditure and the government's share of total health expenditure. Conversely, the HPP would need to be reduced substantially or disinvestment in interventions would be needed if resource levels could not be increased. This costing exercise also suggests that many low-income countries would need to continue relying on development assistance for health as a supplement to public finance for priority conditions, such as HIV/AIDS. Notably, countries from around the world have successfully employed a wide range of public, private, and hybrid financing models to achieve UHC (Reich and others 2016). Financing models are usually path dependent, but the key objective in any case is to divert out-of-pocket payments into pooled and prepayment mechanisms and to establish fairness in risk pooling. In addition, measures such as price negotiation with industry and local health technology assessment are crucial to managing cost escalation and maximizing efficiency of public expenditure (Nicholson and others 2015).

Health Workforce

Short- to medium-run constraints on the health workforce are probably among the most important bottlenecks in implementation of UHC reforms (Reich and others 2016; Stenberg and others 2017). *DCP3* has highlighted numerous examples of task sharing that allow for broader coverage of essential health services, such as the use of midlevel providers and general physicians for basic first-level hospital surgical procedures (Mock and others 2015). At the same time, as health systems become more complex and oriented toward management of NCDs, specialized systems and providers will also be required in many cases (Samb and others 2010). The EUHC and the HPP interventions include a limited number of specialized and referral services that reflect these future needs, but the human and material resources required to deliver these services at any reasonable level of coverage can take years to develop. Hence, low-income countries could consider adding capacity for specialized services that provide good value for money, such as specialized surgery and cancer centers (Gelband and others 2015; Mock and others 2015), as a first step during the SDG period toward more advanced, comprehensive health systems.

Medical Product and Technology Availability

Implementing EUHC will also require greater availability of existing medical products and technologies. Problems and proposed solutions to gaps in access to essential medicines have been reviewed by others and are not dealt with here (Howitt and others 2012; Wirtz and others 2017). However, *DCP3*'s model benefits packages could provide a useful input to the revision of national formularies and essential medicines lists. Procurement bodies and local agencies that regulate and manage supply chains could then be strengthened along the lines of these essential medicines so that they reach the last mile and make UHC truly universal. Additionally, *DCP3* has stressed the importance of using generic medications throughout (Patel and others 2015; Prabhakaran and others 2017). Generic medications nearly always have equivalent clinical effectiveness and can be a major factor ensuring the affordability and sustainability of UHC.

Information and Research

As critical as information and research are to health systems, they are often the most neglected of all health system functions in limited-resource settings. In particular, strong disease surveillance programs can inform the priorities for UHC and track progress. Box 3.2 summarizes some of the major information needs in limited-resource settings, emphasizing disease surveillance.

Although research is often perceived as a global public good rather than a specific national priority for limited-resource settings, a local research agenda could prioritize the validation of interventions and policies that have been tried in other settings but that likely vary significantly in effectiveness and cost-effectiveness because of differences in culture, language, disease epidemiology, and health system arrangements. In the long term, many countries could begin to develop completely novel interventions guided by local experience. Developing local capacity to conduct health technology

Box 3.2

Health System Information and Research Needs in Limited-Resource Settings

Routine, reliable, low-cost, long-term surveillance are vital to maintaining public health and providing effective medical care. Health surveillance systems are also critical to tracking trends in health conditions of the population, detecting new epidemics and outbreaks (such as Ebola and Zika virus infection), evaluating the success of control programs, and improving accountability for health expenditures. Surveillance supports five objectives, although, unfortunately, systems covering all five functions are rare in most LMICs:

- Monitoring of population health status (the most important aspect of which is premature mortality) to guide policy choices
- Efficiency in use of resources
- Disease surveillance to aid control programs
- Epidemic alert to enable rapid response and containment
- Identification of new risk factors or intermediate determinants of disease

Currently, no low-income country has adequate coverage of these key and often quite different surveillance functions. However, effective models have been implemented successfully in some countries, often at low cost. In India, for example, the Registrar General has created the Million Death Study in which a verbal autopsy instrument is added to its Sample Registration System to obtain cause-of-death data, by age, from about 1.4 million nationally representative homes from every state. The overall system costs less than US$1 per person annually. The Million Death Study has transformed disease control in India by enhancing the amount and quality of health data available for public health officials (Jha 2014).

A variety of new approaches could be taken to expand surveillance to support the core goals of UHC and increase the demand for such surveillance. These include increasing global assistance allocations from development agencies, expanding monitoring for NCDs in particular, and promoting international health audit days. More information on these opportunities can be found in annex 3G.

---

assessment and health policy analysis, while still aspirational for a number of LMICs, will ensure that the UHC agenda is realized in the most effective, efficient, and equitable manner possible.

The Role of Priority-Setting Institutions

This chapter has argued that UHC in some form can be realized in nearly every country and that an array of highly cost-effective, currently available interventions can be efficiently employed in limited resource settings to help countries reach most, if not all, of the SDG 3 goals and targets. By using economic tools and evidence, countries can develop health benefits packages that address their major health concerns on the basis of allocative efficiency, equity, and feasibility. Benefits packages designed in this way provide good value for money. By dramatically improving population health, they could also, over time, foster economic development and support other social goals, including poverty reduction.

At the same time, experience from all parts of the world has shown that setting priorities can also evolve in an inefficient and potentially inequitable manner (Kieslich and others 2016). Political calculus, inertia, efforts of prominent disease advocates, and donor priorities, among other influences, can at times create inefficiencies and increase inequalities if not well managed. In contrast, public sector priorities need to account for the preferences and expectations of the local population, which may deviate from what clinicians or technocrats would predict or extrapolate from other settings (Larson and others 2015). Robust, transparent, and publicly accountable priority-setting institutions are essential in all countries, but most LMICs do not yet have these sorts of institutions. Notable country examples from across the development spectrum can provide a template for building local capacity for health policy analysis and health technology assessment in LMICs (Li and others 2016). Academic organizations and partnerships such as the International Decision Support Initiative also play an important role in building local capacity to conduct health technology assessment and policy analysis in lower resource settings.[5]

As resources increase within a country, the possibilities for what a UHC scheme could include will grow as well. Glassman and others (2016) have described the process of defining a health benefits package as cyclical, with iterative improvements and revisions over time as well as expansions in the services offered. At the same time, *Making Fair Choices* argued that, when an existing package of interventions is not yet universally available, it is fairer to focus on achieving full coverage of that package before adding interventions to the package (WHO 2014). In practice, this principle can be difficult to follow, and in some cases, novel interventions are arguably worth considering on efficiency grounds if they result in significant economies of scope. Yet within the context of *DCP3*, the ethical principle suggests that, in general, all countries could first strive to achieve full coverage of the HPP (that is, of the most cost-effective interventions in a given setting), begin to add the EUHC interventions incrementally, and then expand to a broader range of interventions similar to those available in upper-middle-income or high-income settings.

For most low-income countries, implementing and scaling up a package like the HPP would likely be the focus during the SDG period. (Low-income countries that wish to offer a broader set of interventions than what is outlined in the HPP could continue to deliver this set of interventions; however, lower-priority interventions would need to be identified from among this set and financed through copayment or cost recovery mechanisms until public budgets were sufficient to cover the entire set [WHO 2014].) For lower-middle-income countries, the initial focus might be reaching full coverage of the HPP (if full coverage has not already been achieved), then moving toward full EUHC. The focus for most upper-middle-income and high-income countries might be ensuring full EUHC, which in some cases may require disinvesting from interventions and technologies that provide less value for money.

These sorts of actions undoubtedly require strong political commitment and mechanisms for managing special interests (Reich and others 2016). Nevertheless, this chapter argues that EUHC is a relevant and useful notion for all countries regardless of income, because it represents the aspects of health care that are likely to provide the best value for money and thus be the most efficient use of the next health care dollar. For LMICs in particular, EUHC could provide an economically grounded and realistic pathway to UHC and facilitate progress toward a "grand convergence" in global health during the SDG period (Jamison and others 2013).

ACKNOWLEDGMENTS

The authors wish to thank the following individuals for their contributions to the background materials for this chapter: Matthew Schneider and Carol Levin, who contributed to the cost analyses for HIV/AIDS and surgery, respectively; Kjell Arne Johansson and Matthew Coates, who produced the indicators for conditions that affect the worse off; and the volume and series editors of *DCP3* and the Advisory Committee to the Editors, who provided input on the conceptualization of this chapter and—in many cases—critically reviewed draft tables and annexes.

ANNEXES

The following annexes to this chapter are available at http://www.dcp-3.org/DCP.

- Annex 3A: An Essential Package of Interventions to Address Congenital and Genetic Disorders
- Annex 3B: An Essential Package of Interventions to Address Musculoskeletal Disorders
- Annex 3C: Essential Universal Health Coverage: Interventions and Platforms
- Annex 3D: Notes on the Essential UHC Interventions in Annex 3C
- Annex 3E: Methods for Appraisal of Essential UHC Interventions
- Annex 3F: Findings from the Appraisal of Essential UHC Interventions
- Annex 3G: The Role of Surveillance in Achieving UHC

NOTES

World Bank Income Classifications as of July 2014 are as follows, based on estimates of gross national income (GNI) per capita for 2013:

- Low-income countries (LICs) = US$1,045 or less
- Middle-income countries (MICs) are subdivided:
  (a) lower-middle-income = US$1,046 to US$4,125.
  (b) upper-middle-income (UMICs) = US$4,126 to US$12,745.
- High-income countries (HICs) = US$12,746 or more.

1. SDG 3, titled "Good Health and Well-Being," provides the following: "Ensure healthy lives and promote well-being for all at all ages" (UN 2016).
2. The "*Making Fair Choices* consultation" refers to the WHO Consultative Group on Equity and Universal Health Coverage, the author of *Making Fair Choices on the Path to Universal Health Coverage* (WHO 2014).
3. Estimates from Vos and others (2016) were used because similar data were not available from WHO.

4. Current GNI data by country aggregated using the 2014 country classification, see http://data.worldbank.org /indicator/NY.GNP.ATLS.CD?page=1.

5. For more information, see the International Decision Support Initiative website, http://www.idsihealth.org/who-we-are /about-us.

REFERENCES

Akachi, Y., and M. Kruk. 2017. "Quality of Care: Measuring a Neglected Driver of Improved Health." *Bulletin of the World Health Organization* 95 (6): 465–72. doi:http://dx .doi.org/10.2471/BLT.16.180190.

Atun, R., T. de Jongh, F. Secci, K. Ohiri, and O. Adeyi. 2010. "A Systematic Review of the Evidence on Integration of Targeted Health Interventions into Health Systems." *Health Policy and Planning* 25 (1): 1–14.

Black, R. E., R. Laxminarayan, M. Temmerman, and N. Walker, eds. 2016. *Reproductive, Maternal, Newborn, and Child Health.* Volume 2, *Disease Control Priorities* (third edition), edited by D. T. Jamison, R. Nugent, H. Gelband, S. Horton, P. Jha, and R. Laxminarayan. Washington, DC: World Bank.

Boyle, C. F., C. Levin, A. Hatefi, S. Madriz, and N. Santos 2015. "Achieving a 'Grand Convergence' in Global Health: Modeling the Technical Inputs, Costs, and Impacts from 2016 to 2030." *PLoS One* 10 (10): e0140092.

Bump, J., C. Cashin, K. Chalkidou, D. Evans, and others. 2016. "Implementing Pro-Poor Universal Health Care Coverage." *The Lancet Global Health* 4 (1): e14–e16. doi:http://dx.doi .org/10.1016/S2214-109X(15)00274-0.

Busse, R., J. Schreyögg, and C. Gericke. 2007. "Analyzing Changes in Health Financing Arrangements in High-Income Countries: A Comprehensive Framework Approach." HNP Discussion Paper, World Bank, Washington, DC.

Cairns, J. 2016. "Using Cost-Effectiveness Evidence to Inform Decisions as to Which Health Services to Provide." *Health Systems and Reform* 2 (1): 32–38.

Chan, M. 2016. "Making Fair Choices on the Path to Universal Health Coverage." *Health Systems & Reform* 2 (1): 5–7.

Chang, A. Y., S. Horton, and D. T. Jamison. 2018. "Benefit-Cost Analysis in *Disease Control Priorities*, Third Edition." In *Disease Control Priorities* (third edition): Volume 9, *Disease Control Priorities: Improving Health and Reducing Poverty,* edited by D. T. Jamison, H. Gelband, S. Horton, P. Jha, R. Laxminarayanm, C. N. Mock, and R. Nugent. Washington, DC: World Bank.

Ethiopia, Ministry of Health. 2015. "HSTP: Health Sector Transformation Plan, 2015/16–2019/20." Strategy and planning document for Second Growth and Transformation Plan (GTP II), Addis Ababa.

Gelband, H., P. Jha, R. Sankaranarayanan, C. L. Gavreau, and S. Horton. 2015. "Summary." In *Disease Control Priorities* (third edition): Volume 3, *Cancer,* edited by H. Gelband, P. Jha, R. Sankaranarayanan, and S. Horton. Washington, DC: World Bank.

Giedion, U., E. A. Alfonso, and Y. Díaz. 2013. "The Impact of Universal Coverage Schemes in the Developing World: A Review of the Existing Evidence." Universal Health Coverage (UNICO) Studies Series No. 25, World Bank, Washington, DC.

Glassman, A., U. Giedion, Y. Sakuma, and P. C. Smith. 2016. "Defining a Health Benefits Package: What Are the Necessary Processes?" *Health Systems and Reform* 2 (1): 39–50.

Holmes, K. K., S. Bertozzi, B. Bloom, and P. Jha, eds. 2017. *Major Infectious Diseases.* Volume 6, *Disease Control Priorities* (third edition), edited by D. T. Jamison, H. Gelband, S. Horton, P. Jha, and R. Laxminarayan. Washington, DC: World Bank.

Horton, S. 2018. "Cost-Effectiveness Analysis in *Disease Control Priorities,* Third Edition." In *Disease Control Priorities* (third edition): Volume 9, *Disease Control Priorities: Improving Health and Reducing Poverty,* edited by D. T. Jamison, H. Gelband, S. Horton, P. Jha, R. Laxminarayan, C. N. Mock, and R. Nugent. Washington, DC: World Bank.

Howitt, P., A. Darzi, G. Z. Yang, H. Ashrafian, R. Atun, and others. 2012. "Technologies for Global Health." *The Lancet* 380 (9840): 507–35.

Jamison, D. T., A. Alwan, C. N. Mock, R. Nugent, D. A. Watkins, and others. 2018. "Universal Health Coverage and Intersectoral Action for Health: Findings from *Disease Control Priorities,* Third Edition." In *Disease Control Priorities* (third edition): Volume 9, *Disease Control Priorities: Improving Health and Reducing Poverty,* edited by D. T. Jamison, H. Gelband, S. Horton, P. Jha, R. Laxminarayan, C. N. Mock, and R. Nugent. Washington, DC: World Bank.

Jamison, D. T., J. G. Breman, A. R. Measham, G. Alleyne, M. Claeson, D. B. Evans, P. Jha, A. Mills, and P. Musgrove, eds. 2006. *Disease Control Priorities in Developing Countries,* second edition. Washington, DC: World Bank and Oxford University Press.

Jamison, D. T., L. H. Summers, G. Alleyne, K. J. Arrow, S. Berkley, and others 2013. "Global Health 2035: A World Converging within a Generation." *The Lancet* 382 (9908): 1898–55.

Jha, P. 2014. "Reliable Direct Measurement of Causes of Death in Low- and Middle-Income Countries." *BMC Medicine* 12 (19). https://doi.org/10.1186/1741-7015-12-19.

Ji, J. S., and L. Chen. 2016. "UHC Presents Universal Challenges." *Health Systems and Reform* 2 (1): 1–14.

Kieslich, K., J. Bump, O. F. Norheim, S. Tantivess, and P. Littlejohns. 2016. "Accounting for Technical, Ethical, and Political Factors in Priority Setting." *Health Systems and Reform* 2 (1): 51–60.

Kruk, M., A. Chukwuma, G. Mbaruku, and H. H. Leslie. 2017. "Variation in Quality of Primary-Care Services in Kenya, Malawi, Namibia, Rwanda, Senegal, Uganda, and the United Republic of Tanzania." *Bulletin of the World Health Organization* 95 (6): 408–18. doi:http://dx.doi.org/10.2471 /BLT.16.175869.

Kruk M. E., E. Goldmann, S. Galea. 2009. "Borrowing and Selling to Pay for Health Care in Low- and Middle-Income Countries." *Health Affairs* 28 (4): 1056–66.

Larson, E., D. Vail, G. M. Mbaruku, A. Kimweri, L. P. Freedman, and M. E. Kruk. 2015. "Moving toward Patient-Centered

Care in Africa: A Discrete Choice Experiment of Preferences for Delivery Care among 3,003 Tanzanian Women." *PLoS One* 10 (8): e0135621.

Li, R., K. Hernandez-Villafuerte, A. Towse, I. Vlad, and K. Chalkidou. 2016. "Mapping Priority Setting in Health in 17 Countries across Asia, Latin America, and Sub-Saharan Africa." *Health Systems and Reform* 2 (1): 71–83.

Mathers, C., G. Stevens, D. Hogan, A. Mahanani, and J. Ho. 2018. "Global and Regional Causes of Death: Patterns and Trends, 2000–15." In *Disease Control Priorities* (third edition): Volume 9, *Disease Control Priorities: Improving Health and Reducing Poverty,* edited by D. T. Jamison, H. Gelband, S. Horton, P. Jha, R. Laxminarayanm, C. N. Mock, and R. Nugent. Washington, DC: World Bank.

McIntyre, D., F. Meheus, and J. A. Rottingen. 2017. "What Level of Domestic Government Health Expenditure Should We Aspire to for Universal Health Coverage?" *Health Economics Policy and Law* 12 (2): 12–37.

McIntyre, D., M. Thiede, G. Dahlgren, and M. Whitehead. 2006. "What Are the Economic Consequences for Households of Illness and of Paying for Health Care in Low- and Middle-Income Country Contexts?" *Social Science and Medicine* 62 (4): 858–65.

Mills, A. 2014. "Health Care Systems in Low- and Middle-Income Countries." *New England Journal of Medicine* 370: 552–57. doi:10.1056/NEJMra1110897.

Mock, C. N., P. Donkor, A. Gawande, D. T. Jamison, M. E. Kruk, and H. T. Debas. 2015. "Essential Surgery: Key Messages of This Volume." In *Disease Control Priorities* (third edition): Volume 1, *Essential Surgery*, edited by H. T. Debas, P. Donkor, A. Gawande, D. T. Jamison, M. E. Kruk, and C. N. Mock. Washington, DC: World Bank.

Ng, M., N. Fullman, J. L. Dieleman, A. D. Flaxman, C. J. Murray, and S. S. Lim. 2014. "Effective Coverage: A Metric for Monitoring Universal Health Coverage." *PLoS Med* 11 (9): e1001730.

Nicholson, D., R. Yates, W. Warburton, and G. Fontana. 2015. "Delivering Universal Health Coverage: A Guide for Policymakers." Report of the WISH Universal Health Coverage Forum 2015, World Innovation Summit for Health (WISH), Doha, Qatar.

Norheim, O. F., P. Jha, K. Admasu, T. Godal, R. J. Hum, and others. 2015. "Avoiding 40% of the Premature Deaths in Each Country, 2010–30: Review of National Mortality Trends to Help Quantify the UN Sustainable Development Goal for Health." *The Lancet* 385 (9964): 239–52.

Ochalek, J., J. Lomas, and K. Claxton. 2015. "Cost per DALY Averted Thresholds for Low- and Middle-Income Countries: Evidence from Cross Country Data." Centre for Health Economics (CHE) Research Paper 122, University of York, York, U.K. https://www.york.ac.uk/media/che/documents/papers/researchpapers/CHERP122_cost_DALY_LMIC_threshold.pdf.

Patel, V., D. Chisholm, T. Dua, R. Laxminarayan, and M. E. Medina-Mora, eds. 2015. *Mental, Neurological, and Substance Use Disorders*. Volume 4, *Disease Control Priorities* (third edition), edited by D. T. Jamison, R. Nugent, H. Gelband, S. Horton, P. Jha, R. Laxminarayan, and C. N. Mock. Washington, DC: World Bank.

Peabody, J., R. Shimkhada, O. Adeyi, H. Wang, E. Broughton, and M. Kruk. 2018. "Quality of Care." In *Disease Control Priorities* (third edition): Volume 9, *Disease Control Priorities: Improving Health and Reducing Poverty,* edited by D. T. Jamison, H. Gelband, S. Horton, P. Jha, R. Laxminarayan, C. N. Mock, and R. Nugent. Washington, DC: World Bank.

Prabhakaran, D., S. Anand, T. Gaziano, J.-C. Mbanya, Y. Wu, and R. Nugent, eds. 2017. *Cardiovascular, Respiratory, and Related Conditions.* Volume 5, *Disease Control Priorities* (third edition), edited by D. T. Jamison, R. Nugent, H. Gelband, S. Horton, P. Jha, R. Laxminarayan, and C. N. Mock. Washington, DC: World Bank.

Reich, M. R., J. Harris, N. Ikegami, A. Maeda, C. Cashin, and others. 2016. "Moving Towards Universal Health Coverage: Lessons from 11 Country Studies." *The Lancet* 387 (10020): 811–16.

Samb, B., N. Desai, S. Nishtar, S. Mendis, H. Bekedam, and others. 2010. "Prevention and Management of Chronic Disease: A Litmus Test for Health-Systems Strengthening in Low-Income and Middle-Income Countries." *The Lancet* 376 (9754): 1785–97.

Savedoff, W., D. de Ferranti, A. Smith, and V. Fan. 2012. "Political and Economic Aspects of the Transition to Universal Health Coverage." *The Lancet* 3880 (9845): 924–32.

Seshadria, S. R., P. Jha, P. Sati, C. Gauvreau, U. Ram, and R. Laxminarayan. 2015. "Karnataka's Roadmap to Improved Health: Cost Effective Solutions to Address Priority Diseases, Reduce Poverty and Increase Economic Growth." Report for the Government of Karnataka, Azim Premji University, Bangalore.

Stenberg, K., O. Hanssen, T. Edejer, M. Bertram, C. Brindley, and others. 2017. "Financing Transformative Health Systems Towards Achievement of the Health Sustainable Developmenbt Goals: A Model for Projected Resource Needs in 67 Low-Income and Middle-Income Countries." *The Lancet Global Health* 5 (9): e875–e887.

UN (United Nations). 2016. "Sustainable Development Goals: 17 Goals to Transform Our World. Goal 3: Ensure Healthy Lives and Promote Well-Being for All at All Ages." Website, UN, New York. http://www.un.org/sustainabledevelopment/health/.

UN DESA (United Nations Department of Economic and Social Affairs). 2017. "World Population Prospects: 2017 Revision, Key Findings and Advance Tables." Report ESA/P/WP/248, UN DESA Population Division, New York.

Verguet, S., and D. T. Jamison. 2018. "Health Policy Analysis: Applications of Extended Cost-Effectiveness Analysis Methodology in *Disease Control Priorities*, Third Edition." In *Disease Control Priorities* (third edition): Volume 9, *Disease Control Priorities: Improving Health and Reducing Poverty,* edited by D. T. Jamison, H. Gelband, S. Horton, P. Jha, R. Laxminarayan, C. N. Mock, and R. Nugent. Washington, DC: World Bank.

Vos, T., C. Allen, M. Arora, R. M. Barber, Z. A. Bhutta, and others. 2016. "Global, Regional, and National Incidence, Prevalence, and Years Lived with Disability for 310 Acute and Chronic Diseases and Injuries, 1990–2015: A Systematic Analysis for the Global Burden of Disease Study 2015." *The Lancet* 388 (10053): 1545–1602.

Watkins, D. A., O. F. Norheim, P. Jha, and D. T. Jamison. 2017. "Mortality Impact of Achieving Essential Universal Health Coverage in Low- and Lower-Middle-Income Countries." Working Paper 21 for *Disease Control Priorities* (third edition), Department of Global Health, University of Washington, Seattle.

Watkins, D. A., R. A. Nugent, H. Saxenian, G. Yarney, K. Danforth, E. González-Pier, C. N. Mock, P. Jha, A. Alwan, and D. T. Jamison. 2018. "Intersectoral Policy Priorities for Health." In *Disease Control Priorities* (third edition): Volume 9, *Disease Control Priorities: Improving Health and Reducing Poverty*, edited by D. T. Jamison, H. Gelband, S. Horton, P. Jha, R. Laxminarayan, C. N. Mock, and R. Nugent. Washington, DC: World Bank.

Watkins, D. A., J. Qi, and S. E. Horton. 2017. "Costs and Affordability of Essential Universal Health Coverage in Low- and Middle-Income Countries." Working Paper 20 for *Disease Control Priorities* (third edition), Department of Global Health, University of Washington, Seattle.

WHO (World Health Organization). 2007. *Everybody's Business: Strengthening Health Systems to Improve Health Outcomes. WHO's Framework for Action.* Geneva: WHO.

———. 2010. *The World Health Report. Health Systems Financing: The Path to Universal Coverage.* Geneva: WHO.

———. 2011. *Global Status Report on Noncommunicable Diseases 2010.* Geneva: WHO.

———. 2013a. *Global Action Plan for the Prevention and Control of Noncommunicable Diseases 2013–2020.* Geneva: WHO.

———. 2013b. *The World Health Report 2013: Research for Universal Health Coverage.* Geneva: WHO.

———. 2014. *Making Fair Choices on the Path to Universal Health Coverage: Final Report of the WHO Consultative Group on Equity and Universal Health Coverage.* Geneva: WHO.

———. 2016. Global Health Observator database. WHO, Geneva. http://www.who.int/gho/en/.

Wirtz, V. J., H. V. Hogerzeil, A. L. Gray, M. Bigdeli, C. P. de Joncheere, and others. 2017. "Essential Medicines for Universal Health Coverage." *The Lancet* 389 (10067): 403–76.

World Bank. 2016. "Universal Health Coverage Study Series (UNICO)." Studies from 23 countries, World Bank, Washington, DC. http://www.worldbank.org/en/topic/health/publication/universal-health-coverage-study-series.

Xu, K., D. B. Evans, G. Carrin, A. M. Aguilar-Rivera, P. Musgrove, and T. Evans. 2007. "Protecting Households from Catastrophic Health Spending." *Health Affairs* 26 (4): 972–83.

Youngkong, S. 2012. "Multi-Criteria Decision Analysis for Including Health Interventions in the Universal Health Coverage Benefit Package in Thailand." PhD dissertation, Radboud University, Nijmegen, Netherlands.

Part **2**

Problems and Progress

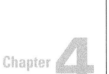

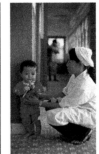

Chapter 4

Global and Regional Causes of Death: Patterns and Trends, 2000–15

Colin Mathers, Gretchen Stevens, Dan Hogan,
Wahyu Retno Mahanani, and Jessica Ho

INTRODUCTION

One of the six core functions of the World Health Organization (WHO) is monitoring the health situation, trends, and determinants in the world. Global, regional, and country statistics on population and health indicators are important for assessing progress toward goals for development and health and for guiding the allocation of resources. Timely data are needed to monitor progress on increasing life expectancy and reducing age- and cause-specific mortality rates. In particular, timely data are needed to monitor progress toward reaching the health-related targets within the Sustainable Development Goals (SDGs), which will require regular reporting on child mortality; maternal mortality; and mortality owing to noncommunicable diseases (NCDs), suicide, air pollution, road traffic injuries, homicide, natural disasters, and conflict.

This chapter summarizes global and regional patterns of causes of death for 2015 and trends for 2000–15 using the 2015 Global Health Estimates (GHE 2015) released by the WHO at the beginning of 2017 (WHO 2017a). The GHE 2015 statistics provide a comprehensive, comparable set of cause-of-death estimates from 2000 onward, consistent with and incorporating estimates from the United Nations (UN) and interagency and the WHO data for population, births, all-cause deaths, and specific causes of death.

The GHE 2015 present results for 183 WHO member states with a population of 90,000 or greater in 2015. The GHE 2015 cause-of-death estimates by country, region, and world for 2000–15 confirm and expand previous WHO analyses of global health trends. In particular, the WHO published an assessment of progress toward achievement of the UN Millennium Development Goals (MDGs) at the end of 2015 (WHO 2015b), followed by the *World Health Statistics 2016: Monitoring Health for the SDGs* (WHO 2016d), which focused on progress and challenges for achieving the SDGs for 2030.

The SDGs expand the focus of health targets from the unfinished MDG agenda for child and maternal mortality and priority infectious diseases to a broader agenda including NCDs, injuries, health emergencies, and health risk factors as well as a strong focus on universal health coverage (UN Statistics Division 2017; WHO 2016d). The GHE 2015 estimates of trends and levels of mortality by cause will contribute to WHO and UN monitoring and reporting of progress toward the SDG health goals and targets.

METHODS

Categories of Analysis

The GHE 2015 provide estimates of the total number of deaths in 2000–15 for 177 detailed categories of disease and injury as well as for all causes. The categories of

Corresponding author: Colin Mathers, Department of Information, Evidence, and Research, World Health Organization, Geneva; mathersc@who.int.

cause are specified in the *International Statistical Classification of Diseases and Related Health Problems* (known as the International Classification of Diseases, or ICD) tenth revision codes (WHO 1990), as shown in annex 4A. Deaths are estimated for the neonatal period (1 to 27 days), the postneonatal period (1 to 11 months), 1 to 4 years, and 5-year age groups starting at age 5 to 85 years and above.

This chapter uses World Bank classifications of national income (gross national income per capita) as of July 2014 to classify countries into four income categories: low, lower middle, upper middle, and high.

All-Cause Mortality

The WHO life tables were revised and updated for 183 member states for 1990–2015 (WHO 2016b), drawing on the *World Population Prospects: 2015 Revision* (UN 2015), recent and unpublished analyses of all-cause mortality and mortality from human immunodeficiency virus/acquired immune deficiency syndrome (HIV/AIDS) for countries with high HIV/AIDS prevalence (Avenir Consulting 2016; UNAIDS 2016), vital registration data (WHO 2016c), and United Nations Inter-agency Group for Child Mortality Estimation estimates of levels and trends for under-age-5 mortality (UN-IGME 2015). Methods and data sources are documented in more detail in annex 4A. The WHO life tables are available in the WHO Global Health Observatory (2016).

Total deaths by age and sex were estimated for each country by applying death rates in the WHO life tables to the estimated de facto resident population prepared by the UN Population Division in its 2015 revision (UN 2015).

Causes of Death

The GHE 2015 are consistent with UN agency, interagency, and WHO estimates for population, births, allcause deaths, and specific causes of death, including the following:

- The most recent vital registration data for all countries where the quality of data is assessed as usable
- UN estimates of levels and trends for all-cause mortality for older children and adults and UN interagency estimates of neonatal, infant, and child mortality
- WHO programs and interagency groups' updated estimates for specific causes of death, including maternal, HIV/AIDS, tuberculosis, malaria, cancers, road traffic injuries, and homicide

- Global Burden of Disease 2015 (GBD 2015) estimates for other causes in countries lacking usable vital registration data or other nationally representative sources of information on causes of death (IHME 2016).

Figure 4.1 provides an overview of the data and processes used to produce the GHE 2015. Annex 4A provides a more detailed summary, which covers the processes involved in the use of death registration data submitted to the WHO Mortality Database (WHO 2016c).

Death Registration Data Used Directly

Death registration data, with medical certification of the cause of death and the cause of death coded using the ICD, are the preferred source of information for monitoring mortality by cause, age, and sex. However, there are major gaps in the coverage of death registration data and persistent issues in the quality of such data. In 2015, nearly half of all deaths worldwide were registered in a national death registration system with information on cause of death (figure 4.2), an improvement from about one-third in 2005. However, only 38 percent of all global deaths are currently reported to the WHO Mortality Database (WHO 2016c). Of these reported deaths, 43 percent are for high-income countries (HICs), 44 percent are for upper-middle-income countries, 13 percent are for lowermiddle-income countries, and less than 1 percent are for low-income countries, (LICs). Only about 28 percent of all global deaths are reported to the WHO by ICD code, and only 23 percent are reported to the WHO with meaningful information on their underlying cause.

Two main dimensions of quality impede the use of death registration data for public health monitoring: (a) low level of completeness and (b) missing, incomplete, or invalid information on the underlying cause of death. "Completeness" is defined as the percentage of all deaths in the de facto resident population that are registered and compiled nationally. The quality of information on underlying cause of death is summarized by the proportion of deaths coded to so-called garbage codes, which do not provide information on valid underlying disease or injury causes of death.

Since 2010, the WHO has been summarizing the usability of death registration data for estimating causes of death in a population with a usability score calculated as follows:

$$(\text{Percentage usable}) = \text{Completeness (\%)} \times (1 - \text{Proportion garbage}). \quad (4.1)$$

Death registration data reported to the WHO were used to estimate causes of death for 69 countries

Figure 4.1 Overview of the Processes Involved in Preparing the Global Health Estimates Dataset for Causes of Death in 183 WHO Member States, 2000–15

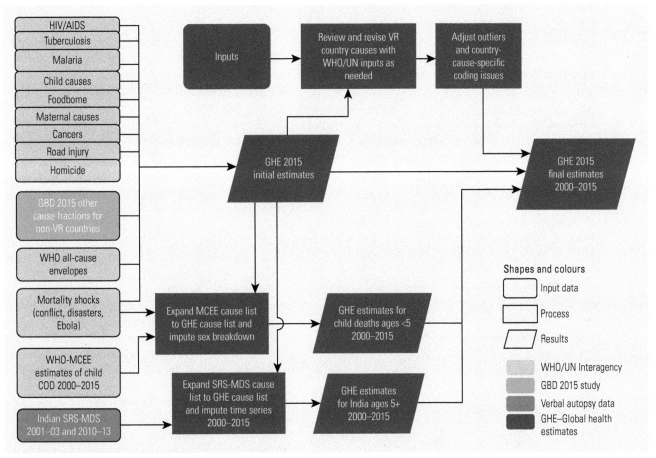

Note: COD = cause of death; GBD 2015 = Global Burden of Disease 2015; GHE 2015 = 2015 Global Health Estimates; HIV/AIDS = human immunodeficiency virus/acquired immune deficiency syndrome; MCEE = Maternal and Child Epidemiology Estimation Collaboration; SRS-MDS = Sample Registration System–Million Death Study; UN = United Nations; VR = vital registration; WHO = the World Health Organization.

meeting the following inclusion criteria: (a) at least five years of data were available during 2005–15, and (b) at least 65 percent of deaths were usable for 2000 to the latest available year (WHO 2016c). The following short list of garbage codes was used to compute the usable percentage:

- Symptoms, signs, and ill-defined conditions (ICD 10 codes R00–R99)
- Injuries undetermined whether intentional or unintentional (ICD 10 Y10–Y34, Y87.2)
- Ill-defined cancers (C76, C80, and C97)
- Ill-defined cardiovascular diseases (I46, I47.2, I49.0, I50, I51.4, I51.5, I51.6, I51.9, and I70.9).

Deaths coded to these and various other garbage codes were redistributed to valid underlying causes of death. Estimates for India were based on WHO analyses of data from the Sample Registration System (SRS) for two

Figure 4.2 Number of Global Deaths in 2015, by Expected Registration or Reporting Status

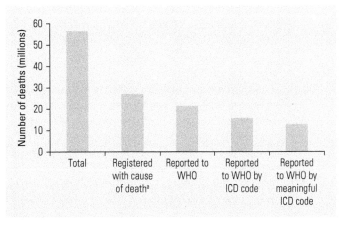

Note: Reports to the World Health Organization (WHO) are projected on the basis of 2010 data to allow for reporting lag. ICD = International Classification of Diseases.
a. Local death registration, in the absence of a state or national system to compile data, is excluded, as is registration with cause of death based on verbal autopsy.

periods: 2001–03 (Registrar General of India 2009) and 2010–13 (Registrar General of India and CGHR 2015). Estimates for China drew on death registration data for 2013 (China CDC 2016) together with IHME analyses of trends in causes of death (GBD 2016).

Causes of Death for Children under Age 5

For countries lacking usable death registration data, neonatal deaths and deaths at age 1–59 months were estimated for 15 major causes identifiable from verbal autopsy studies using methods described by Liu and others (2015). These categories were expanded to the full GHE list of causes using nested cause fraction results predicted from the GBD 2015 study.

For China, estimates of causes of death for children under age 5 were based on a separate analysis of data from the Maternal and Child Health Surveillance System (WHO 2016b). For India, a separate multiple-cause model was used to prepare state-level estimates based on about 40 subnational community-based verbal autopsy studies (WHO and MCEE 2016).

Cause-Specific Estimates from the WHO and UN Agencies

The GHE 2015 incorporate the latest updated WHO and UN interagency assessments of levels and trends for the following specific causes of death:

- Tuberculosis: *Global Tuberculosis Report 2016* (WHO 2016a)
- HIV/AIDS: UNAIDS (2016); WHO (2016b)
- Malaria: *World Malaria Report 2016* (WHO 2016e)
- Vaccine-preventable child causes: Patel and others (2016); WHO (2017b)
- Other major child causes: the WHO and the Maternal and Child Epidemiology Estimation collaboration (WHO and MCEE 2016)
- Foodborne diseases: the WHO Foodborne Disease Burden Epidemiology Reference Group (Torgerson and others 2015)
- Ebola virus infection: WHO estimates of direct deaths owing to infections and indirect deaths owing to measles outbreaks and reduced coverage of treatment for HIV/AIDS and malaria (see annex 4A)
- Maternal mortality: UN Maternal Mortality Estimation Inter-Agency Group (MMEIG 2015)
- Cancers: International Agency for Research on Cancer (Ferlay and others 2013)
- Road injuries: *Global Status Report on Road Safety 2015* (WHO 2015a)
- Homicide: *Global Status Report on Violence Prevention 2014* (WHO 2014a)

- Conflict and natural disasters: the WHO and the Centre for Research on the Epidemiology of Disasters. For methods, see WHO (2016b).

Additional adjustments and revisions were applied to GBD 2015 estimates for schistosomiasis, rabies, leprosy, liver cancer, alcohol use disorders, drug use disorders, and liver cirrhosis, as described in annex 4A.

Other Causes of Death for Countries Lacking Death Registration Data

Estimates of mortality and causes of death were released in 2016 (GBD 2015 Mortality and Causes of Death Collaborators 2016) by the Institute of Health Metrics and Evaluation (IHME) as part of the GBD 2015 study (IHME 2016). The WHO has drawn on the GBD 2015 analyses for selected causes for member states lacking comprehensive death registration data.

For major causes of death except HIV/AIDS and measles, the IHME used ensemble modeling to create a weighted average of many individual covariate-based models (ranging from hundreds to thousands in some cases) for each specific cause. The overall out-of-sample predictive validity of the ensemble is usually not much different from that of the top-ranked model, but ranges of uncertainty are generally much wider and more plausible than for single models. To ensure that the results of all the single-cause models summed to the all-cause mortality estimate for each age-sex-country-year group, the IHME applied a final step to rescale the cause-specific estimates. This step effectively *squeezed* or *expanded* causes with wider uncertainty ranges more than those with narrower uncertainty ranges. The GBD 2015 results (IHME 2016) were resqueezed to the WHO all-cause envelopes to produce a set of so-called prior estimates for the GHE categories of cause by age, sex, country, and year.

Final Adjustments

IHME results for priority causes such as HIV/AIDS, tuberculosis, malaria, cancers, maternal mortality, and child mortality differ to varying degrees from those of the WHO and UN agency partners. In part, these variations reflect not only differences in modeling strategies but also the inclusion by IHME of data from verbal autopsy studies, mapped to ICD categories using IHME-developed computer algorithms. We carried out an adjustment process to ensure that the estimated number of deaths tallied across causes to the estimated total number of deaths by age, sex, country, and year for all countries.

Levels of Evidence and Uncertainty

General guidance on the quality and uncertainty of these cause-of-death estimates for 2000–15 is provided with regard to the quality of data inputs and methods used. Most of the inputs to the GHE 2015 have explicit uncertainty ranges. The two main exceptions are the UN Population Division's *World Population Prospects* 2015 life tables (UN 2015) and the Globocan cancer mortality estimates (IARC 2013). The Globocan 2012 database provides information on sources of data and quality of inputs for seven categories of incidence data and six categories of mortality data as well as six estimation methods for mortality (IARC 2013). The GBD 2015 estimates of deaths by cause, age, sex, country, and year also include estimates of 95 percent uncertainty ranges that take into account some, but not all, sources of uncertainty.

Based on the uncertainty ranges estimated for the inputs, explicit uncertainty ranges for the GHE 2015 are available on the WHO website (see box 4.1).

RESULTS

Broad Patterns of Causes of Death in 2015

In 2015, a total of 56.4 million deaths occurred in the world; of these, 7.0 million occurred in LICs and 20.4 million occurred in lower-middle-income countries. Just under half (46 percent) of all deaths in LICs were caused by Group I conditions, which include communicable diseases, maternal causes, conditions arising during the perinatal period, and nutritional deficiencies (figure 4.3). For HICs that have passed through the epidemiological transition, Group I conditions accounted for less than 7 percent of deaths. For LICs, Group I conditions accounted for 65 percent of deaths in 2000,

and death rates for most diseases and disorders in this group of countries declined substantially between 2000 and 2015.

NCDs caused 70 percent of deaths globally in 2015, with regional figures ranging from 43 percent in LICs to 87 percent in HICs. In terms of the absolute number of deaths, however, 74 percent of global NCD-related deaths occurred in low- and middle-income countries (LMICs).

Injuries claimed nearly 5 million lives in 2015 (8.8 percent of total deaths). More than a quarter (27 percent) of these deaths were due to road traffic injuries. LICs had the highest mortality rate for road traffic injuries, with 25.0 deaths per 100,000 population, compared with a global rate of 18.3. More than 90 percent of road traffic deaths occur in LMICs, which account for 82 percent of the world's population but only 54 percent of the world's registered vehicles. Several factors are at work, including poorly designed or implemented regulations, inadequate road and vehicle quality, and a higher proportion of vulnerable road users (pedestrians, cyclists, and motorcyclists).

Leading Causes of Death in 2015

Figure 4.4 shows the 10 leading causes of death for the world and for country income groups in 2015. The 10 leading causes of death globally were 6 NCDs, 3 infectious diseases, and road injuries, which collectively accounted for more than half of all deaths. Ischemic heart disease (IHD) and stroke killed 15 million people in 2015; these two diseases have been the biggest killers globally in the past 15 years. Whereas 7 of the 10 leading causes in low-income countries were Group I conditions, all but 1 of the

---

Box 4.1

Datasets Available for the WHO Global Health Estimates 2015

The WHO Global Health Estimates provide a number of datasets:

- Regional and country spreadsheets of deaths by cause, age, and sex, 2000–15 (http://www.who .int/healthinfo/global_burden_disease/estimates /en/index1.html)
- Regional and country spreadsheets of disability--adjusted life years, years of life lost, and years lost to disability by cause, age, and sex, 2000–15

(http://www.who.int/healthinfo/global_burden _disease/estimates/en/index2.html)
- Files with uncertainty (http://terrance.who.int /mediacentre/data/ghe/)
- Life expectancy and life tables by country, region, and world (http://www.who.int/gho /mortality_burden_disease/life_tables/en/)
- Global Health Estimates technical paper series (http://www.who.int/healthinfo/global_burden _disease/data_sources_methods/en/).

Figure 4.3 Overall Mortality Rates, by Cause and Country Income Group, 2000 and 2015

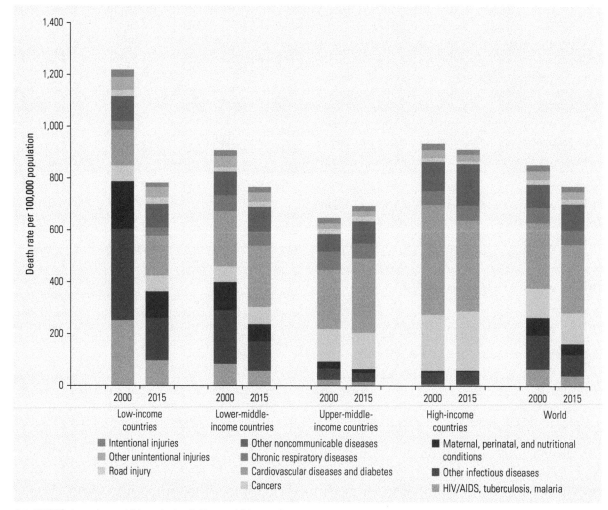

Note: HIV/AIDS = human immunodeficiency virus/acquired immune deficiency syndrome.

10 leading causes of death in HICs were NCDs. Road injuries were among the 10 leading causes of death for countries at all income levels except HICs. The colors of the bars in figure 4.4 indicate causes for which overall death rates are increasing (red) or decreasing (green). Increases in overall (crude) death rates (total deaths divided by total population) may reflect the effect of population aging as well as changes in age-specific risks of death. Population aging is often a dominant factor for diseases with death rates that rise with age, such as most cancers, cardiovascular diseases, and dementia, even when age-specific death rates are falling. One important exception is the substantial decline in the death rates of IHD and stroke in HICs.

Chronic lung disease claimed 3.2 million lives in 2015, while lung cancer (along with tracheal and bronchus cancers) caused 1.7 million deaths. Diabetes killed 1.6 million people in 2015, up from less than

1 million in 2000. Total deaths attributable to diabetes are more than double this number, because diabetes raises the risk of cardiovascular and other diseases. Estimated deaths from dementia more than doubled between 2000 and 2015, making dementia the seventh-leading cause of death globally in 2015. In the case of dementia and diabetes, aging and rising death rates contribute to the rise in overall number of deaths. Rising reported death rates for these two causes may also reflect an increase in diagnosis or recording as an underlying cause of death rather than an increase in the age-specific risk of mortality.

Lower respiratory infections remained the deadliest communicable disease, causing 3.2 million deaths worldwide in 2015. The diarrhea death rate almost halved between 2000 and 2015, but the disease still caused 1.4 million deaths in 2015. Similarly, the tuberculosis death rate fell during the same period, but the

Figure 4.4 The 10 Leading Causes of Death, for the World and by Country Income Group, 2015

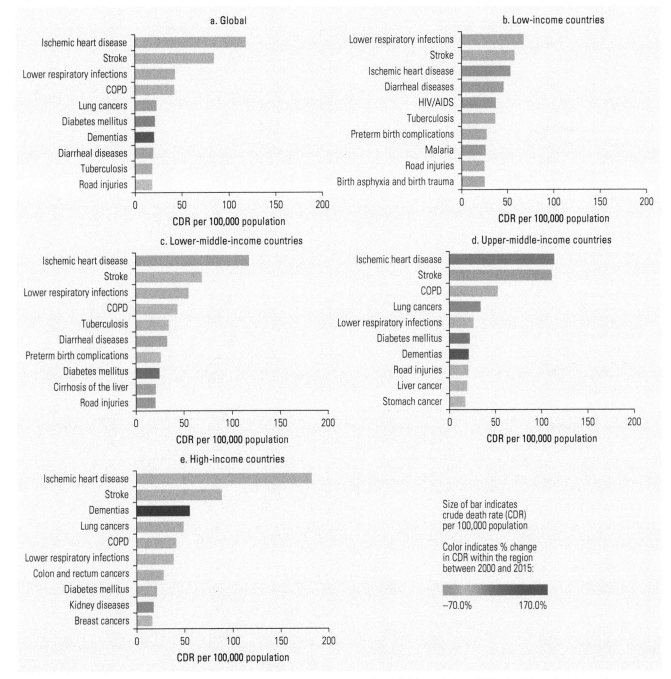

Note: The colors of the bars indicate causes for which overall death rates are increasing (red) or decreasing (green). CDR = crude death rate; COPD = chronic obstructive pulmonary disease; HIV/AIDS = human immunodeficiency virus/acquired immune deficiency syndrome.

disease was still among the top 10 causes of death in 2015, with a death toll of 1.4 million. HIV/AIDS dropped out of the top 10 causes of death globally, falling from 1.5 million deaths in 2000 to just under 1.1 million in 2015. However, it remains the fifth-leading cause of death in LICs.

Cause-Specific Trends from 2000 to 2015

Tables 4.1 to 4.10 provide summary tabulations of deaths by cause, age, and sex for the world and for country income groups for 2000 and 2015. More detailed results at the country and regional levels are also available on the WHO website (see box 4.1).

Table 4.1 Deaths from Selected Causes in the World, by Age and Sex, 2015

thousands

Sex Age group	Both sexes Total	Male Total	Female Total	Both sexes					
				0–4 yrs.	5–14 yrs.	15–29 yrs.	30–49 yrs.	50–69 yrs.	70+ yrs.
Population (millions)	*7,344*	*3,705*	*3,639*	*671*	*1,244*	*1,802*	*1,987*	*1,248*	*393*
All causes	56,441	30,177	26,264	5,992	1,303	2,687	5,780	14,628	26,051
I. Communicable, maternal, perinatal, and nutritional conditions	11,959	6,317	5,642	4,843	638	792	1,525	1,620	2,540
A. Infectious and parasitic diseases	5,706	3,195	2,512	1,452	463	513	1,202	1,115	961
1. Tuberculosis[a]	1,373	927	446	69	28	87	328	513	348
3. HIV/AIDS	1,060	617	443	87	46	134	602	178	13
4. Diarrheal diseases	1,389	684	705	526	103	90	95	207	368
5. Vaccine-preventable diseases[b]	273	139	134	207	34	10	8	9	5
6. Meningitis and encephalitis	405	209	196	116	91	69	44	47	37
7. Acute hepatitis[c]	145	77	68	8	14	24	32	41	28
8. Malaria	439	228	211	312	31	27	29	22	18
9. Other infectious and parasitic diseases	623	314	309	129	116	71	65	97	145
B. Respiratory infections	3,913	2,122	1,791	36	14	36	122	989	2,716
C. Maternal conditions	303	—	303	—	—	155	148	—	—
D. Neonatal conditions	2,311	1,292	1,019	2,311	—	—	—	—	—
1. Preterm birth complications	1,058	586	472	1,058	—	—	—	—	—
2. Birth asphyxia and birth trauma	691	386	305	691	—	—	—	—	—
3. Neonatal sepsis and infections	405	240	166	405	—	—	—	—	—
4. Other neonatal conditions	157	81	76	157	—	—	—	—	—
E. Nutritional deficiencies	439	215	224	160	35	23	26	60	135
II. Noncommunicable diseases	39,544	20,541	19,003	783	312	778	3,049	12,001	22,622
A. Malignant neoplasms	8,763	4,982	3,781	37	49	152	947	3,498	4,080
3. Stomach cancer	754	490	263	—	—	5	64	300	384
4. Colon and rectum cancers	774	418	356	1	1	7	61	267	438
5. Liver cancer	788	554	235	—	2	11	112	347	315
7. Lung cancer	1,695	1,174	521	1	—	4	95	724	870
9. Breast cancer	571	1	570	—	—	8	131	247	185
Other cancers	4,182	2,345	1,836	36	46	117	484	1,611	1,889
C. Diabetes mellitus	1,586	729	856	2	4	18	101	582	879
E. Mental and behavioral disorders	317	233	84	—	—	49	115	109	44
4. Alcohol use disorders[d]	129	108	21	—	—	9	46	59	15
5. Drug use disorders[e]	168	117	51	—	—	39	63	43	23

table continues next page

Table 4.1 Deaths from Selected Causes in the World, by Age and Sex, 2015 (continued)

Sex Age group	Both sexes Total	Male Total	Female Total	Both sexes					
				0–4 yrs.	5–14 yrs.	15–29 yrs.	30–49 yrs.	50–69 yrs.	70+ yrs.
F. Neurological conditions	2,011	812	1,199	17	29	60	66	209	1,629
1. Alzheimer's disease and other dementias	1,542	557	985	—	—	—	2	109	1,432
H. Cardiovascular diseases	17,689	8,850	8,839	39	37	194	1,072	5,136	11,210
3. Ischemic heart disease	8,756	4,603	4,153	2	2	62	528	2,586	5,576
4. Stroke	6,241	2,990	3,250	12	15	57	314	1,845	3,997
I. Respiratory diseases	3,913	2,122	1,791	36	14	36	122	989	2,716
J. Digestive diseases	2,347	1,355	991	27	47	119	386	853	914
2. Cirrhosis of the liver	1,162	762	400	8	20	59	258	517	301
K. Genitourinary diseases	1,382	701	681	18	17	55	134	407	751
1. Kidney diseases	1,129	580	549	12	14	44	113	349	598
N. Congenital anomalies	647	340	307	509	58	34	20	16	10
Other noncommunicable diseases[f]	888	415	473	96	56	62	87	201	388
III. Injuries	4,939	3,319	1,619	366	352	1,118	1,206	1,007	889
A. Unintentional injuries	3,527	2,322	1,204	344	304	646	749	731	752
1. Road traffic injury	1,342	1,014	328	73	70	353	400	307	140
2. Other unintentional injuries	2,184	1,308	877	271	234	293	349	425	612
B. Intentional injuries	1,412	997	415	22	48	472	457	276	137
1. Suicide	788	504	284	—	13	221	241	200	114
2. Homicide and collective violence	624	493	131	22	35	251	216	76	23

Note: — = fewer than 500 deaths are attributable to a specific cause; HIV/AIDS = human immunodeficiency virus/acquired immune deficiency syndrome.

a. Tuberculosis deaths in HIV-negative people. Tuberculosis deaths in HIV-positive people are included in the HIV/AIDS category.

b. Pertussis, diphtheria, measles, and tetanus are included here.

c. Liver cancer and cirrhosis deaths resulting from past hepatitis infection are not included here.

d. Only direct deaths because of alcohol intoxication are included.

e. Only direct deaths because of drug overdose or adverse reaction for licit and illicit drugs are included.

f. Benign neoplasms; endocrine, blood, and immune disorders; sense organ diseases; skin diseases; musculoskeletal diseases; oral conditions; and sudden infant death syndrome are included.

Table 4.2 Deaths from Selected Causes in Low-Income Countries, by Age and Sex, 2015
thousands

Sex Age group	Both sexes Total	Male Total	Female Total	Both sexes					
				0–4 yrs.	5–14 yrs.	15–29 yrs.	30–49 yrs.	50–69 yrs.	70+ yrs.
Population (millions)	*896*	*446*	*449*	*128*	*223*	*249*	*193*	*83*	*20*
All causes	6,997	3,712	3,285	1,902	460	652	945	1,362	1,676
I. Communicable, maternal, perinatal, and nutritional conditions	3,248	1,706	1,542	1,588	265	283	427	334	349
A. Infectious and parasitic diseases	1,730	948	782	569	195	178	329	256	203
1. Tuberculosis[a]	326	222	104	25	10	16	66	119	90
3. HIV/AIDS	334	179	155	35	22	46	177	49	4
4. Diarrheal diseases	413	214	199	177	42	37	32	47	77
5. Vaccine-preventable diseases[b]	103	52	52	78	14	5	3	2	1
6. Meningitis and encephalitis	142	76	66	47	36	27	14	11	8
7. Acute hepatitis[c]	18	10	8	1	2	4	4	4	3
8. Malaria	225	115	110	155	19	17	16	10	9
9. Other infectious and parasitic diseases	171	82	88	51	51	26	17	14	12
B. Respiratory infections	291	155	136	8	5	10	18	85	165
C. Maternal conditions	117	—	117	—	—	61	56	—	—
D. Neonatal conditions	632	359	273	632	—	—	—	—	—
1. Preterm birth complications	242	136	106	242	—	—	—	—	—
2. Birth asphyxia and birth trauma	223	124	99	223	—	—	—	—	—
3. Neonatal sepsis and infections	130	80	50	130	—	—	—	—	—
4. Other neonatal conditions	36	19	17	36	—	—	—	—	—
E. Nutritional deficiencies	160	89	71	80	19	12	9	14	25
II. Noncommunicable diseases	3,014	1,517	1,497	192	90	174	377	932	1,249
A. Malignant neoplasms	549	268	281	8	9	28	124	235	144
3. Stomach cancer	31	18	13	—	—	1	6	15	9
4. Colon and rectum cancers	27	14	13	—	—	1	6	12	8
5. Liver cancer	35	22	13	—	—	2	9	17	7
7. Lung cancer	46	28	17	—	—	—	5	22	17
9. Breast cancer	43	—	43	—	—	2	18	18	6
Other cancers	367	185	183	8	8	23	81	151	97
C. Diabetes mellitus	138	70	68	—	1	4	13	47	73
E. Mental and behavioral disorders	18	14	5	—	—	4	7	5	3
4. Alcohol use disorders[d]	9	8	1	—	—	2	4	3	1
5. Drug use disorders[e]	8	5	3	—	—	3	3	1	2

table continues next page

Table 4.2 Deaths from Selected Causes in Low-Income Countries, by Age and Sex, 2015 (continued)

| Sex
Age group | Both sexes
Total | Male
Total | Female
Total | Both sexes | | | | | |
				0–4 yrs.	5–14 yrs.	15–29 yrs.	30–49 yrs.	50–69 yrs.	70+ yrs.
F. Neurological conditions	116	54	62	6	6	18	10	12	65
1. Alzheimer's disease and other dementias	66	25	42	—	—	—	—	6	60
H. Cardiovascular diseases	1,229	581	648	9	12	39	113	404	653
3. Ischemic heart diseases	474	248	226	—	1	9	43	162	258
4. Stroke	521	236	285	3	4	14	42	174	284
I. Respiratory diseases	291	155	136	8	5	10	18	85	165
J. Digestive diseases	285	170	114	8	13	26	59	96	82
2. Cirrhosis of the liver	146	92	53	2	4	12	36	58	34
K. Genitourinary diseases	107	54	53	5	5	13	15	29	41
1. Kidney diseases	77	39	38	3	4	10	10	21	29
N. Congenital anomalies	156	83	73	119	21	10	4	2	1
Other noncommunicable diseases[f]	124	68	57	30	19	20	15	17	23
III. Injuries	735	489	246	121	105	195	141	95	77
A. Unintentional injuries	583	381	202	115	96	132	96	76	68
1. Road traffic injury	224	158	66	28	21	67	50	36	22
2. Other unintentional injuries	360	223	136	87	76	65	46	40	45
B. Intentional injuries	151	108	43	6	9	63	45	19	10
1. Suicide	66	44	22	—	3	25	18	12	8
2. Homicide and collective violence	85	64	21	6	6	38	26	7	2

Note: — = fewer than 500 deaths are attributable to a specific cause; HIV/AIDS = human immunodeficiency virus/acquired immune deficiency syndrome.

a. Tuberculosis deaths in HIV-negative people. Tuberculosis deaths in HIV-positive people are included in the HIV/AIDS category.

b. Pertussis, diphtheria, measles, and tetanus are included here.

c. Liver cancer and cirrhosis deaths resulting from past hepatitis infection are not included here.

d. Only direct deaths because of alcohol intoxication are included.

e. Only direct deaths because of drug overdose or adverse reaction for licit and illicit drugs are included.

f. Benign neoplasms; endocrine, blood, and immune disorders; sense organ diseases; skin diseases; musculoskeletal diseases; oral conditions; and sudden infant death syndrome are included.

Table 4.3 Deaths from Selected Causes, in Lower-Middle-Income Countries, by Age and Sex, 2015

thousands

Sex Age group	Both sexes Total	Male Total	Female Total	Both sexes					
				0–4 yrs.	5–14 yrs.	15–29 yrs.	30–49 yrs.	50–69 yrs.	70+ yrs.
Population (millions)	*2,669*	*1,361*	*1,307*	*290*	*538*	*717*	*682*	*355*	*87*
All causes	20,422	11,064	9,358	3,308	665	1,317	2,646	5,606	6,880
I. Communicable, maternal, perinatal, and nutritional conditions	6,323	3,339	2,984	2,745	328	420	781	902	1,146
A. Infectious and parasitic diseases	3,143	1,767	1,376	785	238	277	624	663	556
1. Tuberculosis[a]	905	604	301	40	16	63	227	343	218
3. HIV/AIDS	425	252	173	44	17	55	243	62	4
4. Diarrheal diseases	858	413	445	303	56	50	58	147	243
5. Vaccine-preventable diseases[b]	160	82	78	120	20	5	4	6	3
6–7. Meningitis and encephalitis	217	109	107	59	49	37	24	27	20
8. Acute hepatitis[c]	107	55	52	6	11	18	25	28	19
9a. Malaria	199	106	93	146	11	10	12	12	9
Other infectious and parasitic diseases	273	146	126	67	57	39	32	39	40
B. Respiratory infections	1,437	779	658	24	7	17	63	465	862
C. Maternal conditions	165	—	165	—	—	84	81	—	—
D. Neonatal conditions	1,381	766	615	1,381	—	—	—	—	—
1. Preterm birth complications	669	367	302	669	—	—	—	—	—
2. Birth asphyxia and birth trauma	385	216	169	385	—	—	—	—	—
3. Neonatal sepsis and infections	237	137	99	237	—	—	—	—	—
4. Other neonatal conditions	91	46	45	91	—	—	—	—	—
E. Nutritional deficiencies	188	85	104	63	13	9	13	36	54
II. Noncommunicable diseases	12,065	6,383	5,681	389	160	385	1,366	4,330	5,435
A. Malignant neoplasms	1,768	916	852	14	21	62	337	831	503
3. Stomach cancer	116	75	41	—	—	2	21	58	36
4. Colon and rectum cancers	125	69	56	—	—	4	22	56	44
5. Liver cancer	140	94	46	—	1	4	26	69	40
7. Lung cancer	199	147	52	—	—	2	24	110	63
9. Breast cancer	181		180	—	—	4	60	84	32
Other cancers	1,006	530	476	14	19	45	185	455	288
C. Diabetes mellitus	643	292	351	1	2	8	48	263	321
E. Mental and behavioral disorders	76	59	17	—	—	19	28	21	8
4. Alcohol use disorders[d]	26	22	4	—	—	3	10	9	3
5. Drug use disorders[e]	47	36	11	—	—	15	16	11	4

table continues next page

Table 4.3 Deaths from Selected Causes, in Lower-Middle-Income Countries, by Age and Sex, 2015 (continued)

Sex Age group	Both sexes Total	Male Total	Female Total	Both sexes					
				0–4 yrs.	5–14 yrs.	15–29 yrs.	30–49 yrs.	50–69 yrs.	70+ yrs.
F. Neurological conditions	374	169	206	7	16	26	26	52	248
1. Alzheimer's disease and other dementias	261	107	154	—	—	—	1	28	232
H. Cardiovascular diseases	5,640	2,992	2,649	17	18	103	537	2,068	2,897
3. Ischemic heart disease	3,117	1,749	1,368	2	1	35	292	1,162	1,625
4. Stroke	1,813	894	919	6	8	28	142	660	968
I. Respiratory diseases	1,437	779	658	24	7	17	63	465	862
J. Digestive diseases	1,008	589	418	15	31	80	214	369	299
2. Cirrhosis of the liver	545	362	183	6	15	42	147	220	115
K. Genitourinary diseases	538	305	232	9	10	32	78	196	213
1. Kidney diseases	455	259	197	7	8	25	67	172	177
N. Congenital anomalies	310	161	149	257	27	14	6	4	2
Other noncommunicable diseases[f]	270	121	149	45	29	26	28	60	83
III. Injuries	2,034	1,341	693	174	176	512	500	374	298
A. Unintentional injuries	1,479	962	517	163	152	295	314	289	268
1. Road traffic injury	517	404	113	29	31	147	159	109	43
2. Other unintentional injuries	962	558	404	134	121	148	155	180	225
B. Intentional injuries	554	379	176	11	25	218	186	85	30
1. Suicide	298	183	115	—	7	123	99	50	19
2. Homicide and collective violence	257	196	61	11	18	95	87	35	12

Note: — = fewer than 500 deaths are attributable to a specific cause; HIV/AIDS = human immunodeficiency virus/acquired immune deficiency syndrome.

a. Tuberculosis deaths in HIV-negative people. Tuberculosis deaths in HIV-positive people are included in the HIV/AIDS category.

b. Pertussis, diphtheria, measles, and tetanus are included here.

c. Liver cancer and cirrhosis deaths resulting from past hepatitis infection are not included here.

d. Only direct deaths because of alcohol intoxication are included.

e. Only direct deaths because of drug overdose or adverse reaction for licit and illicit drugs are included.

f. Benign neoplasms; endocrine, blood, and immune disorders; sense organ diseases; skin diseases; musculoskeletal diseases; oral conditions; and sudden infant death syndrome are included.

Table 4.4 Deaths from Selected Causes in Upper-Middle-Income Countries, by Age and Sex, 2015

thousands

Sex Age group	Both sexes Total	Male Total	Female Total	Both sexes					
				0–4 yrs.	5–14 yrs.	15–29 yrs.	30–49 yrs.	50–69 yrs.	70+ yrs.
Population (millions)	*2,473*	*1,252*	*1,221*	*179*	*337*	*590*	*747*	*486*	*134*
All causes	17,124	9,343	7,781	693	156	555	1,531	4,963	9,227
I. Communicable, maternal, perinatal, and nutritional conditions	1,606	863	743	465	43	75	248	266	510
A. Infectious and parasitic diseases	617	356	262	95	29	51	204	145	94
1. Tuberculosis[a]	110	77	33	4	2	6	25	43	30
3. HIV/AIDS	248	146	103	7	7	29	151	51	4
4. Diarrheal diseases	84	44	40	45	4	3	5	9	18
5. Vaccine-preventable diseases[b]	10	5	5	8	1	—	—	—	—
6–7. Meningitis and encephalitis	36	19	17	8	6	4	5	7	5
8. Acute hepatitis[c]	15	9	6	—	—	1	3	6	4
9a. Malaria	15	8	8	11	1	1	1	1	1
Other infectious and parasitic diseases	98	48	51	11	7	6	13	29	32
B. Respiratory infections	1,430	781	649	4	2	7	30	314	1,073
C. Maternal conditions	20	—	20	—	—	10	10	—	—
D. Neonatal conditions	261	146	115	261	—	—	—	—	—
1. Preterm birth complications	125	70	54	125	—	—	—	—	—
2. Birth asphyxia and birth trauma	77	42	35	77	—	—	—	—	—
3. Neonatal sepsis and infections	36	21	15	36	—	—	—	—	—
4. Other neonatal conditions	24	13	11	24	—	—	—	—	—
E. Nutritional deficiencies	66	33	33	17	2	2	3	8	34
II. Noncommunicable diseases	14,066	7,476	6,590	164	51	160	887	4,348	8,455
A. Malignant neoplasms	3,474	2,153	1,322	12	16	48	351	1,416	1,631
3. Stomach cancer	417	281	136	—	—	2	28	169	218
4. Colon and rectum cancers	256	143	113	—	—	2	20	90	144
5. Liver cancer	464	339	125	—	1	5	71	206	181
7. Lung cancer	817	580	236	—	—	2	48	338	428
9. Breast cancer	138	—	138	—	—	1	33	64	39
Other cancers	1,383	809	574	12	15	37	150	549	621
C. Diabetes mellitus	532	234	298	—	1	4	31	206	290
E. Mental and behavioral disorders	90	62	28	—	—	10	27	33	20
4. Alcohol use disorders[d]	35	31	4	—	—	2	12	16	5
5. Drug use disorders[e]	43	26	17	—	—	7	12	12	12

table continues next page

Table 4.4 Deaths from Selected Causes in Upper-Middle-Income Countries, by Age and Sex, 2015 (continued)

Sex Age group	Both sexes Total	Male Total	Female Total	Both sexes					
				0–4 yrs.	5–14 yrs.	15–29 yrs.	30–49 yrs.	50–69 yrs.	70+ yrs.
F. Neurological conditions	593	243	350	4	5	11	18	77	477
1. Alzheimer's disease and other dementias	497	190	306	—	—	—	1	51	445
H. Cardiovascular diseases	6,507	3,245	3,262	12	7	39	279	1,837	4,332
3. Ischemic heart disease	2,809	1,426	1,383	—	—	14	125	773	1,897
4. Stroke	2,756	1,380	1,377	3	2	12	103	823	1,813
I. Respiratory diseases	1,430	781	649	4	2	7	30	314	1,073
J. Digestive diseases	617	363	255	4	3	11	79	250	271
2. Cirrhosis of the liver	309	201	108	1	1	5	51	153	99
K. Genitourinary diseases	447	212	235	3	2	10	35	138	259
1. Kidney diseases	375	180	195	2	2	8	30	121	212
N. Congenital anomalies	138	73	65	109	9	7	6	4	3
Other noncommunicable diseases[f]	237	111	126	15	7	13	31	72	99
III. Injuries	1,452	1,005	448	63	62	320	396	349	261
A. Unintentional injuries	988	678	311	59	50	172	252	250	205
1. Road traffic injury	483	367	117	14	16	113	156	130	54
2. Other unintentional injuries	505	311	194	45	34	59	95	121	151
B. Intentional injuries	464	327	137	4	12	148	144	99	56
1. Suicide	228	129	98	—	2	41	60	74	50
2. Homicide and collective violence	236	198	38	4	10	106	84	25	6

Note: — = fewer than 500 deaths are attributable to a specific cause; HIV/AIDS = human immunodeficiency virus/acquired immune deficiency syndrome.

a. Tuberculosis deaths in HIV-negative people. Tuberculosis deaths in HIV-positive people are included in the HIV/AIDS category.

b. Pertussis, diphtheria, measles, and tetanus are included here.

c. Liver cancer and cirrhosis deaths resulting from past hepatitis infection are not included here.

d. Only direct deaths because of alcohol intoxication are included.

e. Only direct deaths because of drug overdose or adverse reaction for licit and illicit drugs are included.

f. Benign neoplasms; endocrine, blood, and immune disorders; sense organ diseases; skin diseases; musculoskeletal diseases; oral conditions; and sudden infant death syndrome are included.

Table 4.5 Deaths from Selected Causes in High-Income Countries, by Age and Sex, 2015

thousands

Sex Age group	Both sexes Total	Male Total	Female Total	Both sexes					
				0–4 yrs.	5–14 yrs.	15–29 yrs.	30–49 yrs.	50–69 yrs.	70+ yrs.
Population (millions)	*1,307*	*645*	*662*	*74*	*146*	*247*	*365*	*324*	*152*
All causes	11,899	6,058	5,841	90	22	164	658	2,698	8,269
I. Communicable, maternal, perinatal, and nutritional conditions	781	409	373	45	2	13	69	118	534
A. Infectious and parasitic diseases	216	124	92	4	1	7	46	51	107
1. Tuberculosis[a]	31	23	8	—	—	2	10	9	11
3. HIV/AIDS	53	41	12	—	—	4	31	17	1
4. Diarrheal diseases	34	13	21	1	—	—	1	4	29
5. Vaccine-preventable diseases[b]	1	—	—	1	—	—	—	—	—
6–7. Meningitis and encephalitis	10	5	5	1	—	—	1	3	3
8. Acute hepatitis[c]	5	3	2	—	—	—	1	2	2
9a. Malaria	—	—	—	—	—	—	—	—	—
Other infectious and parasitic diseases	81	38	44	1	—	1	3	16	61
B. Respiratory infections	755	407	348	—	—	2	11	125	617
C. Maternal conditions	2	—	2	—	—	1	1	—	—
D. Neonatal conditions	37	21	16	37	—	—	—	—	—
1. Preterm birth complications	22	13	10	22	—	—	—	—	—
2. Birth asphyxia and birth trauma	6	3	3	6	—	—	—	—	—
3. Neonatal sepsis and infections	3	2	1	3	—	—	—	—	—
4. Other neonatal conditions	6	3	3	6	—	—	—	—	—
E. Nutritional deficiencies	25	10	15	—	—	—	—	2	21
II. Noncommunicable diseases	10,400	5,165	5,234	37	11	60	420	2,391	7,482
A. Malignant neoplasms	2,972	1,646	1,326	3	4	14	134	1,015	1,803
3. Stomach cancer	189	116	73	—	—	—	9	59	121
4. Colon and rectum cancers	365	192	174	—	—	1	13	109	243
5. Liver cancer	149	98	51	—	—	—	6	56	87
7. Lung cancer	633	418	215	—	—	—	18	253	362
9. Breast cancer	209	1	208	—	—	—	20	81	108
Other cancers	1,426	821	605	2	4	12	68	457	883
C. Diabetes mellitus	273	133	140	—	—	1	10	66	195
E. Mental and behavioral disorders	133	99	34	—	—	16	52	51	14
4. Alcohol use disorders[d]	58	47	12	—	—	2	19	31	6
5. Drug use disorders[e]	70	50	20	—	—	14	32	18	6

table continues next page

Table 4.5 Deaths from Selected Causes in High-Income Countries, by Age and Sex, 2015 (continued)

Sex / Age group	Both sexes Total	Male Total	Female Total	Both sexes 0–4 yrs.	5–14 yrs.	15–29 yrs.	30–49 yrs.	50–69 yrs.	70+ yrs.
F. Neurological conditions	927	347	581	1	2	5	13	68	839
1. Alzheimer's disease and other dementias	718	235	483	—	—	—	—	24	694
H. Cardiovascular diseases	4,313	2,032	2,281	1	1	13	142	827	3,328
3. Ischemic heart disease	2,356	1,180	1,176	—	—	3	67	489	1,796
4. Stroke	1,150	481	669	—	—	2	27	187	933
I. Respiratory diseases	755	407	348	—	—	2	11	125	617
J. Digestive diseases	437	233	204	—	—	2	34	138	262
2. Cirrhosis of the liver	162	107	55	—	—	1	23	85	53
K. Genitourinary diseases	290	130	160	—	—	1	7	44	238
1. Kidney diseases	222	103	119	—	—	1	6	35	180
N. Congenital anomalies	43	23	20	25	2	3	4	6	4
Other noncommunicable diseasesf	257	115	141	6	1	3	13	50	182
III. Injuries	718	484	234	8	8	90	169	189	253
A. Unintentional injuries	476	301	175	7	6	47	87	116	212
1. Road traffic injury	118	85	33	2	2	27	35	33	21
2. Other unintentional injuries	357	216	142	6	4	20	53	84	191
B. Intentional injuries	242	183	59	1	2	44	82	73	41
1. Suicide	196	148	48	—	1	31	63	63	38
2. Homicide and collective violence	46	35	11	1	1	13	18	10	3

Note: — = fewer than 500 deaths are attributable to a specific cause; HIV/AIDS = human immunodeficiency virus/acquired immune deficiency syndrome.

a. Tuberculosis deaths in HIV-negative people. Tuberculosis deaths in HIV-positive people are included in the HIV/AIDS category.

b. Pertussis, diphtheria, measles, and tetanus are included here.

c. Liver cancer and cirrhosis deaths resulting from past hepatitis infection are not included here.

d. Only direct deaths because of alcohol intoxication are included.

e. Only direct deaths because of drug overdose or adverse reaction for licit and illicit drugs are included.

f. Benign neoplasms; endocrine, blood, and immune disorders; sense organ diseases; skin diseases; musculoskeletal diseases; oral conditions; and sudden infant death syndrome are included.

Table 4.6 Deaths from Selected Causes in the World, by Age and Sex, 2000
thousands

Sex Age group	Both sexes Total	Male Total	Female Total	Both sexes					
				0–4 yrs.	5–14 yrs.	15–29 yrs.	30–49 yrs.	50–69 yrs.	70+ yrs.
Population (millions)	*6,122*	*3,082*	*3,040*	*606*	*1,241*	*1,587*	*1,609*	*813*	*266*
All causes	52,135	27,617	24,517	10,063	1,644	2,993	5,937	12,016	19,481
I. Communicable, maternal, perinatal, and nutritional conditions	16,160	8,384	7,776	8,715	901	1,053	1,879	1,617	1,995
A. Infectious and parasitic diseases	8,608	4,615	3,993	3,551	697	717	1,515	1,223	906
1. Tuberculosis[a]	1,667	1,108	559	100	50	133	425	590	369
3. HIV/AIDS	1,463	754	709	222	29	227	788	181	16
4. Diarrheal diseases	2,177	1,061	1,116	1,206	166	115	111	234	345
5. Vaccine-preventable diseases[b]	1,040	527	513	802	172	33	13	13	7
6–7. Meningitis and encephalitis	560	289	271	281	96	65	40	44	33
8. Acute hepatitis[c]	131	71	60	19	16	23	24	30	19
9a. Malaria	859	440	419	749	23	24	26	23	15
Other infectious and parasitic diseases	711	366	345	171	144	97	88	108	102
B. Respiratory infections	3,672	1,976	1,696	61	17	44	157	1,043	2,350
C. Maternal conditions	425	—	425	—	—	220	205	—	—
D. Neonatal conditions	3,232	1,817	1,415	3,232	—	—	—	—	—
1. Preterm birth complications	1,340	731	609	1,340	—	—	—	—	—
2. Birth asphyxia and birth trauma	1,120	637	483	1,120	—	—	—	—	—
3. Neonatal sepsis and infections	540	325	215	540	—	—	—	—	—
4. Other neonatal conditions	232	124	108	232	—	—	—	—	—
E. Nutritional deficiencies	475	234	241	207	43	27	28	53	117
II. Noncommunicable diseases	31,391	16,128	15,263	914	321	778	2,875	9,623	16,880
A. Malignant neoplasms	6,950	3,840	3,110	37	60	149	916	2,789	2,998
3. Stomach cancer	739	460	280	—	—	6	80	303	350
4. Colon and rectum cancers	578	292	285	—	1	6	51	202	318
5. Liver cancer	662	450	212	—	4	14	128	282	233
7. Lung cancer	1,255	886	370	1	—	5	101	556	592
9. Breast cancer	445	2	443	—	—	6	113	185	140
Other cancers	3,272	1,751	1,521	36	55	112	442	1,262	1,365
C. Diabetes mellitus	958	431	527	3	4	17	80	365	489
E. Mental and behavioral disorders	267	206	60	—	—	45	116	81	26
4. Alcohol use disorders[d]	143	119	24	—	—	11	64	56	12
5. Drug use disorders[e]	105	79	26	—	—	31	45	19	9

table continues next page

Sex Age group	Both sexes Total	Male Total	Female Total	Both sexes					
				0–4 yrs.	5–14 yrs.	15–29 yrs.	30–49 yrs.	50–69 yrs.	70+ yrs.
F. Neurological conditions	1,008	437	571	20	30	64	67	130	698
1. Alzheimer's disease and other dementias	654	243	411	—	—	—	1	64	589
H. Cardiovascular diseases	14,425	7,009	7,416	60	43	210	989	4,164	8,958
3. Ischemic heart disease	6,883	3,531	3,352	4	3	67	468	1,989	4,353
4. Stroke	5,407	2,479	2,927	21	17	63	304	1,590	3,412
I. Respiratory diseases	3,672	1,976	1,696	61	17	44	157	1,043	2,350
J. Digestive diseases	1,880	1,110	769	39	47	109	355	655	674
2. Cirrhosis of the liver	905	603	302	12	18	54	230	379	212
K. Genitourinary diseases	898	467	431	23	19	53	110	259	434
1. Kidney diseases	709	368	341	16	15	42	90	212	333
N. Congenital anomalies	687	355	331	575	50	29	16	9	7
Other noncommunicable diseases[f]	647	296	351	97	49	58	69	129	246
III. Injuries	4,583	3,105	1,478	434	422	1,163	1,183	775	606
A. Unintentional injuries	3,228	2,150	1,078	409	375	675	726	544	500
1. Road traffic injury	1,118	829	289	75	90	320	339	200	95
2. Other unintentional injuries	2,110	1,321	789	334	284	356	387	344	405
B. Intentional injuries	1,355	955	400	25	47	488	457	231	106
1. Suicide	748	479	269	—	15	240	245	162	87
2. Homicide and collective violence	607	476	131	25	32	248	212	70	20

Note: — = fewer than 500 deaths are attributable to a specific cause; HIV/AIDS = human immunodeficiency virus/acquired immune deficiency syndrome.

a. Tuberculosis deaths in HIV-negative people. Tuberculosis deaths in HIV-positive people are included in the HIV/AIDS category.

b. Pertussis, diphtheria, measles, and tetanus are included here.

c. Liver cancer and cirrhosis deaths resulting from past hepatitis infection are not included here.

d. Only direct deaths because of alcohol intoxication are included.

e. Only direct deaths because of drug overdose or adverse reaction for licit and illicit drugs are included.

f. Benign neoplasms; endocrine, blood, and immune disorders; sense organ diseases; skin diseases; musculoskeletal diseases; oral conditions; and sudden infant death syndrome are included.

Table 4.7 Deaths from Selected Causes in Low-Income Countries, by Age and Sex, 2000
thousands

Sex Age group	Both sexes Total	Male Total	Female Total	Both sexes					
				0–4 yrs.	5–14 yrs.	15–29 yrs.	30–49 yrs.	50–69 yrs.	70+ yrs.
Population (millions)	*636*	*317*	*319*	*101*	*166*	*176*	*125*	*55*	*12*
All causes	7,735	4,030	3,705	3,145	535	706	1,084	1,162	1,102
I. Communicable, maternal, perinatal, and nutritional conditions	4,998	2,554	2,444	2,856	343	383	689	401	326
A. Infectious and parasitic diseases	3,070	1,599	1,470	1,446	269	258	571	321	203
1. Tuberculosis[a]	380	252	128	34	15	24	86	129	92
3. HIV/AIDS	744	349	396	129	20	101	393	92	9
4. Diarrheal diseases	683	352	330	409	59	44	36	57	78
5. Vaccine-preventable diseases[b]	359	182	177	281	60	11	4	3	1
6–7. Meningitis and encephalitis	200	108	93	120	33	23	11	9	5
8. Acute hepatitis[c]	17	9	8	1	2	5	4	3	2
9a. Malaria	474	241	233	426	12	12	12	7	6
Other infectious and parasitic diseases	212	107	106	47	69	39	25	21	11
B. Respiratory infections	212	111	101	11	6	9	17	72	97
C. Maternal conditions	158	—	158	—	—	82	77	—	—
D. Neonatal conditions	797	451	346	797	—	—	—	—	—
1. Preterm birth complications	306	170	135	306	—	—	—	—	—
2. Birth asphyxia and birth trauma	297	165	132	297	—	—	—	—	—
3. Neonatal sepsis and infections	151	92	59	151	—	—	—	—	—
4. Other neonatal conditions	43	23	20	43	—	—	—	—	—
E. Nutritional deficiencies	202	109	93	86	25	15	14	25	36
II. Noncommunicable diseases	2,087	1,036	1,051	175	79	137	276	691	729
A. Malignant neoplasms	389	177	212	6	7	19	83	183	91
3. Stomach cancer	26	15	11	—	—	1	5	13	7
4. Colon and rectum cancers	18	9	9	—	—	1	4	9	4
5. Liver cancer	26	16	10	—	—	1	6	13	5
7. Lung cancer	28	17	11	—	—	—	3	16	9
9. Breast cancer	29	—	29	—	—	1	12	12	3
Other cancers	262	121	141	6	6	15	54	119	62
C. Diabetes mellitus	70	37	33	—	1	3	8	28	29
E. Mental and behavioral disorders	11	9	2	—	—	3	5	3	1
4. Alcohol use disorders[d]	7	6	1	—	—	2	3	2	1
5. Drug use disorders[e]	4	3	1	—	—	1	1	—	—

table continues next page

Table 4.7 Deaths from Selected Causes in Low-Income Countries, by Age and Sex, 2000 (continued)

Sex Age group	Both sexes Total	Male Total	Female Total	Both sexes					
				0–4 yrs.	5–14 yrs.	15–29 yrs.	30–49 yrs.	50–69 yrs.	70+ yrs.
F. Neurological conditions	79	40	40	6	5	14	7	8	38
1. Alzheimer's disease and other dementias	39	15	24	—	—	—	—	4	35
H. Cardiovascular diseases	803	369	433	9	11	32	83	286	380
3. Ischemic heart diseases	275	142	133	—	1	8	29	102	136
4. Stroke	356	155	201	3	4	11	32	132	174
I. Respiratory diseases	212	111	101	11	6	9	17	72	97
J. Digestive diseases	235	139	96	10	14	25	50	79	57
2. Cirrhosis of the liver	108	66	42	2	4	10	29	42	21
K. Genitourinary diseases	71	38	34	6	5	10	11	19	22
1. Kidney diseases	50	26	24	4	4	8	7	13	14
N. Congenital anomalies	126	66	61	100	15	7	3	1	1
Other noncommunicable diseases[f]	90	51	39	27	16	14	10	12	12
III. Injuries	650	440	210	113	113	186	119	70	48
A. Unintentional injuries	472	311	161	106	96	106	70	52	42
1. Road traffic injury	148	105	43	17	19	47	32	20	11
2. Other unintentional injuries	324	206	118	89	77	59	37	31	30
B. Intentional injuries	178	129	50	7	17	80	50	18	6
1. Suicide	52	34	18	—	3	22	14	9	4
2. Homicide and collective violence	127	95	32	7	14	58	36	9	2

Note: — = fewer than 500 deaths are attributable to a specific cause; HIV/AIDS = human immunodeficiency virus/acquired immune deficiency syndrome.

a. Tuberculosis deaths in HIV-negative people. Tuberculosis deaths in HIV-positive people are included in the HIV/AIDS category.

b. Pertussis, diphtheria, measles, and tetanus are included here.

c. Liver cancer and cirrhosis deaths resulting from past hepatitis infection are not included here.

d. Only direct deaths because of alcohol intoxication are included.

e. Only direct deaths because of drug overdose or adverse reaction for licit and illicit drugs are included.

f. Benign neoplasms; endocrine, blood, and immune disorders; sense organ diseases; skin diseases; musculoskeletal diseases; oral conditions; and sudden infant death syndrome are included.

Table 4.8 Deaths from Selected Causes in Lower-Middle-Income Countries, by Age and Sex, 2000

thousands

Sex Age group	Both sexes Total	Male Total	Female Total	Both sexes					
				0–4 yrs.	5–14 yrs.	15–29 yrs.	30–49 yrs.	50–69 yrs.	70+ yrs.
Population (millions)	*2,103*	*1,072*	*1,032*	*261*	*488*	*582*	*491*	*224*	*57*
All causes	19,067	10,121	8,946	5,414	829	1,352	2,283	4,339	4,850
I. Communicable, maternal, perinatal, and nutritional conditions	8,403	4,329	4,074	4,803	492	521	804	887	897
A. Infectious and parasitic diseases	4,474	2,395	2,079	1,863	381	345	628	709	548
1. Tuberculosis[a]	1,042	684	358	54	28	91	265	381	224
3. HIV/AIDS	383	204	179	59	7	60	203	50	4
4. Diarrheal diseases	1,335	627	708	689	101	67	68	166	243
5. Vaccine-preventable diseases[b]	650	329	321	501	106	21	8	9	5
6–7. Meningitis and encephalitis	294	147	147	134	54	36	22	27	21
8. Acute hepatitis[c]	82	42	40	16	13	16	13	14	9
9a. Malaria	359	187	173	302	10	12	13	15	9
Other infectious and parasitic diseases	329	176	153	107	62	43	37	46	33
B. Respiratory infections	1,272	711	561	41	7	21	80	489	634
C. Maternal conditions	236	—	236	—	—	123	112	—	—
D. Neonatal conditions	1,887	1,052	835	1,887	—	—	—	—	—
1. Preterm birth complications	774	412	361	774	—	—	—	—	—
2. Birth asphyxia and birth trauma	639	367	272	638	—	—	—	—	—
3. Neonatal sepsis and infections	332	199	133	332	—	—	—	—	—
4. Other neonatal conditions	142	74	69	142	—	—	—	—	—
E. Nutritional deficiencies	182	83	99	95	15	9	9	18	36
II. Noncommunicable diseases	8,945	4,683	4,262	419	150	368	1,087	3,184	3,738
A. Malignant neoplasms	1,259	617	642	11	20	51	266	578	333
3. Stomach cancer	102	64	39	—	—	2	20	50	30
4. Colon and rectum cancers	77	40	37	—	—	2	14	34	26
5. Liver cancer	105	67	39	—	1	4	23	48	29
7. Lung cancer	131	97	34	—	—	1	18	72	39
9. Breast cancer	123	—	123	—	—	3	44	55	20
Other cancers	721	349	371	11	19	37	147	319	189
C. Diabetes mellitus	326	151	175	1	2	8	35	141	139
E. Mental and behavioral disorders	54	42	11	—	—	14	21	14	5
4. Alcohol use disorders[d]	23	20	3	—	—	3	10	8	2
5. Drug use disorders[e]	27	21	6	—	—	10	10	5	2

table continues next page

Table 4.8 Deaths from Selected Causes in Lower-Middle-Income Countries, by Age and Sex, 2000 (continued)

Sex Age group	Both sexes Total	Male Total	Female Total	Both sexes					
				0–4 yrs.	5–14 yrs.	15–29 yrs.	30–49 yrs.	50–69 yrs.	70+ yrs.
F. Neurological conditions	254	122	132	6	16	33	32	42	124
1. Alzheimer's diseases and other dementias	136	56	79	—	—	—	1	23	112
H. Cardiovascular diseases	4,147	2,123	2,023	24	19	108	400	1,485	2,111
3. Ischemic heart diseases	2,185	1,190	994	3	1	37	210	786	1,148
4. Stroke	1,441	683	758	10	8	30	111	525	757
I. Respiratory diseases	1,272	711	561	41	7	21	80	489	634
J. Digestive diseases	755	461	294	24	27	66	167	266	205
2. Cirrhosis of the liver	385	261	124	9	13	36	106	145	76
K. Genitourinary diseases	361	208	154	11	11	29	57	121	132
1. Kidney diseases	279	157	122	8	8	23	46	96	98
N. Congenital anomalies	300	151	149	257	22	11	6	2	1
Other noncommunicable diseases[f]	218	98	120	44	24	26	25	45	54
III. Injuries	1,719	1,109	610	192	187	463	393	268	215
A. Unintentional injuries	1,268	808	460	182	171	271	247	203	193
1. Road traffic injury	342	263	79	29	34	101	94	59	26
2. Other unintentional injuries	926	544	381	153	138	170	153	145	168
B. Intentional injuries	451	301	149	10	16	193	146	65	21
1. Suicide	270	165	106	—	7	125	86	40	13
2. Homicide and collective violence	180	137	43	10	9	68	60	25	8

Note: — = fewer than 500 deaths are attributable to a specific cause; HIV/AIDS = human immunodeficiency virus/acquired immune deficiency syndrome.

a. Tuberculosis deaths in HIV-negative people. Tuberculosis deaths in HIV-positive people are included in the HIV/AIDS category.

b. Pertussis, diphtheria, measles, and tetanus are included here.

c. Liver cancer and cirrhosis deaths resulting from past hepatitis infection are not included here.

d. Only direct deaths because of alcohol intoxication are included.

e. Only direct deaths because of drug overdose or adverse reaction for licit and illicit drugs are included.

f. Benign neoplasms; endocrine, blood, and immune disorders; sense organ diseases; skin diseases; musculoskeletal diseases; oral conditions; and sudden infant death syndrome are included.

Table 4.9 Deaths from Selected Causes in Upper-Middle-Income Countries, by Age and Sex, 2000

thousands

Sex Age group	Both sexes Total	Male Total	Female Total	Both sexes					
				0–4 yrs.	5–14 yrs.	15–29 yrs.	30–49 yrs.	50–69 yrs.	70+ yrs.
Population (millions)	*2,184*	*1,106*	*1,078*	*173*	*428*	*575*	*634*	*290*	*84*
All causes	14,130	7,751	6,380	1,369	244	695	1,668	3,828	6,326
I. Communicable, maternal, perinatal, and nutritional conditions	2,053	1,129	924	983	63	134	309	229	334
A. Infectious and parasitic diseases	892	512	380	234	45	104	264	151	94
1. Tuberculosis[a]	193	130	62	12	7	15	55	64	40
3. HIV/AIDS	302	175	126	33	2	63	168	32	3
4. Diarrheal diseases	150	78	72	106	6	4	6	10	17
5. Vaccine-preventable diseases[b]	30	16	14	20	6	1	1	1	1
6–7. Meningitis and encephalitis	53	27	26	25	8	5	6	5	4
8. Acute hepatitis[c]	24	15	9	1	1	2	6	9	5
9a. Malaria	25	12	13	21	1	1	1	1	1
Other infectious and parasitic diseases	117	59	58	16	13	13	22	29	24
B. Respiratory infections	1,548	800	748	9	3	11	45	362	1,117
C. Maternal conditions	29	—	29	—	—	14	15	—	—
D. Neonatal conditions	493	283	211	493	—	—	—	—	—
1. Preterm birth complications	227	129	98	227	—	—	—	—	—
2. Birth asphyxia and birth trauma	175	100	75	175	—	—	—	—	—
3. Neonatal sepsis and infections	51	30	21	51	—	—	—	—	—
4. Other neonatal conditions	40	23	16	40	—	—	—	—	—
E. Nutritional deficiencies	72	35	36	26	3	3	4	8	28
II. Noncommunicable diseases	10,706	5,666	5,039	270	77	201	954	3,366	5,838
A. Malignant neoplasms	2,718	1,612	1,106	17	28	62	386	1,086	1,137
3. Stomach cancer	399	254	146	—	—	3	40	164	192
4. Colon and rectum cancers	164	82	81	—	—	2	18	57	86
5. Liver cancer	410	286	123	—	3	8	91	169	139
7. Lung cancer	543	380	163	—	—	3	52	232	256
9. Breast cancer	99	—	99	—	—	1	31	42	25
Other cancers	1,103	609	494	16	25	45	155	422	439
C. Diabetes mellitus	325	139	186	1	1	5	26	135	158
E. Mental and behavioral disorders	68	50	18	—	—	10	27	21	10
4. Alcohol use disorders[d]	31	27	4	—	—	2	13	12	3
5. Drug use disorders[e]	24	17	8	—	—	7	9	5	4

table continues next page

Table 4.9 Deaths from Selected Causes in Upper-Middle-Income Countries, by Age and Sex, 2000 (continued)

Sex Age group	Both sexes Total	Male Total	Female Total	Both sexes					
				0–4 yrs.	5–14 yrs.	15–29 yrs.	30–49 yrs.	50–69 yrs.	70+ yrs.
F. Neurological conditions	304	133	171	6	6	12	15	41	223
1. Alzheimer's disease and other dementias	233	94	139	—	—	—	—	26	207
H. Cardiovascular diseases	4,637	2,326	2,311	25	11	53	304	1,409	2,835
3. Ischemic heart diseases	1,717	898	819	1	1	17	124	523	1,052
4. Stroke	2,131	1,062	1,069	8	4	18	119	668	1,315
I. Respiratory diseases	1,548	800	748	9	3	11	45	362	1,117
J. Digestive diseases	494	299	194	5	5	15	91	191	186
2. Cirrhosis of the liver	259	173	86	1	1	7	62	118	69
K. Genitourinary diseases	260	129	131	6	3	12	34	83	123
1. Kidney diseases	224	111	113	4	3	10	29	74	104
N. Congenital anomalies	209	112	97	182	11	7	4	2	2
Other noncommunicable diseases[f]	143	67	77	18	8	13	22	36	47
III. Injuries	1,372	955	417	116	104	360	405	234	154
A. Unintentional injuries	933	651	282	109	93	204	256	159	111
1. Road traffic injury	452	334	118	26	32	121	158	82	33
2. Other unintentional injuries	481	317	164	83	61	83	99	77	78
B. Intentional injuries	439	304	135	7	11	155	149	74	42
1. Suicide	222	123	99	—	4	57	70	54	37
2. Homicide and collective violence	217	181	36	7	7	98	79	20	6

Note: — = fewer than 500 deaths are attributable to a specific cause; HIV/AIDS = human immunodeficiency virus/acquired immune deficiency syndrome.

a. Tuberculosis deaths in HIV-negative people. Tuberculosis deaths in HIV-positive people are included in the HIV/AIDS category.

b. Pertussis, diphtheria, measles, and tetanus are included here.

c. Liver cancer and cirrhosis deaths resulting from past hepatitis infection are not included here.

d. Only direct deaths because of alcohol intoxication are included.

e. Only direct deaths because of drug overdose or adverse reaction for licit and illicit drugs are included.

f. Benign neoplasms; endocrine, blood, and immune disorders; sense organ diseases; skin diseases; musculoskeletal diseases; oral conditions; and sudden infant death syndrome are included.

Table 4.10 Deaths from Selected Causes in High-Income Countries, by Age and Sex, 2000

thousands

Sex Age group	Both sexes Total	Male Total	Female Total	Both sexes					
				0–4 yrs.	5–14 yrs.	15–29 yrs.	30–49 yrs.	50–69 yrs.	70+ yrs.
Population (millions)	*1,200*	*588*	*612*	*70*	*158*	*255*	*360*	*244*	*113*
All causes	11,202	5,715	5,487	135	35	241	902	2,686	7,203
I. Communicable, maternal, perinatal, and nutritional conditions	706	371	335	73	3	15	78	100	438
A. Infectious and parasitic diseases	173	110	63	8	2	9	52	41	60
1. Tuberculosis[a]	52	42	11	1	—	4	20	15	13
3. HIV/AIDS	35	26	8	—	—	3	24	7	—
4. Diarrheal diseases	10	4	6	2	—	—	—	1	6
5. Vaccine-preventable diseases[b]	1	1	1	1	—	—	—	—	—
6–7. Meningitis and encephalitis	13	7	6	2	1	2	2	3	3
8. Acute hepatitis[c]	9	5	4	—	—	—	2	3	3
9a. Malaria	1	—	—	1	—	—	—	—	—
Other infectious and parasitic diseases	52	24	28	1	1	1	4	11	35
B. Respiratory infections	641	355	286	1	1	3	15	120	502
C. Maternal conditions	3	—	3	—	—	1	1	—	—
D. Neonatal conditions	55	32	23	55	—	—	—	—	—
1. Preterm birth complications	33	19	14	33	—	—	—	—	—
2. Birth asphyxia and birth trauma	10	6	4	10	—	—	—	—	—
3. Neonatal sepsis and infections	5	3	2	5	—	—	—	—	—
4. Other neonatal conditions	7	4	3	7	—	—	—	—	—
E. Nutritional deficiencies	20	7	13		—	—	1	2	17
II. Noncommunicable diseases	9,654	4,743	4,911	50	15	72	559	2,383	6,575
A. Malignant neoplasms	2,585	1,434	1,150	3	5	17	181	942	1,437
3. Stomach cancer	212	127	84	—	—	1	15	75	121
4. Colon and rectum cancers	319	161	158	—	—	1	15	101	202
5. Liver cancer	121	81	40	—	—	1	9	52	60
7. Lung cancer	554	392	162	—	—	—	29	236	288
9. Breast cancer	194	2	192	—	—	—	27	75	91
Other cancers	1,185	671	514	3	5	14	86	402	675
C. Diabetes mellitus	237	104	133	—	—	2	11	61	163
E. Mental and behavioral disorders	134	105	29	—	—	17	63	43	10
4. Alcohol use disorders[d]	81	65	16	—	—	4	38	34	6
5. Drug use disorders[e]	50	39	11	—	—	13	24	9	3

table continues next page

Table 4.10 Deaths from Selected Causes in High-Income Countries, by Age and Sex, 2000 (continued)

Sex Age group	Both sexes Total	Male Total	Female Total	Both sexes					
				0–4 yrs.	5–14 yrs.	15–29 yrs.	30–49 yrs.	50–69 yrs.	70+ yrs.
F. Neurological conditions	371	143	228	1	3	4	12	38	312
1. Alzheimer's disease and other dementias	246	78	168	—	—	—	—	11	235
H. Cardiovascular diseases	4,838	2,190	2,648	2	2	17	203	983	3,632
3. Ischemic heart diseases	2,706	1,301	1,404	—	—	5	106	578	2,017
4. Stroke	1,479	580	899	—	1	4	42	266	1,166
I. Respiratory diseases	641	355	286	1	1	3	15	120	502
J. Digestive disease	396	211	185	—	—	3	47	119	227
2. Cirrhosis of the liver	153	103	50	—	—	1	33	73	46
K. Genitourinary diseases	205	93	113	—	—	2	9	36	157
1. Kidney diseases	156	73	83	—	—	1	8	29	117
N. Congenital anomalies	51	27	24	35	3	3	4	4	3
Other noncommunicable diseases[f]	196	81	115	8	2	4	13	37	132
III. Injuries	842	601	241	13	17	154	265	203	190
A. Unintentional injuries	555	380	175	12	14	94	153	129	154
1. Road traffic injury	177	127	49	3	5	51	55	38	25
2. Other unintentional injuries	379	253	125	9	9	44	98	91	129
B. Intentional injuries	287	221	66	1	3	60	113	74	37
1. Suicide	204	157	47	—	1	36	76	59	32
2. Homicide and collective violence	83	64	19	1	2	24	37	15	4

Note: — = fewer than 500 deaths are attributable to a specific cause; HIV/AIDS = human immunodeficiency virus/acquired immune deficiency syndrome.

a. Tuberculosis deaths in HIV-negative people. Tuberculosis deaths in HIV-positive people are included in the HIV/AIDS category.

b. Pertussis, diphtheria, measles, and tetanus are included here.

c. Liver cancer and cirrhosis deaths resulting from past hepatitis infection are not included here.

d. Only direct deaths because of alcohol intoxication are included.

e. Only direct deaths because of drug overdose or adverse reaction for licit and illicit drugs are included.

f. Benign neoplasms; endocrine, blood, and immune disorders; sense organ diseases; skin diseases; musculoskeletal diseases; oral conditions; and sudden infant death syndrome are included.

Figure 4.5 displays the trends in global death rates for specific causes from 2000 to 2015, covering NCDs, Group I conditions, and injuries. Trends include those for dementia, already noted; for HIV/AIDS, where the scale-up of antiretroviral treatment coverage has had a significant effect; and for falls, where population aging is driving much of the increase in deaths.

The relative contributions of population growth, aging, and epidemiological change (changes in age-specific death rates) to overall growth in the number of deaths from 2000 to 2015 are summarized in figure 4.6 for HICs and for LMICs. Population growth and epidemiological improvement have been the dominant factors in mortality for LMICs over the past 15 years, acting in opposite directions and resulting in an overall increase of 34 percent for total NCD-related deaths and 13 percent for injury-related deaths. The 28 percent decline in Group I–related deaths is driven by epidemiological improvement. Population aging is an important factor for only NCD mortality, but it is likely to become more important over the next 15 years. For HICs, population

aging and epidemiological change act in opposite directions, resulting in a relatively small increase in the number of deaths overall from Group I causes and NCDs and a decline in deaths from injuries from 2000 to 2015.

Table 4.11 summarizes average annual rates of change for cause-specific death rates over the period 2000 to 2015 for the world and for countries grouped by income. For children under age 15 years, death rates from leading infectious causes have declined for all groups of countries by more than 4 percent per year, while death rates from preterm birth complications have declined in all groups, but at a lower rate of about 2 to 4 percent.

For younger adults ages 15–49 years, death rates from major causes are declining across all income groups, with the exception of road injuries, where rates are almost flat or rising in LMICs and declining significantly in HICs.

For older adults ages 50–69 years, NCD mortality rates are declining slowly in most regions at 1–2 percent per year, with the exception of mortality from IHD, which is increasing in low-income and upper-middle-income countries, and mortality from IHD, stroke,

Figure 4.5 Trends in Global Mortality Rates for Selected Causes, 2000–15

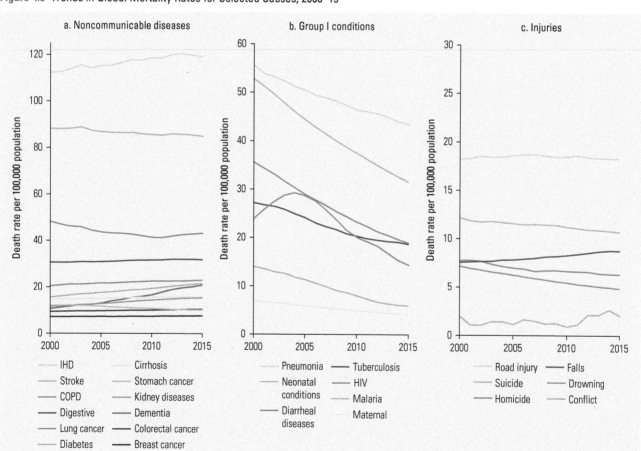

Note: COPD = chronic obstructive pulmonary disease; HIV = human immunodeficiency virus; IHD = ischemic heart disease.

Figure 4.6 Decomposition of Changes in Annual Number of Deaths, by Country Income Group and Major Cause, 2000–15

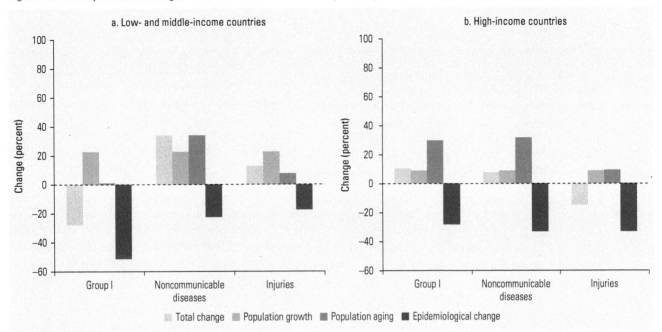

Table 4.11 Average Annual Rate of Change in Cause-Specific Death Rates, by Selected Causes within Age Groups, for the World and by Country Income Group, 2000–15

percent

Age and cause	World	Low income	Lower-middle income	Upper-middle income	High income
Ages 0–14 years					
Diarrheal diseases	–6.0	–6.9	–6.0	–5.8	–5.6
Malaria	–6.3	–8.0	–5.4	–4.4	–6.5
Lower respiratory infections	–4.8	–5.0	–4.7	–6.1	–5.9
Preterm birth complications	–2.2	–3.1	–1.7	–4.1	–2.9
Ages 15–49 years					
HIV/AIDS	–3.2	–7.6	–0.9	–2.3	1.8
Tuberculosis	–3.1	–4.4	–3.1	–5.7	–4.5
Maternal conditions	–3.3	–4.5	–4.1	–3.1	–1.4
Road injury	–0.2	0.0	1.2	–0.9	–3.5
Self-harm	–1.4	–1.2	–1.4	–2.1	–1.1
Interpersonal violence	–1.3	–0.8	–1.3	–0.9	–3.7
Ages 50–69 years					
Malignant neoplasms	–1.0	–0.7	–0.5	–1.3	–0.8
Ischemic heart disease	–1.1	0.9	–0.6	0.2	–2.7
Stroke	–1.7	–0.2	–1.4	–1.5	–3.5
Chronic obstructive pulmonary disease	–2.2	0.2	–1.4	–3.9	–1.1

Note: HIV/AIDS = human immunodeficiency virus/acquired immune deficiency syndrome.

and COPD, which are declining at around 3 to 4 percent per year in HICs.

Gains in Life Expectancy

Figure 4.7 decomposes the gains in life expectancy from 2000 to 2015 to identify the contribution of major causes using the methods of Beltran-Sanchez, Preston, and Canudas-Romo (2008). For LICs, 88 percent of the nine-year increase in life expectancy is due to declines in Group I cause-specific death rates, particularly for HIV/AIDS, tuberculosis, malaria, diarrheal diseases, lower respiratory infections (mainly pneumonia), and neonatal causes (mainly complications of prematurity, birth trauma, and neonatal infections). At the other end of the epidemiological spectrum, in HICs, 96 percent of the 3.7-year gain in life expectancy is associated with a reduction in mortality from NCDs (62 percent) and injuries (33 percent).

Figure 4.7 Gains in Life Expectancy at Birth Because of Improved Outcomes for Major Causes of Death, for the World and by Country Income Group, 2000–15

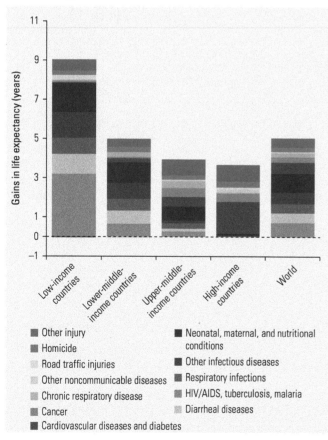

■ Other injury
■ Homicide
■ Road traffic injuries
■ Other noncommunicable diseases
■ Chronic respiratory disease
■ Cancer
■ Cardiovascular diseases and diabetes

■ Neonatal, maternal, and nutritional conditions
■ Other infectious diseases
■ Respiratory infections
■ HIV/AIDS, tuberculosis, malaria
■ Diarrheal diseases

Note: HIV/AIDS = human immunodeficiency virus/acquired immune deficiency syndrome.

DISCUSSION

Globally, life expectancy has been improving at a rate of more than three years per decade since 1950, with the exception of the 1990s (UN 2015). During that period, progress on life expectancy stalled in Africa because of the rising HIV/AIDS epidemic and in Europe because of higher mortality in many former Soviet republics following the collapse of the Soviet Union. Gains in life expectancy accelerated in most regions from 2000 onward, and overall life expectancy rose 5.0 years overall between 2000 and 2015, with an even larger increase of 9.4 years in Sub-Saharan Africa (WHO Global Health Observatory 2016). Almost 90 percent of the increase in life expectancy in Sub-Saharan Africa is the result of lower death rates for Group I causes, the main focus of the MDG health targets and of global health policies over the MDG period. In contrast, the increase of 3.7 years in life expectancy in HICs (corresponding to an average increase of 2.5 years per decade or 6 hours per day) was dominated by decreases in NCD death rates, particularly for cardiovascular disease. Rates of premature deaths (ages 50–69 years) from IHD and stroke decreased 36 percent and 47 percent, respectively, from 2000 to 2015.

The global average increase in life expectancy at birth since 2000 exceeds the overall average increase in life expectancy achieved by the best-performing countries over the past century (Oeppen and Vaupel 2002). The world as a whole is catching up with those countries, and improvements in outcomes for all major causes of death have contributed to these huge gains. The gap between life expectancy for HICs and LICs has narrowed, from 26 years in 2000 to 19 years in 2015, a decrease of 7 years.

Prospects for Accelerated Improvement to Achieve the 2030 Sustainable Development Agenda

The post-2015 SDGs include 13 cause-specific or age-specific mortality targets (WHO 2017c), with many focusing on reducing or ending *preventable* deaths. Achievement of the major SDG targets for child, maternal, and infectious diseases and for NCDs would result in a projected increase in global average life expectancy of about 4 years by 2030. The gap in average life expectancy between HICs and LICs would narrow from about 19 years in 2015 to about 14 years in 2030 (WHO 2014b).

Norheim and others (2015) have proposed an overarching target for health of reducing the number of deaths before age 70 years—both globally and in every country—by 40 percent by 2030. Countries at different stages of development could, depending on their epidemiological priorities, achieve this kind of gain in premature mortality by reducing mortality from HIV/AIDS, malaria, and tuberculosis or reducing causes of child deaths or NCD-related deaths under age 70 years. Concerted action to reduce NCD-related deaths before age 70 years would also reduce NCD death rates for people ages 70 years and over.

Applying the SDG targets to the estimated number of deaths in 2015 by cause, age, and sex can approximate the effect of attaining the SDG health-related targets for number of deaths under age 70 years. In 2015, there were an estimated 30.3 million deaths under age 70 years; if the SDG mortality targets had been achieved in 2015, the number would have been reduced to 19.6 million deaths.[1] This represents a 35 percent reduction (almost 11 million premature deaths averted)—close to the proposed 40 percent target. Of these averted deaths, 5 million from infectious diseases, malnutrition, and child and maternal mortality (the MDG causes) would have been avoided, with a further 5 million from NCDs and 900,000 from injuries also avoided. Figure 4.8 shows the rates of premature deaths (under age 70 years) per 1,000 population in 2015 for the world and for country income groups, together with the estimated number of deaths that would have been averted by achievement of the SDG mortality targets in 2015. The achievement of SDG mortality targets would have dramatically narrowed cross-income variations in the rate of premature deaths.

Uncertainty of Estimates and Limitations

Comparable information about the number of deaths and mortality rates by cause, age, sex, country, and year provides important information for discussing priorities and for monitoring and evaluating progress toward global health goals. However, serious problems exist with the quality and availability of information on levels and causes of death, particularly in LICs, where the mortality burden is highest. For this reason, there is considerable uncertainty in most cause-of-death estimates.

Demographic methods of assessing the completeness of death registration all involve strong assumptions or information about migration and are prone to error resulting from age misstatement in registration or census data and to differential completeness of successive censuses. These errors can result in considerable uncertainty in estimates for countries with partially complete registration systems, even before one considers the quality of cause-of-death assignment.

All-cause mortality estimates in countries without well-functioning death registration systems rely heavily on census and survey data (particularly sibling survival data) and model life tables. Yet no consensus has been reached on the methods for analyzing sibling survival

Figure 4.8 Premature Deaths (under Age 70 Years) That Would Have Been Averted by Achievement of SDG Mortality Targets, for the World and by Country Income Group, 2015

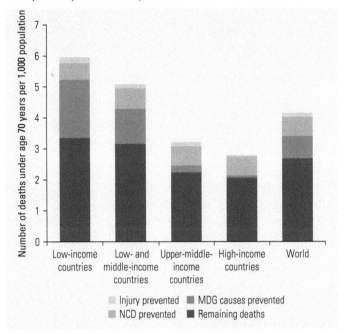

Note: NCD = noncommunicable disease; MDG = Millennium Development Goal.

data or assessing the level of underreporting of deaths in surveys or censuses.

In many low-income countries and lower-middle-income countries, estimates for many causes of death are predicted from available data on causes of death, using covariates such as gross domestic product and educational attainment. Even in HICs with relatively complete health statistics information systems, data quality is problematic for many causes. Approximate estimates of cause-specific uncertainty ranges are available in datasets that can be downloaded from the WHO website (see box 4.1).

Although death registration data are generally the best form of available information on causes of death, such data have considerable limitations, even in well-functioning systems with medical certification of cause of death. The so-called garbage codes represent a substantial proportion of deaths in some countries, and methods for reassigning these deaths to valid causes are highly uncertain and generally not based on empirical data. The assignment of underlying cause of death is both limited by the information provided on the death certificate and quite sensitive to the order in which diagnoses are written. For most causes of death, variability (owing to differences in physician practice when certifying a death) in the assignment of valid underlying causes of death has not been addressed to date.

Additionally, some diseases and injuries have specific problems that create difficulty in judging the underlying cause of death (for example, diabetes and heart disease, Alzheimer's disease and heart disease, and drug or alcohol overdose). Finally, HIV/AIDS and other stigmatized causes of death, such as suicide, are routinely certified incorrectly; incorrect certification rates vary substantially across settings.

For many countries without a functioning death registration system, particularly in Africa, there is strong reliance on verbal autopsy studies. Most studies are not nationally representative samples and, even when conducted well, have substantial limitations with respect to sensitivity and specificity of identifying specific causes of death. Considerable variation also exists in verbal autopsy instruments and in analysis and cause assignment methods. Validation studies are challenging and difficult to generalize to other settings.

The WHO GHE bring together single-cause analyses from several WHO departments, interagency collaborations, and other sources and estimates drawn from the GBD 2015 study. These estimates are updated using different timetables and varying methods and assumptions in some cases. Ensuring consistency across cause analyses that are created by various sources is more difficult than for large comprehensive estimates, such as GBD 2015, that are prepared by a single academic group. In addition, preparing separate estimates of total mortality and cause-specific mortality can lead to incompatible cause-specific and total mortality estimates.

Differences from Other Global Cause-of-Death Assessments

Academic institutions are increasingly publishing estimates in parallel to those of the WHO, using different methods that may result in substantially different results. *The Lancet* has become a regular channel for publication of global, regional, and country statistics on key health indicators and the burden of disease. Rudan and Chan (2015) recently characterized this practice as a competitive situation that is challenging the position of the WHO.

Over recent years, investigation into differences in the estimates for the same indicator has led to improvements in the data inputs and estimation methods used by UN agencies and by the GBD 2015 study. The existence of divergent estimates for the same indicator also has led to increased awareness of major data gaps, especially in LMICs. Lack of reliable data suggests greater use of data from other—often higher-income—countries and covariates to predict country statistics.

The type and complexity of models used for GHE vary widely by research and institutional group and by health estimate. More complex models are necessary to generate more comprehensive uncertainty intervals. These models require greater expertise and time and greater computational resources to run. In cases of available, high-quality data, estimates from different institutions are generally in agreement. Discrepancies are more likely to arise for countries where data are poor and for conditions where data are sparse and potentially biased. This situation is best addressed through improving the primary data.

The WHO and the UN devote considerable attention to estimates for several high-priority areas, including neonatal, child, and maternal mortality; HIV/AIDS; tuberculosis; malaria; major causes of child death; road injuries; homicides; and cancers. In all of these cases, input data for the particular area are scrutinized by specialists in that area, including academic collaborators; household survey technical staff involved with data collection; and country experts, including through the WHO country consultation mechanism.

The GHE 2015 draw on these WHO and UN agency or interagency statistics and place them in a consistent comprehensive context for all causes, drawing on death registration data and GBD 2015 analyses for causes and for countries lacking both death registration data and investment by the UN system in detailed estimates. Over time, some convergence has occurred between GBD and WHO estimates for some causes, although major differences remain in areas such as adult malaria mortality. However, the WHO continues to produce its own GHE, partly because of differences in the estimates of all-cause mortality (envelope) and of mortality for some major causes. In addition, the WHO has been unwilling to rely on third-party statistics for which it is not responsible or accountable to member states and for which it does not have, in many cases, access to the data and methods used.

The GHE 2015 use the latest UN Population Division life tables to provide envelopes, with some adjustments for countries with high HIV/AIDS prevalence and for countries with relatively complete death registration data. The UN life tables are less systematic than the GBD project (which uses its own model life table system), in part because of greater investment both in closely examining and assessing available country data and context and in ensuring consistency of estimated deaths with population, fertility, and migration estimates. For countries with high HIV/AIDS prevalence, the UN Population Division works with the Joint United Nations Programme on HIV/AIDS (UNAIDS) to maximize consistency of HIV/AIDS estimates and all-cause mortality trends and age patterns. In its most recent updates, the GBD 2015 study also uses UNAIDS models and inputs but has modified key assumptions regarding survival owing to antiretroviral treatment. It also models HIV/AIDS mortality as part of its overall model life table analysis in a way that may not adequately account for the complexity of time and age patterns for the HIV/AIDS epidemic.

The GBD model life tables differ most significantly from the UN estimates in three ways:

- Much lower estimates of older child mortality
- Different estimates of all-cause mortality in countries with high HIV/AIDS prevalence
- Slower time trends, with lower mortality rates in the 1990s in some parts of the world.

In the latest update, some of these differences are reduced, but the GBD 2015 estimate of 8.0 million deaths for the WHO African region is still much lower than the UN estimate of GHE 2015 of 9.2 million deaths (table 4.12). The GBD 2015 estimates for African deaths are consistently lower by close to 1.1 million across 1990–2015. In contrast, GHE 2015 and GBD 2015 estimates of deaths in children under age 5 years have converged globally and in most regions. Past GBD estimates have oscillated above and below the UN interagency estimates.

There are also significant differences (at the global, regional, and country levels) for some major causes of death. These differences include HIV/AIDS mortality, for which the GBD 2015 has converged somewhat by using the UNAIDS Spectrum model but has changed some input parameters. The parameters also include malaria mortality, which has seen some convergence for child mortality. However, significant differences remain for adult mortality, with the high GBD 2015 estimates for rates of adult malaria deaths not deemed plausible by many experts in malaria. Some convergence has occurred in other areas, such as maternal mortality, tuberculosis, and causes of child death. Pathogen-specific estimates for diarrhea and pneumonia mortality have also converged, largely as a result of revisions to GBD methods.

There are some more specific causes where the WHO and the GBD assessments differ (for example, road traffic injuries and homicides), in part because of different data inclusion and adjustment criteria. For example, both GBD 2015 and the WHO use death registration data and police or justice system data for homicides. Despite the intense effort put into assessing and adjusting data from incomplete death registration, GBD 2015 has not yet put the same effort into assessing and adjusting data from police or justice systems, resulting in low estimates in some countries (for example, estimated homicide rates are lower for Burkina Faso and Nigeria than for Japan).

Table 4.12 Comparison of Estimates of Total Global Deaths, 1990, 2000, and 2015

millions

Year	1990	2000	2015
World			
Global Health Estimates (WHO)	48.9	52.1	56.4
Global Burden of Disease estimates (IHME)	47.9	52.1	55.8
Africa			
Global Health Estimates (WHO)	7.9	9.8	9.2
Global Burden of Disease estimates (IHME)	6.8	8.5	8.0

Note: GHE 2015; WHO = World Health Organization; IHME = Institute for Health Metrics and Evaluation.

The WHO and other UN agencies will continue to prepare and report on global health indicators to fulfill their mandate from member states and to be accountable to those states through a transparent process, reproducible methods, and country involvement. For many years, this involvement has occurred mainly in the context of WHO or UN expert groups; this work is now also taking place in independent academic research institutions, notably through the IHME's work on the global burden of disease. The resulting debates on data interpretation, methods, and results can be healthy and productive and can lead to improvements in global health statistics, as long as the focus on methodological sophistication does not come at the expense of working together to improve the essential investments in data collection, analysis, and resulting use in LMICs.

CONCLUSIONS

The results presented here document major changes during the MDG era. On the whole, progress toward the MDGs has been remarkable, including, for instance, poverty reduction, improved education, and increased access to improved drinking water. Progress on the three health goals and targets has also been considerable. Globally, the HIV/AIDS, tuberculosis, and malaria epidemics have been "turned around," and child mortality and maternal mortality have decreased greatly (53 percent and 44 percent, respectively, since 1990), despite falling short of the MDG targets. Large reductions in mortality have occurred in Sub-Saharan Africa since the early 2000s, coinciding with increased coverage of HIV/AIDS treatment, methods of malaria control, and scale-up of vaccination coverage. Despite this progress, major challenges remain in achieving further progress on child and maternal mortality and on infectious diseases such as

HIV/AIDS, tuberculosis, malaria, neglected tropical diseases, and hepatitis.

The rate of increase in life expectancy in LICs over the past 15 years has exceeded the rate of growth observed for life expectancy in the countries with the highest life expectancies. Longer life expectancies and population aging have resulted in an increased focus on NCDs and their risk factors in LMICs and in HICs. Three-quarters of NCD-related deaths occurred in LMICs in 2015.

Over the past four decades, death rates from cardiovascular disease and smoking-associated cancers have declined substantially in most HICs, and rates for premature deaths from cardiovascular disease at ages 30 to 69 declined 28 percent in HICs over the period 2000–15, more than three times the decrease seen in LMICs. Public health action to address risk factors such as tobacco smoking and air pollution, along with the scale-up of health system coverage for individual-level risk factor interventions, are important priorities in the SDG era, particularly for LMICs. Weak health systems are a major obstacle in many countries, resulting in major deficiencies in universal health coverage for even the most basic health services and inadequate preparedness for health emergencies.

Lower poverty levels and economic growth have moved many countries to the middle-income categories and enabled an increasing proportion of countries to become self-sufficient in health and even to become aid donors and health technology suppliers (Jamison and others 2013). With enhanced investments to scale up health systems toward universal health coverage and to address major risk factors, continuing and accelerating the convergence of death rates across country income categories will be possible. At the same time, the challenges of population aging may be joined by additional challenges arising from climate change, political instability, and potential new epidemic outbreaks.

ACKNOWLEDGMENTS

The authors thank Doris Ma Fat for her assistance in extracting death registration data from the WHO Mortality Database and mapping them to the cause categories used in this chapter and Dean Jamison for his support and advice. The authors also drew heavily on advice and inputs from other WHO departments, collaborating UN agencies, and WHO expert advisory groups and academic collaborators.

Although we cannot name all those who provided advice, assistance, or data, both inside and outside the WHO, we would particularly like to note the assistance and inputs provided by Bob Black, Ties Boerma, Phillipe Boucher, Louisa Degenhardt, Jacques Ferlay, Patrick Gerland, Prabhat Jha, Joy Lawn, Li Liu, Mary Mahy, Bruno Masquelier, Shefali Oza, Francois Pelletier, Juergen Rehm, John Stover, and Danzhen You. The WHO funded this work.

ANNEXES

The two annexes to this chapter are available at http://www.dcp-3.org/DCP.

- Annex 4A. Global and Regional Causes of Death 2000–15: Data and Methods
- Annex 4B. Global and Regional Burden of Disease 2000–15: Methods and Summary Results

NOTES

World Bank Income Classifications as of July 2014 are as follows, based on estimates of gross national income (GNI) per capita for 2013:

- Low-income countries (LICs) = US$1,045 or less
- Middle-income countries (MICs) are subdivided:
  (a) lower-middle-income = US$1,046 to US$4,125
  (b) upper-middle-income (UMICs) = US$4,126 to US$12,745
- High-income countries (HICs) = US$12,746 or more.

1. Reduction of maternal mortality ratio to 70 per 100,000 live births; reduction of neonatal and under-age-5 mortality rates to 12 and 25 per 1,000 live births, respectively; 90 percent reduction in deaths from HIV/AIDS, tuberculosis, malaria, and neglected tropical diseases; 33 percent reduction in deaths from hepatitis, cancer, diabetes, cardiovascular disease, and chronic respiratory disease; 50 percent reduction in road injury deaths; 50 percent reduction in diarrheal deaths (through achievement of the target for water, sanitation, and hygiene); and 33 percent reduction (arbitrary interpretation of the SDG target of substantial reduction) in deaths from homicide, conflicts, and disasters. These estimated mortality reductions are conservative and do not include the effects of suicide, pollution, and drug and alcohol use on mortality targets (beyond their contribution to NCD mortality).

REFERENCES

Avenir Consulting. 2016. "Provisional Updated Spectrum Modelled Estimates of HIV Mortality for Years 1985–2015." Unpublished results provided by John Stover, Avenir Consulting, Sydney.

Beltran-Sanchez, H., S. H. Preston, and V. Canudas-Romo. 2008. "An Integrated Approach to Cause-of-Death Analysis:

Cause-Deleted Life Tables and Decompositions of Life Expectancy." *Demographic Research* 19 (35): 1323–50.

China CDC (Centre for Disease Control and Prevention). 2016. "Death Registration System." Unpublished tabulations for 2013.

Ferlay, J., I. Soerjomataram, M. Ervik, R. Dikshit, S. Eser, and others. 2013. Globocan 2012 v1.0, Cancer Incidence and Mortality Worldwide: IARC CancerBase No. 11. International Agency for Research on Cancer, Lyon, France. http://globocan.iarc.fr.

GBD 2015 (Global Burden of Disease 2015 Study) Mortality and Causes of Death Collaborators. 2016. "Global, Regional, and National Life Expectancy, All-Cause Mortality, and Cause-Specific Mortality for 249 Causes of Death, 1980–2015: A Systematic Analysis for the Global Burden of Disease Study 2015." *The Lancet* 388 (10053): 1459–544.

IARC (International Agency for Research on Cancer). 2013. "Globocan 2012: Data Sources and Methods." Lyon, France: IARC. http://globocan.iarc.fr/Pages/DataSource _and_methods.aspx.

IHME (Institute for Health Metrics and Evaluation). 2016. "Global Health Data Exchange: GBD Results Tool." Seattle, WA: IHME. http://ghdx.healthdata.org/gbd-results-tool.

Jamison, D. T., L. H. Summers, G. A. Alleyne, K. J. Arrow, S. Berkley, and others. 2013. "Global Health 2035: A World Converging within a Generation." *The Lancet* 382 (9908): 1898–955.

Liu, L., S. Oza, D. Hogan, J. Perin, I. Rudan, and others. 2015. "Global, Regional, and National Causes of Child Mortality in 2000–2013 with Projections to Inform Post-2015 Priorities: An Updated Systematic Analysis." *The Lancet* 385 (9966): 430–40.

MMEIG (Maternal Mortality Estimation Inter-Agency Group). 2015. *Trends in Maternal Mortality: 1990 to 2015.* Geneva: World Health Organization (WHO) on behalf of WHO, United Nations Children's Fund, United Nations Population Fund, World Bank, and United Nations Population Division.

Norheim, O. F., P. Jha, K. Admasu, T. Godal, R. J. Hum, and others. 2015. "Avoiding 40% of the Premature Deaths in Each Country, 2010–30: Review of National Mortality Trends to Help Quantify the UN Sustainable Development Goal for Health." *The Lancet* 385 (9964): 239–52. http://www.thelancet.com/journals/lancet/article /PIIS0140-6736%2814%2961591-9/fulltext.

Oeppen, J., and J. W. Vaupel. 2002. "Demography: Broken Limits to Life Expectancy." *Science* 296 (5570): 1029–31.

Patel, M. K., M. Gacic-Dobo, P. M. Strebel, A. Dabbagh, M. M. Mulders, and others. 2016. "Progress towards Regional Measles Elimination—Worldwide, 2000–2015." *Weekly Epidemiological Record* 65 (44): 1228–33.

Registrar General of India. 2009. "Causes of Death in India in 2001–2003." Registrar General of India, New Delhi.

Registrar General of India and CGHR (Centre for Global Health Research). 2015. "Causes of Death Statistics 2010–2013." Joint report, India Ministry of Home Affairs, Sample Registration System, New Delhi. http://www.censusindia.gov .in/2011-common/Sample_Registration_System.html.

Rudan, I., and K. Y. Chan. 2015. "Global Health Metrics Needs Collaboration and Competition." *The Lancet* 385 (9963): 92–94.

Torgerson, P. R., B. Devleesschauwer, N. Praet, N. Speybroeck, A. L. Willingham, and others. 2015. "World Health Organization Estimates of the Global and Regional Disease Burden of 11 Foodborne Parasitic Diseases, 2010: A Data Synthesis." *PLoS Medicine* 12 (12): e1001920.

UN (United Nations). 2015. *World Population Prospects: 2015 Revision.* New York: UN, Department of Economic and Social Affairs, Population Division.

UNAIDS (Joint United Nations Programme on HIV/AIDS). 2016. "HIV Estimates with Uncertainty Bounds 1990–2015." UNAIDS, Geneva. http://www.unaids.org/en/resources /documents/2016/HIV_estimates_with_uncertainty _bounds_1990-2015.

UN-IGME (United Nations Inter-agency Group for Child Mortality Estimation). 2015. *Levels and Trends in Child Mortality: Report 2015.* New York: United Nations Children's Fund on behalf of UN-IGME.

UN Statistics Division. 2017. "Revised List of Global Sustainable Development Goal Indicators." In *Report of the Inter-agency and Expert Group on Sustainable Development Goal Indicators,* annex III. New York: UN. https://unstats.un.org /sdgs/indicators/Official%20Revised%20List%20of%20 global%20SDG%20indicators.pdf.

WHO (World Health Organization). 1990. *International Statistical Classification of Diseases and Related Health Problems: 10th Revision.* Geneva: WHO.

———. 2014a. *Global Status Report on Violence Prevention 2014.* Geneva: WHO.

———. 2014b. "An Overarching Health Indicator for the Post-2015 Development Agenda: Brief Summary of Some Proposed Candidate Indicators." Background paper for Expert Consultation, December 11–12, WHO, Geneva. http://www.who.int/healthinfo/indicators/hsi _indicators_SDG_TechnicalMeeting_December2015 _BackgroundPaper.pdf?ua=1.

———. 2015a. *Global Status Report on Road Safety 2015.* Geneva: WHO.

———. 2015b. *Health in 2015: From MDGs to SDGs.* Geneva: WHO. http://www.who.int/gho/publications /mdgs-sdgs/en/.

———. 2016a. *Global Tuberculosis Report 2016.* Geneva: WHO. http://www.who.int/tb/publications/global_report/en/.

———. 2016b. "WHO Methods and Data Sources for Life Tables 1990–2015." Global Health Estimates Technical Paper WHO/HIS/IER/GHE/2016.2, WHO, Geneva. http:// www.who.int/healthinfo/statistics/LT_method.pdf.

———. 2016c. WHO Mortality Database. WHO, Geneva. http://www.who.int/healthinfo/mortality_data/en/.

———. 2016d. *World Health Statistics 2016: Monitoring Health for the SDGs.* Geneva: WHO. http://who.int/gho /publications/world_health_statistics/2016/en.

———. 2016e. *World Malaria Report 2016.* Geneva: WHO. http://www.who.int/malaria/publications/world -malaria-report-2016/en/.

———. 2017a. Global Health Estimates. http://www.who.int /healthinfo/global_burden_disease/en/.

———. 2017b. "Immunization Surveillance, Assessment, and Monitoring." WHO, Geneva. http://www.who.int /immunization/monitoring_surveillance/en/.

———. 2017c. World Health Statistics 2017: Monitoring Health for the SDGs. Geneva: WHO. http://who.int/gho /publications/world_health_statistics/2017/en/.

WHO Global Health Observatory. 2016. "Life Tables by WHO Region." WHO, Geneva. http://apps.who.int/gho/data /node.main.LIFEREGION?lang=en.

WHO and MCEE (Maternal and Child Epidemiology Estimation). 2016. "MCEE-WHO Methods and Data Sources for Child Causes of Death 2000–2015." WHO, Geneva. http://www.who.int/healthinfo/global_burden _disease/ChildCOD_method_2000_2015.pdf?ua=1.

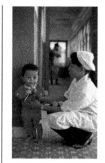

Chapter 5

Annual Rates of Decline in Child, Maternal, Tuberculosis, and Noncommunicable Disease Mortality across 109 Low- and Middle-Income Countries from 1990 to 2015

Osondu Ogbuoji, Jinyuan Qi, Zachary D. Olson, Gavin Yamey,
Rachel Nugent, Ole Frithjof Norheim, Stéphane Verguet, and
Dean T. Jamison

INTRODUCTION

A country's performance in health is typically defined by how much better or worse it performs with respect to a particular outcome (for example, life expectancy) compared with what would be expected in light of certain contextual attributes (for example, income and education) (Jamison and Sandbu 2001). In *Good Health at Low Cost*, Halstead, Walsh, and Warren (1985) used a case study approach to assess country performance in levels of mortality, examining why three countries and one Indian state had low levels of mortality despite scant resources. Later analyses also quantified performance with respect to levels of mortality and fertility (Wang and others 1999).

The number of deaths is affected strongly by long-standing country-level determinants. Essentially, a country that starts with a low level of mortality is likely to continue to have lower mortality, whereas a country that begins with a high level of mortality might improve substantially but still have comparatively high mortality. Examining alterations in the number of deaths or annual rate of change in mortality is useful for understanding

how a country's health performance might relate to adjustments in policy. Most published work on country performance is based on estimates of mortality levels, but some studies investigate rates of change (Bhutta and others 2010; Croghan, Beatty, and Ron 2006; Kassebaum and others 2014; Lozano and others 2011; Muennig and Glied 2010; Munshi, Yamey, and Verguet 2016; Verguet and Jamison 2013a, 2013b, 2014; Wang and others 2014). To the extent that rates of change respond to the introduction of health policies (for example, a new immunization program), rates of decline in mortality offer a dependent variable with which to understand the effect on performance of social and system determinants. Nevertheless, the measure—like any one-dimensional metric—still has weaknesses. Notably, large declines from high levels of mortality may still leave an unacceptably large number of deaths. Therefore, rates of change complement rather than replace the important information conveyed by estimates of mortality levels.

The need to measure progress in health was especially apparent when assessing whether countries were on track

Corresponding author: Osondu Ogbuoji, Department of Global Health and Population, Harvard T. H. Chan School of Public Health, Boston, Massachusetts, United States, oogbuoji@mail.harvard.edu.

to achieve the Millennium Development Goals (Bhutta and others 2010; Kassebaum and others 2014; Lozano and others 2011; Wang and others 2014). Measuring progress is also crucial to determining whether countries can achieve the next set of post-2015 Sustainable Development Goals (SDGs) that were adopted by United Nations (UN) member states in 2015. The SDGs include health goals with an associated set of targets; the *Lancet* Commission on Investing in Health proposed a target of achieving a "grand convergence in global health" by 2035, defined as reducing infectious, maternal, and child deaths to universally low levels, similar to today's rates in the best-performing middle-income countries, such as Chile and Turkey (Jamison and others 2013). Other targets were proposed by the Global Investment Framework for Women's and Children's Health (Stenberg and others 2014), the United Nations Children's Fund (UNICEF 2013), the Sustainable Development Solutions Network (SDSN 2013), and the High-Level Panel on the post-2015 development agenda (Norheim and others 2015; Peto, Lopez, and Norheim 2014; UN 2013). All of these proposals were debated before adoption of the SDGs by all UN member states.

Studying historical rates of change (rates of decline) in mortality across countries over recent decades can be helpful for testing the feasibility of these different proposals and the SDGs, which include ambitious targets for child, maternal, tuberculosis, human immunodeficiency virus/acquired immune deficiency syndrome (HIV/AIDS), and noncommunicable disease (NCD) mortality that would require high rates of decline from 2015 to 2030. Such targets for mortality can be tested for their feasibility by looking at whether high rates of decline in mortality have ever been achieved by any low- or middle-income country (LMIC) and whether similar declines could be achieved in 2016–30.

Assessing a country's health performance with respect to changes in rates of decline in mortality is, therefore, valuable for studying the effects of policy and for testing the feasibility of proposed post-2015 health goals. This chapter updates a previous study (Verguet and others 2014) that examined changes in the annual rate of decline of key mortality indicators for 109 LMICs by expanding the period to cover 1990–2015. In addition, we examine annual rates of decline in NCD mortality (the probability of dying between ages 50 and 69 years from NCDs in the presence of other causes) over 1993–2013.

METHODS

Verguet and others (2014) analyzed the rates of decline for under-five, maternal, tuberculosis, and HIV/AIDS-related mortality. The analysis in this chapter is restricted to four indicators—under-five mortality rates (5q0),

maternal mortality ratios, tuberculosis mortality rates, and NCD mortality rates in persons between ages 50 and 69 years. These indicators feature prominently in SDG 3, and updated data became available since the last analysis. We assessed the annual rates of decline in the chosen mortality indicators for 109 LMICs, as defined in the World Bank income classifications for 2014, with populations greater than 1 million people (Zeileis 2015). We used the 2013 World Bank income group classification to ensure that all of the countries in the original paper were covered. Annex 5B presents the countries and regional groupings included in the analysis.

We estimated rates of decline in under-five mortality rates (number of children who die after birth and before age five years per 1,000 live births), maternal mortality ratios (number of pregnant women who die per 100,000 live births), tuberculosis mortality ratios (number of deaths from tuberculosis per 100,000 population per year), and NCD mortality rates (probability of dying between ages 50 and 69 years from an NCD in the presence of other causes). Depending on the availability of data, we used a 1990–2015 time series for under-five mortality rates (UNICEF and others 2015), a 1990–2015 time series for maternal mortality ratios (WHO 2016b), a 1990–2014 time series for tuberculosis mortality rates (WHO 2016a), and a 1993–2013 time series for NCD mortality rates from UN-DESA (2015) life tables and IHME (2015) cause-of-death data. We used several time anchor points for every indicator: 1990, 1995, 2000, 2005, 2010, and 2015 for under-five mortality rates and maternal mortality ratios; 1990, 1995, 2000, 2005, 2010, and 2014 for tuberculosis mortality rates; and 1993, 1998, 2003, 2008, and 2013 for NCD mortality rates. Thus, our calculations differ from annualized rates of reduction computed using different time frames. We calculated 95 percent uncertainty intervals around the estimates and used R software for all analyses.

We calculated the average annual rates of decline from levels of the first three indicators for every five-year interval from 1990 to 2015 and the average annual rates of decline in NCD mortality rates for every five-year interval from 1993 to 2013 (equations 5.1 to 5.4). In total, we have five estimates for the annual rate of decline in under-five mortality rates, maternal mortality ratios, and tuberculosis mortality rates, and for estimates for the annual rate of decline in NCD mortality rates for every country included in the study: 1990–94, 1995–99, 2000–04, 2005–09, and 2010–15 (six-year interval) for under-five mortality rates and maternal mortality ratios; 1990–94, 1995–99, 2000–04, 2005–09, and 2010–14 for tuberculosis mortality rates; and 1993–98, 1998–2003, 2003–08, and 2008–13 (mid-year estimate) for NCD mortality rates.

Equations (5.1)–(5.4) are used to perform the estimates:

$$R(t) = \frac{L_{t+1} - L_t}{L_t}, \tag{5.1}$$

$$R(p) = \frac{1}{n}\sum_{t=1}^{n} R(t), \tag{5.2}$$

$$RCR(p) = \frac{R_{p+1} - R_p}{R_p}, \tag{5.3}$$

$$RCR(p)_t = \frac{1}{n}\sum_{p=1}^{n} \frac{R_{p+1} - R_p}{R_p}, \tag{5.4}$$

where $R(t)$ is the annual rate of decline; L represents levels of under-five mortality rates, maternal mortality ratios, tuberculosis mortality rates, and NCD mortality rates; $R(p)$ is the average $R(t)$ for each period; $RCR(p)$ is the rate of change in the rate of decline (acceleration or deceleration) from one period to the next; $RCR(p)_t$ is the period average of annual rate of change (acceleration or deceleration) in the rate of decline; t represents time intervals; and n represents the number of time intervals in a period.

We calculated the annual rate of change in the decline (either an acceleration or a deceleration) for every transition from one five-year period to the next between 1990 and 2015 (equations 5.3 and 5.4). In total, we have four values for the rate of change in decline for each country using equation 5.3 for the first three mortality indicators, three values using equation 5.3 for NCD mortality rates, and five values using equation 5.4 for under-five and maternal mortality ratios. For acceleration between periods in equation 5.3, we use the rates of decline from two consecutive five-year periods (for example, 1995–99 and 2000–05) to estimate the rate of change in decline for the transition between those two periods. For simplicity, we present results obtained using equations 5.1, 5.2, and 5.4.

For every mortality indicator, we estimated the year by which the *Lancet* Commission on Investing in Health target (Jamison and others 2013) and SDG target (UN 2016) would be achieved (figures 5.1–5.4). We obtained estimates for every country's aspirational best-performer rate of decline (90th percentile for all countries) and every region's aspirational rate of decline (90th percentile for each region).

Figure 5.1 Year by Which the Global Targets for Under-Five Mortality Rates Will Be Reached at Aspirational Rates of Decline, Disaggregated by Geographic Region, 2015–50

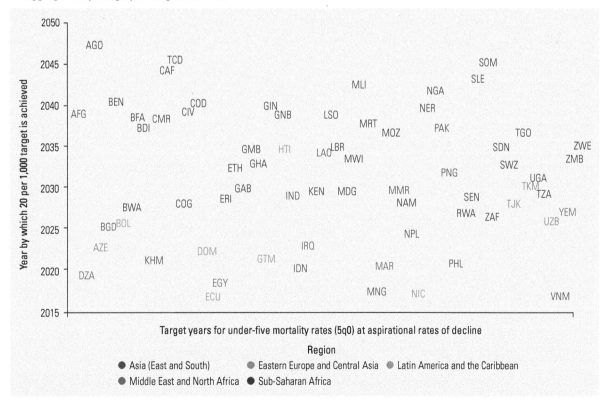

Figure 5.2 Year by Which the Global Targets for Maternal Mortality Ratios Will Be Reached at Aspirational Rates of Decline, Disaggregated by Geographic Region, 2015–50

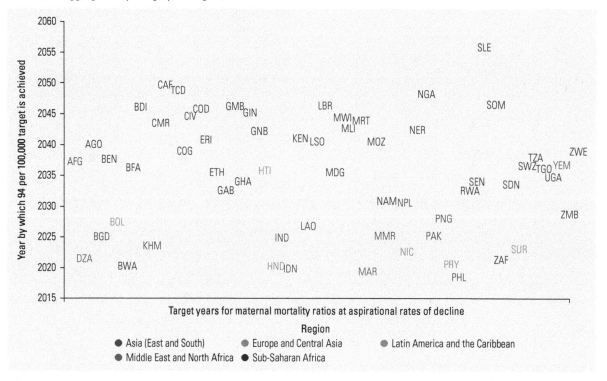

Figure 5.3 Year by Which the Global Targets for Tuberculosis Mortality Rates Will Be Reached at Aspirational Rates of Decline, Disaggregated by Geographic Region, 2015–50

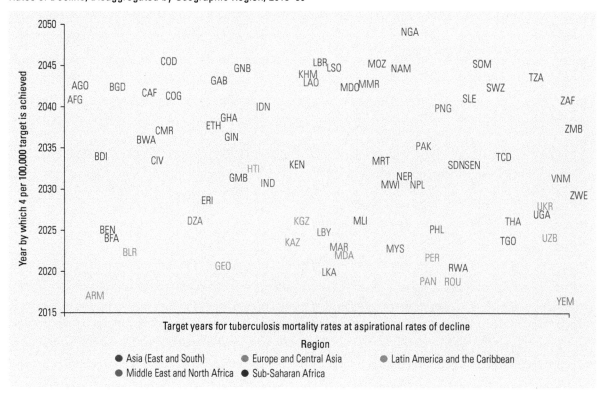

Figure 5.4 Year by Which the Global Targets for NCD Mortality Rates Will Be Reached at Aspirational Rates of Decline, Disaggregated by Geographic Region, 2015–40

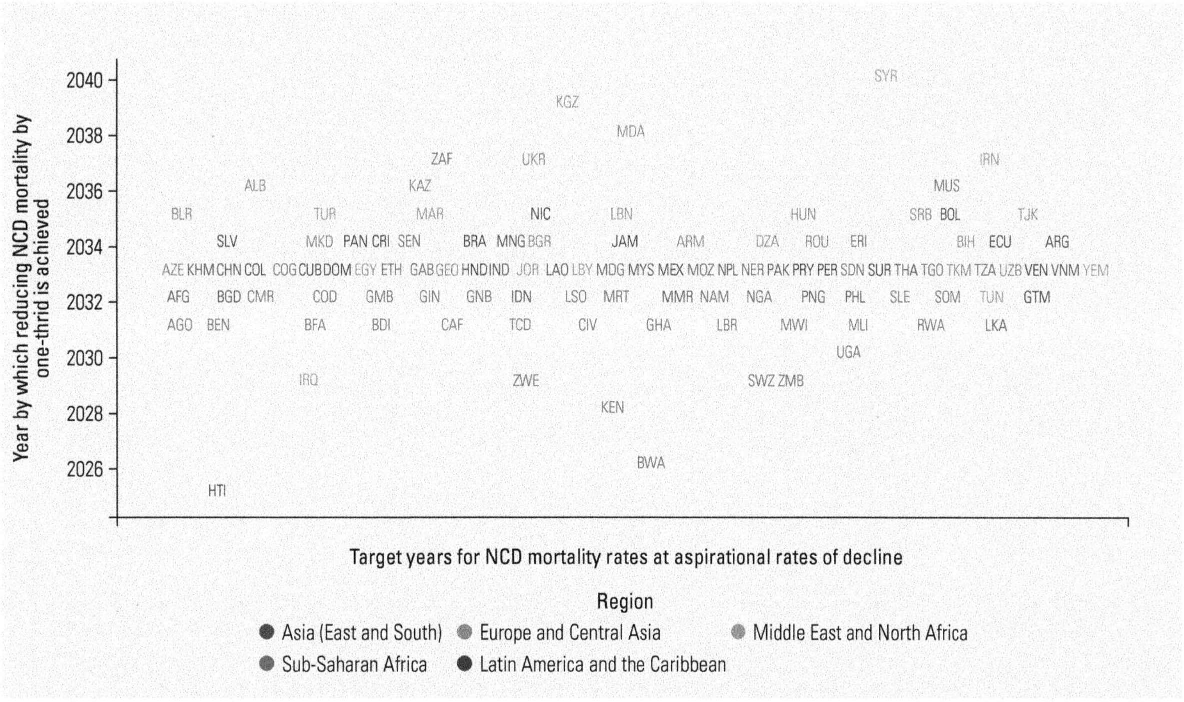

Year by which reducing NCD mortality by one-third is achieved

2040	SYR
2038	KGZ; MDA
2036	ZAF UKR IRN; ALB KAZ MUS
2034	BLR TUR MAR NIC LBN HUN SRB BOL TJK; SLV MKD PAN CRI SEN BRA MNG BGR JAM ARM DZA ROU ERI BIH ECU ARG; AZE KHM CHN COL COG CUB DOM EGY ETH GAB GEO HND IND JOR LAO LBY MDG MYS MEX MOZ NPL NER PAK PRY PER SDN SUR THA TGO TKM TZA UZB VEN VNM YEM
2032	AFG BGD CMR COD GMB GIN GNB IDN LSO MRT MMR NAM NGA PNG PHL SLE SOM TUN GTM; AGO BEN BFA BDI CAF TCD CIV GHA LBR MWI MLI RWA LKA
2030	UGA
2028	IRQ ZWE SWZ ZMB; KEN
2026	BWA; HTI

Target years for NCD mortality rates at aspirational rates of decline

Region
- Asia (East and South)
- Europe and Central Asia
- Middle East and North Africa
- Sub-Saharan Africa
- Latin America and the Caribbean

Note: NCD = noncommunicable disease.

RESULTS

Tables 5.1–5.4 show the rates of decline in mortality indicators and highlight the best and worst performers (top-five and bottom-five rates of decline). For under-five mortality and NCD mortality rates, the distribution of rates of decline among the 109 LMICs is narrow (annex 5C) and becomes narrower in the most recent 10-year period (2005–15 and 2003–13, respectively), while the distribution of rates of decline in maternal mortality ratios and tuberculosis mortality rates starts out wide and becomes more narrow in recent periods; notably, several countries had very high or very low rates of decline in maternal mortality ratios. For under-five mortality rate, in 2010–15, the mean rate of decline was 3.5 percent per year; the aspirational rate was 6.5 percent per year, with some variation across regions (3.9 percent for South-East Asia, 4.2 percent for Sub-Saharan Africa, 3.8 percent for Middle East and North Africa, 4.8 percent for Europe and Central Asia, and 3.5 percent for Latin America and the Caribbean). The top two performers between 2010 and 2015 were Haiti and the former Yugoslav Republic of Macedonia, with rates of 14.8 and 11.1 percent per year,

respectively (table 5.1). Between 1990 and 2004, countries with the worst performance for under-five mortality rate had zero or negative rates of decline (that is, mortality remained the same or increased) and, with the exception of Sri Lanka, were largely in Southern Africa. Some countries (for example, FYR Macedonia, Peru, and Serbia in 1990–99; Cambodia and Rwanda in 2001–15) maintained very high rates of decline in under-five mortality rates, above 6.0 percent per year.

For maternal mortality ratio, in 2010–15, the mean rate of decline was 2.7 percent per year; the aspirational rate was 6.6 percent per year, with some variation across regions (4.3 percent for South-East Asia, 2.7 percent for Sub-Saharan Africa, 1.6 percent for North Africa and the Middle East, 2.1 percent for Eastern Europe and Central Asia, and 1.9 percent for Latin America and the Caribbean). The top performers in 2010–15 were Kazakhstan, the Lao People's Democratic Republic, and Ethiopia, with rates of 10.0, 7.6, and 7.6 percent per year, respectively (table 5.2). In all periods assessed, the five worst performers had negative rates of decline, while the five top performers had high rates, greater than 7.0 percent per year.

Table 5.1 Top-Five and Bottom-Five Country Performers in Rate of Decline for Under-Five Mortality Rate (5q0), 1990–2015

	1990–94		1995–99		2000–04		2005–09		2010–15	
	Country	Rate of decline per year (%)	Country	Rate of decline per year (%)	Country	Rate of decline per year (%)	Country	Rate of decline per year (%)	Country	Rate of decline per year (%)
Best performers										
1	Macedonia, FYR	7.6	Bosnia and Herzegovina	9.5	Rwanda	9.6	Rwanda	10.3	Haiti	14.8
2	Serbia	7.0	Serbia	8.5	Cambodia	9.6	Congo, Rep.	8.7	Macedonia, FYR	11.1
3	Peru	6.3	Macedonia, FYR	8.2	Moldova	8.8	Belarus	8.3	Rwanda	8.2
3	Hungary	6.3	Peru	7.7	China	8.2	China	8.1	Kazakhstan	8.2
4	Turkey	5.8	Brazil	7.1	Belarus	8.0	Cambodia	8.0	Cambodia	7.8
Worst performers										
1	Rwanda	−14.4	Swaziland	−5.8	Sri Lanka	−6.5	Haiti	−29.4	Brazil	0.2
2	Swaziland	−5.4	South Africa	−3.9	Lesotho	−1.1	Costa Rica	0.4	Costa Rica	1.0
3	Botswana	−5.2	Botswana	−3.5	Swaziland	−0.3	Malaysia	0.5	Algeria	1.4
4	Zimbabwe	−4.7	Lesotho	−3.4	Somalia	0.0	Mauritius	0.6	Moldova	1.7
5	Moldova	−2.9	Congo, Rep.	−2.5	South Africa	0.0	Myanmar	1.5	Dominican Republic	1.8

Table 5.2 Top-Five and Bottom-Five Country Performers in Rate of Decline for Maternal Mortality Ratios, 1990–2015

	1990–94		1995–99		2000–04		2005–09		2010–15	
	Country	Rate of decline per year (%)	Country	Rate of decline per year (%)	Country	Rate of decline per year (%)	Country	Rate of decline per year (%)	Country	Rate of decline per year (%)
Best performers										
1	South Africa	10.4	Dominican Republic	15.2	Belarus	13.0	Belarus	16.8	Kazakhstan	10.0
2	Thailand	9.9	Tajikistan	11.9	Rwanda	11.0	Turkey	16.5	Lao PDR	7.6
3	Uzbekistan	9.7	Azerbaijan	10.8	Mongolia	10.1	Kazakhstan	13.9	Ethiopia	7.6
4	Honduras	9.4	Iran, Islamic Rep.	8.7	Lebanon	8.3	Botswana	9.3	Afghanistan	7.5
5	Romania	9.1	Ukraine	7.9	Libya	8.3	Cambodia	8.5	Brazil	7.3
Worst performers										
1	Suriname	−7.1	Suriname	−7.9	South Africa	−5.8	Dominican Republic	−8.9	Dominican Republic	−12.5
2	Azerbaijan	−6.8	South Africa	−6.5	Uzbekistan	−4.2	Mauritius	−8.7	Syrian Arab Republic	−6.5
3	Moldova	−5.5	Zimbabwe	−5.6	Kyrgyz Republic	−3.2	South Africa	−6.5	Hungary	−1.8
4	Tajikistan	−4.8	Botswana	−5.6	Lesotho	−2.8	Panama	−3.2	Libya	−1.8
5	Nicaragua	−4.3	Lesotho	−4.4	Honduras	−2.5	Georgia	−1.6	Serbia	−1.6

Table 5.3 Top-Five and Bottom-Five Country Performers in Rate of Decline for Tuberculosis Mortality Rates, 1990–2014

	1990–94		1995–99		2000–04		2005–09		2010–14	
	Country	Rate of decline per year (%)	Country	Rate of decline per year (%)	Country	Rate of decline per year (%)	Country	Rate of decline per year (%)	Country	Rate of decline per year (%)
Best performers										
1	Zimbabwe	16.5	Syrian Arab Republic	14.0	Azerbaijan	12.7	Azerbaijan	34.4	Azerbaijan	24.1
2	Mauritius	15.3	Morocco	13.6	Mongolia	11.6	Tajikistan	16.4	Turkmenistan	22.8
3	Kenya	14.2	Lebanon	13.2	Georgia	11.1	Turkmenistan	15.2	Philippines	20.9
4	Lesotho	13.2	Cuba	11.6	Ecuador	11.0	Honduras	13.7	Egypt, Arab Rep.	18.1
5	Libya	12.9	Mongolia	11.5	Turkey	11.0	Kazakhstan	13.5	Syrian Arab Republic	16.7
Worst performers										
1	Cameroon	−23.8	Mauritius	−19.3	Suriname	−26.2	Lebanon	−16.4	Albania	−17.7
2	Kazakhstan	−20.7	Lesotho	−15.3	Mauritius	−19.7	Suriname	−16.0	Libya	−15.9
3	Burundi	−19.3	Albania	−14.1	Jamaica	−10.8	Cuba	−8.8	Mauritius	−11.1
4	Azerbaijan	−16.6	Tajikistan	−11.9	Lebanon	−8.7	Libya	−8.6	Lebanon	−9.8
5	Moldova	−16.2	Thailand	−11.1	Congo, Rep.	−7.6	Georgia	−7.9	Kenya	−8.9

Table 5.4 Top-Five and Bottom-Five Performers in Rate of Decline for Noncommunicable Disease Mortality Rates, 1993–2013

	1993–98		1998–2003		2003–08		2008–13		1993–13	
	Country	Rate of decline per year (%)	Country	Rate of decline per year (%)	Country	Rate of decline per year (%)	Country	Rate of decline per year (%)	Country	Rate of decline per year (%)
Best performers										
1	Rwanda	10.3	Botswana	7.1	Haiti	8.0	Syrian Arab Republic	4.5	Rwanda	3.6
2	Malawi	4.9	Zimbabwe	6.0	Lebanon	3.6	Kyrgyz Republic	4.0	Malawi	2.5
3	Eritrea	4.4	Sri Lanka	4.6	South Africa	3.4	Moldova	3.7	South Africa	2.5
4	Uganda	3.3	Albania	4.1	Lesotho	3.0	Iran, Islamic Rep.	3.3	Syrian Arab Republic	2.3
5	Burundi	3.2	Kenya	3.6	Mongolia	2.7	South Africa	3.2	Algeria	2.2
Worst performers										
1	Kazakhstan	−3.8	Liberia	−3.8	Eritrea	−3.0	Haiti	−7.3	Burkina Faso	−0.7
2	Belarus	−2.9	Guinea	−1.7	Zambia	−1.2	Botswana	−5.1	Guinea	−0.6
3	Sri Lanka	−2.6	Bosnia and Herzegovina	−1.3	Central African Republic	−1.2	Kenya	−3.1	Côte d'Ivoire	−0.6
4	Kyrgyz Republic	−2.6	Burkina Faso	−0.7	Albania	−1.1	Zambia	−2.7	Ghana	−0.4
5	Lesotho	−2.0	Senegal	−0.6	Burkina Faso	−1.1	Zimbabwe	−2.5	Central African Republic	−0.3

In contrast to under-five and maternal mortality ratios, rates of decline for tuberculosis mortality rates were distributed more widely and showed little change over time (annex 5C). During 2010–14, the mean rate of decline was 3.5 percent per year; the aspirational rate was 6.5 percent per year, with substantial variation across regions (4.6 percent for South-East Asia, 1.0 percent for Sub-Saharan Africa, 3.7 percent for North Africa and the Middle East, 6.9 percent for Eastern Europe and Central Asia, and 5.0 percent for Latin America and the Caribbean). The top performers in 2010–14 were Azerbaijan, Turkmenistan, and the Philippines, with rates of 24.1, 22.8, and 20.9 percent per year, respectively (table 5.3). In all periods assessed, the worst performers had high negative rates, with more than half of them having rates of less than −15 percent per year. In the last three periods Azerbaijan ranked as the best performer, with rates above 10 percent (12.7 percent in 2000–04, 34.4 percent in 2005–09, and 24.1 percent in 2010–14).

For NCD mortality rates, the distribution of rates of decline varied greatly across World Bank income groups (annex 5C). From 1993 to 2013, the mean rate of decline was 0.51 percent per year for low-income countries and 0.48 percent per year for lower-middle-income countries. For upper-middle-income and high-income countries, the mean rate of decline over 20 years was much higher, at 1.43 and 1.71 percent per year, respectively. Low- and lower-middle-income countries are off-track to achieve the SDG target of reducing premature mortality from NCDs by one-third by 2030 (UN 2016). LMICs exhibit wide distribution in the rates of decline, with NCD mortality rates rising in some countries. Over the periods assessed, the worst performers were Burkina Faso and Guinea, with mean rates of decline per year of −0.7 and −0.6 percent, respectively, and the best performers were Rwanda (3.6 percent), Malawi (2.5 percent), and South Africa (2.5 percent), with mean annual rates of decline of more than 2 percent (table 5.4).

Based on the change in the rate of decline, it is possible to identify rapid transitions in performance over time (annex 5D, tables 5D.1 to 5D.3). For under-five mortality rates, most countries had small rates of acceleration or deceleration (0 percent ± 3 percent) for all periods; when the estimates were larger, they were not significant, with uncertainty intervals spanning zero. Likewise, for tuberculosis mortality rates, the point estimates were small, ranging from 2 percent per year to −3.4 percent per year. However, unlike for under-five mortality rates, many of the point estimates for rates of change in tuberculosis mortality rates were significant. For maternal mortality ratio, although many of the point estimates were large, none was found to be significant.

A country's performance with respect to the rate of change in mortality differs greatly from its performance with respect to death rate. Examining rates of decline versus number of deaths for under-five and maternal mortality from 1990 to 2015, we found little correlation between the two indicators (annex 5D, figure 5D.1). Our findings show that high rates of decline in mortality can be achieved even at low levels of mortality.

For under-five mortality rates, 36 of 109 countries (33 percent) have already achieved the interim 2030 target of 20 deaths per 1,000 live births and 73 have not. At current rates of mortality decline, none of these 73 countries will achieve the target between 2030 and 2050. With an aspirational best-performer rate of decline (at the 90th percentile), 38 (35 percent) of the 73 countries will achieve the target by 2030 and the remaining 35 countries (32 percent) will achieve it over 2030–50 (figure 5.1). With regional aspirational rates, 37 of the 73 countries (34 percent) will achieve the target by 2030, and the remaining 36 countries (33 percent) will achieve it between 2030 and 2050 (annex 5E).

For maternal mortality ratios, 46 of 109 countries (42 percent) have already achieved the interim 2030 target of 94 deaths per 100,000 live births and 63 have not. At current rates, none of these 63 countries will achieve the target by 2050. At the aspirational rate, 21 countries (19 percent) will achieve the target by 2030, 41 countries (38 percent) will achieve it between 2030 and 2050, and one country (Sierra Leone) will achieve it after 2050 (figure 5.2). At regional aspirational rates, 21 (19 percent) of these 63 countries will achieve the target by 2030, 28 countries (26 percent) will achieve it between 2030 and 2050, and 14 countries (13 percent) will achieve the target after 2050 (annex 5E).

For tuberculosis mortality rates, 36 (33 percent) of 108 countries have already achieved the *Lancet* Commission's target of 4 deaths per 100,000 population per year and 72 have not. At current rates, none of these 72 countries will achieve the target by 2050. At the aspirational rate, 27 countries (25 percent) will achieve the target by 2030, and the remaining 45 countries (42 percent) will achieve it between 2030 and 2050 (figure 5.3). At regional aspirational rates, 25 countries (23 percent) will achieve the target by 2030, 46 countries (43 percent) will achieve it between 2030 and 2050, and the remaining country (Nigeria) will achieve it in 2054 (annex 5E).

For NCD mortality rates between age 50 and 69, we estimated the 2016 (January) NCD mortality level as the starting point to achieve the SDG target of one-third lower NCD mortality in 2030. At current rates, 30 countries have increasing rates of NCD mortality; only 6 countries will achieve the target by 2030, and 27 countries will achieve it by 2050. At the aspirational rate, all countries will achieve the target by 2040 (figure 5.4). At regional aspirational rates, 30 countries (28 percent) will achieve the target by 2030, and 24 countries (22 percent) will achieve it between 2030 and 2050 (Annex 5C, figure 5C.4). Countries in South-East Asia and Sub-Saharan Africa have much lower rates of decline.

DISCUSSION

We studied the historical rates of decline in rates of under-five, maternal, tuberculosis, and NCD mortality for 109 LMICs. Annex 5A of this chapter provides a graphical overview of our findings by country income group. We also identified countries with the best and worst performance and regions in which performance had changed rapidly, either improving or deteriorating.

Analysis of rates of change in health is useful because rapid alterations in rates of decline—whether accelerations or decelerations—can point to a potential effect of policy changes and provide a mechanism for understanding what constitutes good policy. We noted almost no correlation between number of deaths and rate of decline in mortality indicators (annex 5D, figure 5D.1), which suggests that rates of change augment the information conveyed by mortality estimates but cannot replace the examination of number of deaths, particularly with regard to capturing the underlying intensity of country-level mortality.

As in our original analysis (Verguet and others 2014), this update reveals some interesting patterns. Rates of decline in child mortality indicate the severe effect of the HIV/AIDS epidemic in Southern Africa. In this region, large increases were recorded in child mortality over 1995–99, but the number of deaths fell rapidly beginning in 2000, reaching a peak rate of decline of 6.3 percent per year in 2005–09. This is probably linked to the rollout of antiretroviral therapy for the prevention of mother-to-child transmission of HIV/AIDS (UNAIDS 2013; WHO 2011). Likewise, rates of decline in maternal and tuberculosis mortality rates deteriorated during 1990–99 in many Central Asian countries after the collapse of the Soviet Union in 1991, and rates of decline in under-five mortality rates dropped abruptly in Rwanda during 1990–99, probably because of the genocide in 1994. Low rates of decline in NCD mortality rates between ages 50 and 69 years for low- and lower-middle-income countries over the 20 years between 1993 and 2013 suggest lack of effective health interventions (screening, prevention, treatment) and rising risk factors (smoking, alcohol consumption, high-calorie processed food).

A few countries have sustained high rates of decline—for example, under-five mortality rates in Turkey from 1990 to 2015, maternal mortality ratios in Cambodia from 1990 to 2015, and NCD mortality rates in Rwanda from 1993 to 2003. Did unusual circumstances or specific policies account for these changes in mortality? Indeed, subsequent assessments could control for contextual determinants (for example, income) and exceptional events (for example, natural disasters, political instability) and try to identify the contributions of specific policies implemented. For instance, Turkey's high rates of decline in under-five mortality rates coincide with substantial economic growth, political stability, and the introduction of the Health Transformation Program, which rapidly expanded access to health care services (Atun and others 2013). Cambodia's progress in maternal mortality can probably be attributed to socioeconomic improvements, better primary education, and specific policies leading to increases in skilled birth attendance (Liljestrand and Sambath 2012).

We used the rates of decline in mortality to test the feasibility of achieving SDGs, with a particular focus on the 2030 targets proposed by the *Lancet* Commission on Investing in Health. Because post-2015 goals present ambitious targets for levels of mortality, meeting them will require high (aspirational) rates of mortality decline from 2015 to 2030. Hence, we used historical rates of decline—including best-performer aspirational rates—to identify how many countries will achieve these ambitious targets if they achieve similar rates of decline over 2015–30. If all LMICs are able to achieve aspirational best-performer rates of decline in mortality, some countries will meet the targets for under-five, maternal, and tuberculosis mortality by 2030, but the majority will reach their targets by 2050. However, meeting the SDG target of reducing premature mortality from NCDs by one-third by 2030 requires a 2.7 percent annual rate of decline. Only Lebanon and South Africa had average annual rates of decline greater than 2.7 percent during most of the 15 years between 1998 and 2013, and a few countries maintained rates greater than 2 percent in the same period, including Algeria, the Islamic Republic of Iran, Malawi, Rwanda, and the Syrian Arab Republic. The majority of LMICs will not reach the NCD target by 2030.

Similar methods have been used to assess the feasibility of other post-2015 targets. Norheim and others (2015) have suggested setting (in addition to specific subtargets for under-five mortality) an overarching goal of reducing premature (under age 70) deaths by 40 percent in 2030 from what they were in 2010.

Our analysis has three key limitations. First, for some countries with poor data, the mortality estimates were predicted largely from past trends. Many countries, particularly those with high mortality, do not have strong registration systems for vital statistics, so mortality estimates are not always reliable. In view of the large number of countries and distinct mortality indicators analyzed, some findings might also be attributable to poor quality of data. We used mortality estimates from the UN, UNICEF, World Health Organization (WHO), and Institute for Health Metrics and Evaluation to draw general lessons, but our findings could be strengthened further by incorporating additional sources of data (IHME 2015; Jamison, Murphy, and Sandbu 2016; Kassebaum and others 2014; Liu and others 2012; Lozano and others 2013; Murray and others 2014; UN-DESA 2015; Wang and others 2014).

Second, in contrast to our original analysis, where we used five-year intervals, we used annual estimates for this update. Although this may improve the accuracy of the estimates, it may also produce too much noise and mask changes or reveal only small changes that may not be relevant for policy. Despite this noise, annual outcomes could isolate inflection points that capture times when countries make performance transitions and help identify seasonal variations or cyclical patterns that longer intervals (for example, every five years) might not flag.

The final limitation is that other modeling techniques could be used to forecast rates of decline in mortality and to ascertain whether countries would achieve targets by 2030. For instance, specific explanatory variables related to declines in mortality could be used, and regression models could be fitted to mortality time series to make future predictions. However, it is the purpose of our analyses to provide specific performance indicators to be explained, rather than explanations. As such, they provide a starting point. Further research focusing on individual countries can elucidate the reasons for these differences in the rates of change.

ANNEXES

This chapter has one accompanying print annex:

- Annex 5A: Cross-Country Variation in Rates of Decline for Mortality Indicators, 1998–2013

The online annexes to this chapter are as follows. They are available at http://www.dcp-3.org/DCP.

- Annex 5B: Countries and Regional Groupings in the Analysis

- Annex 5C: Distribution of Country-Level Rates of Decline in Mortality Indicators, by Period
- Annex 5D: Rate of Change in Decline for Mortality Indicators
- Annex 5E: Reaching Global Targets for Mortality Indicators under Regional Best-Performer Rates of Decline.

NOTES

Large portions of this chapter have been reproduced from: Verguet, S., O. F. Norheim, Z. D. Olson, G. Yamey, and D. T. Jamison. 2014. "Annual Rates of Decline in Child, Maternal, HIV, and Tuberculosis Mortality across 109 Countries of Low and Middle Income from 1990 to 2013: An Assessment of the Feasibility of Post-2015 Goals." *The Lancet Global Health* 2 (12): e698–709.

World Bank Income Classifications as of July 2014 are as follows, based on estimates of gross national income (GNI) per capita for 2013:

- Low-income countries (LICs) = US$1,045 or less
- Middle-income countries (MICs) are subdivided:
  (a) lower-middle-income = US$1,046 to US$4,125
  (b) upper-middle-income (UMICs) = US$4,126 to US$12,745
- High-income countries (HICs) = US$12,746 or more.

ANNEX 5A: CROSS-COUNTRY VARIATION IN RATES OF DECLINE FOR MORTALITY INDICATORS, 1998–2013

For under-five mortality rates, tuberculosis mortality rates, and maternal mortality ratios, we calculated the average annual rate of decline over a 15-year period (1998–2013). We also calculated separate average rates of decline for the World Bank's low-income, lower-middle-income, and upper-middle-income countries. For NCD mortality, we calculated the mean rate of decline over the same 15-year period and average rates of change for all four World Bank income groups, including high income.

For each of the four mortality indicators, we graph the distribution of rates of decline separately for the three income groups (four income groups for NCDs). Each graph also displays the mean for its income group and the rate of decline for a populous country in the group (China, Ethiopia, India, United States).

Annex Figure 5A.1 Cross-country variation in rates of decline of under-five mortality rates (5q0)

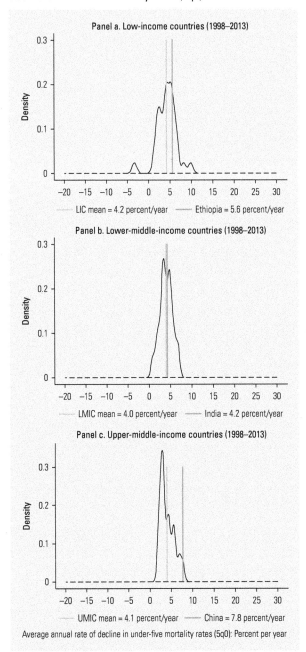

Note: LIC = low-income countries; LIMC = lower-middle-income countries; UMIC = upper-middle-income countries.

Annex Figure 5A.2 Cross-country variation in rates of decline of maternal mortality ratios

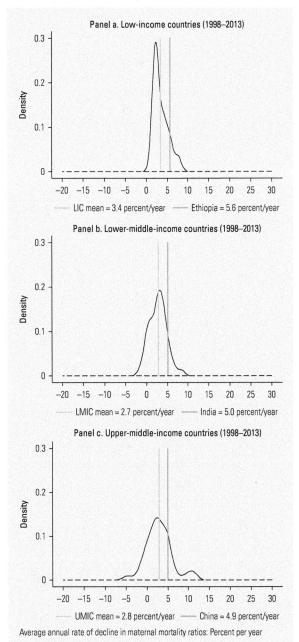

Note: LIC = low-income countries; LIMC = lower-middle-income countries; UMIC = upper-middle-income countries.

Annex Figure 5A.3 Cross-country variation in rates of decline of tuberculosis mortality rates

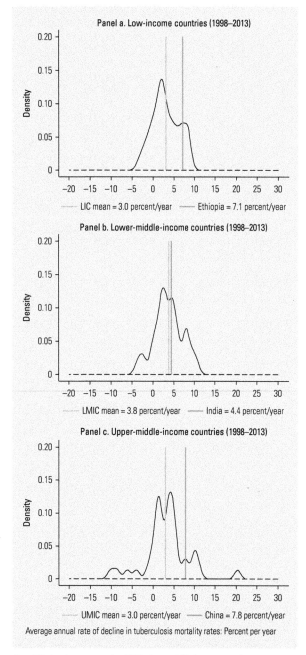

Panel a. Low-income countries (1998–2013)

LIC mean = 3.0 percent/year —— Ethiopia = 7.1 percent/year

Panel b. Lower-middle-income countries (1998–2013)

LMIC mean = 3.8 percent/year —— India = 4.4 percent/year

Panel c. Upper-middle-income countries (1998–2013)

UMIC mean = 3.0 percent/year —— China = 7.8 percent/year

Average annual rate of decline in tuberculosis mortality rates: Percent per year

Note: LIC = low-income countries; LIMC = lower-middle-income countries; UMIC = upper-middle-income countries.

Annex Figure 5A.4 Cross-country variation in rates of decline in mortality rates age 50-69 from noncommunicable diseases

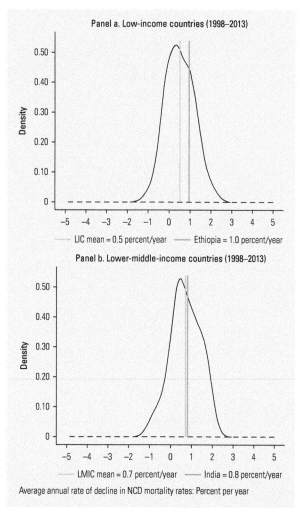

Panel a. Low-income countries (1998–2013)

LIC mean = 0.5 percent/year —— Ethiopia = 1.0 percent/year

Panel b. Lower-middle-income countries (1998–2013)

LMIC mean = 0.7 percent/year —— India = 0.8 percent/year

Average annual rate of decline in NCD mortality rates: Percent per year

figure continues next page

Annex Figure 5A.4 (continued)

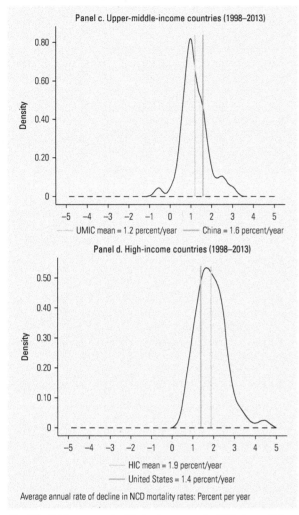

Panel c. Upper-middle-income countries (1998–2013)

——— UMIC mean = 1.2 percent/year   ——— China = 1.6 percent/year

Panel d. High-income countries (1998–2013)

——— HIC mean = 1.9 percent/year

——— United States = 1.4 percent/year

Average annual rate of decline in NCD mortality rates: Percent per year

Note: HIC = high-income countries; LIC = low-income countries; LIMC = lower-middle-income countries; NCD = noncommunicable diseases; UMIC = upper-middle-income countries.

REFERENCES

Atun, R., S. Aydın, S. Chakraborty, S. Sümer, M. Aran, and others. 2013. "Universal Health Coverage in Turkey: Enhancement of Equity." *The Lancet* 382 (9886): 65–99.

Bhutta, Z. A., M. Chopra, H. Axelson, P. Berman, T. Boerma, and others. 2010. "Countdown to 2015 Decade Report (2000–10): Taking Stock of Maternal, Newborn, and Child Survival." *The Lancet* 375 (9730): 2032–44.

Croghan, T. W., A. Beatty, and A. Ron. 2006. "Routes to Better Health for Children in Four Developing Countries." *Milbank Quarterly* 84 (2): 333–58.

Halstead, S. B., J. A. Walsh, and K. S. Warren. 1985. *Good Health at Low Cost.* New York: Rockefeller Foundation.

IHME (Institute for Health Metrics and Evaluation). 2015. "GBD Compare." IHME, University of Washington, Seattle, WA.

Jacobs, R., P. C. Smith, and A. Street. 2006. *Measuring Efficiency in Health Care: Analytic Techniques and Health Policy.* Cambridge, U.K.: Cambridge University Press.

Jamison, D. T., S. M. Murphy, and M. E. Sandbu. 2016. "Why Has Under-5 Mortality Decreased at Such Different Rates in Different Countries?" *Journal of Health Economics* 48: 16-25.

Jamison, D. T., and M. E. Sandbu. 2001. "WHO Ranking of Health System Performance." *Science* 293 (5535): 1595–96.

Jamison, D. T., L. H. Summers, G. Alleyne, K. J. Arrow, S. Berkley, and others. 2013. "Global Health 2035: A World Converging within a Generation." *The Lancet* 382 (9908): 1898–955.

Kassebaum, N. J., A. Bertozzi-Villa, M. S. Coggeshall, K. A. Shackelford, C. Steiner, and others. 2014. "Global, Regional, and National Levels and Causes of Maternal Mortality during 1990–2013: A Systematic Analysis for the Global Burden of Disease Study 2013." *The Lancet* 384 (9947): 980–1004.

Liljestrand, J., and M. R. Sambath. 2012. "Socio-Economic Improvements and Health System Strengthening of Maternity Care Are Contributing to Maternal Mortality Reduction in Cambodia." *Reproductive Health Matters* 20 (39): 62–72.

Liu, L., H. L. Johnson, S. Cousens, J. Perin, S. Scott, and others. 2012. "Global, Regional, and National Causes of Child Mortality: An Updated Systematic Analysis for 2010 with Time Trends since 2000." *The Lancet* 379 (9832): 2151–61.

Lozano, R., M. Naghavi, K. Foreman, S. Lim, K. Shibuya, and others. 2013. "Global and Regional Mortality from 235 Causes of Death for 20 Age Groups in 1990 and 2010: A Systematic Analysis for the Global Burden of Disease Study 2010." *The Lancet* 380 (9859): 2095–128.

Lozano, R., H. Wang, K. J. Foreman, J. K. Rajaratnam, M. Naghavi, and others. 2011. "Progress towards Millennium Development Goals 4 and 5 on Maternal and Child Mortality: An Updated Systematic Analysis." *The Lancet* 378 (9797): 1139–65.

Muennig, P. A., and S. A. Glied. 2010. "What Changes in Survival Rates Tell Us about US Health Care." *Health Affairs* 29 (11): 2105–13.

Murray, C. J. L., K. F. Ortblad, C. Guinovart, S. S. Lim, T. M. Wolock, and others. 2014. "Global, Regional, and National Incidence and Mortality for HIV, Tuberculosis, and Malaria during 1990–2013: A Systematic Analysis for the Global Burden of Disease Study 2013." *The Lancet* 384 (9947): 1005–70.

Munshi, V., G. Yamey, and S. Verguet. 2016. "Trends In State-Level Child Mortality, Maternal Mortality, and Fertility Rates in India." *Health Affairs* 35 (10): 1759–63.

Norheim, O. F., P. Jha, K. Admasu, T. Godal, R. J. Hum, and others. 2015. "Avoiding 40% of the Premature Deaths in Each Country, 2010–30: Review of National Mortality Trends to Help Quantify the UN Sustainable Development Goal for Health." *The Lancet* 385 (9964): 239–52.

Peto, R., A. D. Lopez, and O. F. Norheim. 2014. "Halving Premature Death." *Science* 345 (6202): 1272–72.

SDSN (Sustainable Development Solutions Network). 2013. "An Action Agenda for Sustainable Development." SDSN, Paris.

Stenberg, K., H. Axelson, P. Sheehan, I. Anderson, A. M. Gülmezoglu, and others. 2014. "Advancing Social and

Economic Development by Investing in Women's and Children's Health: A New Global Investment Framework." *The Lancet* 383 (9925): 1333–54.

UN (United Nations). 2013. "A New Global Partnership: Eradicate Poverty and Transform Economies through Sustainable Development." UN High-Level Panel, New York.

———. 2016. "Sustainable Development Knowledge Platform." UN, New York. https://sustainabledevelopment.un.org/sdg3.

UNAIDS (Joint United Nations Programme on HIV/AIDS). 2013. *UNAIDS Report on the Global AIDS Epidemic 2013.* Geneva: UNAIDS.

UN-DESA (United Nations Department of Economic and Social Affairs). 2015. *World Population Prospects: The 2015 Revision.* DVD ed. New York: UN-DESA, Population Division.

UNICEF (United Nations Children's Fund). 2013. "UNICEF Key Asks on the Post-2015 Development Agenda." UNICEF, New York.

UNICEF (United Nations Children's Fund), WHO (World Health Organization), World Bank, and UN-DESA (United Nations Department of Economic and Social Affairs), Population Division. 2015. *Levels and Trends in Child Mortality Report 2015.* New York: UNICEF.

Verguet, S., and D. T. Jamison. 2013a. "Improving Life Expectancy: How Many Years Behind Has the USA Fallen? A Cross-National Comparison among High-Income Countries from 1958 to 2007." *British Medical Journal Open* 3 (7): e002814.

———. 2013b. "Performance in Rate of Decline of Adult Mortality in the OECD, 1970–2010." *Health Policy* 109 (2): 137–42.

———. 2014. "Estimates of Performance in the Rate of Decline of Under-Five Mortality for 113 Low- and Middle-Income Countries, 1970–2010." *Health Policy and Planning* 29 (2): 151–63.

Verguet, S., O. F. Norheim, Z. D. Olson, G. Yamey, and D. T. Jamison. 2014. "Annual Rates of Decline in Child, Maternal, HIV, and Tuberculosis Mortality across 109 Countries of Low and Middle Income from 1990 to 2013: An Assessment of the Feasibility of Post-2015 Goals." *The Lancet Global Health* 2 (12): e698–709.

Wang, H., C. A. Liddell, M. M. Coates, M. D. Mooney, C. E. Levitz, and others. 2014. "Global, Regional, and National Levels of Neonatal, Infant, and Under-5 Mortality during 1990–2013: A Systematic Analysis for the Global Burden of Disease Study 2013." *The Lancet* 384 (9947): 957–79.

Wang, J., D. T. Jamison, E. Bos, A. Preker, and J. Peabody. 1999. *Measuring Country Performance on Health: Selected Indicators for 115 Countries.* Washington, DC: World Bank.

WHO (World Health Organization). 2011. *Global HIV/AIDS Response: Epidemic Update and Health Sector Progress towards Universal Access.* Progress report, WHO, Geneva.

———. 2016a. "Tuberculosis Burden Estimates." WHO, Geneva.

———. 2016b. "WHO GHO Maternal Mortality Data." WHO, Geneva. http://apps.who.int/gho/data/node.main.15?lang=en.

Zeileis, A. 2015. "pwt8: Penn World Table (Version 8.x)." R package version 8.1-0. http://CRAN.R-project.org/package=pwt8.

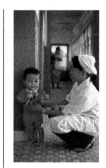

Chapter 6

Economic Burden of Chronic Ill Health and Injuries for Households in Low- and Middle-Income Countries

Beverley M. Essue, Tracey-Lea Laba, Felicia Knaul,
Annie Chu, Hoang Van Minh, Thi Kim Phuong Nguyen,
and Stephen Jan

INTRODUCTION

The *World Health Report 2000: Health Systems: Improving Performance* (WHO 2000); the World Health Organization (WHO) resolution on sustainable health financing, universal health coverage, and social health insurance (WHO 2005); and the *World Health Report: Health Systems Financing: The Path to Universal Coverage* (WHO 2010) all highlighted the substantial economic burden faced by individuals with no access to affordable, high-quality health care. These reports placed the need to address the economic effect of illness—in particular, catastrophic and impoverishing health expenditure—on the global health policy agenda.

Financial protection—a core element of universal health coverage—aims to ensure that people receive the health care services they require without facing financial ruin (WHO 2010). Devising strategies to protect populations from financial risk has become a major focus of global health policy development (WHO and World Bank 2014).

Affordable access to high-quality health care is now considered a basic human right and a critical step to the achievement of sustainable economic and social development and the elimination of poverty (Sustainable Development Solutions Network 2014; WHO 2015). This imperative is reflected in the third Sustainable Development Goal, which sets a target for achieving universal health coverage, including financial risk protection; access to high-quality essential health care services; and access to safe, effective, high-quality, and affordable essential medicines and vaccines for all (UN General Assembly 2015). This commitment is echoed in the World Bank's recent call to eradicate impoverishment owing to health care expenditures by 2030 (Kim 2014).

A lack of both prepayment mechanisms and the means and resources to pool risks has limited the capacity of many health care systems to provide access to high-quality health care services. As a result, for decades, many health systems, particularly in low- and middle-income countries (LMICs), have relied heavily on private payments in the form of out-of-pocket costs to fund health care. In 2014, 18 percent of total health expenditure globally came from out-of-pocket payments (WHO 2014). The burden is even greater in LMICs. In 2014, out-of-pocket payments equaled approximately 39 percent of total health expenditure for low-income countries, 56 percent for lower-middle-income countries, and 30 percent for upper-middle-income countries (WHO 2016).

Corresponding author: Beverley Essue, University of Sydney, Sydney, Australia; beverley.essue@sydney.edu.au.

Relying on out-of-pocket costs to finance health care is both inefficient and inequitable and places a major financial strain on individuals and households (WHO 2010). Out-of-pocket costs can perpetuate poverty and lead many individuals to delay or forgo necessary care (Peters and others 2008; van Doorslaer and others 2006). This link, where the household's investment in health further impoverishes that household, can lead to a continuous cycle of poor health and poverty (Knaul, Wong, and Arreola-Ornelas 2012).

This burden is of particular concern for persons with chronic diseases, for whom repeated and lifelong costs are associated with the management and treatment of illness (Kankeu and others 2013). For example, in some countries, a household may have to pay as much as eight days' worth of wages to purchase one month's supply of only one of the multiple medicines required for the optimal treatment of cardiovascular disease (CVD) or diabetes (Cameron and others 2009; Gelders and others 2006). In more extreme cases, the costs of treatment for chronic and long-term conditions such as human immunodeficiency virus/acquired immune deficiency syndrome (HIV/AIDS) and surgery for some cancers have kept patients confined to hospitals indefinitely pending payment to the hospitals or forced them to stop treatment altogether (Human Rights Watch 2006). Although households, even those that are already impoverished, may be able to manage a one-time shock and recover in the short run (for example, over a period of a week or a month), they may not be able to withstand the ongoing costs of treatment for chronic diseases.

Furthermore, LMICs are undergoing a protracted epidemiological transition (Frenk and others 1989). Underfunded and weak health systems continue to face a backlog of acute diseases and conditions associated with poverty, together with the onslaught of costly and chronic noncommunicable diseases (NCDs), conditions that affect the entire population at all income levels. This situation inevitably results in competing priorities about which services to include in essential packages of care and which to cover through national insurance funds (Beaglehole and others 2011). However, evidence is lacking on the household-level economic burden associated with certain categories of disease, particularly chronic diseases. Such evidence would inform global health policy development by highlighting where the greatest gains in financial protection might be realized (Shrime and others 2015) and help governments prioritize the measures needed to move toward universal health coverage.

This chapter estimates the burden of catastrophic health expenditure (CHE) associated with chronic ill health and injuries in LMICs and describes the broader economic effects on households. It is organized as follows.

We begin by estimating the population-level burden of CHE—the most common indicator of the household economic burden of health expenditure—and draw on empirical research of specific chronic diseases and injuries to estimate the prevalence of CHE associated with seven categories of conditions: cancers, CVDs, chronic infectious diseases, endocrine diseases, injuries, renal diseases, and respiratory diseases. We then draw on a review of NCDs in LMICs to describe the broader household economic effects associated with ill health, including impoverishing health expenditure, productivity effects, distressed financing, and treatment discontinuation. We discuss implications of the results for improving financial protection and offer directions for future research.

POPULATION-LEVEL ESTIMATES OF CATASTROPHIC AND IMPOVERISHING HEALTH EXPENDITURES

Catastrophic and impoverishing health expenditures, also referred to as *medical impoverishment*, continue to challenge health systems around the world and pose a key barrier to improving economic and social well-being (Knaul, Wong, and Arreola-Ornelas 2012). Very conservative estimates suggest that, globally, at least 150 million people a year face financial catastrophe and 100 million are driven into poverty by expenditure on health care (Xu and others 2007).

CHE and impoverishing health expenditure are interrelated, but distinct, concepts (figure 6.1). Consensus is lacking on the definition of what constitutes a

Figure 6.1 Definition of Catastrophic and Impoverishing Health Expenditures

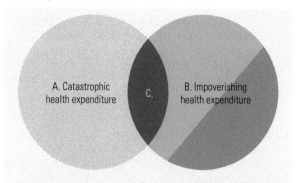

A. Health care expenditure is defined as catastrophic using any of the conventional definitions.
B. Impoverishing health expenditure results at any level of expenditure:
 • Darker shaded area: for the population already in poverty, any level of spending further entrenches social disadvantage, and there is a high likelihood of forgoing care.
C. Health care expenditure is catastrophic and impoverishes the household.

catastrophic level of expenditure for households and the most appropriate denominator for measuring CHE: expenditure, income, or consumption (Knaul, Wong, and Arreola-Ornelas 2012; O'Donnell and others 2007). Box 6.1 distinguishes between these two concepts.

The economic burden associated with ill health extends beyond paying for care (table 6.1). Household members cope with the onset of illness in various ways, and the response can influence their treatment-seeking behavior (McIntyre and others 2006; Okoli and Cleary 2011; Sauerborn, Adams, and Hien 1996; Xu and others 2007). When faced with ill health, particularly unexpected events, the household must mobilize resources to pay for health care, often by borrowing money, using limited savings, and selling assets—all of which can negatively affect the long-term economic well-being of the household, including its ability to deal with ongoing health care needs and future health shocks (Kruk, Goldmann, and Galea 2009; McIntyre and others 2006; Peters and others 2008; Russell 2004). Ill health can also affect the productivity of both the sick individual and a family caregiver, leading to loss of paid employment or educational opportunities. All these factors severely impair the family's capacity to earn income in both temporary and longer-term ways.

Financial protection through tax-financed social health insurance programs is a major pillar of efforts by national governments to achieve universal health coverage. Indeed, there is evidence of the extent to which health insurance–based measures effectively provide financial protection by curbing the burden of

medical expenditure (Essue and others 2015; Knaul, Arreola-Ornelas, and Méndez-Carniado 2016). Although progress has been made at a population level, research shows variations in the financial protection afforded to different subgroups (box 6.2).

Box 6.1

Conceptual Relationship between Catastrophic Health Expenditure and Impoverishing Health Expenditure

Conceptually, catastrophic health expenditure is a measure of the burden of health care expenditure (that is, out-of-pocket costs) on a household's available resources. It can result from sizable and unpredictable one-off payments and from a steady flow of unbudgeted medical bills, including relatively small payments (Knaul and others 2006; Schoenberg and others 2007; Thuan and others 2006).

Impoverishing health expenditure is defined as expenditure on health care that results in a household falling below the prevailing poverty line or deepening its impoverishment if it is already poor (Knaul, Wong, and Arreola-Ornelas 2012; Xu 2005). Such impoverishment is also linked to employment, because loss of income owing to ill health can drive households into poverty (Gertler and Gruber 2002).

Table 6.1 Indicators Used to Measure the Household Economic Burden of Ill Health

Indicator	Definition	Advantages	Limitations
Catastrophic health expenditure	Total health care expenditure (out-of-pocket costs) as a percentage of household resources (O'Donnell and others 2007; Xu and others 2003). The denominator, household resources, is measured as discretionary expenditure (also referred to as *capacity to pay* or *nonfood expenditure*), total expenditure, or household income.	• Provides objective measure of the drain on available household resources caused by health care expenditure • Is the most commonly used indicator and widely endorsed	• Has wide variation in the threshold and denominator used and the categories of health care expenditure included, which makes it difficult to use as a benchmark across studies • Does not capture forgone care owing to unaffordable health care costs • Arbitrary threshold: implicitly assumes that the given level of expenditure will impose the same burden across the population
Impoverishing health expenditure (also referred to as *medical impoverishment*)	The outcome when total health care expenditure subtracted from baseline income results in the household's income falling below the prevailing poverty line (Wagstaff and van Doorslaer 2003)	• Provides a measure of the effect of illness on the household's economic well-being and potentially the national economy	• Does not account well for the poorest households, for whom any level of expenditure further entrenches their poverty

table continues next page

Table 6.1 Indicators Used to Measure the Household Economic Burden of Ill Health (continued)

Indicator	Definition	Advantages	Limitations
Economic hardship or financial stress	A measure of the potential consequences for the household of health care expenditure. It captures instances in which the household is unable to meet the costs of essential payments (housing, food, heating, child care, transport, health care). It is most commonly defined as an instance of missing any one of the specified payments (Essue and others 2011).	• Takes account of the opportunity costs associated with health care expenditure and potential economic consequences for households	• Has wide variation in the definition and categories of expenses included, which limits its generalizability • Does not account well for instances in which households were unable to meet essential bills before the onset of illness • Tends to be measured in cross-sectional studies, which are unable to assess the effect and recurrence of these consequences over time
Distressed financing	A measure of the strategies used by the household to pay for health care expenses, often including savings, borrowed funds (either through formal or informal loan or through credit schemes), or sale of assets. It is a descriptive measure that accounts for the percentage of households using each of the financing strategies (Kruk, Goldmann, and Galea 2009; McIntyre and others 2006).	• Accounts for the economic consequences of health care expenditure for household economies • Offers insights into potentially effective informal strategies for dealing with health care costs	• Has wide variation in the distressed financing categories included, which limits its generalizability • Tends to be measured in cross-sectional studies, which are unable to assess the effect of using these strategies over time

---

Box 6.2

Monitoring Universal Health Coverage: Achieving Financial Protection in Asia

Universal health coverage entails everyone having access to needed health services without financial hardship. In the Western Pacific region, several countries have made progress toward achieving universal health coverage and protecting their populations from financial risk.

Country-specific studies on the equity of health service use and financial protection have been conducted in Mongolia (Tsilaajav, Nanzad, and Ichinnorov 2015), the Philippines (Ulep and dela Cruz 2013), and Vietnam (Minh and Phuong 2016). These studies examined health service use, out-of-pocket health expenditures, catastrophic health expenditure, impoverishing health expenditure, and their determinants over time. Data were from nationally representative surveys—socioeconomic or income and expenditure surveys—containing information on health service use and health expenditure. The method used to calculate out-of-pocket, catastrophic, and impoverishing

health expenditure followed the WHO methodology in all four countries (Xu 2005).

Annual household out-of-pocket health expenditures ranged from US$144 in Mongolia to US$190 in Vietnam. Medicines were a major component of out-of-pocket health expenditures in Mongolia and the Philippines. The average proportion of households that incurred catastrophic health expenditure (CHE) ranged from 0.9 percent in Mongolia to 2.3 percent in Vietnam (figure B6.2.1). Across expenditure quintiles, the proportion of households that incurred CHE increased in Mongolia and the Philippines but decreased in Vietnam as the expenditure quintile increased. Over time, the proportion of households incurring CHEs increased in the Philippines, but it fell in Mongolia and Vietnam.

Impoverishment resulting from health expenditures was highest in the lowest and second-to-lowest

box continues next page

Box 6.2 (continued)

Figure B6.2.1 Proportion of Households with Catastrophic Health Expenditure in Selected Asian Countries, by Expenditure Quintile, Various Years

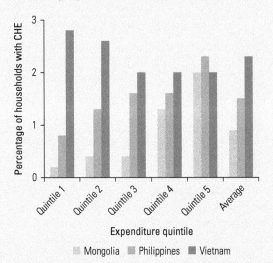

Figure B6.2.2 Proportion of Households Impoverished Owing to Health Expenditures in Selected Asian Countries, by Expenditure Quintile, Various Years

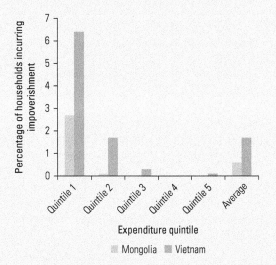

Sources: Tsilaajav, Nanzad, and Ichinnorov 2015, based on data from the 2012 Mongolia Household Socio-Economic Survey; Ulep and dela Cruz 2013, based on data from the 2012 Philippines Family and Income Expenditure Survey; Minh and Phuong 2016, based on data from the 2014 Vietnam Living Standards Survey.

Sources: Tsilaajav, Nanzad, and Ichinnorov 2015, based on data from the 2012 Mongolia Household Socio-Economic Survey; Ulep and dela Cruz 2013, based on data from the 2012 Philippines Family and Income Expenditure Survey; Minh and Phuong 2016, based on data from the 2014 Vietnam Living Standards Survey. *Note:* For the Philippines, the national average proportion of impoverishment owing to health expenditures was 1.0 percent. Analyses by quintile are not available.

expenditure quintiles, with Vietnam at 6.4 percent and Mongolia at 2.3 percent in the lowest expenditure quintile (figure B6.2.2).

Given differences in the data sources, methods, recall periods, and survey years, there are limitations comparing results across countries. However, these country-specific studies offer evidence for monitoring the effects of universal health coverage, including health service use and financial protection. Further research and cross-country comparisons should focus on examining the shock and cumulative effects of the burden of health payments, particularly for poor and vulnerable populations and for households with members who are aging or have chronic diseases, where the effect of these outcomes is likely greater.

The poorest quintile of populations and older adults continue to be at greater risk than the general population (Goeppel and others 2016).

Much of the work in this field has focused on describing the burden associated with catastrophic and impoverishing health expenditure at the population level, illuminating the problem, and mobilizing support for population-wide initiatives such as universal health coverage. A limitation of the research to date is its use of population-based data that lack detailed indicators of the health status, including specific diseases, of individuals in the households under study. Research on the economic burden associated with particular diseases is needed to understand how specific diseases, especially those that are chronic, affect the economic well-being of households.

Population-based estimates of CHE using data from household surveys have been found to vary substantially from research in populations with chronic diseases. For instance, in Vietnam, population-level surveys found that 2.3 percent of all households had CHE in 2014 (box 6.2), whereas studies of individuals with diabetes (Smith-Spangler, Bhattacharya, and Goldhaber-Fiebert 2012), acute myocardial infarction (Jan and others 2016), and HIV/AIDS (Tran and others 2013) found that 8 percent, 38 percent, and 35 percent, respectively, had CHE. In China, population-level surveys found that 13 percent of all households had CHE in 2008 (Y. Li and others 2012), whereas studies of individuals with stroke (Heeley and others 2009), diabetes (Smith-Spangler, Bhattacharya, and Goldhaber-Fiebert 2012), and acute myocardial infarction (Jan and others 2016) found that 71 percent, 80 percent, and 15 percent, respectively, had CHE. This difference between population-level and disease-related estimates of CHE has also been found in both high-income countries (Essue and others 2011; Essue and others 2014; Schoen and others 2010) and other LMICs (Huffman and others 2011; Saito and others 2014; Xu and others 2003).

The household economic burden of ill health is not simply a population-level problem; it is also highly influenced by the disease course of individual conditions. Understanding variations in outcomes within populations can help decision makers identify the highest-risk populations, account for the ways in which different conditions affect patients and their households, and generate economic incentives for preventing and managing disease.

PREVALENCE ESTIMATES OF CATASTROPHIC HEALTH EXPENDITURE ASSOCIATED WITH CHRONIC ILL HEALTH AND INJURIES IN LMICS

This section analyzes the prevalence of CHE related to chronic ill health and injuries in LMICs and the way it differs among regions. The analysis is based on a systematic search of studies that reported rates of CHE associated with the treatment and management of seven conditions:

- *Cancers:* Breast, uterine, cervical, colorectal, mouth, pharynx, ovarian, stomach and tracheal, and bronchial or lung
- *CVDs:* CVD (undefined), angina, heart disease, acute coronary syndrome, acute myocardial infarction, stroke, cerebrovascular disease (undefined), and ischemic heart disease
- *Chronic infectious diseases:* HIV/AIDS, malaria, tuberculosis, and hepatitis B
- *Endocrine diseases:* Diabetes and endocrine disease (undefined, but not diabetes)
- *Injuries:* Injuries caused by assault, blunt objects, burns, falls, road traffic accidents, and sharp objects
- *Renal diseases:* Chronic kidney disease and kidney disease (undefined).
- *Respiratory diseases:* Asthma, chronic obstructive pulmonary disease, and pulmonary disease (undefined).

Table 6.2 Global Burden of Disease, by Category of Disease, 2012

Disease category	Percentage of total global burden of disease[a]
Infectious diseases	15.8
Cardiovascular diseases	14.4
Injuries	11.1
Cancers	8.2
Respiratory diseases	5.0
Endocrine diseases	2.2
Renal diseases	1.1
Total	57.8

Source: WHO 2014.
a. Measured using disability-adjusted life year.

We initially included maternal, infant, and childhood conditions and mental illnesses in the search, but excluded them from the analysis, because too few studies reported rates of CHE for these conditions. From a broader perspective, the remaining seven categories of disease constitute almost 60 percent of the total global burden of disease, as shown in table 6.2.

Methodology

This discussion is based on a systematic search of studies that reported rates of CHE associated with the treatment and management of chronic ill health and injuries. The detailed search strategy and the equations used for the calculations are described in online annex 6A, along with the characteristics of the studies identified in the search.

One issue that arose is the lack of consensus in the measurement of CHE. A commonly used approach is to measure the household's total annual expenditure on health care or health-related expenses (for example, transport) as a proportion of the household's resources, measured in terms of income, expenditure, or consumption (O'Donnell and others 2007). Household resources as the denominator in this equation may involve a measure of either nondiscretionary expenditure (Wagstaff and van Doorslaer 2003) or capacity to pay (Xu and others 2003), both of which define CHE in terms of nonfood expenditure. In this analysis, we note the CHE definitions and thresholds used in each study but nonetheless include each as essentially the same outcome when calculating the prevalence of CHE associated with each condition.

Summary of Findings

The systematic search identified 41 studies (42 published papers) that reported rates of disease-related CHE.

Most studies used a cross-sectional design (30), recruiting either a convenience sample (22) or a random sample (18) from either a health care facility or a hospital (26) or from households in the community (14); 1 study used administrative data. The studies were conducted between 1997 and 2013, with 14 conducted between 2010 and 2013. Of these 41 studies, 7 were conducted in high-income countries (2 in Australia, 1 in Greece, 2 in the Republic of Korea, and 2 in the United States). This analysis focuses only on LMICs.

Most of the studies were conducted in middle-income countries, clustered in South and East Asia; the greatest numbers were conducted in China (8) and India (6) (map 6.1). Endocrine diseases and CVDs were the most studied conditions (table 6.3), which is reasonably consistent with the 20 leading causes of disease burden (Global Burden of Disease Study 2013 Collaborators 2015). Data coverage from the systematic search was best for countries in the upper-middle-income group; the greatest gaps were for research on renal and respiratory diseases (see online annex 6A, table 6A.4).

Map 6.1 Density of Studies on Disease-Related Catastrophic Health Expenditure

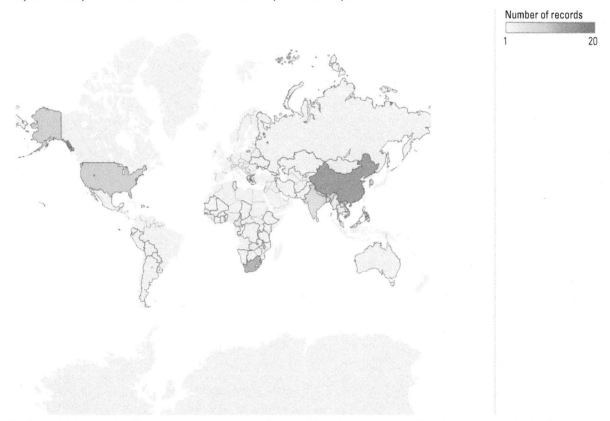

Number of records

1   20

Note: The map includes studies found for all country income categories. For multicountry studies, each country is represented in the figure so the total number of studies depicted exceeds the number of studies identified in the systematic search.

Table 6.3 Density of Conditions for the Study of Disease-Related Catastrophic Health Expenditure, by Country Income Group

Disease	Country income group		
	Low-income	Lower-middle-income	Upper-middle-income
Endocrine diseases	7	17	10
Cardiovascular diseases	5	9	7
Cancers	1	5	5

table continues next page

Table 6.3 Density of Conditions for the Study of Disease-Related Catastrophic Health Expenditure, by Country Income Group **(continued)**

Disease	Country income group		
	Low-income	Lower-middle-income	Upper-middle-income
Chronic infectious diseases	3	4	6
Injuries	1	2	—
Maternal, infant, and childhood conditions	—	2	1
Renal diseases	—	—	1
Respiratory diseases	—	1	—
Mental illnesses	—	1	—
Multiple conditions	—	—	1

Note: The number in each cell is the count of studies of each condition identified in the review. Some studies included multiple conditions and different countries, and thus the total count in this table exceeds the total number of articles reviewed. — = none.

All studies collected data on out-of-pocket payments for direct medical expenses, although the categories of expenses collected varied somewhat. Where specified, most studies collected data on medicines (30), and more than half collected data on hospitalizations (24) and medical consultations (27). Nonmedical costs (travel, accommodation, care expenses) were taken into account in 19 studies and lost productivity in 4 studies.

CHE was most commonly measured in terms of a household's capacity to pay, defined as total expenditure net of food expenses (Xu and others 2003), followed by income thresholds and total expenditure (figure 6.2). By condition category, the ranges in CHE rates were as follows:

- **Cancers:** 6.2 percent (cancer, undefined, Republic of Korea) to 67.9 percent (cancer, undefined, the Islamic Republic of Iran)
- **CVDs:** 0.05 percent (heart disease, Nepal) to 84.3 percent (CVD, Tanzania)
- **Chronic infectious diseases:** 7.1 percent (malaria, South Africa) to 90.0 percent (HIV/AIDS, the Lao People's Democratic Republic)
- **Endocrine diseases:** 1.0 percent (diabetes, Nepal) to 26.6 percent (diabetes, Ecuador)
- **Injuries:** 0.8 percent (injury, undefined, Nepal) to 46 percent (road traffic injury, India).
- **Maternal, infant, and childhood conditions:** 1.0 percent (rotavirus, Malaysia) to 44.8 percent (rotavirus, Bolivia)
- **Mental illnesses:** 5.5 percent (depressive disorders, India)
- **Renal diseases:** 9.8 percent (kidney disease, the United States) to 71.0 percent (chronic kidney disease, Australia)
- **Respiratory diseases:** 3.0 percent (asthma, Myanmar) to 46.0 percent (chronic obstructive pulmonary disease, Australia).

Rates of CHE from studies based on samples from hospitals or health care facilities were significantly higher than those from studies based on samples from households or communities for each World Bank income category (low-income: $\bar{x}_{diff}$, 56.2; t = 5.00, p = 0.007; lower-middle-income: $\bar{x}_{diff}$, 27.1; t = 4.97, p < 0.0001; upper-middle-income: $\bar{x}_{diff}$, 26.5; t = 3.75, p < 0.0001). This difference is not surprising, because hospitals are not an unbiased source of population data on health expenditure.

Overall, across all LMICs, the largest population experiencing CHE comprised persons with renal diseases (187.7 million), followed by CVDs (138.4 million), chronic infectious diseases (101.9 million), endocrine diseases (46.0 million), cancers (14.3 million), respiratory diseases (9.6 million), and injuries (0.9 million). In upper-middle-income countries, the largest population experiencing CHE comprised persons with renal diseases (100.6 million), followed by CVDs (78.2 million), chronic infectious diseases (74.2 million), endocrine diseases (22.4 million), cancers (11.9 million), respiratory diseases (8.2 million), and injuries (0.5 million). In lower-middle-income countries, the largest population experiencing CHE comprised persons with renal diseases (83.3 million), followed by CVDs (59.9 million), endocrine diseases (23.3 million), and chronic infectious diseases (6.2 million). In low-income countries, chronic infectious diseases were associated with the greatest burden of CHE (21.4 million), followed by renal diseases (3.8 million), CVDs (0.4 million), and endocrine diseases (0.3 million) (figure 6.3).

In a sensitivity analysis, we calculated the populations with CVD-related CHE using only studies that measured CHE defined as health care expenditures in excess of 40 percent of the household's capacity to pay. We found

Figure 6.2 Catastrophic Health Expenditure Rates, by Source and Disease Category

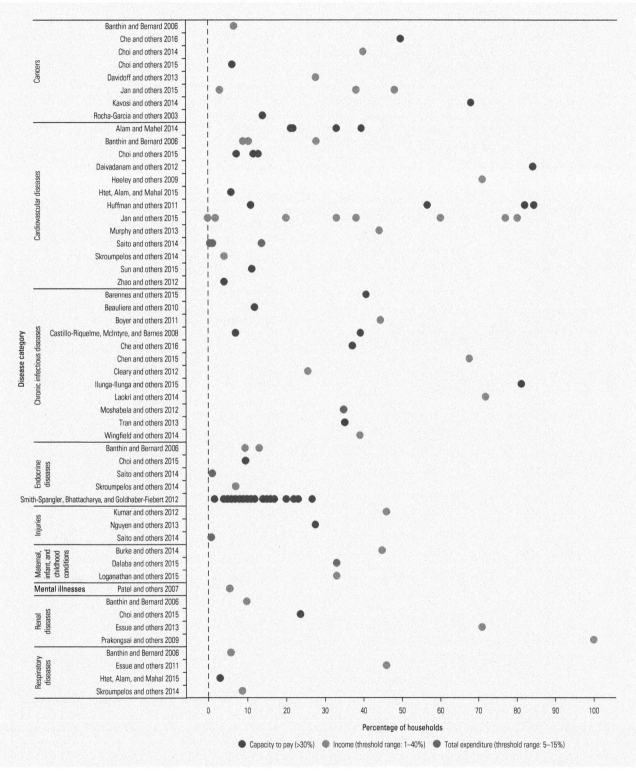

Note: For most studies, capacity to pay was defined as in Xu and others (2003). Different data were used to calculate the denominator for each catastrophic health expenditure (CHE) outcome (capacity to pay, income, total expenditure), so standardizing the estimates to a common benchmark was not possible. Each threshold of CHE was used to denote an event of catastrophic significance for the individual patient or household under investigation. Because they are linked through a common conceptual construct and as a way to allow for comparisons of the burden of CHE across the range of diseases, the varying thresholds used in each study are noted here but are treated as essentially the same outcome in this analysis. The CHE rate of 100 percent, reported for renal replacement therapy in Thailand (Prakongsai and others 2009), was excluded from the calculation of the case catastrophe rate for renal diseases.

no significant difference in case catastrophe rates and the prevalence of CVD-related CHE for all regions when the analysis was limited to studies using this common definition (table 6.4).

Figure 6.4 summarizes the case catastrophe rate relative to the prevalence of each category of condition. The case catastrophe rate is the population-weighted average CHE rate for each condition and World Bank income category. The large estimated burden of CHE predicted to be associated with renal diseases is explained by the high prevalence of disease and the high case catastrophe rate in populations with prevalent disease; renal diseases affect many individuals and are associated with a high burden because of the type of care required. Those circumstances also apply to chronic infectious

diseases and CVDs. The case catastrophe rate for injuries is lower in low-income countries than in the other country income groups, despite the high prevalence of injuries. This variation is in contrast to cancers, where the prevalence of disease is relatively lower, so the main driver of the prevalence of cancer-related CHE is the high case catastrophe rate associated with the treatment and management of these conditions in all national income groups.

OTHER MEASURES OF HOUSEHOLD-LEVEL ECONOMIC EFFECT OF CHRONIC ILL HEALTH AND INJURIES IN LMICS

In this section, we report data from a review of the disease-related burden associated with indicators other than CHE: impoverishing health expenditure, productivity effects, distressed financing, and treatment discontinuation (table 6.1). These indicators supplement and complement the measurement of CHE, because they help describe the effect of ill health on a household's economic well-being (Moreno-Serra, Millett, and Smith 2011; Ruger 2012), including the way households respond, opportunity costs, and the effect of forgone income. The indicators also tend to focus on the effect of ill health on the poorest of the poor, who may be omitted from other measures, including CHE, because their income is so low.

We did not estimate the disease-related prevalence associated with each indicator, as done for CHE, given insufficient data. We thus restrict this discussion to a descriptive analysis. The populations affected by these other measures are not mutually exclusive, so there is significant overlap with the population estimates of disease-related CHE reported in the previous section.

A systematic review of 47 LMIC studies was conducted to evaluate the household economic effect of NCDs.

Figure 6.3 Estimated Population with Catastrophic Health Expenditures Related to Chronic Ill Health and Injuries, by Disease Category and Country Income Group

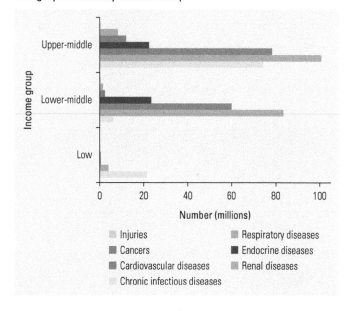

Legend:
- Injuries
- Cancers
- Cardiovascular diseases
- Chronic infectious diseases
- Respiratory diseases
- Endocrine diseases
- Renal diseases

Table 6.4 Sensitivity Analysis: Comparison of Case Catastrophe Rates and the Projected Population with Cardiovascular Disease–Related Catastrophic Health Expenditure

Country income level	All definitions of CHE[a]		Definition limited to CHE as > 40% of household's capacity to pay	
	Case catastrophe rate (%)	Population with CVD-related CHE	Case catastrophe rate (%)	Population with CVD-related CHE
Low	8.1	162,163	6.6	131,398
Lower-middle	21.2	22,065,683	21.0	21,829,842
Upper-middle	51.9	78,153,956	46.9	70,665,614

Note: CHE = catastrophic health expenditure; CVD = cardiovascular disease.

a. Catastrophic health expenditure was defined as (a) more than 40 percent of household capacity to pay (or nonfood expenditure); (b) more than 10 percent of household expenditure; (c) more than 40 percent of effective income; or (d) more than 30 percent of household income in the published studies.

Figure 6.4 Rate of Catastrophic Health Expenditure Relative to Average Prevalence of Each Condition, by Country Income Group

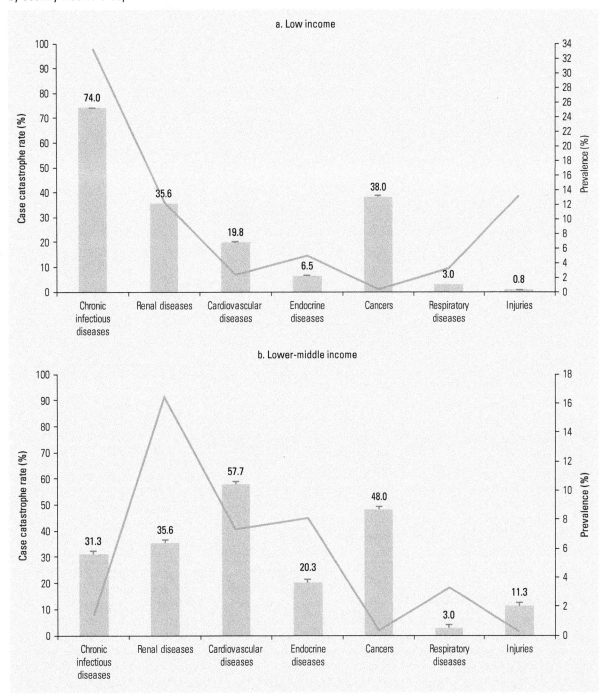

figure continues next page

Figure 6.4 (continued)

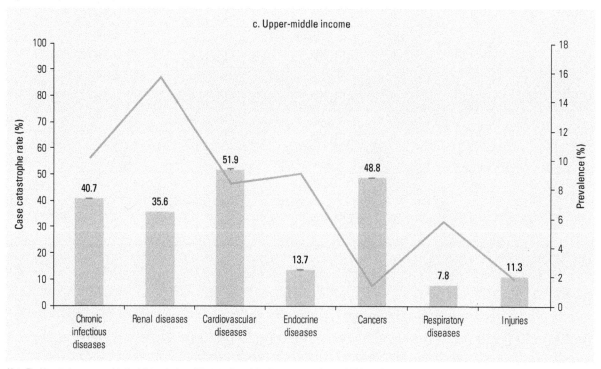

Note: The blue stacks correspond to the left-hand axis and illustrate the weighted case catastrophe rate (%) for each condition, in each country income category. The blue line corresponds to the right-hand axis and illustrates the average weighted prevalence of each condition, in each country income category. The t-bars illustrate the 95 percent confidence intervals for the weighted case catastrophe rates, in cases where they could be calculated.

The methods are described in annex 6B. The systematic review synthesized evidence from studies in populations of patients with NCDs. Of the 47 studies identified, 11 overlapped with the studies identified in the previously described systematic search. CHE was the most commonly measured outcome. However, several studies also incorporated additional indicators of the economic burden of NCDs on households.

Impoverishing Health Expenditure

Although impoverishing health expenditure is now routinely investigated in many population-based studies, including alongside CHE, few studies have investigated the disease-related burden. In the review of NCD studies in LMICs, seven studies measured the rate of NCD-related impoverishing health expenditure. Across the studies, the rate of impoverishment was below 15 percent. However, in a study conducted among Chinese people experiencing hypertension, stroke, or coronary heart disease, the incidence of impoverishment hovered around 50 percent and was not statistically different after implementation of the national health insurance scheme (J. Wang and others 2012; figure 6.5).

Productivity Changes

Six studies examined the effect of chronic diseases, particularly CVDs, on an individual's capacity to maintain usual working status. In some settings, more than 80 percent of patients affected by CVDs reported having to limit their usual work activities and more than 60 percent reported having to work less. In addition to the effect on individuals' productivity, one study conducted across four countries also found that family members had to increase their work activities or find new work. Whether such changes in productivity are different for households that are experiencing disease than for those that are not is unclear. For instance, a study conducted in India found that the decreases in workforce participation of individuals experiencing angina were not significantly different from those of households not experiencing disease (Alam and Mahal 2014).

By contrast, a study by Zhang, Chongsuvivatwong, and Geater (2006) found that the presence of major chronic illness resulted in a 6.5 percent decrease in the probability of remaining in paid work in China. Similarly, although the workforce participation rates of cancer-affected households were significantly lower than those

Figure 6.5 Proportion of Households with Noncommunicable Diseases Experiencing Impoverishing Health Expenditure, by Disease Category and Country Income Group

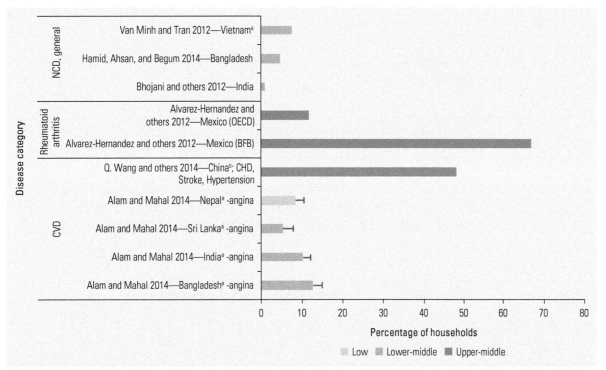

Note: BFB = the proportion of households was calculated using the basic food basket method as the threshold; CVD = cardiovascular disease; NCD = noncommunicable disease; OECD = the proportion of households was calculated using the Organisation for Economic Co-operation and Development definition for poverty as the threshold. The t-bars illustrate the 95 percent confidence intervals for the estimate (percentage of households), in cases where they could be calculated.
a. Statistically significant difference was found between those with and those without disease.
b. No statistically significantly difference was found between those with and those without disease

of non-cancer-affected households, when an individual with cancer was removed from consideration, there were no discernible differences between households with and without disease. In spite of this finding, although the incidence of work-related changes was captured, very few studies valued these changes in monetary terms (figure 6.6).

Distressed Financing

Six studies attempted to quantify the financing strategies used to pay for health care for NCDs, including CVDs and cancers. Whereas in one study, almost all households relied on savings to finance their health care (Bhojani and others 2013), more commonly, households reported selling assets or calling on family and friends. This circumstance was especially evident in the most socioeconomically disadvantaged households (Huffman and others 2011). The few studies that compared households with and without disease found that these strategies were needed more often in households confronted with chronic disease (Alam and Mahal 2014; figure 6.7).

Treatment Discontinuation

An obvious consequence of unaffordable health care is treatment attrition or abandonment (Arora, Eden, and Pizer 2007; Israels and others 2008; Jan and others 2015). For example, in a study of CVD patients in Argentina, China, India, and Tanzania, up to 99 percent of households reported not taking CVD medications because of the cost (Huffman and others 2011). Similarly, in a study conducted among diabetes-affected households across 35 LMICs, less than 30 percent of individuals were in possession of medications in 71 percent of countries (Smith-Spangler, Bhattacharya, and Goldhaber-Fiebert 2012). This outcome was not routinely examined within studies of NCD-related CHE. The relationship between CHE and treatment discontinuation is important for discerning whether trends in health care expenditure, and CHE in particular, have been affected by the discontinuation or avoidance of necessary health care by households or individuals when faced with unaffordable costs. This is highly relevant for the treatment of chronic conditions in cases where treatment attrition or abandonment can lead to further deterioration of health and higher health care costs.

Figure 6.6 Proportion of Households with Noncommunicable Diseases Reporting Productivity Effects, by Disease Category and Country Income Group

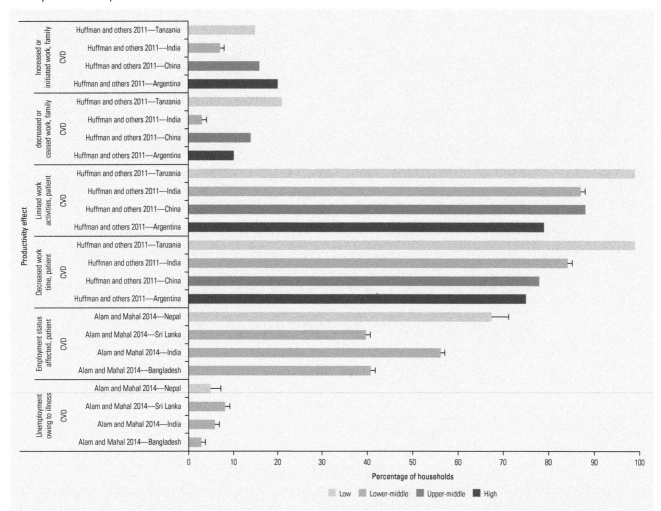

Note: CVD = cardiovascular disease. The t-bars illustrate the 95 percent confidence intervals for the estimate (percentage of households), in cases where they could be calculated.

DISCUSSION

Patients with chronic conditions and injuries in LMICs face a substantial economic burden as a result of paying for health care. Chronic conditions such as renal, cardiovascular, and endocrine diseases account for the largest populations with CHE. However, in low-income countries individuals with chronic infectious diseases such as HIV/AIDS, tuberculosis, and malaria are the largest populations with CHE.

The factors underlying these estimates are both prevalence of disease and rates of CHE associated with each category of conditions. For example, the comparatively higher burden associated with renal conditions in all settings is likely explained by the fact that renal disease is an end product of other NCDs, notably diabetes and CVDs. These precursory NCDs are undertreated (Khatib and

others 2016; Lange and others 2004; W. Li and others 2016), and the costs associated with treating renal disease are high, including the costs of medicines and dialysis (Teerawattananon and others 2016; White and others 2008).

The high costs of treatment for different conditions are due to factors such as place of treatment and out-of-pocket costs for different types of treatment. For example, out-of-pocket costs associated with hospitalization for an acute event may be high, as for conditions such as stroke in China (Heeley and others 2009) and acute myocardial infarction in both China and India (Jan and others 2016). However, paying for treatment that is required on an ongoing basis can also lead to a high cost burden, whether the payments are marginal, such as paying for medicines or, at a more extreme end, the cost of regular dialysis for managing chronic kidney

Figure 6.7 Proportion of Households with Noncommunicable Disease Using Distressed Financing Strategies, by Disease Category and Country Income Group

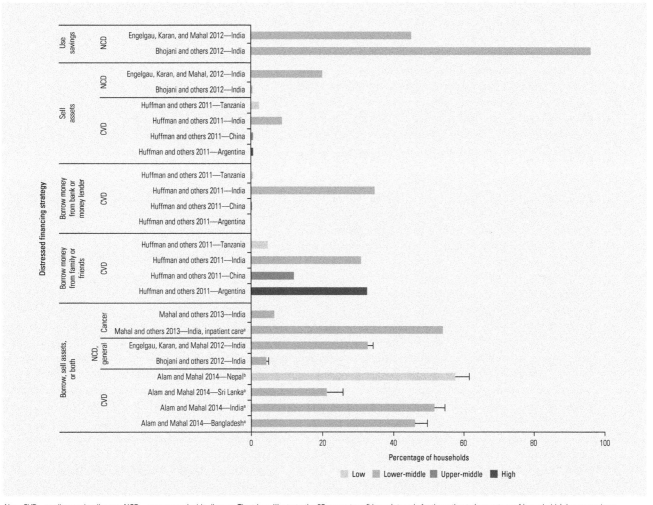

Note: CVD = cardiovascular disease; NCD = noncommunicable disease. The t-bars illustrate the 95 percent confidence intervals for the estimate (percentage of households), in cases where they could be calculated.

a. Statistically significant difference was found between those with and those without disease.

b. No statistically significantly difference was found between those with and those without disease.

disease (Prakongsai and others 2009; Ramachandran and Jha 2013).

Endocrine diseases and injuries in low-income settings both have relatively high prevalence but comparatively lower rates of CHE. For injuries, although the costs associated with treating an acute episode in either a hospital or a community health setting may be high, ongoing health care costs after recovery may be minimal. However, if the severity of the injury affects the individual's ability to continue in paid work, the household may still experience negative economic consequences from this loss of income, which is not captured in the CHE measures. In addition, in low-income countries, survival rates from injuries such as those resulting

from traffic accidents are lower (Dalal and others 2013), so the risk of incurring CHE is lower.

HIV/AIDS, like other long-term illnesses, is associated with a relatively higher rate of CHE, likely because of the ongoing costs of medicines in settings where access to free antiretroviral treatment is suboptimal. For cancers, the prevalence of disease is relatively lower, both overall and in each country income category, but the cost burden is comparatively high because of treatment costs associated with chemotherapy, radiation, and surgery (Aggarwal and Sullivan 2014; Pramesh and others 2014).

In the context of an increasing prevalence of multiple morbidity, estimated at 7.8 percent in LMICs (Afshar and others 2015), such high levels of expenditure associated with one condition would potentially compromise an individual's ability to afford the range of care that is required when faced with multiple morbidity. This circumstance could lead to trade-offs, including a prioritization of treatment for acute conditions over chronic care, especially in cases where conditions are asymptotic.

There is substantial variation in the cost burden and risk of CHE associated with chronic conditions and injuries in cases where expenditures are often repeated and continuous. Curbing the rates of CHE will require targeting financial risk protection to cover elements of treatment for conditions with high risk of CHE and high prevalence, such as renal diseases and CVDs. In low-income settings, additional protection might be required for major infectious diseases. Identifying the elements of treatment that impose the greatest cost burden, which may be common across various disease categories, will help achieve the greatest gains in mitigating the risk of CHE at a population level.

Global work, especially from the WHO, has highlighted the significant household economic burden that is associated with accessing and using health care services, particularly in LMICs. In addition, it has been a driving force in efforts to implement effective financial protection mechanisms to mitigate this burden. Comparability of our results with WHO global estimates of the prevalence of CHE depends on the relative distribution of chronic diseases, injuries, and comorbidity within the population-level data used to generate the estimates. The rates of CHE are much higher when measured in the population with disease than in the population as a whole. Our analysis, which uses samples of persons with disease, shows that many more people in LMICs and globally are at risk of CHE than previously estimated (Xu and others 2007). Furthermore, the estimates reported here for each category of conditions are not cumulative, given the high prevalence of multiple morbidity overall and the overlapping of comorbid conditions between disease categories included in this analysis.

LIMITATIONS OF THE RESEARCH

Comparability among Countries and Health Care System Contexts

The economic burden associated with health care expenses is context specific. Differences in the financing and service provision arrangements among health care systems in each country may influence the populations and the breadth of services covered, the mix of private and publicly funded services, and the out-of-pocket costs associated with health care use. In addition, despite advances in evidence-based medicine and its contribution toward mitigating variations in health care practice among settings, the disease-specific treatment options that are available and that constitute best practice may vary among (and within) countries. These differences ultimately influence the generalizability and interpretation of the individual estimates.

Differences in Measurement of CHE

The studies consulted measured CHE using different definitions, thresholds, and categories of expenditure included as out-of-pocket costs, different data sources, and different recall periods, which potentially introduced measurement error. However, the findings from a sensitivity analysis indicated that our results were robust despite the combining of varied estimates.

Differences in Quality and Breadth of Evidence

Given the lack of comprehensive evidence on the level of CHE in different populations, estimates for one setting sometimes were based on data extrapolated from studies conducted in other settings. In cases where data on the prevalence of CHE for any particular country income category were missing, we applied a conservative strategy of using the estimate from the next-highest income category. In addition, the results describe the relative burden of disease-related CHE between conditions and country-income categories but not the potential distributional burden within the populations in each category.

Much of the evidence on the disease-related burden of CHE is from cross-sectional studies that lack a control group and cannot capture repeat expenditures, so they are limited in their ability to attribute CHE directly to the disease or injuries. In addition, the smaller, clinic-based studies may not be fully representative of the population with disease in each country. Despite their limitations, these studies are the sole source of evidence and provide a starting point from which to investigate differences in the burden of CHE among different categories of chronic conditions.

The evidence also tends to come from smaller studies of cohorts recruited from hospitals or health care facilities, which can lead to higher estimates of health care expenditure than those based on community or household samples (Lavado, Brooks, and Hanlon 2013; Raban, Dandona, and Dandona 2013). Hospital expenses may explain some of this difference, because the samples in hospitals are a biased (nonrandom) sample of the population. Moreover, household samples were asked to report costs associated with previous hospitalizations, which suggests that recall bias may be stronger in the community-based studies than in the clinic- or hospital-based studies.

POLICY DIRECTIONS FOR IMPROVING FINANCIAL PROTECTION

As the epidemiological transition progresses over the next few decades, the double burden of infectious diseases and NCDs will continue to challenge health care systems in LMICs, which will be confronted with caring for older and more costly populations. Catastrophic and impoverishing health expenditure will increase globally unless action is taken to offer deeper packages of financial protection that include the treatment of chronic disease and injury. In formulating measures to address this issue, policy makers focus on universal health coverage, which aims to provide population-wide protection through various social health protection mechanisms. However, given severe resource constraints, such programs are often able to provide only limited protection of certain diseases and treatments; achieving comprehensive financial protection will inevitably be a long-term goal. The design of the package of entitlements and covered services should take into account both the populations most at risk and the diseases and conditions that drive catastrophic and impoverishing health expenditure. Country examples exist of how to implement this through progressive universalism (Gwatkin and Ergo 2011; Jamison and others 2013); one example, about which much has been written, is the catastrophic expenditure fund of Mexico's Seguro Popular (Knaul, Arreola-Ornelas, and Méndez-Carniado 2016).

In this study, we identify significant variation in the household economic burden by condition. The high burden observed for many chronic conditions such as renal diseases indicates potential areas where targeted programs could be developed to address the populations currently experiencing the greatest financial burden. These results suggest that universal health coverage should be developed as part of a multipronged strategy that addresses not only system-level drivers of the household economic burden but also disease-specific drivers. For individual diseases, basic packages should include specific interventions that are shown to be effective—for example, low-cost dialysis (Liyanage and others 2015) and polypill treatments for CVD (Webster and Rodgers 2016) as well as disease management and prevention strategies.

The research on disease-related CHE tends to be clustered in areas that do not necessarily reflect the diseases that have the greatest burden and largest household economic effect. Under-researched areas such as mental illness should not be overlooked when developing strategies to improve financial risk protection.

This study has important implications for the design of benefit packages. The conventional approach has been to place cost-effectiveness or best buys as the overriding consideration in designing benefit packages (Chisholm and others 2012; Evans and Etienne 2010; WHO and World Economic Forum 2011). The rationale for this approach is strong: given severe resource constraints, priority needs to be given to funding programs that deliver the greatest health outcomes for the dollar. However, although this approach promotes the objective of health maximization, it does not directly address the problem that such benefit packages are designed to address—that is, financial protection. This study provides evidence to guide policy makers in the design of benefit packages and entitlements. It demonstrates the need to prioritize the relative financial burden across disease areas and in different settings to ensure coverage of the disease-specific health care and health-related services that are most associated with catastrophic and impoverishing health expenditure (Jamison and others 2013).

This research also highlights the need for an ongoing focus on and investment in prevention. The most effective way to reduce disease-related CHE is to prevent such conditions. This prevention is particularly critical in LMICs, where the double burden of infectious diseases and NCDs continues to place a major strain on health care systems. Evidence from the extended cost-effectiveness literature has demonstrated the gains to be made in strengthening financial protection through investment in prevention. Public financing of programs such as vaccination for human papillomavirus infection and management of risk factors, such as obesity for diabetes and hypertension for CVD, have been shown to have the potential to curb catastrophic and impoverishing health expenditure significantly, thereby enhancing financial protection across populations (Levin and others 2015; Verguet and others 2015).

Addressing the factors that lead to and perpetuate entrenched poverty will also produce the greatest gains in mitigating the economic burden of chronic ill health experienced by households. Rates of catastrophic and impoverishing health expenditure should decline over time as universal health coverage is implemented alongside other poverty reduction strategies, including efforts to meet the Sustainable Development Goals. These efforts should reduce the burden of disease overall and improve the capacity of households to access and use required health care services. In monitoring progress, including the effect of efforts to reach the Sustainable Development Goals, priority should be given to evaluating changes in financial protection among the population as a whole as well as within subgroups most at risk of catastrophic and impoverishing health expenditure.

FUTURE RESEARCH DIRECTIONS

More prospective longitudinal studies are needed to examine the extent to which households can recover from the burden of catastrophic and impoverishing health expenditure. These types of studies, although few, have helped identify the determinants of recovery from an illness shock as well as factors that potentially enhance resilience to such shocks (Essue and others 2012; Heeley and others 2009; Jan and others 2015; Jan and others 2016; Kimman and others 2015). Prospective studies will also help distinguish between the effect and consequences of one shock versus cumulative expenditure as well as the potential for health interventions to improve household economic circumstances (Essue and others 2014; Kuper and others 2010).

Longitudinal research is also needed to monitor progress in mitigating CHE and impoverishing health expenditure. Monitoring progress using different cross-sections of population data over time cannot account well for the fact that new households may encounter CHE, while others may become nonspenders because they are no longer able to pay for care. Therefore, declines over time do not necessarily mean that health care has become more affordable for all.

Furthermore, the long-term effect on households of impoverishing health expenditure, distressed financing arrangements, changes in workforce participation, and treatment discontinuation are poorly understood. More multidimensional assessments of the household economic burden of chronic ill health are needed using routinely measured indicators along with CHE and impoverishing health expenditure (Moreno-Serra, Millet, and Smith 2011; Ruger 2012). Such studies would support the design of financial protection programs and improve the targeting of interventions, because these indicators provide greater insights into the effect of illness and health care expenditure on the household economy.

More research is needed to understand the link back to health. Although the effect of the social determinants of health is well understood (Friel and Marmot 2011), longer-term cohort studies are needed to assess how these economic consequences perpetuate the cycle of chronic ill health and social disadvantage (van Doorslaer and others 2006). Evidence on the link between the economic burden of disease, health outcomes, and social disadvantage would strengthen the economic case for improving access to affordable care.

CONCLUSIONS

In this chapter, we estimate the economic burden associated with seven categories of chronic conditions as well as injuries. We find that most CHE is due to renal, cardiovascular, and chronic infectious diseases and that the global burden of CHE is much higher than previously estimated.

Meeting the global commitment to enhance financial protection of populations, including the World Bank's goal of eliminating impoverishing health expenditure by 2030, requires a concerted effort to address the main drivers of CHE in all settings. In designing financial protection programs, policy makers need to give priority to covering populations and conditions associated with the greatest economic burden. Furthermore, needed health care services still remain out of reach for millions with disease who live in poverty. Strategies to enhance financial protection need to be implemented alongside broader poverty alleviation efforts, which collectively will generate the greatest gains in mitigating the household-level economic burden of chronic ill health globally.

ANNEXES

The annexes to this chapter are as follows. They are available at http://www.dcp-3.org/DCP.

- Annex 6A. Description of Data Sources and Search Strategy.
- Annex 6B. Search Strategy for Prospectively Designed Studies of Household Economic Effect of Chronic Disease.

NOTE

World Bank Income Classifications as of July 2014 are as follows, based on estimates of gross national income (GNI) per capita for 2013:

- Low-income countries (LICs) = US$1,045 or less
- Middle-income countries (MICs) are subdivided:
  (a) lower-middle-income = US$1,046 to US$4,125
  (b) upper-middle-income (UMICs) = US$4,126 to US$12,745
- High-income countries (HICs) = US$12,746 or more.

ACKNOWLEDGMENTS

The authors are grateful to Ke Xu for the input received on the structure and scope of this chapter early on as well as to the teams in Mongolia, the Philippines, and Vietnam for their contribution to the case studies presented in box 6.2. Financial protection information from Mongolia was taken from a WHO-commissioned report on catastrophic health payments and benefit incidence of government expenditure in Mongolia conducted by Tsolmongerel Tsilaajav, Oyungerel Nanzad, and Enkhbaatar Ichinnorov, under the coordination of Erdenechimeg Enkhee of the Office of the WHO Representative in Mongolia. We also acknowledge the contribution of Melanie Bisnauth, who provided research assistance to support the analysis in this chapter.

REFERENCES

Afshar, S., P. J. Roderick, P. Kowal, B. D. Dimitrov, and A. G. Hill. 2015. "Multimorbidity and the Inequalities of Global Ageing: A Cross-Sectional Study of 28 Countries Using the World Health Surveys." *BMC Public Health* 5 (776): 1–10. doi:10.1186/s12889-015-2008-7.

Aggarwal, A., and R. Sullivan. 2014. "Achieving Value in Cancer Care: The Case of Low- and Middle-Income Countries." *American Journal of Managed Care* 20 (12): 292–94.

Alam, K., and A. Mahal. 2014. "The Economic Burden of Angina on Households in South Asia." *BMC Public Health* 14 (February): 179.

Alvarez-Hernandez, E., I. Pelaez-Ballestas, A. Boonen, J. Vázquez-Mellado, A. Hernández-Garduño, and others. 2012. "Catastrophic Health Expenses and Impoverishment of Households of Patients with Rheumatoid Arthritis." *Reumatología Clínica* 8 (4): 168–73.

Arora, R. S., T. Eden, and B. Pizer. 2007. "The Problem of Treatment Abandonment in Children from Developing Countries with Cancer." *Pediatric Blood and Cancer* 49 (7): 941–46.

Banthin, J. S., and D. M. Bernard. 2006. "Changes in Financial Burdens for Health Care: National Estimates for the Population Younger than 65 Years, 1996 to 2003." *Journal of the American Medical Association* 296 (22): 2712–19.

Barennes, H., A. Frichittavong, M. Gripenberg, and P. Koffi. 2015. "Evidence of High Out-of-Pocket Spending for HIV Care Leading to Catastrophic Expenditure for Affected Patients in Lao People's Democratic Republic." *PLoS One* 10 (9): e0136664.

Beaglehole, R., R. Bonita, R. Horton, C. Adams, G. Alleyne, and others. 2011. "Priority Actions for the Non-Communicable Disease Crisis." *The Lancet* 377 (9775): 1438–47.

Beauliere, A., S. Toure, P. K. Alexandre, K. Koné, A. Pouhé, and others. 2010. "The Financial Burden of Morbidity in HIV-Infected Adults on Antiretroviral Therapy in Côte d'Ivoire." *PLoS One* 5 (6): e11213.

Bhojani, U., T. S. Beerenahalli, R. Devadasan, C. M. Munegowda, N. Devadasan, and others. 2013. "No Longer Diseases of the Wealthy: Prevalence and Health-Seeking for Self-Reported Chronic Conditions among Urban Poor in Southern India." *BMC Health Services Research* 13 (August): 1–10.

Bhojani, U., B. Thriveni, R. Devadasan, C. M. Munegowda, N. Devadasan, and others. 2012. "Out-of-Pocket Healthcare Payments on Chronic Conditions Impoverish Urban Poor in Bangalore, India." *BMC Public Health* 12 (990): 1–13.

Boyer, S., M. Abu-Zaineh, J. Blanche, S. Loubiere, R. C. Bonono, and others. 2011. "Does HIV Services Decentralization Protect Against the Risk of Catastrophic Health Expenditures? Some Lessons from Cameroon." *Health Services Research* 46 (6): 2029–56.

Burke, R. M., E. R. Smith, R. M. Dahl, P. A. Rebolledo, C. Calderón Mdel, and others. 2014. "The Economic Burden of Pediatric Gastroenteritis to Bolivian Families: A Cross-Sectional Study of Correlates of Catastrophic Cost and Overall Cost Burden." *BMC Public Health* 14 (June): 642.

Cameron, A., M. Ewen, D. Ross-Degnan, D. Ball, and R. Laing. 2009. "Medicine Prices, Availability, and Affordability in 36 Developing and Middle-Income Countries: A Secondary Analysis." *The Lancet* 373 (9659): 240–49.

Castillo-Riquelme, M., D. McIntyre, and K. Barnes. 2008. "Household Burden of Malaria in South Africa and Mozambique: Is there a Catastrophic Impact?" *Tropical Medicine and International Health* 13 (1): 108–22.

Che, Y. H., V. Chongsuvivatwong, L. Li, H. Sriplung, Y. Y. Wang, and others. 2016. "Financial Burden on the Families of Patients with Hepatitis B Virus–Related Liver Diseases and the Role of Public Health Insurance in Yunnan Province of China." *Public Health* 130 (January): 13–20.

Chen, S., H. Zhang, Y. Pan, Q. Long, L. Xiang, and others. 2015. "Are Free Anti-Tuberculosis Drugs Enough? An Empirical Study from Three Cities in China." *Infectious Diseases of Poverty* 4 (October): 47.

Chisholm, D., R. Baltussen, D. B. Evans, G. Ginsberg, J. A. Lauer, and others. 2012. "What Are the Priorities for Prevention and Control of Non-Communicable Diseases and Injuries in Sub-Saharan Africa and South East Asia?" *British Medical Journal* 344 (March): e586.

Choi, J.-W., K. H. Cho, Y. Choi, K. T. Han, J. A. Kwon, and others. 2014. "Changes in Economic Status of Households Associated with Catastrophic Health Expenditures for Cancer in South Korea." *Asian Pacific Journal of Cancer Prevention* 15 (6): 2713–17.

Choi, J.-W., J.-W. Choi, J.-H. Kim, K.-B. Yoo, and E.-C. Park. 2015. "Association between Chronic Disease and Catastrophic Health Expenditure in Korea." *BMC Health Services Research* 15 (1): 464–78.

Cleary, S. M., S. Birch, M. Moshabela, and H. Schneider. 2012. "Unequal Access to ART: Exploratory Results from Rural and Urban Case Studies of ART Use." *Sexually Transmitted Infections* 88 (2): 141–46.

Daivadanam, M., K. R. Thankappan, P. S. Sarma, and S. Harikrishnan. 2012. "Catastrophic Health Expenditure and Coping Strategies Associated with Acute Coronary Syndrome in Kerala, India." *Indian Journal of Medical Research* 136 (4): 585–92.

Dalaba, M. A., P. Akweongo, R. A. Aborigo, H. P. Saronga, J. Williams, and others. 2015. "Cost to Households in Treating Maternal Complications in Northern Ghana: A Cross-Sectional Study." *BMC Health Services Research* 15 (January): 34.

Dalal, K., Z. Lin, M. Gifford, and L. Svanström. 2013. "Economics of Global Burden of Road Traffic Injuries and Their Relationship with Health System Variables." *International Journal of Preventive Medicine* 4 (12): 1442–50.

Davidoff, A. J., M. Erten, T. Shaffer, J. S. Shoemaker, I. H. Zuckerman, and others. 2013. "Out-of-Pocket Health Care Expenditure Burden for Medicare Beneficiaries with Cancer." *Cancer* 119 (6): 1257–65.

Engelgau, M. M., A. Karan, and A. Mahal. 2012. "The Economic Impact of Non-Communicable Diseases on Households in India." *Globalization and Health* 8 (1): 9.

Essue, B. M., M. Hackett, Q. Li, N. Glozier, R. Lindley, and others. 2012. "How Are Household Economic Circumstances Affected after a Stroke? The Psychosocial Outcomes In StrokE (POISE) Study." *International Journal of Stroke* 7 (September): 36.

Essue, B. M., P. Kelly, M. Roberts, S. Leeder, and S. Jan. 2011. "We Can't Afford My Chronic Illness! The Out-of-Pocket Burden Associated with Managing Chronic Obstructive Pulmonary Disease in Western Sydney, Australia." *Journal of Health Services Research and Policy* 16 (4): 226–31.

Essue, B. M., M. Kimman, N. Svenstrup, K. L. Kjoege, T. L. Laba, and others. 2015. "The Effectiveness of Interventions to Reduce the Household Economic Burden of Illness and Injury: A Systematic Review." *Bulletin of the World Health Organization* 93 (2): 102–12B.

Essue, B. M., Q. Li, M. L. Hackett, L. Keay, B. Lezzi, and others. 2014. "A Multicenter Prospective Cohort Study of Quality of Life and Economic Outcomes after Cataract Surgery in Vietnam: The VISIONARY Study." *Ophthalmology* 121 (11): 2138–46.

Essue, B. M., G. Wong, J. Chapman, Q. Li, and S. Jan. 2013. "How Are Patients Managing with the Costs of Care for Chronic Kidney Disease in Australia? A Cross-Sectional Study." *BMC Nephrology* 14 (January): 5.

Evans, D. B., and C. Etienne. 2010. "Health Systems Financing and the Path to Universal Coverage." *Bulletin of the World Health Organization* 88 (6): 402.

Frenk, J., J. L. Bobadilla, J. Sepuúlveda, and M. Cervantes. 1989. "Health Transition in Middle-Income Countries: New Challenges for Health Care." *Health Policy and Planning* 4 (1): 29–39.

Friel, S., and M. G. Marmot. 2011. "Action on the Social Determinants of Health and Health Inequities Goes Global." *Annual Review of Public Health* 32 (April): 225–36.

Gelders, S., M. Ewen, N. Noguchi, and R. Laing. 2006. *Price, Availability, and Affordability: An International Comparison of Chronic Disease Medicines.* Cairo: World Health Organization Regional Office for the Eastern Mediterranean and Health Action International.

Gertler, P., and J. Gruber. 2002. "Insuring Consumption against Illness." *American Economic Review* 92 (March): 51–70.

Global Burden of Disease Study 2013 Collaborators. 2015. "Global, Regional, and National Incidence, Prevalence, and Years Lived with Disability for 301 Acute and Chronic Diseases and Injuries in 188 Countries, 1990–2013: A Systematic Analysis for the Global Burden of Disease Study 2013." *The Lancet* 386 (9995): 743–800.

Goeppel, C., P. Frenz, L. Grabenhenrich, T. Keil, and P. Tinnemann. 2016. "Assessment of Universal Health Coverage for Adults Aged 50 Years or Older with Chronic Illness in Six Middle-Income Countries." *Bulletin of the World Health Organization* 94 (4): 276–85C.

Gwatkin, D. R., and A. Ergo. 2011. "Universal Health Coverage: Friend or Foe of Health Equity?" *The Lancet* 377 (9784): 2160–61.

Hamid, S. A., S. M. Ahsan, and A. Begum. 2014. "Disease-Specific Impoverishment Impact of Out-of-Pocket Payments for Health Care: Evidence from Rural Bangladesh." *Applied Health Economics and Health Policy* 12 (4): 421–33.

Heeley, E., C. A. Anderson, Y. Huang, S. Jan, Y. Li, and others. 2009. "Role of Health Insurance in Averting Economic Hardship in Families after Acute Stroke in China." *Stroke* 40 (6): 2149–56.

Htet, S., K. Alam, and A. Mahal. 2015. "Economic Burden of Chronic Conditions among Households in Myanmar: The Case of Angina and Asthma." *Health Policy and Planning* 30 (9): 1173–83.

Huffman, M. D., K. D. Rao, A. Pichon-Riviere, D. Zhao, S. Harikrishnan, and others. 2011. "A Cross-Sectional Study of the Microeconomic Impact of Cardiovascular Disease Hospitalization in Four Low- and Middle-Income Countries." *PLoS One* 6 (6): e20821.

Human Rights Watch. 2006. "A High Price to Pay: Detention of Poor Patients in Burundian Hospitals." Human Rights Watch, September 7.

Ilunga-Ilunga, F., A. Leveque, S. Laokri, and M. Dramaix. 2015. "Incidence of Catastrophic Health Expenditures for Households: An Example of Medical Attention for the Treatment of Severe Childhood Malaria in Kinshasa Reference Hospitals, Democratic Republic of Congo." *Journal of Infection and Public Health* 8 (2): 136–44.

Israels, T., C. Chirambo, H. Caron, J. de Kraker, E. Molyneux, and others. 2008. "The Guardians' Perspective on Paediatric Cancer Treatment in Malawi and Factors Affecting Adherence." *Pediatric Blood and Cancer* 51 (5): 639–42.

Jamison, D. T., L. H. Summers, G. Alleyne, K. J. Arrow, S. Berkley, and others. 2013. "Global Health 2035: A World Converging within a Generation." *The Lancet* 382 (9908): 1898–955.

Jan, S., M. Kimman, S. A. E. Peters, and M. Woodward. 2015. "Financial Catastrophe, Treatment Discontinuation, and Death Associated with Surgically Operable Cancer in South-East Asia: Results from the ACTION Study." *Surgery* 157 (6): 971–82.

Jan, S., S. W. L. Lee, J. P. S. Sawhney, T. K. Ong, C. T. Chin, and others. 2016. "Catastrophic Health Expenditure on Acute Coronary Events in Asia: A Prospective Study." *Bulletin of the World Health Organization* 94 (3): 193–200.

Kankeu, H. T., P. Saksena, K. Xu, and D. B. Evans. 2013. "The Financial Burden from Non-Communicable Diseases in Low- and Middle-Income Countries: A Literature Review." *Health Research Policy and Systems* 11 (August): 1–12.

Kavosi, Z., H. Delavari, A. Keshtkaran, and F. Setoudehzadeh. 2014. "Catastrophic Health Expenditures and Coping Strategies in Households with Cancer Patients in

Shiraz Namazi Hospital." *Middle East Journal of Cancer* 5 (1): 13–22.

Khatib, R., M. McKee, H. Shannon, C. Chow, S. Rangarajan, and others. 2016. "Availability and Affordability of Cardiovascular Disease Medicines and their Effect on Use in High-Income, Middle-Income, and Low-Income Countries: An Analysis of the PURE Study Data." *The Lancet* 387 (10013): 61–69.

Kim, J. Y. 2014. "Speech by World Bank Group President Jim Yong Kim on Universal Health Coverage in Emerging Economies." Conference on Universal Health Coverage in Emerging Economies, Center for Strategic and International Studies, Washington, DC, January 14.

Kimman, M., S. Jan, C. H. Yip, H. Thabrany, S. A. Peters, and others. 2015. "Catastrophic Health Expenditure and 12-Month Mortality Associated with Cancer in Southeast Asia: Results from a Longitudinal Study in Eight Countries." *BMC Medicine* 13 (August): 190.

Knaul, F. M., H. Arreola-Ornelas, and O. Méndez-Carniado. 2016. "Protección financiera en salud: Actualizaciones para México a 2014." *Salud Pública de México* 58 (3): 341–50.

Knaul, F. M., H. Arreola-Ornelas, O. Méndez-Carniado, C. Bryson-Cahn, J. Barofsky, and others. 2006. "Evidence Is Good for Your Health System: Policy Reform to Remedy Catastrophic and Impoverishing Health Spending in Mexico." *The Lancet* 368 (9549): 1828–41.

Knaul, F. M., R. Wong, and H. Arreola-Ornelas, eds. 2012. *Household Spending and Impoverishment*. Vol. 1, *Financing Health in Latin America*. Cambridge, MA: Harvard Global Equity Initiative, Mexican Health Foundation, and International Development Research Centre.

Kruk, M. E., E. Goldmann, and S. Galea. 2009. "Borrowing and Selling to Pay for Health Care in Low- and Middle-Income Countries." *Health Affairs* 28 (4): 1056–66.

Kumar, G. A., T. R. Dilip, L. Dandona, and R. Dandona. 2012. "Burden of Out-of-Pocket Expenditure for Road Traffic Injuries in Urban India." *BMC Health Services Research* 12 (August): 285.

Kuper, H., S. Polack, W. Mathenge, C. Eusebio, Z. Wadud, and others. 2010. "Does Cataract Surgery Alleviate Poverty? Evidence from a Multi-Centre Intervention Study Conducted in Kenya, the Philippines, and Bangladesh." *PLoS One* 5 (11): e15431.

Lange, S., C. Diehm, H. Darius, R. Haberl, J. R. Allenberg, and others. 2004. "High Prevalence of Peripheral Arterial Disease and Low Treatment Rates in Elderly Primary Care Patients with Diabetes." *Experimental and Clinical Endocrinology and Diabetes* 112 (10): 566–73.

Laokri, S., M. Dramaix-Wilmet, F. Kassa, S. Anagonou, and B. Dujardin. 2014. "Assessing the Economic Burden of Illness for Tuberculosis Patients in Benin: Determinants and Consequences of Catastrophic Health Expenditures and Inequities." *Tropical Medicine and International Health* 19 (10): 1249–58.

Lavado, R. F., B. P. Brooks, and M. Hanlon. 2013. "Estimating Health Expenditure Shares from Household Surveys." *Bulletin of the World Health Organization* 91 (7): 519–24.

Levin, C. E., M. Sharma, Z. Olson, S. Verguet, J. F. Shi, and others. 2015. "An Extended Cost-Effectiveness Analysis of Publicly Financed HPV Vaccination to Prevent Cervical Cancer in China." *Vaccine* 33 (24): 2830–41.

Li, W., H. Gu, K. K. Teo, J. Bo, Y. Wang, and others. 2016. "Hypertension Prevalence, Awareness, Treatment, and Control in 115 Rural and Urban Communities Involving 47,000 People from China." *Journal of Hypertension* 34 (1): 39–46.

Li, Y., Q. Wu, L. Xu, D. Legge, Y. Hao, and others. 2012. "Factors Affecting Catastrophic Health Expenditure and Impoverishment from Medical Expenses in China: Policy Implications of Universal Health Insurance." *Bulletin of the World Health Organization* 90 (9): 664–71.

Liyanage, T., T. Ninomiya, V. Jha, B. Neal, H. M. Patrice, and others. 2015. "Worldwide Access to Treatment for End-Stage Kidney Disease: A Systematic Review." *The Lancet* 385 (9981): 1975–82.

Loganathan, T., W. S. Lee, K. F. Lee, M. Jit, and C. W. Ng. 2015. "Household Catastrophic Healthcare Expenditure and Impoverishment Due to Rotavirus Gastroenteritis Requiring Hospitalization in Malaysia." *PLoS One* 10 (5): e0125878.

Mahal, A., A. Karan, V. Y. Fan, and M. Engelgau. 2013. "The Economic Burden of Cancers on Indian Households." *PLoS One* 8 (8): e71853.

McIntyre, D., M. Thiede, G. Dahlgren, and M. Whitehead. 2006. "What Are the Economic Consequences for Households of Illness and of Paying for Health Care in Low- and Middle-Income Country Contexts?" *Social Science and Medicine* 62 (4): 858–65.

Minh, H. V., and N. T. P. Phuong. 2016. "Burden of Household Out-of-Pocket Health Expenditures in Vietnam." Working Paper, Hanoi School of Public Health, Hanoi.

Moreno-Serra, R., C. Millett, and P. C. Smith. 2011. "Towards Improved Measurement of Financial Protection in Health." *PLoS Medicine* 8 (9): e1001087.

Moshabela, M., H. Schneider, S. P. Silal, and S. M. Cleary. 2012. "Factors Associated with Patterns of Plural Healthcare Utilization among Patients Taking Antiretroviral Therapy in Rural and Urban South Africa: A Cross-Sectional Study." *BMC Health Services Research* 12 (July): 182.

Murphy, A., A. Mahal, E. Richardson, and A. E. Moran. 2013. "The Economic Burden of Chronic Disease Care Faced by Households in Ukraine: A Cross-Sectional Matching Study of Angina Patients." *International Journal for Equity in Health* 12 (May): 38.

Nguyen, H., R. Ivers, S. Jan, A. Martiniuk, and C. Pham. 2013. "Catastrophic Household Costs Due to Injury in Vietnam." *Injury* 44 (5): 684–90.

O'Donnell, O., E. van Doorslaer, A. Wagstaff, and M. Lindelow, eds. 2007. *Analyzing Health Equity Using Household Survey Data: A Guide to Techniques and Their Implementation.* Washington, DC: World Bank Group.

Okoli, C. I., and S. M. Cleary. 2011. "Socioeconomic Status and Barriers to the Use of Free Antiretroviral Treatment for HIV/AIDS in Enugu State, South-Eastern Nigeria." *African Journal of AIDS Research* 10 (2): 149–55.

Patel, V., D. Chisholm, B. R. Kirkwood, and D. Mabey. 2007. "Prioritizing Health Problems in Women in Developing Countries: Comparing the Financial Burden of Reproductive Tract Infections, Anaemia, and Depressive Disorders in a Community Survey in India." *Tropical Medicine and International Health* 12 (1): 130–39.

Peters, D. H., A. Garg, G. Bloom, D. G. Walker, W. R. Brieger, and others. 2008. "Poverty and Access to Health Care in Developing Countries." *Annals of the New York Academy of Sciences* 1136 (October): 161–71.

Prakongsai, P., N. Palmer, P. Uay-Trakul, V. Tangcharoensathien, and A. Mills. 2009. "The Implications of Benefit Package Design: The Impact on Poor Thai Households of Excluding Renal Replacement Therapy." *Journal of International Development* 21 (2): 291–308.

Pramesh, C. S., R. A. Badwe, B. B. Borthakur, M. Chandra, E. Hemanth Raj, and others. 2014. "Delivery of Affordable and Equitable Cancer Care in India." *The Lancet Oncology* 15 (6): e223–33.

Raban, M. Z., R. Dandona, and L. Dandona. 2013. "Variations in Catastrophic Health Expenditure Estimates from Household Surveys in India." *Bulletin of the World Health Organization* 91 (10): 726–35.

Ramachandran, R., and V. Jha. 2013. "Kidney Transplantation Is Associated with Catastrophic Out-of-Pocket Expenditure in India." *PLoS One* 8 (7): e67812.

Rocha-Garcia, A., P. Hernandez-Pena, S. Ruiz-Velazco, L. Avila-Burgos, T. Marin-Palomares, and others. 2003. "Out-of-Pocket Expenditures during Hospitalization of Young Leukemia Patients with State Medical Insurance in Two Mexican Hospitals [Spanish]." *Salud Pública de México* 45 (4): 285–92.

Ruger, J. P. 2012. "An Alternative Framework for Analyzing Financial Protection in Health." *PLoS Medicine* 9 (8): e1001294.

Russell, S. 2004. "The Economic Burden of Illness for Households in Developing Countries: A Review of Studies Focusing on Malaria, Tuberculosis, and Human Immunodeficiency Virus/Acquired Immunodeficiency Syndrome." *American Journal of Tropical Medicine and Hygiene* 71 (Suppl 2): 147–55.

Saito, E., S. Gilmour, M. M. Rahman, G. S. Gautam, P. K. Shrestha, and others. 2014. "Catastrophic Household Expenditure on Health in Nepal: A Cross-Sectional Survey." *Bulletin of the World Health Organization* 92 (10): 760–67.

Sauerborn, R., A. Adams, and M. Hien. 1996. "Household Strategies to Cope with the Economic Costs of Illness." *Social Science and Medicine* 43 (3): 291–301.

Schoen, C., R. Osborn, D. Squires, M. M. Doty, R. Pierson, and others. 2010. "How Health Insurance Design Affects Access to Care and Costs, by Income, in Eleven Countries." *Health Affairs* 29 (12): 2323–34.

Schoenberg, N. E., H. Kim, W. Edwards, and S. T. Fleming. 2007. "Burden of Common Multiple-Morbidity Constellations on Out-of-Pocket Medical Expenditures among Older Adults." *Gerontologist* 47 (4): 423–37.

Shrime, M. G., A. J. Dare, B. C. Alkire, K. O'Neill, and J. G. Meara. 2015. "Catastrophic Expenditure to Pay for Surgery Worldwide: A Modelling Study." *The Lancet Global Health* 3 (Suppl 2): S38–44.

Skroumpelos, A., E. Pavi, S. Pasaloglou, and J. Kyriopoulos. 2014. "Catastrophic Health Expenditures and Chronic Condition Patients in Greece." *Value in Health* 17 (7): A501–02.

Smith-Spangler, C. M., J. Bhattacharya, and J. D. Goldhaber-Fiebert. 2012. "Diabetes, Its Treatment, and Catastrophic Medical Spending in 35 Developing Countries." *Diabetes Care* 35 (2): 319–26.

Sun, J., T. Liabsuetrakul, Y. Fan, and E. McNeil. 2015. "Protecting Patients with Cardiovascular Diseases from Catastrophic Health Expenditure and Impoverishment by Health Finance Reform." *Tropical Medicine and International Health* 20 (12): 1846–54.

Sustainable Development Solutions Network. 2014. "Health in the Framework of Sustainable Development: Technical Report for the Post-2015 Development Agenda." Thematic Group on Health for All, Sustainable Development Solutions Network, New York.

Teerawattananon, Y., A. Luz, S. Pilasant, S. Tangsathitkulchai, S. Chootipongchaivat, and others. 2016. "How to Meet the Demand for Good Quality Renal Dialysis as Part of Universal Health Coverage in Resource-Limited Settings?" *Health Research Policy and Systems* 14 (March): 21.

Thuan, N. T., C. Lofgren, N. T. Chuc, U. Janlert, and L. Lindholm. 2006. "Household Out-of-Pocket Payments for Illness: Evidence from Vietnam." *BMC Public Health* 6 (November): 283.

Tran, B. X., A. T. Duong, L. T. Nguyen, J. Hwang, B. T. Nguyen, and others. 2013. "Financial Burden of Health Care for HIV/AIDS Patients in Vietnam." *Tropical Medicine and International Health* 18 (2): 212–18.

Tsilaajav, T., O. Nanzad, and E. Ichinnorov. 2015. "Analysis of Catastrophic Health Payments and Benefit Incidence of Government Spending for Health in Mongolia." Paper commissioned for the World Health Organization, Western Pacific Regional Office, Manila.

Ulep, G. T., and N. A. O. dela Cruz. 2013. "Analysis of Out-of-Pocket Expenditures in the Philippines." *Philippine Journal of Development* 40 (1–2d).

UN (United Nations) General Assembly. 2015. "Seventieth Session. Resolution A/RES/70/1: Transforming Our World: The 2030 Agenda for Sustainable Development." UN, New York, October 21.

van Doorslaer, E., O. O'Donnell, R. P. Rannan-Eliya, A. Somanathan, S. R. Adhikari, and others. 2006. "Effect of Payments for Health Care on Poverty Estimates in 11 Countries in Asia: An Analysis of Household Survey Data." *The Lancet* 368 (9544): 1357–64.

Van Minh, H., and B. X. Tran. 2012. "Assessing the Household Financial Burden Associated with the Chronic Non-Communicable Diseases in a Rural District of Vietnam." *Global Health Action* 5 (December): 1–7.

Verguet, S., Z. D. Olson, J. B. Babigumira, D. Desalegn, K. A. Johansson, and others. 2015. "Health Gains and Financial Risk Protection Afforded by Public Financing of Selected Interventions in Ethiopia: An Extended Cost-Effectiveness Analysis." *The Lancet Global Health* 3 (5): e288–96.

Wagstaff, A., and E. van Doorslaer. 2003. "Catastrophe and Impoverishment in Paying for Health Care: With Applications to Vietnam 1993–1998." *Health Economics* 12 (11): 921–34.

Wang, J., H. W. Zhou, Y. X. Lei, and X. W. Wang. 2012. "Financial Protection under the New Rural Cooperative Medical Schemes in China." *Medical Care* 50 (8): 700–04.

Wang, Q., H. Liu, Z. X. Lu, Q. Luo, and J. A. Liu. 2014. "Role of the New Rural Cooperative Medical System in Alleviating Catastrophic Medical Payments for Hypertension, Stroke, and Coronary Heart Disease in Poor Rural Areas of China." *BMC Public Health* 14 (1): 907.

Webster, R., and A. Rodgers. 2016. "Polypill Treatments for Cardiovascular Diseases." *Expert Opinion on Drug Delivery* 13 (1): 1–6.

White, S. L., S. J. Chadban, S. Jan, J. R. Chapman, and A. Cass. 2008. "How Can We Achieve Global Equity in Provision of Renal Replacement Therapy?" *Bulletin of the World Health Organization* 86 (3): 229–37.

WHO (World Health Organization). 2000. *World Health Report 2000: Health Systems: Improving Performance.* Geneva: WHO.

———. 2005. "World Health Assembly: Sustainable Health Financing, Universal Coverage, and Social Health Insurance." WHA58.33, WHO, Geneva.

———. 2010. *The World Health Report: Health Systems Financing: The Path to Universal Coverage.* Geneva: WHO.

———. 2014. "Global Health Estimates." WHO, Geneva.

———. 2015. "Health and Human Rights." Fact Sheet 323, WHO, Geneva.

———. 2016. Global Health Expenditure Database. WHO, Geneva (accessed August 29, 2016), http://apps.who.int/nha/database.

WHO (World Health Organization) and World Bank. 2014. "Monitoring Progress towards Universal Health Coverage at Country and Global Levels: Framework, Measures, and Targets." WHO, Geneva; World Bank, Washington, DC.

WHO (World Health Organization) and World Economic Forum. 2011. *From Burden to "Best Buys": Reducing the Economic Impact of Non-Communicable Diseases in Low- and Middle-Income Countries.* Geneva: WHO.

Wingfield, T., D. Boccia, M. Tovar, A. Gavino, K. Zevallos, and others. 2014. "Defining Catastrophic Costs and Comparing Their Importance for Adverse Tuberculosis Outcome with Multi-Drug Resistance: A Prospective Cohort Study, Peru." *PLoS Medicine* 11 (7): e1001675.

Xu, K. 2005. "Distribution of Health Payments and Catastrophic Expenditures: Methodology." Discussion Paper 2-2005, WHO, Geneva.

Xu, K., D. B. Evans, G. Carrin, A. M. Aguilar-Rivera, P. Musgrove, and others. 2007. "Protecting Households from Catastrophic Health Spending." *Health Affairs* 26 (4): 972–83.

Xu, K., D. B. Evans, K. Kawabata, R. Zeramdini, J. Klavus, and others. 2003. "Household Catastrophic Health Expenditure: A Multicountry Analysis." *The Lancet* 362 (9378): 111–17.

Zhang, J., V. Chongsuvivatwong, and A. Geater. 2006. "Clinical Severity and Financial Burden among Road Traffic Injury Patients in Kunming, China." *Southeast Asian Journal of Tropical Medicine and Public Health* 37 (5): 1034–39.

Zhao, D., W. Wang, J. Liu, M. Wang, J. Sun, and others. 2012. "The Impact of Cardiovascular Disease on Household Economic Well-Being in Chinese Population." *Circulation* 125 (19): e677–78.

Part **3**

Economic Evaluation Results from *Disease Control Priorities*, Third Edition

Chapter 7

Cost-Effectiveness Analysis in *Disease Control Priorities*, Third Edition

Susan Horton

INTRODUCTION

League tables, which rank the cost-effectiveness of health interventions, are a useful input for prioritizing health expenditures, especially for national health budgets. They have been used as policy tools for high-income countries (HICs), including a comprehensive analysis for Australia (Vos and others 2010) and a similar analysis for cancer across HICs (Greenberg and others 2010). Some low- and middle-income countries (LMICs), such as Mexico, have also used league tables in their policy-making process (Salomon and others 2012).

For LMICs as a group, two major reviews of cost-effectiveness have informed strategies to achieve the Millennium Development Goals (MDGs) (Evans and others 2005; Laxminarayan, Chow, and Shahid-Salles 2006). However, cost-effectiveness is not the only important criterion for policy choice; sustainability, equity, and affordability, among others, also matter. Nevertheless, cost-effectiveness provides a useful and comprehensible reference point.

As strategies and priorities are set for the Sustainable Development Goals and countries consider the transition to universal health coverage, updating the previous reviews for LMICs is appropriate. This chapter synthesizes the results from recent analyses in six different disease areas to provide a comprehensive, updated comparison across a broad range of conditions; to examine changes during the past 10–12 years; and to highlight research gaps.

METHODS

A database of cost and cost-effectiveness results was constructed for the first six volumes of the *Disease Control Priorities*, third edition (*DCP3*) (Black and others 2016; Debas and others 2015; Gelband and others 2015; Holmes and others 2017a; Patel and others 2015; Prabhakaran and others 2017). Systematic searches were conducted in six major health areas, supplemented by expert surveys and existing published systematic surveys and reviews (Gaziano and others 2017; Holmes and others 2017b; Horton and Gauvreau 2015; Horton and Levin 2016; Levin and Chisholm 2015; Prinja and others 2015). The surveys covered literature from 2000 to mid-2013 published in English, because the literature before 2000 had been reviewed previously (Laxminarayan, Chow, and Shahid-Salles 2006).

The searches undertaken employed keywords associated with economic outcomes, the names of all LMICs and regions, and the main disease conditions relevant for each major health area. In this chapter, we report the results per disability-adjusted life year (DALY) averted. In most *DCP3* volumes, studies were also graded according to the Drummond checklist to assess the quality of the economic analysis (Drummond and others 2005). Further details of the searches and summaries of the findings for the six major health areas are available (Gaziano and others 2017; Holmes and others 2017b; Horton and Gauvreau 2015; Horton and Levin 2016; Levin and Chisholm 2015; Prinja and others 2015).

Summary information about each of the 93 health interventions analyzed and full references for the 149 published studies are provided in annex 7A.

All costs were converted to 2012 U.S. dollars by adjusting prices to 2012 values in the original currency of the relevant country and then converting those amounts to U.S. dollars using the exchange rate for 2012. The costs for one group of studies were expressed in international dollars of a World Health Organization (WHO) region (Evans and others 2005) and could not be readily converted, because consumer price indices and exchange rates with the U.S. dollar are not publicly available for those regional aggregates. Although methods exist to make an approximate conversion, the additional information required is not always readily available from the original study, namely, the proportion of all costs (both of the intervention itself and, where relevant, of those costs averted by the intervention) accounted for by tradable and nontradable inputs.

We opted to use exchange rate conversions rather than purchasing power parity (PPP) conversions. Studies using the Choosing Interventions that are Cost-Effective (WHO-CHOICE) methodology (Evans and others 2005) have often used PPP conversions, which assume that health interventions have the same mix of tradable and nontradable inputs as the economy does overall. However, health interventions vary considerably, from those involving behavior change communication by community health workers (relying heavily on nontradable inputs) to vaccine delivery or use of rapid diagnostic tests (relying heavily on tradable inputs); no single conversion method is perfect. We opted for the exchange rate method because it is more readily understood by noneconomists, and it allows comparison with the earlier *Disease Control Priorities* work (Laxminarayan, Chow, and Shahid-Salles 2006). Using market exchange rates, however, can be problematic if they do not respond immediately to differential rates of inflation between countries.

The cost-effectiveness rankings from individual volumes were aggregated to provide two sets of league tables—one for adults and one for children. In a few cases where no study using DALYs was available for an important intervention—for example, human papillomavirus (HPV) vaccination—a study using quality-adjusted life years (QALYs) was used instead, and this substitution is indicated. A natural logarithmic scale was used for cost in the figures because small differences in cost per outcome are less important for the least cost-effective interventions, that is, those with the highest cost per outcome. For some interventions, a single study provided a point estimate for cost-effectiveness; for other interventions, multiple studies were available,

or the individual study provided a range of estimates. In the figures, the geometric mean of the endpoints of the range was the point estimate used. This approach works better for a natural log scale axis and is more appropriate when the ranges are very different.

The WHO has issued guidelines on thresholds for acceptable costs per DALY averted. The recommendation is that anything costing less than the per capita gross national income (GNI) per DALY averted is "very cost-effective" (WHO 2001); anything costing less than three times per capita GNI is "cost-effective." Recent research suggests that health budget constraints are too tight to be able to afford everything, even those items that are very cost-effective according to the WHO threshold. Accordingly, thresholds should be lower (Claxton and others 2015). Deriving a more appropriate threshold—for example, using the marginal health gain with the existing health budget—requires country-specific data. A recent analysis suggests that a threshold of approximately one-half of GNI per capita would be more appropriate for LMICs than the WHO-suggested threshold and better reflects funds that taxpayers in those countries are able and willing to spend from the public budget (Ochalek, Claxton, and Lomas 2016).

In our review, a lower threshold of US$200 per DALY is used to identify priority interventions for consideration in low-income countries (LICs); all but three countries in the World Bank database had per capita income above US$400 in 2014. A higher threshold of US$500 is used to identify priority interventions for consideration in lower-middle-income countries, all of which had per capita GNI above US$1,045 in 2014. Other considerations, such as equity, affordability, and feasibility will also be important in priority setting for individual countries, depending on the context.

RESULTS

We identified cost-effectiveness estimates for 93 interventions and contexts (figures 7.1–7.4), drawn from 149 studies. We excluded cost-effectiveness studies of tax and subsidy policies. Although broad national policy changes are very important, estimating their costs is more difficult, and their cost-effectiveness is not readily compared with that of individual health interventions.

In a few cases, the same intervention appears more than once in different contexts, with different costs per DALY averted. For example, the cost-effectiveness of HPV vaccination has been estimated at two different prices per vaccinated girl: the lower price from Gavi— the Vaccine Alliance (Gavi) is available to some lower-middle-income countries—and the usually higher price applies to countries ineligible for Gavi support.

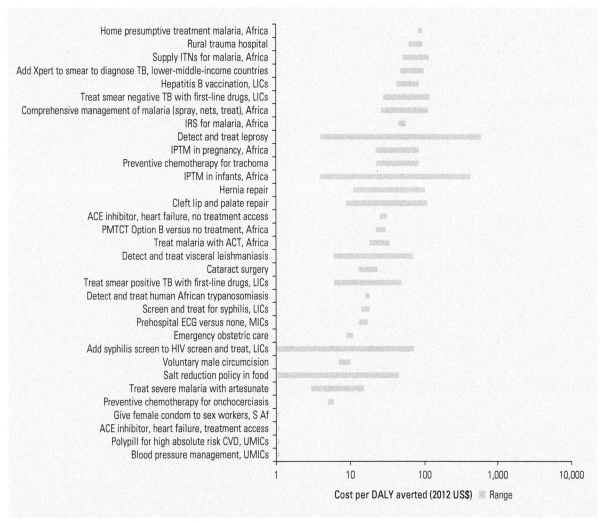

Cost per DALY averted (2012 US$) ▨ Range

Note: ACE = angiotensin converting enzyme; ACT = artemisinin-based combination therapy; CVD = cardiovascular disease; ECG = electrocardiogram; IPTM = intermittent preventive treatment for malaria; IRS = indoor residual spraying; ITNs = insecticide-treated nets; LICs = low-income countries; mgt = management; MICs = middle-income countries; Option B = use of two-drug regime for pregnancy for PMTCT; PMTCT = Prevention of Mother-to-Child Transmission of HIV; S Af = South Africa; TB = tuberculosis; UMICs = upper-middle-income countries.

Gavi has used its ability to undertake bulk purchases and multiyear commitments for vaccines to obtain favorable prices. However, only those countries eligible for Gavi support have access to these prices; other countries must negotiate prices with manufacturers.

Where relevant, the economic level of the country where the study was conducted is identified (for example, LICs as compared to lower-middle-income countries and UMICs) because human resource costs vary significantly and disease patterns are different. In other cases, particularly for the human immunodeficiency virus/acquired immune deficiency syndrome (HIV/AIDS), the epidemiologic context is identified.

The results from southern Africa, which faces a generalized epidemic in a few countries, differ from those of other countries, where the epidemic is more concentrated in certain population groups. If no context is identified, the results are expected to be generally applicable in LMICs.

Of the 93 cost-effectiveness estimates, 37 percent relate to interventions for reproductive, maternal, newborn, and child health interventions and 24 percent relate to interventions for major infectious diseases—HIV/AIDS, tuberculosis, malaria, and neglected tropical diseases (NTDs). This finding is not surprising, given that the MDGs focused on these areas of health.

Figure 7.2 Interventions Costing between US$100 and US$999 per DALY Averted for Adults

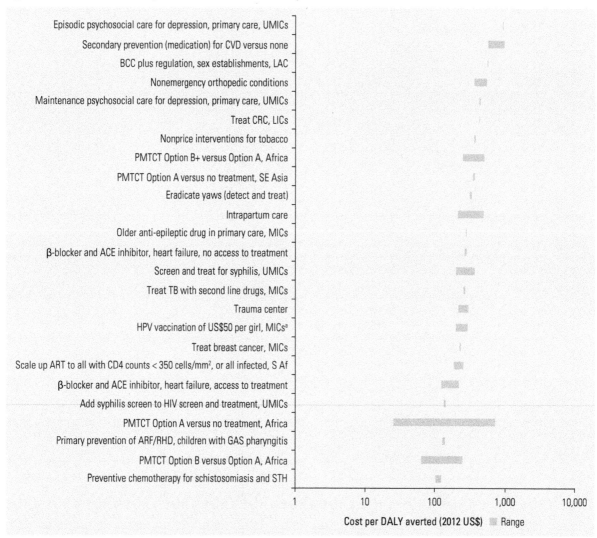

Note: ACE = angiotensin converting enzyme; ARF/RHD = acute respiratory failure/rheumatic heart disease; ART = antiretroviral therapy; BCC = behavior change communication; CRC = colorectal cancer; CVD = cardiovascular disease; HPV = human papillomavirus; LAC = Latin America and the Caribbean; LICs = low-income countries; MICs = middle-income countries; Option A = use of single-drug regime for pregnancy for PMTCT; Option B = use of two-drug regime for pregnancy for PMTCT; Option B+ = use of two-drug regime during pregnancy and then lifelong for PMTCT; PMTCT = Elimination of Mother-to-Child Transmission of HIV; STH = soil-transmitted helminths; TB = tuberculosis; UMICs = upper-middle-income countries.

a. Denotes outcome in QALYs (quality-adjusted life years).

International organizations, such as Gavi and the Global Fund to Fight AIDS, Tuberculosis, and Malaria, mobilized significant resources, leading to considerable interest in, and funding for, cost-effectiveness studies in these health areas. Far fewer economic studies are available for each of the other four areas considered: cancer, cardiovascular disease, mental health, and surgery.

Studies are typically conducted where new policy measures are being considered, such as new vaccines,

new guidelines for treatment, and new diagnostic tools. Hence, no new studies were found for well-established interventions, such as the original Expanded Program of Immunization with six vaccines. Pre-2000 studies of some of these established interventions exist. In other cases, for example, emergency appendectomy, the importance of the intervention was established long before cost-effectiveness estimates became common for LMICs, and thus, no studies were found.

Figure 7.3 Interventions Costing US$1,000 or More per DALY Averted for Adults

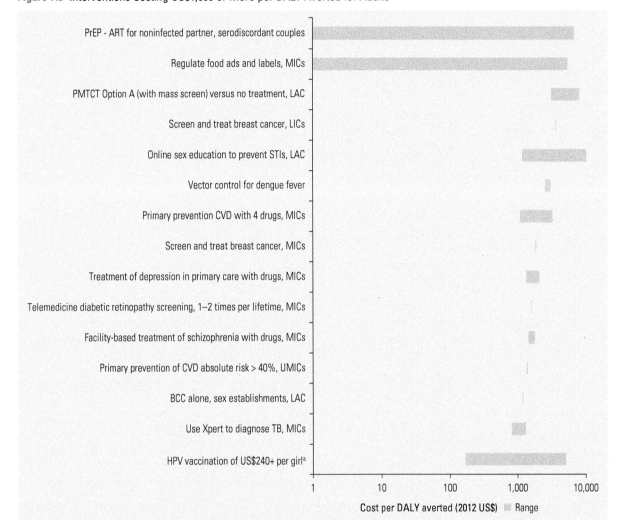

Note: ART = antiretroviral therapy; BCC = behavior change communication; CVD = cardiovascular disease; HPV = human papillomavirus; LAC = Latin America and the Caribbean; LICs = low-income countries; MICs = middle-income countries; Option A = use of single-drug regime for pregnancy for EMTCT; PrEP = pre-exposure prophylaxis; PMTCT = Prevention of Mother-to-Child Transmission of HIV; STIs = sexually transmitted infections; TB= tuberculosis; UMICs = upper-middle-income countries.
a. Denotes outcome in QALYs (quality-adjusted life years).

More than half of the interventions in figures 7.1–7.4 cost less than US$200 per DALY averted. These interventions could be considered for publicly funded health care in LICs and include the following:

- *Treatment of various, primarily infectious diseases*: Treatment for malaria, tuberculosis (including tuberculosis that is resistant to first-line drugs), HIV/AIDS, syphilis, and four of the NTDs; basic treatment using medication for heart failure
- *Prevention of various, primarily infectious diseases:* Male circumcision; intermittent preventive treatment in pregnant women and in infants against malaria, as well as insecticide-treated nets and indoor residual spraying; antiretroviral therapy for pregnant women; hepatitis B vaccinations; and HPV vaccination at US$50 per fully vaccinated girl
- *Pneumococcus, rotavirus, and* **Haemophilus influenza** *type b (Hib) vaccines in LICs*
- *Selected basic surgical interventions*: Basic trauma surgery and emergency obstetric care; surgery for cataracts, hernia, and cleft lip and palate
- *Other miscellaneous interventions*: Training traditional birth attendants and general practitioners for births; community-based neonatal care.

Figure 7.4 Interventions for Children

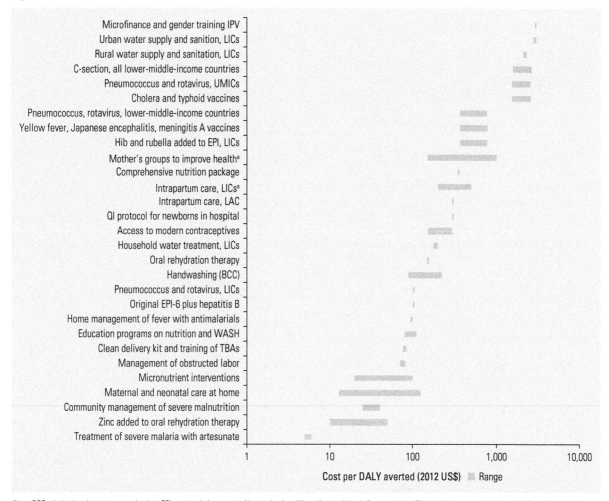

Note: BCC = behavior change communication; EPI = expanded program of immunization; Hib = *Haemophilus influenza* type b; IPV = intimate partner violence; LAC = Latin America and the Caribbean; LICs = low-income countries; QI = quality improvement; TBAs = traditional birth attendants; UMICs = upper-middle income countries; WASH = water, sanitation, and hygiene.

a. Denotes outcome in QALYs (quality-adjusted life years).

Those interventions costing US$200–US$500 per DALY averted could be considered for lower-middle-income countries in addition to the items listed. These include the following:

- Surgery for selected nonemergency orthopedic conditions
- Selected interventions for mental health in primary care settings
- Treatment of one additional NTD
- Various nutrition interventions.

Examples of interventions costing more than US$500 per DALY averted and potentially appropriate for consideration in upper-middle-income countries include the following:

- Secondary and primary prevention of cardiovascular disease with medication
- Additional mental health interventions
- Pre-exposure prophylaxis as antiretroviral treatment of uninfected partners of HIV-infected individuals
- Selected behavior-change interventions
- Provision of balanced protein–energy supplements in pregnancy.

DISCUSSION

A similar analysis to the one reported here was conducted for *Disease Control Priorities in Developing Countries* (second edition; Jamison and others 2006).

It covered studies through the year 2000 (Laxminarayan, Chow, and Shahid-Salles 2006) and provided an informative source of comparison for the current results that date from 2000 through part of 2013. The differences are not only in the results of cost-effectiveness studies but are also—tellingly—in the topics studied.

About half of the interventions appear in both the pre- and post-2000 compilations; the remainders represent some significant changes. Some new interventions that were not in widespread use before 2000—many of them related to substantial investments in new technologies and new methods to change behavior over the MDG period—have been evaluated. For some interventions, substantial reductions in prices have occurred that have made previously unaffordable interventions less costly and more cost-effective. This is particularly true for vaccines, in cases where efforts by Gavi and others have led to lower vaccine prices, and for malaria and AIDS treatments, in cases where efforts by the Global Fund to Fight AIDS, Tuberculosis, and Malaria and Médecins sans Frontières, among others, have similarly led to reduced drug prices. Some new areas of health care, particularly those not involving MDG targets, have been studied, making more detailed cost-effectiveness data available beyond the areas of maternal and child health and major infectious diseases. Some interventions have changed priorities, either as the disease context has changed or as experience has led to a revision of what was expected, based on pilot programs.

Finally, some interventions no longer appear on the list, despite being found to be cost-effective in the previous study. This may be because they have been mainstreamed and either no further need exists to estimate or update cost-effectiveness or they have been superseded by other more effective or more cost-effective interventions. Examples in each of these categories are given in the following sections.

New Technologies and Methods

New interventions for which cost-effectiveness data have become available for LMICs include treating severe malaria with rectal or injected artesunate, which can be done before hospital arrival; adding GeneXpert testing to sputum-smear testing to diagnose disease and determine antibiotic susceptibility; and HPV vaccination for girls to prevent cervical cancer. These all fall into the range of less than US$200 per DALY averted in the appropriate contexts. However, other new technologies, such as pre-exposure prophylaxis, have a relatively high cost per DALY averted in most cases.

Changes in Prices

Reduced prices of pneumococcal and rotavirus vaccines are examples of changes in costs that dramatically change the cost-effectiveness of the interventions. These interventions were high cost per DALY averted in the pre-2000 review, but at current Gavi prices for LICs, the cost is now less than US$100 per DALY averted. Another major example is the NTDs. Following the 2012 London Declaration (Uniting to Combat NTDs Coalition 2016), the key drugs to combat NTDs have been donated by the manufacturers, which has moved the elimination of NTDs by prevention and treatment substantially higher up the priority list in terms of cost-effectiveness in the past decade.

New Health Areas

Efforts by the surgical community (for example, the *Lancet* Commission on Global Surgery and the *DCP3* volume 1 on surgery [Debas and others 2015]) have increased the interest in and emphasis on cost-effectiveness of surgery. Several surgical interventions cost less than US$200 per DALY averted. In urgent cases, these same interventions can be implemented in a first-level hospital with a general surgeon (for example, emergency obstetric care and basic trauma care); in nonurgent cases, they can be implemented in a specialized facility with high volume and modest cost (for example, cataract surgery or repair of cleft lip and cleft palate). Similar efforts are underway in the global cancer community. One study suggests that treatment of early-stage breast cancer falls in the category of less than US$200 per DALY averted for middle-income countries (although not in LICs, where screen-and-treat approaches cost more than US$200 per DALY averted).

Interventions That Have Changed Priority

School-based adolescent health and nutrition programs appeared as a high priority because of their low cost per DALY averted in 2006. This was not the case in 2016, because more recent studies are much more cautious about whether these programs will have long-term positive effects.

Interventions That Are No Longer on the List

Changing technology also means that some previously cost-effective interventions have been superseded or have become usual care. This is particularly evident for HIV/AIDS. In the pre-2000 compilation, eight interventions appeared in the highest-priority list. Peer and education programs for high-risk groups; condom promotion and distribution; voluntary counseling and testing without treatment; diagnosis and treatment of sexually transmitted infections; blood and needle safety; tuberculosis coinfection prevention and treatment; opportunistic infection treatment; and prevention of mother-to-child transmission were included among the most cost-effective interventions (using less than US$150 per DALY averted in 2001 U.S. dollars, roughly comparable to less than US$200 per DALY averted in 2012 U.S. dollars). A decade later, with treatment with antiretroviral agents on the highest priority list, all but two of the other interventions fell off the list; the remaining two are prevention of mother-to-child transmission and testing for and treatment of other sexually transmitted infections. Most of the interventions had become usual care, but voluntary counseling and testing without treatment had been superseded by test-and-treat approaches.

A major limitation of the cost-effectiveness literature, particularly acute in LMICs, is its bias toward the diseases of greatest interest during the period under study. In the current study, the literature overrepresents infectious conditions and childbirth, because these have been prioritized by international donors. Drugs and vaccines tend to be overrepresented relative to behavior change interventions, because manufacturers use cost-effectiveness data as part of the adoption process.

Measurement Issues

The ability to conduct a large comparative study such as this relies on use of common methodologies by individual study authors. For effectiveness studies, progress has been made applying standard guidelines for systematic reviews and using explicit criteria for evaluating evidence. For economics studies, the fairly recent adoption of a common set of reporting standards (Husereau and others 2013) and the development of a reference case for conducting economic evaluations in LMICs (NICE International 2014) are moves in the same direction.

A larger issue is the common metric for cost-effectiveness. The DALY has been the predominant health outcome metric used for studies of LMICs over the past decade or more. It has the advantage over the QALY for work in multiple countries in that a single set of disability weights is used across countries, whereas QALY weightings are, in theory, country specific, and generating QALY weights can be a costly process.

Recent concerns about the DALY relate to the issue of discounting costs and health benefits further in the future. Although this issue is very much accepted by economists, some health specialists find it more problematic. The Institute for Health Metrics and Evaluation has begun using undiscounted DALYs to measure global burden of disease (Murray and others 2012) but without using a new term to differentiate these undiscounted DALYs. This approach is already causing confusion.

The DALY measure itself has limitations. Using the DALY measure tends to underrepresent interventions where outcomes are not readily measured in this metric, such as family planning, and interventions in nutrition where the outcomes are improved cognition rather than improved health, more readily measured with benefit:cost analysis ratios.

On the cost side, studies predominantly use market exchange rates to compare across different currencies. However, an influential body of work from the WHO, the WHO-CHOICE study, used international dollars for WHO subregions rather than countries. International dollars make cross-country comparisons somewhat easier to understand by adjusting for salary differences as a component of costs. The downside is that international dollars make comparison more difficult with other studies not using international dollars. One does not simply use the US$/PPP exchange rate, because having information about cost structure is necessary. A further complication is the lack of published indices for PPP exchange rates of regions.

The advantage of WHO-CHOICE was the ability to compare many interventions at one time, when the MDG strategies were being evaluated, and to compare the outcome of combinations of interventions. The disadvantage is that funding to replicate such a large comprehensive evaluation is difficult to attain. The use of simpler methods, such as market exchange rates, allows the synthesis of many smaller, individually directed studies.

CONCLUSIONS

Cost-effectiveness is not the only criterion by which to choose health priorities, but it is useful for identifying what is given up when a less cost-effective intervention is prioritized. It is also a useful tool for advocacy for increased health budgets. This review has used cost-effectiveness measures from several hundred studies for LMICs to help identify candidates for priority health packages, which may assist policy makers considering how to move to universal health coverage.

This review has identified some of the gaps where future research on cost-effectiveness is needed:

- Given the ongoing decline in infectious disease burden and the growing burden of NCDs, more analyses for NCDs are needed for LMICs. Achieving the goal of health convergence within a generation will not be possible without initiating interventions to reduce NCDs, where the lag between intervention and outcomes is often much longer than for infectious diseases.
- The review highlights the lack of any study of cost-effectiveness for childhood cancer and the dearth of information on cost-effective interventions for mental health in LMICs.
- Another area for future work includes the cost-effectiveness of resource-appropriate treatment of early-stage cancers, such as breast and cervical cancers.
- Given the growth of obesity worldwide, cost-effectiveness studies of interventions to change patterns of diet and inactivity in urban areas are needed.

A publicly available online global database of cost-effectiveness studies using DALY outcomes will make future updates easier (Tufts University 2016).

The major changes in ranking of health priorities over the past decade underscore the need for periodic repetition of league table exercises such as this one.

ACKNOWLEDGMENTS

The authors wish to thank the following individuals for their excellent assistance: Elizabeth Brouwer at the University of Washington for her work in organizing the cost and cost-effectiveness databases; Vittoria Lutje, from the Cochrane Infectious Diseases Group, for conducting extensive literature searches; Emily Thacher and Julian Frare-Davis from the University of Washington for extracting the literature and creating the databases; and Daphne Wu at the University of Waterloo for working on the databases and providing research support for the final analysis presented here.

ANNEX

The annex to this chapter is as follows. It is available at http://www.dcp-3.org/DCP.
- Annex 7A. Details of Interventions Included in figures 7.1, 7.2, 7.3, and 7.4, by Increasing Cost per DALY Averted.

NOTE

World Bank Income Classifications as of July 2014 are as follows, based on estimates of gross national income (GNI) per capita for 2013:

- Low-income countries (LICs) = US$1,045 or less
- Middle-income countries (MICs) are subdivided:
  (a) lower-middle-income = US$1,046 to US$4,125
  (b) upper-middle-income (UMICs) = US$4,126 to US$12,745
- High-income countries (HICs) = US$12,746 or more.

REFERENCES

Black, R. E., R. Laxminarayan, M. Temmerman, and N. Walker, eds. 2016. *Disease Control Priorities* (third edition): Volume 2, *Reproductive, Maternal, Newborn, and Child Health*. Washington, DC: World Bank.

Claxton, K., S. Martin, S. Soares, N. Rice, E. Spackman, and others. 2015. "Methods for the Estimation of the National Institute for Health and Care Excellence Cost-Effectiveness Threshold." *Health Technology Assessment* 19 (14): 1–503. doi:10.3310/hta19140.

Debas, H. T., P. Donkor, A. Gawande, D. T. Jamison, M. E. Kruk, and C. N. Mock, eds. 2015. *Disease Control Priorities* (third edition): Volume 1, *Essential Surgery*. Washington, DC: World Bank.

Drummond, M. F., M. J. Schulpher, G. W. Torrance, D. J. O'Brien, and G. L. Stoddart. 2005. *Methods for the Economic Evaluation of Health Care Programmes*. 3rd ed. New York: Oxford University Press.

Evans, D. B., S. S. Lim, T. Adam, and T. Tan-Torres Edejer. 2005. "Achieving the Millennium Development Goals for Health: Evaluation of Current Strategies and Future Priorities for Improving Health in Developing Countries." *BMJ* 331 (7530): 1457–61.

Gaziano, T., M. Suhrcke, E. Brouwer, C. Levin, I. Nikolic, and R. Nugent. 2017. "Summary of Costs and Cost-Effectiveness of Interventions and Policies to Prevent and Treat Cardiometabolic Diseases." In *Disease Control Priorities* (third edition): Volume 5, *Cardiovascular, Respiratory, and Related Diseases*, edited by D. Prabhakaran, S. Anand, T. Gaziano, Y. F. Wu, J. C. Mbanya, and R. Nugent. Washington, DC: World Bank.

Gelband, H., P. Jha, R. Sankaranarayanan, and S. Horton, eds. 2015. *Disease Control Priorities* (third edition): Volume 3, *Cancer*. Washington, DC: World Bank.

Greenberg, D., C. Earle, C. H. Fang, A. Eldar-Lissai, and P. J. Neumann. 2010. "When Is Cancer Care Cost-Effective? A Systematic Overview of Cost-Utility Analyses in Oncology." *Journal of the National Cancer Institute* 102 (2): 82–88.

Holmes, K. K., S. Bertozzi, B. Bloom, and P. Jha, eds. 2017a. *Disease Control Priorities* (third edition): Volume 6, *Major Infectious Diseases*. Washington, DC: World Bank.

Holmes, K. K., S. Bertozzi, B. Bloom, P. Jha, R. Nugent, H. Gelband, and others. 2017b. "Major Infectious Diseases: Key Messages from *Disease Control Priorities*, Third Edition."

In *Disease Control Priorities* (third edition): Volume 6, *Major Infectious Diseases*, edited by K. K. Holmes, S. Bertozzi, B. Bloom, and P. Jha. Washington, DC: World Bank.

Horton, S., and C. L. Gauvreau. 2015. "Cancer in Low and Middle-Income Countries: Economic Overview." In *Disease Control Priorities* (third edition): Volume 3, *Cancer*, edited by H. Gelband, P. Jha, R. Sankaranarayanan, and S. Horton. Washington, DC: World Bank.

Horton, S., and C. Levin. 2016. "Cost-Effectiveness of Interventions for Reproductive, Maternal, Neonatal, and Child Health." In *Disease Control Priorities* (third edition): Volume 2, *Reproductive, Maternal, Newborn, and Child Health,* edited by R. E. Black, R. Laxminarayan, M. Temmerman, and N. Walker. Washington, DC: World Bank.

Husereau, D., M. Drummond, S. Petrou, C. Carswell, D. Moher, and others. 2013. "Consolidated Health Economic Evaluation Reporting Standards (CHEERS): Explanation and Elaboration: A Report of the ISPOR Health Economic Evaluation Publication Guidelines Good Reporting Practices Task Force." *Value Health* 1 (2): 231–50.

Jamison, D. T., J. G. Breman, A. R. Measham, G. Alleyne, M. Claeson, D. B. Evans, P. Jha, A. Mills, and P. Musgrove, eds. 2006. *Disease Control Priorities in Developing Countries*, Second edition. Washington, DC: World Bank and Oxford University Press. Laxminarayan, R., J. Chow, and S. A. Shahid-Salles. 2006. "Intervention Cost-Effectiveness: Overview of Main Messages." In *Disease Control Priorities in Developing Countries* (second edition), edited by D. T. Jamison, J. G. Breman, A. R. Measham, G. Alleyne, M. Claeson, D. B. Evans, P. Jha, A. Mills, and P. Musgrove. Washington, DC: World Bank and Oxford University Press.

Levin, C., and D. Chisholm. 2015. "Cost-Effectiveness and Affordability of Interventions, Policies, and Platforms for the Prevention and Treatment of Mental, Neurological, and Substance Use Disorders." In *Disease Control Priorities* (third edition): Volume 4, *Mental, Neurological, and Substance Use Disorders,* edited by V. Patel, D. Chisholm, T. Dua, R. Laxminarayan, and M. E. Medina-Mora. Washington, DC: World Bank.

Murray, C. J. L., T. Vos, R. Lozano, M. Naghavi, A. D. Flaxman, and others. 2012. "Disability-Adjusted Life Years (DALYs) for 291 Diseases and Injuries in 21 Regions, 1991–2010: A Systematic Analysis for the Global Burden of Disease Study 2010." *The Lancet* 380 (9859): 2197–233.

NICE International. 2014. "The Gates Reference Case: What It Is, Why It's Important, and How to Use It." Nice International, London. https://www.nice.org.uk/Media /Default/About/what-we-do/NICE-International/projects /Gates-Reference-case-what-it-is-how-to-use-it.pdf.

Ochalek, J., K. Claxton, and J. Lomas. 2016. "Cost per DALY Averted Thresholds for Low- and Middle-Income Countries: Evidence from Cross Country Data." CHE Research Paper 122, Centre for Health Economics, University of York, York, U.K. http://www.idsihealth.org/knowledge_base/cost -per-daly-averted-thresholds-for-low-and-middle-income -countries-evidence-from-cross-country-data/.

Patel, V., D. Chisholm, T. Dua, R. Laxminarayan, and M. E. Medina-Mora, eds. 2015. *Disease Control Priorities* (third edition): Volume 4, *Mental, Neurological, and Substance Use Disorders.* Washington, DC: World Bank.

Prabhakaran, D., S. Anand, T. Gaziano, Y. F. Wu, J. C. Mbanya, and R. Nugent, eds. 2017. *Disease Control Priorities* (third edition): Volume 5, *Cardiovascular, Respiratory, and Related Disorders.* Washington, DC: World Bank.

Prinja, S., A. Nandi, S. Horton, C. Levin, and R. Laxminarayan. 2015. "Costs, Effectiveness, and Cost-Effectiveness of Selected Surgical Procedures and Platforms." In *Disease Control Priorities* (3rd edition): Volume 1: *Essential Surgery*, edited by H. T. Debas, P. Donkor, A. Gawande, D. T. Jamison, M. E. Kruk, and C. N. Mock. Washington, DC: World Bank.

Salomon, J. A., N. Carvalho, C. Gutiérrez-Delgado, R. Orozco, A. Mancuso, and others. 2012. "Intervention Strategies to Reduce the Burden of Non-Communicable Diseases in Mexico: Cost Effectiveness Analysis." *BMJ* 344: e355.

Tufts University. 2016. Global Health Cost-Effectiveness Analysis Registry database. http://healtheconomics .tuftsmedicalcenter.org/orchard.

Uniting to Combat NTDs Coalition. 2016. "Reaching the Unreached: Fourth Progress Report of the London Declaration." http://unitingtocombatntds.org/report/fourth -report-reaching-unreached.

Vos, T., R. Carter, J. Barendregt, C. Mihalopoulos, L. Veerman, and others. 2010. *Assessing Cost-Effectiveness in Prevention.* University of Queensland, Brisbane, and Deakin University, Melbourne. https://public-health.uq.edu.au/files/571/ACE -Prevention_final_report.pdf.

WHO (World Health Organization). 2001. *Macroeconomics and Health: Investing in Health for Economic Development.* Geneva: WHO.

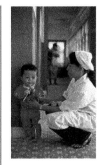

Chapter 8

Health Policy Analysis: Applications of Extended Cost-Effectiveness Analysis Methodology in *Disease Control Priorities*, Third Edition

Stéphane Verguet and Dean T. Jamison

INTRODUCTION

Multiple criteria are involved in making decisions and prioritizing health policies (Baltussen and Niessen 2006). Potential trade-offs between efficiency and equity are among these criteria and have long been emphasized in the treatment and prevention of human immunodeficiency virus/acquired immune deficiency syndrome (HIV/AIDS) (for example, Cleary 2010; Kaplan and Merson 2002; Verguet 2013). Notably, several mathematical frameworks, including mathematical programming, have proposed incorporating equity into resource allocation decisions in the public sector (Birch and Gafni 1992; Bleichrodt, Diecidue, and Quiggin 2004; Epstein and others 2007; Segall 1989; Stinnett and Paltiel 1996). The worldwide application of benefit-cost analysis provided for "distributional weights" as early as the 1970s.

Protection from financial risks associated with health care expenses is emerging as a critical component of national health strategies in many low- and middle-income countries (LMICs). The World Health Organization's *World Health Reports* of 1999 and 2000 included the provision of financial risk protection (FRP) as one criterion of good performance for health systems (WHO 1999, 2000). Reducing these financial risks is one objective of health policy instruments such as universal public finance (UPF), that is, full public finance irrespective of whether services are provided privately or publicly. Indeed, out-of-pocket (OOP) medical payments can lead to impoverishment in many countries, with households choosing from among many coping strategies (borrowing from friends and relatives, selling assets) to manage health-related expenses (Kruk, Goldmann, and Galea 2009; van Doorslaer and others 2006; Xu and others 2003). Absent other financing mechanisms, household medical expenditures can often be *catastrophic* (Wagstaff 2010; Wagstaff and van Doorslaer 2003), defined as exceeding a certain fraction of total household expenditures. A large literature documents the significance of medical impoverishment, but far less is known about the medical conditions responsible for it. Essue and others (2017), in chapter 6 of this volume, review and extend that literature, and Verguet, Memirie, and Norheim (2016) provide a framework for assessing the global burden of medical impoverishment by cause, applying it to a case study of a systematic categorization by disease in Ethiopia. In the literature on medical impoverishment, attenuating such impoverishment is considered a significant objective of health policy, but surprisingly little analysis has been

Corresponding author: Stéphane Verguet, Department of Global Health and Population, Harvard T. H. Chan School of Public Health, Boston, Massachusetts, United States; verguet@hsph.harvard.edu

performed of efficient ways to address the problem. The method of Extended cost-effectiveness analysis (ECEA) was initially developed for *DCP3* by Verguet, Laxminarayan, and Jamison (2015).

Traditionally, economic evaluations of health interventions (cost-effectiveness analyses [CEAs]) have focused on improvements in health and estimated an intervention cost per health gain in dollar per death averted or dollar per disability-adjusted life year (DALY) averted (Jamison and others 2006). However, arguments have been developed for some time that CEA in health should be extended to explicitly consider the multiple dimensions of outcome. Jamison (2009), for example, argued that CEAs can be extended to include FRP on the outcome side and use of scarce health system capacity on the cost side (figure 8.1). Specific methods for advancing this agenda were first proposed and applied in assessments of the consequences of two alternative policies—public finance and improved access to credit—for extending coverage of tuberculosis treatment in India (Verguet, Laxminarayan, and Jamison 2015). That study and other early ECEAs (Verguet 2013; Verguet, Gauvreau, and others 2015; Verguet, Olson, and others 2015) supplemented traditional economic evaluation with evaluation of nonhealth benefits (such as FRP and equity), with the broad objective of providing valuable guidance in the design of health policies.[1]

ECEA in this respect builds on the existing frameworks of cost-benefit analysis and cost-consequence analysis that tabulate disaggregated results (Mauskopf and others 1998) and on analytical frameworks that incorporate equity and FRP concerns into economic evaluations (Asaria and others 2015; Brown and Finkelstein 2008; Cookson, Drummond, and Weatherly 2009; Finkelstein and McKnight 2008; Fleurbaey and

others 2013; McClellan and Skinner 2006; Sassi, Archard, and Le Grand 2001; Smith 2007, 2013). It enables the design of benefits packages that quantify both health and nonhealth benefits for a given expenditure on specific health policies, based on the quantitative inclusion of how much nonhealth benefits are being bought as well as how much health benefits are being bought with a given investment in an intervention or policy. In this respect, ECEA can answer some of the policy questions raised by the *World Health Reports* for 2010 and 2013 (WHO 2010, 2013) regarding how to select and sequence the health services to be provided on the path toward universal health coverage. This chapter first describes the ECEA approach and then summarizes findings of ECEAs undertaken in the context of the third edition of *Disease Control Priorities* (*DCP3*; http://www.dcp-3.org).

APPROACH

Consider the implementation of a given health policy (*HP*) in a given population (*P*). Policy examples include public finance for a package of vaccines, taxation on tobacco products, legislation to enforce the mandatory use of helmets, and so forth. *P* can be divided into subgroups, which can be denoted P_k (with $1 \leq k \leq n$) per socioeconomic status according to five income quintiles, per region according to geographic location (state, region, county), and per gender.

HP entails a given coverage (*Cov*) and given effectiveness (*Eff*) for preventing disease burden (*D*) in the population as well as a net cost (*C*). The ECEA methodology quantifies both health benefits (B_H) and nonhealth benefits (B_{NH}) in *P* for a given increment in public (or private) expenditure (figure 8.2).

Health Benefits

With the introduction of *HP*, health benefits (B_H) are procured—for example, quantified by the sum of the burden of disease averted in each subgroup (P_k)—with a specific effectiveness of the policy (Eff_k) assumed to be constant per subgroup.

In this respect, ECEA estimates the distributional health consequences—in particular, benefits (mortality, morbidity averted, disability-adjusted life years averted, quality-adjusted life years gained)—per population strata, whether socioeconomic group or geographic setting (figure 8.3).

Nonhealth Benefits

With *HP*, nonhealth benefits ($B_{NH,j}$) are procured, with $1 \leq j \leq m$, where *j* indicates the type of nonhealth benefits (FRP, number of school days gained). For example, if

Figure 8.1 Intervention Costs and Effects: A More General View

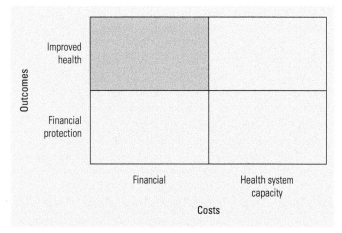

Source: Jamison 2009, by permission of Oxford University Press.
Note: The shaded box represents the domain of traditional cost-effectiveness analysis.

we consider FRP, given a preexisting burden of illness-related impoverishment due to medical expenses, direct nonmedical costs such as transportation costs, and indirect costs such as wages lost, the related nonhealth benefits could be expressed by the sum of the burden of illness-related impoverishment averted in each population subgroup.

Specifically, the ECEA approach goes beyond the societal perspective in traditional economic evaluations (Drummond and others 2015) to examine the perspective of households in estimating the amount of OOP expenditures (direct medical costs, direct nonmedical costs, indirect costs) that could be affected by a specific policy (figure 8.4).

Subsequently, once the amount of OOP private expenditures borne by households that may be "crowded out" has been estimated, ECEA can be used to scale the amount of OOP household expenditures by households' disposable income to estimate FRP—in other words, to account for the fact that a household with annual income of US$100,000 and OOP expenditures of US$10 is much less severely affected than a household with annual income of US$100. The crowding out of private health expenditures will often be an objective as well as a consequence of health policy.

Several metrics can be used to estimate FRP (Flores and others 2008; Wagstaff 2010; Verguet, Laxminarayan, and Jamison 2015), including the following:

- Number of catastrophic health expenditures averted, estimating the number of households no longer crossing a catastrophic threshold (for example, 10 percent, 20 percent, 40 percent of income or capacity to pay) from OOP expenditures
- Number of poverty cases averted, estimating the number of households no longer crossing a poverty line (for example, US$1.25 per day) because of OOP expenditures
- Number of instances of forced asset sales or forced borrowing averted
- A money-metric value of insurance provided, quantifying the willingness to pay or risk premium associated with the policy (figure 8.5).

Equity Benefits

With HP, equity benefits (B_{Eq}), estimated here in terms of health distribution, can be procured. For example, if HP provides more health benefits to poorer than to richer segments of the population, the policy could be deemed equity enhancing (figure 8.3). There are several ways to quantify B_{Eq}, including $\dfrac{B_{H,w}}{B_H}$, where $B_{H,w}$ and B_H are the health benefits procured by HP among the worst-off group and the total sum of health benefits in all groups, respectively.

Figure 8.2 Objective of Extended Cost-Effectiveness Analysis: Efficient Purchase of Health and Nonhealth Benefits

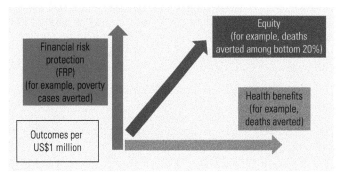

Note: Similar to CEA measures in, say, US$ per death averted, estimate the efficient purchase of FRP in, say, US$ per FRP provided. CEA = cost-effectiveness analysis; FRP = financial risk protection.

Figure 8.3 Distribution of Under-Five Deaths Averted with Universal Public Finance (UPF) of Pneumonia Treatment at a Coverage Level 20 Percent Higher Than the Current Level and UPF of Combined Pneumonia Treatment and Pneumococcal Vaccination at 20 Percent Coverage Level in Ethiopia

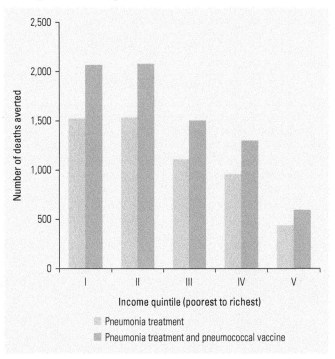

Source: Verguet and others 2016.

"Efficient Purchase" of Health and Nonhealth Benefits

The net cost of the policy is C. For that net cost, HP "efficiently" purchases health benefits (B_H) but also nonhealth benefits (B_{NH})—for example, B_{FRP}. As in CEA, we can then define a usual incremental cost-effectiveness ratio (ICER)—ICER = C/B_H—but we can also define an ICER for each of the nonhealth benefits: for FRP, $ICER_{FRP} = C/B_{FRP}$. In this respect, ECEA can help quantify the efficient purchase of

Figure 8.4 Distribution of Household Private Expenditures Averted with Universal Public Finance (UPF) of Pneumonia Treatment at a Coverage Level 20 Percent Higher Than the Current Level and UPF of Combined Pneumonia Treatment and Pneumococcal Vaccination at 20 Percent Coverage Level in Ethiopia

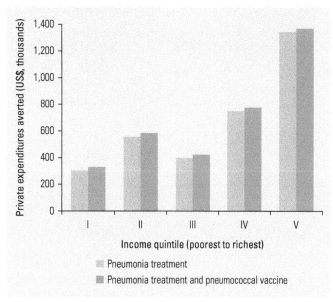

Figure 8.5 Distribution of Financial Risk Protection (Measured by a Money-Metric Value of Insurance Provided) with Universal Public Finance (UPF) of Pneumonia Treatment at a Coverage Level 20 Percent Higher Than the Current Level and UPF of Combined Pneumonia Treatment and Pneumococcal Vaccination at 20 Percent Coverage Level in Ethiopia

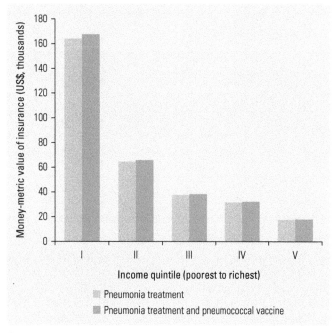

both equity and FRP in addition to health. It also can help generate the evidence base to support informed trade-offs among the partially competing objectives of improved health, improved FRP, and improved equity. Figure 8.6 provides an illustration from Ethiopia.

APPLICATIONS

ECEAs Completed to Date

ECEA was developed for *DCP3* and has been used in health policy assessments for a variety of both policies and settings (table 8.1). The policies include public finance, excise taxes, legislation, regulation, conditional cash transfers, task shifting, and education.

ECEAs are context specific and depend substantially on the epidemiology of the setting (endemicity, distribution of specific diseases), local health system infrastructure (presence and distribution of health facilities), wealth of the location (low-income, lower-middle-income, upper-middle-income country), and financial arrangements (presence of social health insurance, community-based insurance). In total, more than 20 ECEAs have been published (or accepted for publication) as of May 2017. Of these, nine are included in one of *DCP3*'s nine volumes.

Example: Use of Dashboard

We now illustrate ECEA in considering the example of UPF for tuberculosis treatment in India in a population composed of five income quintiles totaling 1 million people (200,000 people per income quintile), drawing on the first completed ECEA (Verguet, Laxminarayan, and Jamison 2015).

Notably, we assume an average incidence of tuberculosis of $p_0 = 100$ per 100,000 per year, with incidence highest in the lowest income quintile. The cost of tuberculosis treatment (that is, directly observed treatment, short course) is US$100 per person. We also assume income in the population is distributed following a Gamma distribution based on a mean income of US$1,500 and a Gini coefficient of 0.33, as produced by an algorithm given by Salem and Mount (1974; see also Kemp-Benedict 2001).

The total number of deaths averted would be about 80 a year. The health benefits would be concentrated among the bottom income quintile (50 percent) because tuberculosis has a higher incidence among this subgroup. The total amount of private OOP expenditures averted by universal public funding would be about US$29,000. The bottom income quintile would benefit from about 20 percent of the private expenditures averted. The total incremental treatment costs incurred by the public sector would be about US$65,000. The total FRP afforded by UPF, estimated here using a money-metric value of insurance, would be about US$9,000, 60 percent of which would be among the bottom quintile (table 8.2).

Examining the efficient purchase of health and non-health benefits, we find the following: ICER = US$800 per death averted, and $ICER_{FRP}$ = US$7 per dollar of insurance value provided. For each US$1 million spent, about 1,200 deaths are averted, 600 of which are in the bottom income quintile, and the money-metric value of insurance is US$140,000, of which 60 percent is in the bottom income quintile.

In addition to examining UPF, the ECEA study for India examined the consequences of improving access to borrowing to cover treatment costs. It found that it was plausible that such policies substantially reduce TB mortality among the poor but—relative to UPF—it would generate high burdens of lingering debt.

Poverty Reduction Benefits of Health Policies and Design of the Benefits Package

ECEA stresses the potential poverty reduction benefits of health policies. Specifically, ECEA explicitly quantifies the FRP benefits or the poverty reduction benefits of policies. In this respect, it fulfills two major objectives. First, it provides a quantitative tool that enables intersectoral comparison of health policies with other sectors (education and transport), which is of particular relevance for

Figure 8.6 Financial Risk Protection Afforded (Poverty Cases Averted) Versus Health Gains (Deaths Averted) per US$100,000 Spent (in 2011 U.S. Dollars) for Interventions Provided through Universal Public Finance in Ethiopia

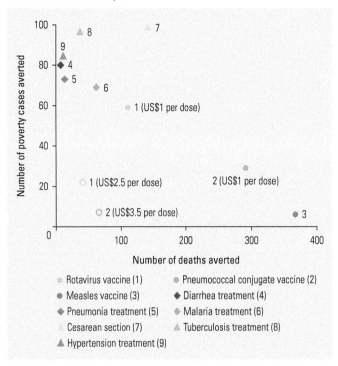

Source: Verguet, Olson, and others 2015.

Table 8.1 Extended Cost-Effectiveness Analyses for *Disease Control Priorities*

a. ECEAs in DCP3

DCP3 Volume	Chapter and topic	Policy instrument	Country	Authors and other relevant publications (if any)
1	19. Expanding surgical access	Task sharing, public finance	Ethiopia	Shrime and others 2015; Shrime and others 2016
2	18. Universal home-based neonatal care package in rural India	Public finance	India	Ashok, Nandi, and Laxminarayan 2015; Nandi, Colson, and others 2016
	19. Diarrhea and pneumonia treatment	Public finance	Ethiopia	Verguet, Pecenka, and others 2016; Johansson, Pecenka, and others 2015; Pecenka and others 2015; Verguet, Murphy, and others 2013
3	18. Human papillomavirus vaccination to prevent cervical cancer	Public finance	China	Levin and others 2015a; Levin and others 2015b
4	13. Universal coverage for mental, neurological, and substance use disorders	Public finance	Ethiopia, India	Chisholm and others 2015; Johansson, Bjerkreim Strand, and others 2016; Megiddo and others 2016; Raykar and others 2016

table continues next page

Table 8.1 Extended Cost-Effectiveness Analyses for *Disease Control Priorities* (continued)

DCP3 Volume	Chapter and topic	Policy instrument	Country	Authors and other relevant publications (if any)
5	20. Selected ECEAs for cardiovascular diseases	Public finance of interventions, tobacco taxation, regulation of salt	China, Ethiopia, South Africa	Watkins, Nugent, and Verguet 2017; Verguet, Gauvreau, and others 2015; Verguet, Olson, and others 2015; Watkins and others 2015
7	11. Motorcycle helmet laws	Regulation	Vietnam	Olson and others 2016; Olson and others 2017
	12. Use of liquefied petroleum gas and other clean energy sources in household	Commodity subsidy	India	Pillarisetti, Jamison, and Smith 2017
8	28. Postponing adolescent parity	Education	India, Niger	Verguet, Nandi, and Bundy 2016; Verguet, Nandi, and others 2017

b. Other published ECEAs (including those accepted for publication)

	Topic	Policy instrument	Country	Reference
	Tuberculosis treatment	Universal public finance; policies to improve ease of borrowing for treatment costs	India	Verguet, Laxminarayan, and Jamison 2015
	Measles vaccine	Conditional cash transfers	Ethiopia	Driessen and others 2015
	Universal immunization	Public finance	India	Megiddo and others 2014
	Water and sanitation	Clean piped water and improved sanitation	India	Nandi, Megiddo, and others 2016
	Tobacco	Taxation	Lebanon/Armenia	Verguet, Gauvreau, and others 2015; Salti, Brouwer, and Verguet 2016; Postolovska and others 2017
	Palliative care	Public finance	Vietnam	Krakauer and others 2017
	Tutorial		Not applicable	Verguet, Kim, and Jamison 2016
	Rotavirus vaccine	Public finance	Malaysia	Loganathan and others 2016
	Malaria vaccine	Public finance	Zambia	Liu, True, and others, forthcoming

Note: ECEA = extended cost-effectiveness analysis. These two papers reference the same study.

Table 8.2 Extended Cost-Effectiveness Analysis Results for Universal Public Finance of Tuberculosis Treatment in India to 90 Percent Current Coverage (per Million Population)

		Income Quintile				
Outcome	Total	I	II	III	IV	V
Tuberculosis deaths averted	80	40	25	12	3	0
Private expenditures averted (US$)	29,000	6,000	6,000	7,000	6,000	4,000
Insurance value (US$)	9,000	5,000	2,000	1,000	1,000	0

Source: Reproduced from table III of Verguet, Laxminarayan, and Jamison 2015.
Note: Financial risk protection is measured as a money-metric value of insurance.

Figure 8.7 Use of Extended Cost-Effectiveness Analysis in Decision Making with the Inclusion of One Health Domain (Deaths Averted by Policy) and One Nonhealth Domain (Financial Risk Protection Provided by Policy) per Dollar Expenditure

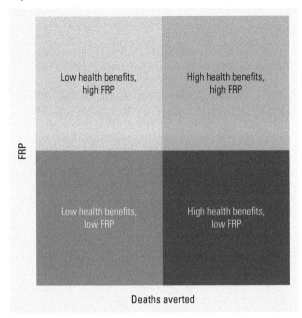

Note: FRP = financial risk protection. As a simplification, the decision-making space can be divided into four quadrants: high health benefits and high FRP, high health benefits and low FRP, low health benefits and high FRP, and low health benefits and low FRP.

ministries of finance in LMICs (figure 8.7). In this context, ECEAs may yield surprising results. Salti and others (2016) found that tobacco taxation not only differentially benefited the health of the poor, but it protected them from financial consequences of illness and thereby constituted a progressive tax. Second, it enables policy makers to assemble a basic benefits package that takes into account how much health and how much FRP they can buy when designing the package. Depending on the preferences of policy makers and users, they can directly choose and optimize the benefits packages.

DISCUSSION

This chapter presents detailed methods for the broader economic evaluation of health policies. ECEAs build on CEAs by assessing consequences in both the health and nonhealth domains.

The ECEA approach is novel in that it includes equity and nonhealth benefits (FRP) in the economic evaluation of health policies, which enables multiple criteria to be included in the decision-making process. More important,

the ECEA approach enables the design of benefits packages, such as essential universal health coverage and the highest-priority package discussed in chapter 3 in this volume (Watkins and others 2018), based on the quantitative inclusion of information about how much nonhealth benefits can be bought, in addition to how much health can be bought, per dollar expenditure on health care (figures 8.6 and 8.7).

Some health policies will rank higher on one metric relative to another. ECEA allows policy makers to take both health and nonhealth outcomes into account when making decisions and thus to target scarce health care resources more effectively toward specific policy objectives.

NOTES

Large parts of this chapter have been reproduced and adapted from the following *PharmacoEconomics* publication: Verguet, S., J. J. Kim, and D. T. Jamison. 2016. "Extended Cost-Effectiveness Analysis for Health Policy Assessment: A Tutorial." *PharmacoEconomics* 34 (9): 913–23. Licensed under Creative Commons Attribution (CC BY 4.0) available at: https://creativecommons.org/licenses/by/4.0/

World Bank Income Classifications as of July 2014 are as follows, based on estimates of gross national income (GNI) per capita for 2013:

- Low-income countries (LICs) = US$1,045 or less
- Middle-income countries (MICs) are subdivided:
  (a) lower-middle-income = US$1,046 to US$4,125
  (b) upper-middle-income (UMICs) = US$4,126 to US$12,745
- High-income countries (HICs) = US$12,746 or more.

1. Kim and others (2006) analyzed the effects of health system constraints on optimal resource allocation, and Rheingans, Atherly, and Anderson (2012) examined the distributional impact of rotavirus immunization.

REFERENCES

Asaria, M., S. Griffin, R. Cookson, S. Whyte, and P. Tappenden. 2015. "Distributional Cost-Effectiveness Analysis of Health Care Programmes: A Methodological Study of the UK Bowel Cancer Screening Programme." *Health Economics* 24 (6): 742–54.

Ashok, A., A. Nandi, and R. Laxminarayan. 2015. "The Benefits of a Universal Home-Based Neonatal Care Package in Rural India: An Extended Cost-Effectiveness Analysis." In *Disease Control Priorities* (third edition): Volume 2, *Reproductive, Maternal, Newborn, and Child Health*, edited by R. E. Black, R. Laxminarayan, M. Temmerman, and N. Walker. Washington, DC: World Bank.

Baltussen, R., and L. Niessen. 2006. "Priority Setting of Health Interventions: The Need for Multi-Criteria Decision Analysis." *Cost Effectiveness and Resource Allocation* 4 (August 21): 14.

Birch, S., and A. Gafni. 1992. "Cost-Effectiveness/Utility Analyses: Do Current Decisions Lead Us to Where We Want to Be?" *Journal of Health Economics* 11 (3): 279–96.

Bleichrodt, H., E. Diecidue, and J. Quiggin. 2004. "Equity Weights in the Allocation of Health Care: The Rank-Dependent QALY Model." *Journal of Health Economics* 23 (1): 157–71.

Brown, J. R., and A. Finkelstein. 2008. "The Interaction of Public and Private Insurance: Medicaid and the Long-Term Care Insurance Market." *American Economic Review* 98 (3): 1083–102.

Chisholm, D., K. A. Johansson, N. Raykar, I. Meggido, A. Nigam, and others. 2015. "Universal Health Coverage for Mental, Neurological, and Substance Use Disorders: An Extended Cost-Effectiveness Analysis." In *Disease Control Priorities* (third edition): Volume 4, *Mental, Neurological, and Substance Use Disorders*, edited by V. Patel, D. Chisholm, T. Dua, R. Laxminarayan, and M. Medina-Mora. Washington, DC: World Bank.

Cleary, S. 2010. "Equity and Efficiency in Scaling Up Access to HIV-Related Interventions in Resource-Limited Settings." *Current Opinion in HIV and AIDS* 5 (3): 210–14.

Cookson, R., M. Drummond, and H. Weatherly. 2009. "Explicit Incorporation of Equity Considerations into Economic Evaluation of Public Health Interventions." *Health Economics, Policy, and Law* 4 (2): 231–45.

Driessen, J. R., Z. D. Olson, D. T. Jamison, and S. Verguet. 2015. "Comparing the Health and Social Protection Effects of Measles Vaccination Strategies in Ethiopia: An Extended Cost-Effectiveness Analysis." *Social Science and Medicine* 139 (August): 115–22.

Drummond, M. F., M. J. Sculpher, K. Claxton, G. L. Stoddart, and G. W. Torrance. 2015. *Methods for the Economic Evaluation of Health Care Programmes*. 4th ed. Oxford: Oxford University Press.

Epstein, D., Z. Chalabi, K. Claxton, and M. Sculpher. 2007. "Efficiency, Equity, and Budgetary Policies: Informing Decisions Using Mathematical Programming." *Medical Decision Making* 27 (2): 128–37.

Essue, B., T. Laba, F. M. Knaul, A. Chu, H. Van Minh, and others. 2018. "The Economic Burden of Chronic Ill-Health and Injuries for Households in Low- and Middle-Income Countries." In *Disease Control Priorities* (third edition): Volume 9, *Disease Control Priorities: Improving Health and Reducing Poverty*, edited by D. T. Jamison, H. Gelband, S. Horton, P. Jha, R. Laxminarayan, C. N. Mock, and R. Nugent. Washington, DC: World Bank.

Finkelstein, A., and R. McKnight. 2008. "What Did Medicare Do? The Initial Impact of Medicare on Mortality and Out of Pocket Medical Spending." *Journal of Public Economics* 92 (7): 1644–68.

Fleurbaey, M., S. Luchini, C. Muller, and E. Schokkaert. 2013. "Equivalent Income and Fair Evaluation of Healthcare." *Health Economics* 22 (6): 711–29.

Flores, G., J. Krishnakumar, O. O'Donnell, and E. van Doorslaer. 2008. "Coping with Health-Care Costs: Implications for the Measurement of Catastrophic Expenditures and Poverty." *Health Economics* 17 (12): 1393–412.

Jamison, D. T. 2009. "Cost Effectiveness Analysis: Concepts and Applications." In *Oxford Textbook of Public Health*, Vol. 2, edited by R. Detels, J. McEwen, R. Beaglehole, and H. Tanaka. 5th ed. Oxford: Oxford University Press.

Jamison, D. T. 2018. "Disease Control Priorities: Improving Health and Reducing Poverty." In *Disease Control Priorities* (third edition): Volume 9, *Disease Control Priorities: Improving Health and Reducing Poverty*, edited by D. T. Jamison, H. Gelband, S. Horton, P. Jha, R. Laxminarayan, C. N. Mock, and R. Nugent. Washington, DC: World Bank.

Jamison, D. T., J. G. Breman, A. R. Measham, G. Alleyne, M. Claeson, D. B. Evans, P. Jha, A. Mills, and P. Musgrove, eds. 2006. *Disease Control Priorities in Developing Countries*, second edition. Washington, DC: World Bank.

Johansson, K. A., K. Bjerkreim Strand, A. Fekadu, and D. Chisholm. 2016. "Health Gains and Financial Protection Provided by the Ethiopian Mental Health Strategy: An Extended Cost-Effectiveness Analysis." *Health Policy and Planning* 1–8. doi:10.1093/heapol/czw134.

Johansson, K. A., C. Pecenka S. T. Memirie, D. T. Jamison, and S. Verguet. 2015. "Health Gains and Financial Protection from Pneumococcal Vaccination and Pneumonia Treatment in Ethiopia: Results from an Extended Cost-Effectiveness Analysis." *PLoS One* 10 (12): e0142691.

Kaplan, E. H., and M. H. Merson. 2002. "Allocating HIV-Prevention Resources: Balancing Efficiency and Equity." *American Journal of Public Health* 92 (12): 1905–7.

Kemp-Benedict, E. 2001. "Income Distribution and Poverty Methods for Using Available Data in Global Analysis." PoleStar Technical Note 4, Stockholm Environment Institute of the Global Scenario Group. http://gdrs.sourceforge.net /docs/PoleStar_TechNote_4.pdf.

Kim, J. J., J. A. Salomon, M. C. Weinstein, and S. J. Goldie. 2006. "Packaging Health Services When Resources Are Limited: The Example of a Cervical Cancer Screening Visit." *PLoS Medicine* 3 (11): e34.

Krakauer, E., Z. Ali, H. Arreola, A. Bhadelia, S. Connor and others. 2018. "Palliative Care in response to the Global Burden of Remediable Suffering." In *Disease Control Priorities* (third edition): Volume 9, *Disease Control Priorities: Improving Health and Reducing Poverty*, edited by D. T. Jamison, R. Nugent, H. Gelband, S. Horton, P. Jha, R. Laxminarayan, and C. N. Mock. Washington, DC: World Bank.

Kruk, M. E., E. Goldmann, and S. Galea. 2009. "Borrowing and Selling to Pay for Health Care in Low- and Middle-Income Countries." *Health Affairs* 28 (4): 1056–66.

Levin, C. L., M. Sharma, Z. Olson, S. Verguet, J. F. Shi, and others. 2015a. "An Extended Cost-Effectiveness Analysis of Publicly Financed HPV Vaccination to Prevent Cervical Cancer in China." In *Disease Control Priorities* (third edition): Volume 3, *Cancer*, edited by H. Gelband, P. Jha, R. Sankaranarayanan, and S. Horton. Washington, DC: World Bank.

Levin, C. L., M. Sharma, Z. Olson, S. Verguet, J. F. Shi, and others. 2015a. "An Extended Cost-Effectiveness Analysis of Publicly Financed HPV Vaccination to Prevent Cervical Cancer in China." *Vaccine* 33 (24): 2830–41.

Liu, L., Z. True, G. Fink, and S. Verguet. Forthcoming. "Estimating the Household Health and Financial Benefits of Malaria Vaccine in Zambia: An Extended Cost-Effectiveness Analysis."

Loganathan, T., M. Jit, R. Hutubessy, C. W. Ng, W. S. Lee, and others. 2016. "Rotavirus Vaccines Contribute towards Universal Health Coverage in a Mixed Public-Private Healthcare System." *Tropical Medicine and International Health* (August 24).

Mauskopf, J. A., J. E. Paul, D. M. Grant, and A. Stergachis. 1998. "The Role of Cost-Consequence Analysis in Healthcare Decision-Making." *PharmacoEconomics* 13 (3): 277–88.

McClellan, M., and J. Skinner. 2006. "The Incidence of Medicare." *Journal of Public Economics* 90 (1–2): 257–76.

Megiddo, I., A. R. Colson, D. Chisholm, T. Dua, A. Nandi, and others. 2016. "Health and Economic Benefits of Public Financing of Epilepsy Treatment in India: An Agent-Based Simulation Model." *Epilepsia* 57 (3): 464–74.

Megiddo, I., A. R. Colson, A. Nandi, S. Chatterjee, S. Prinja, and others. 2014. "Analysis of the Universal Immunization Programme and Introduction of a Rotavirus Vaccine in India with IndiaSim." *Vaccine* 32 (S1): A151–61.

Nandi, A., A. R. Colson, A. Verma, I. Megiddo, A. Ashok, and others. 2016. "Health and Economic Benefits of Scaling Up a Home-Based Neonatal Care Package in Rural India: A Modeling Analysis." *Health Policy and Planning* 31 (5): 634–44.

Nandi, A., I. Megiddo, A. Ashok, A. Verma, and R. Laxminarayan. 2016. "Reduced Burden of Childhood Diarrheal Diseases through Increased Access to Water and Sanitation in India: A Modeling Analysis." *Social Science and Medicine.* http://dx.doi.org/10.1016/j.socscimed.2016.08.049.

Olson, Z. D., J. A. Staples, C. Mock, N. P. Nguyen, A. M. Bachani, and others. 2016. "Helmet Regulation in Vietnam: Impact on Health, Equity, and Medical Impoverishment." *Injury Prevention* 22 (4): 233–38.

Olson, Z. D., J. A. Staples, C. N. Mock, N. P. Nguyen, A. M. Bachani, and others. 2017. "Helmet Regulation in Vietnam: Impact on Health, Equity, and Medical Impoverishment." In *Disease Control Priorities* (third edition): Volume 7, *Injury Prevention and Environmental Health*, edited by C. N. Mock, O. Kobusingye, R. Nugent, and K. R. Smith. Washington, DC: World Bank.

Pecenka, C., K. A. Johansson, S. T. Memirie, D. T. Jamison, and S. Verguet. 2015. "Health Gains and Financial Risk Protection in Ethiopia: Assessing the Benefits of Diarrhea Treatment and Prevention." *PLoS One* 10 (12): e0142691.

Pillarisetti, A., D. T. Jamison, and K. R. Smith. 2017. "Effect of Household Energy Interventions on Health and Finances in Haryana, India: An Extended Cost-Effectiveness Analysis." In *Disease Control Priorities* (third edition): Volume 7, *Injury Prevention and Environmental Health*, edited by C. N. Mock, O. Kobusingye, R. Nugent, and K. R. Smith. Washington, DC: World Bank.

Postolovska, I., R. Lavado, G. Tarr, and S. Verguet. 2017. "Estimating the Distributional Impact of Increasing Taxes on Tobacco Productions in Armenia: Results from an Extended Cost-Effectiveness Analysis." Report. World Bank, Washington, DC.

Raykar N., A. Nigam, and D. Chisholm. 2016. "An Extended Cost-Effectiveness Analysis of Schizophrenia Treatment in India under Universal Public Finance." *Cost Effectiveness and Resource Allocation* 14: 9.

Rheingans, R. D., D. Atherly, and J. Anderson. 2012. "Distributional Impact of Rotavirus Vaccination in 25 GAVI Countries: Estimating Disparities in Benefits and Cost-Effectiveness." *Vaccine* 30 (Suppl 1): A15–23.

Salem, A. B. Z., and T. D. Mount. 1974. "A Convenient Descriptive Model of Income Distribution: The Gamma Density." *Econometrica* 42 (6): 1115–27.

Salti, N., E. D. Brouwer, and S. Verguet. 2016. "The Health, Financial, and Distributional Consequences of Increases in the Tobacco Excise Tax among Smokers in Lebanon." *Social Science and Medicine* 170: 161–69.

Sassi, F., L. Archard, and J. Le Grand. 2001. "Equity and the Economic Evaluation of Healthcare." *Health Technology Assessment* 5 (3): 1–138.

Segall, R. S. 1989. "Some Nonlinear Optimization Modeling for Planning Objectives of Large Market-Oriented Systems: With an Application to Real Health Data." *Applied Mathematical Modelling* 13 (4): 203–14.

Shrime, M. G., S. Verguet, K. A. Johansson, D. Desalegn, D. T. Jamison, and M. E. Kruk. 2015. "Task-Sharing or Public Finance for Expanding Surgical Access in Rural Ethiopia: An Extended-Cost Effectiveness Analysis." In *Disease Control Priorities* (third edition): Volume 1, *Essential Surgery*, edited by H. T. Debas, P. Donkor, A. Gawande, D. T. Jamison, M. E. Kruk, and C. N. Mock. Washington, DC: World Bank.

Shrime, M. G., S. Verguet, K. A. Johansson, D. Desalegn, D. T. Jamison, and others. 2016. "Task-Sharing or Public Finance for the Expansion of Surgical Access in Rural Ethiopia: An Extended Cost-Effectiveness Analysis." *Health Policy and Planning* 31 (6): 706–16.

Smith, P. C. 2007. "Provision of a Public Benefit Package alongside Private Voluntary Health Insurance." In *Private Voluntary Health Insurance in Development: Friend or Foe?* edited by A. Preker, R. M. Scheffer, and M. C. Bassett. Washington, DC: World Bank.

———. 2013. "Incorporating Financial Protection into Decision Rules for Publicly Financed Healthcare Treatments." *Health Economics* 22 (2): 180–93.

Stinnett, A. A., and D. A. Paltiel. 1996. "Mathematical Programming for the Efficient Allocation of Health Care Resources." *Journal of Health Economics* 15 (5): 641–53.

van Doorslaer, E., O. O'Donnell, R. P. Rannan-Eliya, A. Somanathan, S. R. Adhikari, and others. 2006. "Effect of Payments for Health Care on Poverty Estimates in 11 Countries in Asia: An Analysis of Household Survey Data." *The Lancet* 368 (9544): 1357–64.

Verguet, S. 2013. "Efficient and Equitable HIV Prevention: A Case Study of Male Circumcision in South Africa." *Cost Effectiveness and Resource Allocation* 11 (December): 1.

Verguet, S., C. L. Gauvreau, S. Mishra, M. MacLennan, S. M. Murphy, and others. 2015. "The Consequences of Tobacco Tax on Household Health and Finances in Rich and Poor Smokers in China: An Extended Cost-Effectiveness Analysis." *The Lancet Global Health* 3 (4): e206–16.

Verguet, S., J. J. Kim, and D. T. Jamison. 2016. "Extended Cost-Effectiveness Analysis for Health Policy Assessment: A Tutorial." *PharmacoEconomics* 34 (9): 913–23.

Verguet, S., R. Laxminarayan, and D. T. Jamison. 2015. "Universal Public Finance of Tuberculosis Treatment in India: An Extended Cost-Effectiveness Analysis." *Health Economics* 24 (3): 318–32.

Verguet, S., S. T. Memirie, and O. F. Norheim. 2016. "Assessing the Burden of Medical Impoverishment by Cause: A Systematic Breakdown by Disease in Ethiopia." *BMC Medicine* 14 (1): 164.

Verguet, S., S. M. Murphy, B. Anderson, K. A. Johansson, R. Glass, and others. 2013. "Public Finance of Rotavirus Vaccination in India and Ethiopia: An Extended Cost-Effectiveness Analysis." *Vaccine* 31 (42): 4902–10.

Verguet, S., A. Nandi, V. Filippi, and D. A. P. Bundy. 2016. "Maternal-Related Deaths and Impoverishment among Adolescent girls in India and Niger: Findings from a Modelling Study." *BMJ Open* 6: e011586.

Verguet, S., A. Nandi, V. Filippi, and D. A. P. Bundy. 2017. "Maternal Deaths and Impoverishment Averted by Postponing Adolescent Parity in Developing Countries through Education: An Extended Cost-Effectiveness Analysis." In *Disease Control Priorities* (third edition): Volume 8, *Child and Adolescent Health and Development*, edited by D. A. P. Bundy, N. de Silva, S. Horton, D. T. Jamison, and G. C. Patton. Washington, DC: World Bank.

Verguet, S., Z. D. Olson, J. B. Babigumira, D. Desalegn, K. A. Johansson, and others. 2015. "Health Gains and Financial Risk Protection Afforded by Public Financing of Selected Interventions in Ethiopia: An Extended Cost-Effectiveness Analysis." *The Lancet Global Health* 3 (5): e288–96.

Verguet, S., C. Pecenka, K. A. Johansson, S. T. Memirie, I. K. Friberg, and others. 2016. "Health Gains and Financial Risk Protection Afforded by Treatment and Prevention of Diarrhea and Pneumonia in Ethiopia: An Extended Cost-Effectiveness Analysis." In *Disease Control Priorities* (third edition): Volume 2, *Reproductive, Maternal, Newborn, and Child Health*, edited by R. Black, R. Laxminarayan, M. Temmerman, and N. Walker. Washington, DC: World Bank.

Wagstaff, A. 2010. "Measuring Financial Protection in Health." In *Performance Measurement for Health System Improvement*, edited by P. C. Smith, E. Mossialos, I. Papanicolas, and S. Leatherman. Cambridge, U.K.: Cambridge University Press.

Wagstaff, A., and E. van Doorslaer. 2003. "Catastrophe and Impoverishment in Paying for Health Care: Its Applications to Vietnam 1993–1998." *Health Economics* 12 (11): 921–34.

Watkins, D. A., R. Nugent, and S. Verguet. 2017. "Extended Cost-Effectiveness Analyses of Cardiovascular Risk Factor Reduction Policies." In *Disease Control Priorities* (third edition): Volume 5, *Cardiovascular, Respiratory and Related Disorders*, edited by D. Prabhakaran, S. Anand, T. Gaziano, J. C. Mbanya, Y. Wu, and R. Nugent. Washington, DC: World Bank.

Watkins, D. A., D. T. Jamison, A. Mills, C. N. Mock, R. Nugent, and others. 2018. "Essential Universal Health Coverage." In *Disease Control Priorities* (third edition): Volume 9, *Disease Control Priorities: Improving Health and Reducing Poverty*, edited by D. T. Jamison, H. Gelband, S. Horton, P. Jha, R. Laxminarayan, C. N. Mock, and R. Nugent. Washington, DC: World Bank.

Watkins, D. A., Z. D. Olson, S. Verguet, R. Nugent, and D. T. Jamison. 2015. "Cardiovascular Disease and Impoverishment Averted due to a Salt Reduction Policy in South Africa: An Extended Cost-Effectiveness Analysis." *Health Policy and Planning* (April 3). doi:10.1093/heapol/czv023.

WHO (World Health Organization). 1999. *World Health Report 1999: Making a Difference.* Geneva: WHO.

———. 2000. *World Health Report 2000: Health Systems: Improving Performance.* Geneva: WHO.

———. 2010. *World Health Report 2010: Health Systems Financing, the Path to Universal Coverage.* Geneva: WHO.

———. 2013. *World Health Report 2013: Research for Universal Health Coverage.* Geneva: WHO.

Xu, K., D. B. Evans, K. Kawabata, R. Zeramdini, J. Klavus, and others. 2003. "Household Catastrophic Health Expenditure: A Multicountry Analysis." *The Lancet* 362 (9378): 111–17.

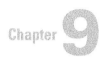
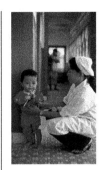

Chapter 9

Benefit-Cost Analysis in *Disease Control Priorities*, Third Edition

Angela Y. Chang, Susan Horton, and Dean T. Jamison

INTRODUCTION: ROLE OF BENEFIT-COST ANALYSIS IN THE HEALTH SECTOR

A variety of economic methods is used for analysis in the health sector. Other chapters in this volume summarize the findings from *Disease Control Priorities* (third edition) (*DCP3*) concerning cost-effectiveness analysis (CEA) and extended cost-effectiveness analysis (ECEA) (Horton 2018; Verguet and Jamison 2018). This chapter summarizes the findings concerning benefit-cost analysis (BCA).

BCA has long been used for the analysis of public policy. The U.S. Secretary of the Treasury first used it in 1808, and its use became mandatory for the U.S. Army Corps of Engineers in 1936. The U.S. Bureau of the Budget first issued guidelines for its use in 1952. Mills, Lubell, and Hanson (2008) suggest that BCA became less well used for analysis of malaria eradication around 1980, when CEA methods were becoming well developed. More recently, there has been a resurgence of interest in applying BCA to assess the viability of public investment programs and to set priorities among a list of interventions (Jha and others 2015; Ozawa and others 2016).

BCA tends to be relatively readily understood by the general public, because the private sector uses analogous concepts. However, BCA also tends to raise controversies because it assigns monetary values to outcomes (such as small changes in annual mortality probabilities) that cannot be monetized according to many individuals.

We observe that BCA and CEA in the health sector represent two distinct cultures. The metric for value in CEA can accommodate real health outcomes, such as child deaths averted, and aggregate measures, such as quality-adjusted life years (QALYs) or disability-adjusted life years (DALYs), as well as more granular measures, such as malaria cases correctly treated. When health benefits are measured in life years, both the ages of the individuals and their remaining life expectancies are implicitly factored into the analysis. In contrast, in BCA, health benefits are often measured in terms of the number of statistical lives; ages and remaining life expectancy of individuals are often not considered. BCA involves an additional step of assigning monetary value to health benefits; analysts are required to explicitly assume a certain relationship between the proportional change in this monetary value and the differences in countries' income levels, namely, income elasticity. This factor is often not considered in CEA.

The choice of applying CEA or BCA to evaluate economic benefits depends on the type of outcomes produced by the health interventions. For some interventions, the main benefits include reduced mortality, improved quality of life, or reduced morbidity or disability. For these outcomes, CEA works well and allows comparisons with other health interventions. Many health interventions also affect future health care requirements; preventive interventions, in particular, can reduce future health care costs. In CEA, these future

Corresponding author: Angela Y. Chang, Harvard T. H. Chan School of Public Health, Boston, Massachusetts, United States; angela.chang@mail.harvard.edu.

cost reductions can be subtracted from current costs of the intervention before comparing net costs to the health benefits.

Other interventions may improve health, but their key outcomes are more easily expressed in monetary terms. For example, supplementation or food fortification with iron or iodine produces modest health benefits in the form of reduced anemia and cretinism. However, the most pervasive benefits accrue via improved human capital—in this case, cognition and education—and thus BCA is more appropriate. The eradication of a disease, such as smallpox, improves health but can also save a substantial amount of money through elimination of future prevention and treatment costs. Hence, BCA may be the most effective way to provide evidence of and advocate for this as a policy intervention.

A third group of interventions undertaken in sectors outside health (for example, improvements in road safety, safety regulations for vehicles, or water and sanitation) are more naturally assessed by BCA methods. The investment decisions are made in sectors that are accustomed to using BCA, and the investments with health benefits are being compared to other investments with outcomes that are assessed by BCA. CEA is more frequently used for comparisons within the health sector; it has been refined for specific policy purposes, such as the decision whether to allow insurance coverage of a particular new drug, technique, health technology, or diagnostic test within a country, or for the prioritization of the use of donor funds when international assistance is involved. (For alternative approaches incorporating noneconomic considerations, see also Norheim and others 2017.)

BCA, CEA, and ECEA are complementary techniques; each has value in addressing specific circumstances or specific policy questions. This chapter summarizes the BCA findings from *DCP3*. It then examines the existing methods for valuing life and considers possible improvements and ends with concluding comments.

CONTRIBUTION OF *DISEASE CONTROL PRIORITIES* (THIRD EDITION) TO BCA IN THE HEALTH SECTOR

The approaches in the *DCP3* chapters and *DCP*-supported literature take many forms. Some directly report benefit-cost ratios from existing literature, while others conduct their own BCA using primary data. Key BCA findings and the methods applied are summarized in tables 9.1 and 9.2.

Most of the benefit-cost ratios reported in tables 9.1 and 9.2 range from 1 to 10. Only one reported ratio is below 1 (likely owing to publication bias), a small number are in the 11–30 range, and a few outliers have higher ratios. In part, this variation in results may stem from variations in the methodologies adopted. Some studies use methods of value per statistical life (VSL) based on willingness to pay (for example, Alkire, Vincent, and Meara 2015; Cropper and others 2017). Others assign dollar values to morbidity and mortality averted (for example, Jamison and others 2013; Jha and others 2013; Stenberg and others 2016) or to mortality risk reduction (Fan, Jamison, and Summers 2018; Jamison, Summers, and others 2013), using productivity or cost of illness averted to value years of life lost. Of those assigning a value to mortality averted, only Stenberg and others (2016) include an explicit intrinsic value to life in excess of an assumed contribution to, or share of, GDP. These methods are described in more detail in the next section.

Several studies examine health interventions that improve human capital and value the outcome according to higher wages. These include interventions in early child development and preschool (Horton and Black 2017), school feeding and deworming (Fernandes and Aurino 2017) and programs to educate school-age children and adolescents in health prevention (Horton and others 2017). Other studies include future wages and averted future health care costs in regard to malaria elimination (for example, Mills, Lubell, and Hanson 2008) and improvements in sanitation (Hutton 2013; Whittington and others 2009).

BCA findings were not surveyed and analyzed systematically in all volumes (unlike CEAs), and thus we can draw only tentative conclusions as to the areas where BCA is used most often. It is widely used in injury prevention and environmental health areas, and volume 7 (Mock and others 2017) has very few examples of CEA. Similarly, the analyses of pandemics and elimination or eradication of infectious diseases lend themselves to BCA. BCA is underrepresented in volume 2, because space did not permit the inclusion of BCAs on nutrition, an area with many BCAs already (Black and others 2016). BCAs are scarcely visible in volume 3 (Gelband and others 2015) and volume 5 (Prabhakaran and others 2017). The focus of these particular areas of noncommunicable diseases is on health interventions more relevant to individuals than populations and on treatment and screening of those individuals, which may make CEA methods more appropriate.

The next section considers the issues around the variation in methodology and associated effects on the magnitudes of BCA reported.

Table 9.1 Economic Burden of Disease, BCA, and Investment Cases in *DCP3*

Subject	*DCP3* reference	Summary of key findings	Method of valuing health or changes in mortality
Essential Surgery	Volume 1, chapter 21 (Alkire, Vincent, and Meara 2015)	• B/C of cleft lip and palate repair were 42 (income elasticity = 1.0) and 12 (income elasticity = 1.5), respectively. • The median B/C of cesarean-section delivery for obstructed labor across countries is 4.0 (income elasticity = 1.5), ranging from 0.3 for the Democratic Republic of Congo to 76 for Gabon.	• The base VSL was set at $7.4 million (2006 US$), and income elasticities of 1.0 and 1.5 were applied when extrapolating to other countries. Age adjustment was applied, with the highest value of VSLY occurring at two-thirds of life expectancy. A 3 percent discount rate was applied.
Reproductive, Maternal, Newborn, and Child Health	Volume 2, chapter 16 (Stenberg and others 2016)	• Additional investments of $5 (2011 US$) per person per year in 74 countries with 95 percent of the global maternal and child mortality burden would yield a B/C of 8.7 by 2035. • B/C in low-, lower-middle-, and upper-middle-income (excluding China) countries are 7.2, 11.3, and 6.1, respectively, at 3 percent discount rate	Values for changes in mortality and morbidity and in consequences of decline in fertility and unintended pregnancies were estimated using human capital methods. No age adjustment was applied. • Mortality averted: The authors assigned an average benefit of 1.0 times the GDP per capita for the direct economic benefits in terms of increased labor supply and productivity and an additional 0.5 times the GDP per capita for the social value of a life year. • Morbidity averted: A morbidity-to-mortality ratio of disability weights (namely, severity) was applied to estimate the social value of morbidity averted. • Positive economic and social consequences of decreases in fertility and reductions in unintended pregnancies: The economic benefit (expressed as percentage of GDP per capita) of this category was calculated by assuming different levels of decline in total fertility rate (TFR) and applying the model by Ashraf, Weil, and Wilde (2013) to calculate the effect of TFR reduction on GDP per capita.
Major Infectious Diseases: Malaria	Volume 6, chapter 12 (Shretta and others 2017)	• B/C of malaria elimination programs surveyed by Mills, Lubell and Hanson (2008) range from 2.4 in the Philippines to 4.1 and 9.2 for control in India, 17.1 for elimination in Greece to almost 150 in Sri Lanka. • B/C of global malaria reduction and elimination between 2013 and 2015 is estimated at 6.1 (Purdy and others 2013) • B/C of malaria eradication efforts between 2015 and 2040 is estimated to be 17 (Gates and Chambers 2015).	Various methods are used to value benefits (varies by study): • Elimination of costs required to control malaria • Productivity gains (labor, land, or both) • Modeled macroeconomic growth benefits
Major Infectious Diseases: NTDs	Volume 6, chapter 17 (Fitzpatrick and others 2017)	• B/C of interventions to end NTDs is 25 between 1990 and 2030. The benefits include health expenditure and lost wages averted, estimated at around $657 billion (international dollars) between 2011 and 2030. Total cost of the investment is estimated at US$27 billion. A discount rate of 3 percent per annum was applied for both benefits and costs	• The benefits of the interventions include only health expenditure and lost wages averted. No value was assigned to the intrinsic value of mortality risk reduction.

table continues next page

Table 9.1 Economic Burden of Disease, BCA, and Investment Cases in *DCP3* (continued)

Subject	*DCP3* reference	Summary of key findings	Method of valuing health or changes in mortality
Injury Prevention and Environmental Health: Environment	Volume 7, chapter 9 (Hutton and Chase 2017)	B/C from Hutton (2013) and Whittington and others (2009): • Networked water and sewerage services: 0.7 • Deep borehole with public hand pump: 4.6 • Total sanitation campaign (South Asia): 3.0 • Household water treatment (biosand filters): 2.5 • Improved water supply: 2.0 • Improved sanitation: 5.5	• Health estimates based on direct health costs (treatment of water- and sanitation-related disease), productivity losses during illness, and mortality losses were measured using human capital. • Estimates also include reduced travel and access time for water and sanitation owing to improvements.
Injury Prevention and Environmental Health: Environment	Volume 7, chapter 13 (Cropper and others 2017)	B/C of installing flue-gas desulfurization units at every coal-fired power plant in India is greater than 1, for all reasonable VSL estimates applied	• Empirical estimates of the VSL in India range widely, from US$50,600 (Bhattacharya, Alberini, and Cropper 2007) to US$362,000 (Madheswaran 2007) (2007 US$). • Transferring the U.S. VSL to India at current exchange rates, using an income elasticity of 1, suggests a VSL of US$250,000 (2006 US$).
Child and Adolescent Health and Development: Early childhood	Volume 8, chapter 24 (Horton and Black 2017)	B/C for the following interventions: • Videos on early childhood development shown to parents with children age 2 years and younger waiting in health centers, followed by group discussion: 5.3 (Walker and others 2015) • Responsive stimulation and nutrition intervention (sprinkles) for children age 2 years and younger: 1.5 (López Boo, Palloni, and Urzua 2014) • Home visiting program that educates mothers with children age 2 years and younger in child development: 2.6–3.6 (Berlinski and Schady 2015) • Preschool programs for children ages 3 to 5 years: generally exceed 3 (Berlinski and Schady 2015) • Nutritional add-on to preschool: 77 (Psacharopoulos 2014) • Overall, B/C of a well-designed and well-implemented early childhood program is in the range of 2 to 5.	• Benefits include improved cognition and greater school grade attainment, which translate into higher wages and employment. Same pathway exists for all interventions (except sprinkles, which reduce anemia and then also has same effects). • Psacharopoulos (2014) study does not fully incorporate the cost of all interventions, hence the incredibly high B/C ratio.

table continues next page

Table 9.1 Economic Burden of Disease, BCA, and Investment Cases in *DCP3* (continued)

Subject	*DCP3* reference	Summary of key findings	Method of valuing health or changes in mortality
Child and Adolescent Health and Development: school-age children	Volume 8, chapter 25 (Fernandes and Aurino 2017)	• School feeding programs with micronutrient fortification had estimated B/C of 3 and 7 for low- and lower-middle-income countries, respectively (2012 US$, discount rate 3 percent). The average cost of school feeding is US$56 in low- and lower-middle-income countries	• Benefits are assumed to be gained through improved education outcomes over the lifetime of targeted children and to translate into improved productivity and contributions to GDP. No intrinsic value of health improvements was included.
Child and Adolescent Health and Development: adolescents	Volume 8, chapter 26 (Horton and others 2017)	B/C for adolescent health in high-income countries is as follows: • Education sessions with children ages 11–12 years and parents and other interventions for alcohol use in the United States: range of 5 to 100 (McDaid and others 2014) • School-based smoking programs in Germany: 3.6 (McDaid and others 2014) • Programs to promote mental well-being in the United States: range of 5 to 28 (McDaid and others 2014) • Programs for reduced drug dependency, smoking, and delinquency in the United States: 25 (McDaid and others 2014)	• Benefits included health care costs averted, human capital gains (via education, reduced mortality), and reduced costs of crime (for alcohol and drug interventions).
Disease Control Priorities: Improving Health and Reducing Poverty: Pandemic flu	Volume 9, chapter 18 (Fan, Jamison, and Summers 2018)	• The total cost of a pandemic is presented as a sum of its effect on income and the intrinsic value of lives prematurely lost and illness suffered (Fan, Jamison, and Summers, 2018). • For the first dimension, the authors estimated the expected annual income losses globally of US$16 billion for moderately severe pandemics and US$64 billion for severe pandemics. • For the second dimension, they estimated the expected annual loss for the whole world from the intrinsic cost as 0.6 percent of global income and variation by income group, from 0.3 percent in high-income countries to 1.6 percent in lower-middle-income countries. • In total, the expected annual inclusive cost, reflecting both dimensions above, amounts to about 0.7 percent (US$570 billion per year) of global income, with income losses accounting for a small fraction of inclusive costs (12 percent) for severe pandemics, but a larger fraction (40 percent) for moderately severe pandemics.	• The values of a 1-in-10,000 mortality risk reduction for one year for a person age 35 years were set at 0.7, 1.0, 1.3, and 1.6 percent of income per capita for low-, lower-middle-, upper-middle-, and high-income countries, respectively. This amount was then adjusted for ages other than age 35 years in proportion to the ratio of life expectancies at those ages to life expectancy at age 35 years.

Note: B/C = benefit/cost; GDP = gross domestic product; NTDs = neglected tropical diseases; VSL = value per statistical life; VSLY = value per statistical life year.

Table 9.2 Economic Burden of Disease, BCA, and Investment Cases Supported by *DCP3*

Subject	Reference	Summary of key findings	Method of valuing health or changes in mortality
Global Health 2035 grand convergence	Jamison, Summers, and others (2013)	• The recommended set of investments to scale up health technologies and systems in LMICs, compared to a scenario of stagnant investment and no improvements in technology, would yield a B/C of 9 in lower-income countries and 20 in lower-middle-income countries over a 20-year period.	• The value of a 1-in-10,000 mortality risk reduction for one year for a 35-year-old person was set at 1.8 percent of income per capita, assuming an income elasticity of 1.0. This was then adjusted for ages other than age 35 years in proportion to the ratio of life expectancies at those ages to life expectancy at age 35 years, using the historical Japanese life table. • Four different age adjustment scenarios were applied: no adjustment, reducing progress in children under age 4 years by 50 percent, excluding all children under age 10 years from the calculation, and excluding over-70 mortality. Under the second age adjustment scenario, the value of a life year is 2.3 times the per person income.
Infectious disease and maternal health	Jamison, Jha, and others (2013)	Recommended investment solutions and B/Cs are as follows: 1. Tuberculosis: Appropriate case finding and treatment, including dealing with MDR TB—15 2. Malaria: Subsidy for appropriate treatment via Affordable Medicines Facility—malaria—35 3. Childhood diseases: Expanded immunization coverage—20 4. HIV: Accelerated vaccine development—11 5. Essential surgery: Management of difficult childbirth, trauma, and other—10 6. Deworming of schoolchildren—10	• US$1,000 per DALY was applied to value the health benefits gained; it roughly equals the lower end of the proposed value of a statistical life year of 2 to 4 times per capita income of low-income countries. US$5,000 per DALY was used for sensitivity analysis. • The DALYs were discounted at 3 percent, and the DALY cost of a typical death under age 5 years was reduced by 50 percent. For DALYs accrued near the time of birth, a smoothing formula using the concept of acquisition of life potential was applied to assign greater weights to DALYs resulting from deaths of a fetus.

table continues next page

Table 9.2 Economic Burden of Disease, BCA, and Investment Cases Supported by *DCP3* (continued)

Subject	Reference	Summary of key findings	Method of valuing health or changes in mortality
NCDs	Jha and others (2013)	Key investment priorities and B/Cs are as follows: 1. Tobacco taxation: 40 2. Acute management of heart attacks with low-cost drugs: 25 3. Salt reduction: 20 4. Hepatitis B immunization: 10 5. Secondary prevention of heart attacks and strokes with 3–4 drugs in a *generic risk pill*: 4	• Same method as the Copenhagen Consensus on infectious disease (Jamison and others 2013b) was applied.
Rheumatic heart disease	Watkins and Chang (2017)	Economic burden of RHD found to be approximately US$64.8 billion, or an average of US$ 360,000 per preventable death in low- and middle-income countries	• The value of a 1-in-10,000 mortality risk reduction for one year for a 35-year-old person in the United States was set at $900. These were adjusted downward for low- and middle-income countries based on average GDP per capita in each region, assuming an income elasticity of 1.0. This was then adjusted for ages other than age 35 years in proportion to the ratio of region-specific life expectancies at those ages to life expectancy at age 35 years. • Sensitivity analyses conducted for income elasticity (0.6 and 1.5), anchoring age (from age 35 years to ages with remaining life expectancy of 45 years).

Note: DALY = disability-adjusted life year; HIV = human immunodeficiency disease; MDR = multidrug-resistant; NCDs = noncommunicable diseases; RHD = rheumatic heart disease; TB = tuberculosis.

USE OF THE VALUE PER STATISTICAL LIFE IN ESTIMATING BCA IN THE HEALTH SECTOR

Several of the *DCP3* chapters and related articles build on the concept of the VSL to estimate the intrinsic value of health improvements. The VSL is defined as the marginal rate of substitution between money and mortality risk in a defined time period. It is typically calculated by dividing individuals' willingness to pay for a small change in their own risks in a defined time period by the risk change. For example, individuals have a VSL of US$9 million if they are willing to pay US$900 for a 10^{-4} reduction in mortality risk in the current year. Note that money is used as a measure to reflect the trade-offs individuals are willing to make, and it is not itself important. Jamison, Summers, and others (2013) argue that terminology should be used in cases where the risk change units are close to those actually measured so that one avoids the occasionally contentious interpretations of value of life (Chang and others 2017). They propose that risk be measured in source measure units (SMUs), or units of 10^{-4}. Rather than referring to the value of a statistical life, they propose referring to the value of an SMU (VSMU). In the example just provided, the risk change was 1 SMU and the associated VSMU was US$900. Most published VSL studies focus on the risks of accidental deaths, mainly among adult populations in high-income settings (Lindhjem and others 2011; Robinson and Hammitt 2015b; Viscusi 2015; Viscusi and Aldy 2003).

Far fewer VSL studies are conducted in low- and middle-income countries (LMICs), and the quality of the papers varies widely (Bhattacharya, Alberini, and Cropper 2007; Guo and Hammitt 2009; Hammitt and Zhou 2006; Hoffmann and others 2012; Shanmugam 2001; Simon and others 1999; Tekeşin and Ara 2014; Vassanadumrongdee and Matsuoka 2005; Viscusi and Masterman 2017a). Under this limitation, analyses that value health improvements in LMICs often rely on studies from high-income countries (HICs) as their base VSL estimates, and these are adapted on the basis of some characteristics of the population of interest. This section discusses the common practices, as well as the challenges, that analysts face in using previously established values for another setting of interest (also known as *benefit transfer*) and provides an alternative to existing methods.

Current Practice of Benefit Transfer in Global Health

Selection of Base VSL or VSL-to-Income Ratio
Benefit transfer often begins with selecting a base VSL or a VSL-to-income ratio (VSLr). We consider the VSL estimates produced by major U.S. regulatory agencies and the Organisation for Economic Co-operation and Development (OECD) as two reasonable starting points. In the United States, a simple average of the values applied by three regulatory agencies is US$9.3 million (Robinson and Hammitt 2015b; U.S. DOT 2015; U.S. EPA 2014), which translates into a VSLr of roughly 180. OECD (2012, 2014) proposed a VSL of US$3.6 million and a VSLr of roughly 100, which is much lower than the U.S. estimates.

Several considerations need to be made when extrapolating existing estimates to other populations. The VSL is expected to vary, depending on the characteristics of those affected (for example, health status, age, life expectancy, and income) and the characteristics of the risks (for example, latency, morbidity before death, voluntariness, and controllability). However, the effects of many of these characteristics need further research. There are significant inconsistencies and gaps in the available literature, even for HICs (Hammitt 2017, Robinson and Hammitt 2015b; Viscusi and Masterman 2017b). The most commonly adjusted characteristic is income, possibly because both theoretical and empirical evidence are readily available (although consensus on the magnitude of adjustments one should make between countries with varying income levels is still lacking). Other important characteristics, such as the average age or remaining life expectancy of those affected, are often ignored.

Relationship to Income
Research on the relationship between income and the VSL generally indicates that the VSL increases as income increases. However, the proportional change in the VSL in response to a change in real income—its income elasticity—is uncertain (Robinson and Hammitt 2015a). Income elasticity is of particular importance in estimating the VSL for lower-income countries because changing the elasticity can affect the resulting VSL by orders of magnitude (equations 9.1 and 9.2) (Hammitt and Robinson 2011). (In equations 9.1 and 9.2, r = ratio of VSL to GDP per capita and pc = per capita.)

$$\text{VSL}_{\text{country x}} = \text{VSL}_{\text{US}} \times \left(\frac{\text{GDP per capita}_{\text{x}}}{\text{GDP per capita}_{\text{US}}} \right)^{\text{elasticity}} \quad (9.1)$$

$$\begin{aligned} \text{VSL}_{\text{r}} &= \frac{\text{VSL}_{\text{country x}}}{\text{GDP per capita}_{\text{country x}}} \\ &= \frac{\text{VSL}_{\text{US}} \times \left(\frac{\text{GDPpc}_{\text{country x}}}{\text{GDPpc}_{\text{US}}} \right)^{\text{elasticity}}}{\text{GDPpc}_{\text{country x}}} \quad (9.2) \\ &= \text{VSL}_{\text{US}} \times \frac{\text{GDPpc}_{\text{country x}}^{(\text{elasticity}-1)}}{\text{GDPpc}_{\text{US}}^{\text{elasticity}}} \end{aligned}$$

Empirical studies comparing VSL estimates from HICs and middle-income countries (MICs), as well as between higher- and lower-income groups in the United States, support the use of elasticity greater than 1.0 when applying VSL across income levels (Biausque 2012; Costa and Kahn 2004; Hammitt and Ibarrarán 2006; Kniesner, Viscusi, and Ziliak 2010). However, similar research has not been conducted in low-income countries (LICs). Nevertheless, the global meta-analysis in Lindhjem and others (2011) and OECD (2012) for OECD countries yielded the estimate of 0.8 (range 0.7–0.9). Figure 9.1 illustrates the relationship between VSLr and income when an income elasticity of 1.2 is applied across countries, using the U.S. VSLr of 180 as the base. If elasticity of 1 were applied, all countries would face the same VSLr of 180. With greater income elasticity, countries with greater GDP per capita will behave a higher VSLr, with the highest occurring in Qatar at 217. For LMICs, the VSLr drops exponentially, with the lowest VSLr occurring in the Central African Republic at 73.

One issue with extrapolating the VSL from a higher- to a lower-income setting is that the VSL may fall below the expected income or consumption in the relevant period in the lower-income country. Theory suggests that the VSL will exceed the present value of future earnings and of future consumption, both of which vary by age, because it reflects the intrinsic value of living in addition to an individual's productivity or consumption. Accordingly, the VSL is expected to at least equal the present value of future income, as well as consumption, discounted to the age at which the risk reduction occurs (Hammitt and Robinson 2011).

Relationship to Age and Life Expectancy
Because the VSL cannot be directly estimated from market measures such as earnings or consumption, researchers instead rely on revealed or stated preference studies. The former estimates the value of risk reductions based on related market transactions or behavior, often on the relationship between wages and occupational risks in the case of the VSL. Some of these studies found an inverse U-shaped relationship; the VSL increased in young adulthood, peaked in middle age, and then declined, consistent with the patterns of income and consumption predicted under the lifecycle models (Rosen 1988; Shepard and Zeckhauser 1982, 1984). Others found that the values for older adults decrease or remain constant (Evans and Smith 2006; Krupnick 2007). One limitation of the revealed preference method is that it addresses only working age populations. Stated preference methods instead involve surveying respondents to determine their willingness to pay for risk reductions of various types. Some stated preference studies suggest that adult

Figure 9.1 VSLr, with VSL Extrapolated from the U.S. VSL with Income Elasticity of 1.2

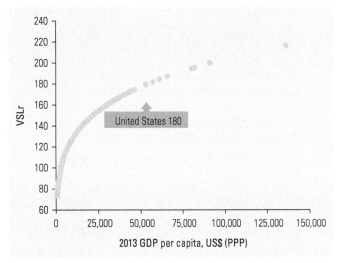

Note: GDP = gross domestic product; PPP = purchasing power parity; VSLr = value per statistical life-to-income ratio.

willingness to pay to reduce risks to children is likely to be larger than the value adults place on reducing risks to themselves, although the magnitude of the difference varies across studies. For example, Hammitt and Haninger (2010) found that willingness to pay for risk reduction is nearly twice as large for children than for adults. To date, we are unaware of a general consensus in the BCA community on how to adjust the value of risk change for differences in age.

Age and life expectancy are related but distinct concepts. As Sanderson and Scherbov (2007) stated, a person has two different ages: the retrospective age, which is a measure of how many years one has already lived, and the prospective age—remaining life expectancy—which reflects how many years a person will live. For example, a person age 35 years in 1960 and a person age 35 years in 2015 likely would have different levels of willingness to pay for mortality risk reduction, because they would have had different perceptions of how much longer they will live. This distinction is important in transferring base VSL from an HIC to an LIC. Comparing the remaining life expectancies of persons at age 35 years in 2015 in Lesotho (the lowest life expectancy at birth), the United States, and Japan (the highest life expectancy at birth), one finds that the average person in Lesotho faced a 26-year life expectancy, while a person in the United States and Japan faced 45 years and 49 years, respectively (UNDP 2015). Intuitively, all else equal, we would expect lower willingness to pay among people in Lesotho, given the lower number of years remaining. However, no empirical data support this claim.

As an illustration, in figure 9.2 we estimate the VSLr for all countries, based on the ratio of the remaining life expectancy at age 35 years of persons of a selected country and of the United States (equation 9.3). (In equation 9.3, r = ratio of VSL to GDP per capita.) The figure shows a narrower range of the VSLr across countries, because the differences among remaining life expectancies are smaller than among income levels. The lowest VSLr occurs in Lesotho, the country with the lowest life expectancy, at a VSLr of 101, and highest in Japan, at 194.

$$VSL_{r\,country\,x} = VSL_{r\,US} \times \left(\frac{\text{remaining life expectancy} \, (35)_{country\,x}}{\text{remaining life expectancy} \, (35)_{US}} \right)$$

(9.3)

Alternative Approaches

Given the limited theoretical and empirical evidence on the appropriate framework to account for transferring the value of mortality risk reduction to populations with different characteristics, we propose five simple and defensible alternative approaches to incorporate these key characteristics. We start with the two VSLr described earlier as the starting point (VSLr = 180 and 100), and we estimate the VSLr for each World Bank income group in table 9.3.[1]

The first approach ([1] in table 9.3) is to not apply any adjustments based on income or age and to assume that the VSLr remains the same across all populations.

The second approach ([2] in table 9.3) makes income adjustments by applying an elasticity of 0.8 for HICs and 1.2 for all other countries, based on equation 9.2, to the VSLr. We use 2013 GDP per capita in U.S. dollars (PPP) for each income group.

The third approach applies age and life expectancy adjustment ([3] in table 9.3) by assuming that the value decreases proportional to remaining life expectancy. This method reflects common practices in the health economics literature, and specifically in CEA in the health sector, in which the units of health benefits are in life years, rather than, for example, lives saved. These analyses implicitly assume that the VSL decreases in proportion to remaining life expectancy and that

Figure 9.2 VSLr Extrapolated with the Ratio of Remaining Life Expectancies at Age 35 Years for Persons in Selected Countries and the United States

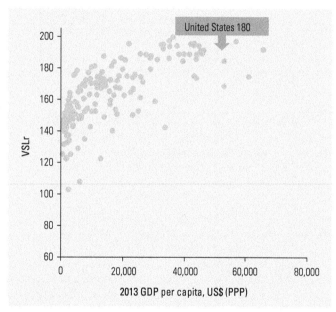

Note: GDP = gross domestic product; PPP = purchasing power parity; VSLr = value per statistical life–to–income ratio.

Table 9.3 Estimated VSLr for Four Alternative Approaches, World Bank Income

Anchor VSL	Alternative options	HICs	UMICs	LMICs	LICs
US 180	[1] No adjustment	180	180	180	180
US 180	[2] Income adjustment	191	137	115	88
US 180	[3] Age adjustment	80	81	104	117
US 180	[4] Income and age adjustment	85	62	66	57
OECD 100	[1] No adjustment	100	100	100	100
OECD 100	[2] Income adjustment	101	80	67	51
OECD 100	[3] Age adjustment	44	45	58	65
OECD 100	[4] Income and age adjustment	45	36	39	33

Note: HICs = high-income countries; LICs = low-income countries; LMICs = lower-middle-income countries; OECD = Organisation for Economic Co-operation and Development; UMICs = upper-middle-income countries; VSL = value per statistical life; VSLr = VSL-to-income ratio.

saving the life of a younger person with higher remaining life expectancy has a greater yield than saving the life of an older person. To estimate the changes in VSLr, we first collected the most recent (2010–15) age-specific death rates for all four income groups (UNDP 2015) and used the 2015 world population distribution to create age-standardization for the distribution of deaths. Assuming that the value of risk reduction decreases proportional to remaining life expectancy, we then applied a ratio of the remaining life expectancy at that age and at age 35 years for each age group (equation 9.4).

Age-adjusted $\text{VSLr}_j = \text{Base VSLr}$

$$\times \frac{\sum_{i=0}^{21} \text{world population size}_i \times \text{death rate}_{ij} \times \dfrac{e(a)_{ij}}{e(35)_j}}{\sum_{i=0}^{21} \text{world population size}_i \times \text{death rate}_{ij}}$$

(9.4)

where j is income group, i is age group (0, 1–4, 5–9, and so on up to 95+), $e(a)_{ij}$ is the remaining life expectancy at age a in age group i in the jth income group, and $e(35)_j$ is the remaining life expectancy of 35 year olds in the jth income group.

The fourth approach combines the second and third approach to adjust for both differences in income and in age and life expectancy ([4] in table 9.3).

The fifth and final approach involves using an alternative functional form that incorporates different characteristics. This varies substantially from the previous four approaches, which are all built on the same functional form commonly applied in the VSL literature (equation 9.2). In searching for an appropriate functional form to calculate the VSLr for countries, we set the following criteria that we consider important when transferring VSLr from one country to another:

1. The base VSLr is set roughly at the U.S. average of 180 or the OECD's estimate at 100 (for purpose of illustration, we use the former in the calculation that follows equation 9.5).
2. Following the income elasticity literature, we apply an elasticity of roughly 0.8 for HICs and 1.2 for LMICs.
3. All VSLr should be above the income floor, namely, the VSLr should not be lower than the discounted remaining life expectancy.

We found that the sine function can approximately meet these criteria and could therefore be an appropriate functional form to represent the relationship between VSLr and income. For example, one function form that meets the criteria is as follows:

$$\text{VSLr}(y) = 115 + 70 \sin(y_n) \tag{9.5}$$

where y_n is the normalized 2013 GDP per capita in U.S. dollars (PPP).

$$y_n = \frac{x - a}{b - a} \tag{9.6}$$

where x is the country's income level. We set a (where $\sin(y_n) = 0$) as the average income of upper-middle-income countries and b as the average income of non-OECD HICs. We excluded the following small countries with very high income levels to simplify the analysis: Qatar, Luxembourg, Kuwait, and Singapore. We present this relationship between VSLr and income level under the scenario in figure 9.3 and the implied VSL as a function of income under this analysis in figure 9.4. We constrained the U.S. VSLr to be approximately at 180. The lowest VSLr occurs in the Central African Republic, an LIC with a 2013 GDP per capita of US\$603, and the highest VSLr occurs in several HICs, including Iceland and the Netherlands, with the 2013 GDP per capita ranging from US\$42,000 to US\$46,000. Under this formulation, the income elasticities in LMICs and HICs are approximately 1.2 and 0.9, respectively.

Figure 9.3 VSLr Extrapolated with the Sine Function

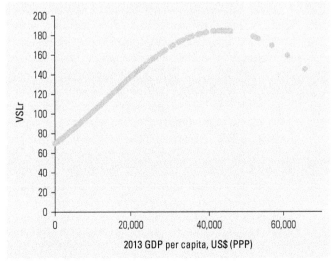

Note: GDP = gross domestic product; PPP = purchasing power parity; VSLr = value per statistical life–to–income ratio.

Figure 9.4 Implied VSL, Based on the Sine Function Extrapolation of the VSLr

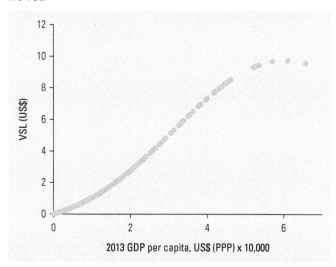

Note: GDP = gross domestic product; PPP = purchasing power parity; VSLr = value per statistical life–to–income ratio.

CONCLUSIONS

This chapter reviews estimates of B/C ratios from *DCP3* and illustrates the large number of applications of the technique to the health sector. Two major streams of methods are used within the health sector for B/C estimation in *DCP3*. One uses willingness to pay and the VSL concept. The other uses a human capital measure, analyzing costs of lost productivity because of morbidity and mortality or improved productivity associated with improved cognition. The literature on VSL is evolving, and we have presented current thinking on how that evolution might continue. The following research priorities are recommended for future examination.

First, standardization of the assumptions within each methodology would be useful. Currently, actual differences across alternative interventions are obscured by variations in methods and assumptions. Disagreements about how the VSL should vary with population characteristics are built on both empirical and normative arguments. The human capital side lacks consistency of rules for valuing future years of human life: Do we use current GDP? Do we use rates of actual growth per capita of countries? Do we use a common measure of expected growth, for example, 2 percent per capita per annum? This lack of consistency makes the comparison of estimates challenging. Estimates made in different sectors with different traditions is part of the problem. The development of a reference case would help. Such a reference case is being supported by the Bill & Melinda Gates Foundation, in part as a follow-up to *DCP3*.

A possible proposal is that each BCA (or economic burden of disease assessment) would select its own values for key parameters while also reporting standardized sensitivity analyses to enable accumulation of comparative knowledge.

Second, more empirical VSL estimates from low- and middle-income countries are needed. The current practice of benefit transfer does not adequately reflect the different characteristics between populations, and we believe this inadequacy leads to inaccurate estimations of the population's willingness to pay. Having empirical estimates of VSL from a diverse set of populations will fill an important research gap in this field.

Third, advances in BCA also need to be harmonized with the evolution in thinking about thresholds for cost-effectiveness. We know that VSL methods tend to assign large values to health because they focus on willingness to pay without specific reference to ability to pay. At the same time, recent studies (Claxton and others 2015; Ochalek, Lomas, and Claxton 2015) have shown that the public tends to undervalue public dollars spent on health care, acting as if a DALY (one year of enjoyment of full health) is worth only 50 percent of per capita at the margin. If this methodological issue is not resolved, health policy makers will overspend on health interventions assessed by BCA (for example, environmental interventions, injury prevention, and human capital promotion) and underspend on those assessed primarily by CEA (used to decide between many curative interventions). This is an important area for future work.

Finally, both CEA and BCA entail implicit ethical judgments. An approach using BCA that incorporates considerations of future wages gives a larger weight to individuals who are of working age, to those with higher labor force participation rates (men compared to women), and to urban populations as compared to rural populations. These same groups (working-age population, men, urban residents) also tend to have higher health-care expenditures and, hence, also receive greater weight in benefit calculations of future health expenditures averted. Because benefits measured in CEA are denominated in years of health, they are less subject to bias by gender, higher income, and residence. However, they share similar ethical concerns as do measures of the global burden of disease. Years of life saved for someone who suffers from a disability or mental illness are valued less than those for someone who is free of disability, for example. For these reasons, a common compromise between CEA and BCA methods is to assign the same VSL to everyone within a country. These topics may be usefully examined in future research.

NOTES

World Bank Income Classifications as of July 2014 are as follows, based on estimates of gross national income (GNI) per capita for 2013:

- Low-income countries (LICs) = US$1,045 or less
- Middle-income countries (MICs) are subdivided:
  (a) lower-middle-income = US$1,046 to US$4,125
  (b) upper-middle-income (UMICs) = US$4,126 to US$12,745
- High-income countries (HICs) = US$12,746 or more.

1. These scenarios build on conversations among an informal group of researchers interested in developing standardized VSL sensitivity analyses to enhance the comparability of assessments of global health and development issues. The group was initially convened by Dean Jamison and Maureen Cropper in February 2016 and ultimately grew to include over 30 participants as of April 2016. Major contributors included Kenneth Arrow, Nils Axel Braathen, Angela Y. Chang, Rob Dellink, James K. Hammitt, Michael Holland, Alan Krupnick, Elisa Lanzi, Urvashi Narain, Ståle Navrud, Lisa A. Robinson, Rana Roy, and Christopher Sall, among others. The analysis presented here uses these discussions as a starting point, but it has not been reviewed or approved by that group.

REFERENCES

Alkire, B. C., J. R. Vincent, and J. G. Meara. 2015. "Benefit-Cost Analysis for Selected Surgical Interventions in Low- and Middle-Income Countries." In *Disease Control Priorities* (third edition): Volume 1, *Essential Surgery*, edited by H. Debas, P. Donkor, A. Gawando, D. T, Jamison, M. Kruk, and C. N. Mock. Washington, DC: World Bank.

Ashraf, Q., D. Weil, and J. Wilde. 2013. "The Effect of Fertility Reduction on Economic Growth." *Population and Development Review* 39 (1): 97–130.

Berlinski, S., and N. Schady, eds. 2015. *The Early Years: Child Well-Being and the Role of Public Policy*. Washington, DC: Inter-American Development Bank.

Bhattacharya, S., A. Alberini, and M. L. Cropper. 2007. "The Value of Mortality Risk Reductions in Delhi, India." *Journal of Risk and Uncertainty* 34 (1): 21–47.

Biausque, V. 2012. "The Value of Statistical Life: A Meta-Analysis." Report ENV/EPOC/WPNEP(2010)9/FINAL, Working Party on National Environmental Policies, Organisation for Economic Development and Co-operation. http://www.oecd.org/officialdocuments/publicdisplaydocumentpdf/?cote=ENV/EPOC/WPNEP(2010)9/FINAL&doclanguage=en.

Black, R., R. Laxminarayan, M. Temmerman, and N. Walker. 2016. *Disease Control Priorities* (third edition): Volume 2, *Reproductive, Maternal, Newborn, and Child Health*. Washington, DC: World Bank.

Chang, A. Y., L. A. Robinson, J. K. Hammitt, and S. C. Resch. 2017. "Economics in 'Global Health 2035': A Sensitivity Analysis of the Value of a Life Year Estimates." *Journal of Global Health* 7 (1). doi:10.7189/jogh.07.010401.

Claxton, K., S. Martin, M. Soares, N. Rice, E. Spackman, and others. 2015. "Methods for the Estimation of the National Institute for Health and Care Excellence Cost-Effectiveness Threshold." *Health Technology Assessment* 19 (14): 1–503. doi:10.3310/hta19140.

Costa, D. L., and M. E. Kahn. 2004. "Changes in the Value of Life, 1940–1980." *Journal of Risk and Uncertainty* 29 (2): 159–80.

Cropper, M., S. Guttikunda, P. Jawahar, K. Malik, and I. Partridge. 2017. "Costs and Benefits of Installing Scrubbers at Coal-Fired Power Plants in India." In *Disease Control Priorities* (third edition): Volume 7, *Injury Prevention and Environmental Health,* edited by C. N. Mock, O. Kobusingye, R. Nugent, and K. Smith. Washington, DC: World Bank.

Evans, M. R., and V. K. Smith. 2006. "Do We Really Understand the Age-VSL Relationship?" *Resource and Energy Economics* 28 (3): 242–61.

Fan, V. Y., D. T. Jamison, and L. H. Summers. 2018. "The Inclusive Loss from Pandemic Influenza Risk." In *Disease Control Priorities* (third edition): Volume 9, *Disease Control Priorities: Improving Health and Reducing Poverty*, edited by D. T. Jamison, H. Gelband, S. Horton, P. Jha, R. Laxminarayan, C. N. Mock, and R. Nugent. Washington, DC: World Bank.

Fernandes, M., and E. Aurino. 2017. "Identifying an Essential Package for School-Age Child Health: Economic Analysis." In *Disease Control Priorities* (third edition): Volume 8, *Child and Adolescent Health and Development*, edited by D. A. P. Bundy, N. de Silva, S. Horton, D. T. Jamison, and G. Patton. Washington, DC: World Bank.

Fitzpatrick, C., U. Nwankwo, E. Lenk, S. J. de Vlas, and D. A. P. Bundy. 2017. "An Investment Case for Ending Neglected Tropical Diseases." In *Disease Control Priorities* (third edition): Volume 6, *Major Infectious Diseases*, edited by K. K. Holmes, S. Bertozzi, B. Bloom, and P. Jha. Washington, DC: World Bank.

Gates, B., and R. Chambers. 2015. "From Aspiration to Action: What Will It Take to End Malaria?" United Nations, New York, and the Bill & Melinda Gates Foundation, Seattle, WA. https://www.mmv.org/sites/default/files/uploads/docs/publications/Aspiration-to-Action.pdf.

Gelband, H., P. Jha, R. Sankaranarayanan, and S. Horton, eds. 2015. *Disease Control Priorities* (third edition): Volume 3, *Cancer*. Washington, DC: World Bank.

Guo, X., and J. K. Hammitt. 2009. "Compensating Wage Differentials with Unemployment: Evidence from China." *Environmental and Resource Economics* 42 (2): 187–209. doi:10.1007/s10640-008-9217-9.

Hammitt, J. K. 2017. "Extrapolating the Value per Statistical Life between Populations: Theoretical Implications." *Journal of Benefit-Cost Analysis* 8 (2), forthcoming.

Hammitt, J. K., and K. Haninger. 2010. "Valuing Fatal Risks to Children and Adults: Effects of Disease, Latency, and Risk Aversion." *Journal of Risk and Uncertainty* 40 (1): 57–83.

Hammitt, J. K., and M. E. Ibarrarán. 2006. "The Economic Value of Fatal and Non-Fatal Occupational Risks in Mexico City Using Actuarial- and Perceived-Risk Estimates." *Health Economics* 15 (12): 1329–35. doi:10.1002/hec.1137.

Hammitt, J. K., and L. A. Robinson. 2011. "The Income Elasticity of the Value per Statistical Life: Transferring Estimates between High and Low Income Populations." *Journal of Benefit-Cost Analysis* 2 (1): 1–29.

Hammitt, J. K., and Y. Zhou. 2006. "The Economic Value of Air-Pollution-Related Health Risks in China: A Contingent Valuation Study." *Environmental and Resource Economics* 33 (3): 399–423. doi:10.1007/s10640-005-3606-0.

Hoffmann, S., P. Qin, A. Krupnick, B. Badrakh, S. Batbaatar, and others. 2012. "The Willingness to Pay for Mortality Risk Reductions in Mongolia." *Resource and Energy Economics* 34 (4): 493–513. doi:10.1016/j.reseneco.2012.04.005.

Horton, S. 2018. "Cost-Effectiveness in *Disease Control Priorities*, Third Edition." In *Disease Control Priorities* (third edition): Volume 9, *Disease Control Priorities: Improving Health and Reducing Poverty*, edited by D. T. Jamison, H. Gelband, S. Horton, P. Jha, R. Laxminarayan, C. N. Mock, and R. Nugent. Washington, DC: World Bank.

Horton, S., and M. Black. 2017. "Identifying an Essential Package for Early Child Development: Economic Analysis." In *Disease Control Priorities* (third edition): Volume 8, *Child and Adolescent Health and Development*, edited by D. A. P. Bundy, N. de Silva, S. Horton, D. T. Jamison, and G. Patton. Washington, DC: World Bank.

Horton, S., J. Waldfogel, E. De la Cruz Toledo, J. Mahon, and J. Santelli. 2017. "Economic Factors in Defining the Adolescence Package." In *Disease Control Priorities* (third edition): Volume 8, *Child and Adolescent Health and Development*, edited by D. A. P. Bundy, N. de Silva, S. Horton, D. T. Jamison, and G. Patton. Washington, DC: World Bank.

Hutton, G. 2013. "Global Costs and Benefits of Reaching Universal Coverage of Sanitation and Drinking-Water Supply." *Journal of Water and Health* 11 (1): 1–12.

Hutton, G., and C. Chase 2017. "Water Supply, Sanitation, and Hygiene." In *Disease Control Priorities* (third edition): Volume 7, *Injury Prevention and Environmental Health*, edited by C. N. Mock, O. Kobusingye, R. Nugent, and K. Smith. Washington, DC: World Bank.

Jamison D. T., P. Jha, V. Malhotra, and S. Verguet. 2013. "Human Health: The Twentieth-Century Transformation of Human Health: Its Magnitude and Value." In *How Much Have Global Problems Cost the World?*, ed. by B. Lomborg. Cambridge University Press.

Jamison, D. T., L. H. Summers, G. Alleyne, K. J. Arrow, S. Berkley, and others. 2013. "Global Health 2035: A World Converging within a Generation." *The Lancet* 382 (9908): 1898–955.

Jha, P., K. Jordan, R. Hum, and C. Gauvreau. 2015. "Health." Copenhagen Consensus Center, Copenhagen. http://www.copenhagenconsensus.com/publication/post-2015-consensus-health-assessment-jha-et-al.

Jha, P., R. Nugent, S. Verguet, D. Bloom, and R. Hum. 2013. "Chronic Disease." In *Global Problems, Smart Solutions: Costs and Benefits*, edited by B. Lomborg, 137–69. Cambridge, U.K.: Cambridge University Press.

Kniesner, T., W. K. Viscusi, and J. P. Ziliak. 2010. "Policy Relevant Heterogeneity in the Value of Statistical Life: New Evidence from Panel Data Quantile Regressions." *Journal of Risk and Uncertainty* 40 (1): 15–31. doi:10.1007/s11166-009-9084-y.

Krupnick, A. 2007. "Mortality-Risk Valuation and Age: Stated Preference Evidence." *Review of Environmental Economics and Policy* 1 (2): 261–82.

Lindhjem, H., S. Navrud, N. A. Braathen, and V. Biausque. 2011. "Valuing Mortality Risk Reductions from Environmental, Transport, and Health Policies: A Global Meta-Analysis of Stated Preference Studies." *Risk Analysis* 31 (9): 1381–407. doi:10.1111/j.1539-6924.2011.01694.

López Boo, F. L., G. Palloni, and S. Urzua. 2014. "Cost-Benefit Analysis of a Micronutrient Supplementation and Early Childhood Stimulation Program in Nicaragua." *Annals of the New York Academy of Sciences* 1308: 139–48.

Madheswaran, S. 2007. "Measuring the Value of Statistical Life: Estimating Compensating Wage Differentials among Workers in India." *Social Indicators Research* 84 (1): 83–96.

McDaid, D., A.-L. Park, C. Currie, and C. Zanotti. 2014. "Investing in the Wellbeing of Young People: Making the Economic Case." In *The Economics of Wellbeing*: Vol. 5, *Wellbeing: A Complete Reference Guide*, edited by D. McDaid and C. L. Cooper, 181–214. Oxford: Wiley-Blackwell.

Mills, A., Y. Lubell, and K. Hanson. 2008. "Malaria Eradication: The Economic, Financial and Institutional Challenge." *Malaria Journal* 7 (Supp 1): S11.

Mock, C. N., O. Kobusingye, R. Nugent, and K. R. Smith, eds. 2017. *Disease Control Priorities* (third edition): Volume 7, *Injury Prevention and Environmental Health*. Washington, DC: World Bank.

Norheim, O. F., E. Emanuel, D. T. Jamison, K. A. Johansson, J. Millum, and others. 2017. *Global Health Priority-Setting: Beyond Cost-Effectiveness*. New York: Oxford University Press.

Ochalek, J., J. Lomas, and K. Claxton. 2015. "Cost per DALY Averted Thresholds for Low- and Middle-Income Countries: Evidence from Cross Country Data." CHE Research Paper 122, Centre for Health Economics, University of York, York, U.K.

OECD (Organisation for Economic Co-operation and Development). 2012. *Mortality Risk Valuation in Environment, Health and Transport Policies*. Paris: OECD Publishing. http://www.oecd.org/env/tools-evaluation/mortalityriskvaluationinenvironmenthealthandtransportpolicies.htm.

———. 2014. *The Cost of Air Pollution: Health Impacts of Road Transport*. OECD Publishing. http://www.oecd.org/env/the-cost-of-air-pollution-9789264210448-en.htm.

Ottersen, T., J. Millum, J. Prah Ruger, S. Verguet, K. A. Johansson, and others. 2017. "The Future of Priority Setting in Global Health." In *Global Health Priority-Setting: Beyond Cost-Effectiveness*, edited by O. F. Norheim and others. New York: Oxford University Press.

Ozawa, S., S. Clark, A. Portnoy, S. Grewal, L. Brenzel, and D. G. Walker. 2016. "Return on Investment from Childhood Immunization in Low- and Middle-Income Countries, 2011–20." *Health Affairs* 35 (2): 199–207.

Prabhakaran, D., S. Anand, T. Gaziano, J.-C. Mbanya, Y. Wu, and R. Nugent. 2017. *Disease Control Priorities* (third edition): Volume 5, *Cardiovascular, Respiratory, and Related Disorders*. Washington, DC: World Bank.

Psacharopoulos, G. 2014. "Education Assessment Paper: Benefits and Costs of the Education Targets for the Post-2015 Development Agenda." Copenhagen Consensus Center, Tewksbury, MA. http://www.copenhagenconsensus .com/publication/post-2015-consensus-education-assess ment-psacharopoulos.

Purdy, M., M. Robinson, K. Wei, and D. Rublin. 2013. "The Economic Case for Combating Malaria." *American Journal of Tropical Medicine and Hygiene* 89 (5): 819–23.

Robinson, L. A., and J. K. Hammitt. 2015a. "The Effect of Income on the Value of Mortality and Morbidity Risk Reductions." Prepared for Industrial Economics, Inc., Cambridge, MA, on behalf of the U.S. Environmental Protection Agency, Washington, DC. https://yosemite.epa.gov/sab/SABPRODUCT .NSF/0/0CA9E925C9A702F285257F380050C842/$File/IEc_ Income%20elasticity%20Report%20_final.pdf.

———. 2015b. "Valuing Reductions in Fatal Illness Risks: Implications of Recent Research." *Health Economics* 25 (8): 1039–52. doi:10.1002/hec.3214.

Rosen, S. 1988. "The Value of Changes in Life Expectancy." *Journal of Risk and Uncertainty* 1 (3): 285–304.

Sanderson, W. C., and S. Scherbov. 2007. "A New Perspective on Population Aging." *Demographic Research* 16 (January): 27–58. doi:10.4054/DemRes.2007.16.2.

Shanmugam, K. R. 2001. "Self Selection Bias in the Estimates of Compensating Differentials for Job Risks in India." *Journal of Risk and Uncertainty* 22 (3): 263–75.

Shepard, D. S., and R. Zeckhauser. 1982. "Life-Cycle Consumption and Willingness to Pay for Increased Survival." Institute for Research on Poverty, University of Wisconsin-Madison, WI.

———. 1984. "Survival versus Consumption." *Management Science* 30 (4): 423–39.

Shretta, R., J. Liu, C. Cotter, J. Cohen, C. Dolenz, and others. 2017. "Malaria Elimination and Eradication." In *Disease Control Priorities* (third edition): Volume 6, *Major Infectious Diseases*, edited by K. K. Holmes, S. Bertozzi, B. Bloom, and P. Jha. Washington, DC: World Bank.

Simon, N. B., M. L. Cropper, A. Alberini, and S. Arora. 1999. "Valuing Mortality Reductions in India: A Study of Compensating Wage Differentials." Policy Research Working Paper 2078, World Bank, Washington, DC. http://documents .worldbank.org/curated/en/582261468751139383/pdf/multi -page.pdf.

Stenberg, K., K. Sweeney, H. Axelson, M. Temmerman, and P. Sheehan. 2016. "Returns on Investment in the Continuum of Care for Reproductive, Maternal, Newborn, and Child Health." In *Disease Control Priorities* (third edition): Volume 2, *Reproductive, Maternal, Newborn and Child Health*,

edited by R. E. Black, R. Laxminarayan, M. Temmerman, and N. Walker. Washington, DC: World Bank.

Tekeşin, C., and S. Ara. 2014. "Measuring the Value of Mortality Risk Reductions in Turkey." *International Journal of Environmental Research and Public Health* 11 (7): 6890–922. doi:10.3390/ijerph110706890.

UNDP (United Nations Population Division). 2015. *2015 Revision of World Population Prospects*. New York: UNDP. http://esa.un.org/unpd/wpp/.

U.S. DOT (U.S. Department of Transportation). 2015. "Guidance on Treatment of the Economic Value of a Statistical Life (VSL) in Departmental Analyses—2015 Adjustment. Memorandum to Secretarial Officers and Modal Administrators from K. Thomson, General Counsel, and C. Monje, Assistant Secretary for Policy." U.S. DOT, Washington, DC.

U.S. EPA (U.S. Environmental Protection Agency). 2014. *Guidelines for Preparing Economic Analyses*. Washington, DC: U.S. EPA.

Vassanadumrongdee, S., and S. Matsuoka. 2005. "Risk Perceptions and Value of a Statistical Life for Air Pollution and Traffic Accidents: Evidence from Bangkok, Thailand." *Journal of Risk and Uncertainty* 30 (3): 261–87.

Verguet, S., and D. T. Jamison. 2018. "Health Policy Assessment: Applications of Extended Cost-Effectiveness Analysis Methodology in *Disease Control Priorities*." In *Disease Control Priorities* (third edition): Volume 9, *Disease Control Priorities: Improving Health and Reducing Poverty*, edited by D. T. Jamison, H. Gelband, S. Horton, P. Jha, R. Laxminarayan, C. N. Mock, and R. Nugent. Washington, DC: World Bank.

Viscusi, W. K. 2015. "The Role of Publication Selection Bias in Estimates of the Value of a Statistical Life." *American Journal of Health Economics* 1 (1): 27–52.

Viscusi, W. K., and J. E. Aldy. 2003. "The Value of a Statistical Life: A Critical Review of Market Estimates throughout the World." *Journal of Risk and Uncertainty* 27 (1): 5–76.

Viscusi, W. Kip, and Clayton J. Masterman. 2017a. "Income Elasticities and Global Values of a Statistical Life." *Journal of Benefit-Cost Analysis*: 1–25.

Viscusi, W. K., and C. J. Masterman. 2017b. "Anchoring Biases in International Estimates of the Value of a Statistical Life." *Journal of Risk and Uncertainty* 54 (2): 103–28. doi:10.1007 /s11166-017-9255-1.

Walker, S. P., C. Powell, S. M. Chang, H. Baker-Henningham, S. Grantham-McGregor, and others. 2015. "Delivering Parenting Interventions through Health Services in the Caribbean: Impact, Acceptability and Costs." Working Paper IDB-WP-642, Inter-American Development Bank, Washington, DC.

Watkins, D. A., and A. Chang. 2017. "The Economic Impact of Rheumatic Heart Disease in Low- and Middle-Income Countries." Working Paper 19, *DCP3* Working Paper Series, World Bank, Washington, DC.

Whittington, D., W. M. Hanemann, C. Sadoff, and M. Jeuland. 2009. "The Challenge of Improving Water and Sanitation Services in Less Developed Countries." *Foundations and Trends in Microeconomics* 4 (6): 469–607.

Part **4**

Health System Topics from *Disease Control Priorities*, Third Edition

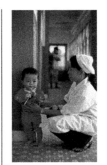

Chapter **10**

Quality of Care

John Peabody, Riti Shimkhada, Olusoji Adeyi, Huihui Wang,
Edward Broughton, and Margaret E. Kruk

INTRODUCTION

Just after dawn, Vivej arrives at the hospital with her newborn under her arm to see you. She is 21 years old, two days postpartum, and exhausted after 36 hours of protracted labor. She is worried because she cannot get her firstborn, Esmile, to breastfeed. You learn that she delivered at a birthing clinic near her home and tells you that, even after her water broke, it took more than a day before the birth attendant could deliver her son. Your examination reveals a dire clinical picture: Esmile is lethargic and hypotonic, he has a poor suck reflex, his temperature is 39.8°C, his pulse is 180, and his breathing is labored. You check his white blood count, confirming leukocytosis. A spinal tap shows pleocytosis. You start him on fluids and antibiotics for neonatal sepsis with likely meningitis and quickly turn your attention to Vivej. Her situation is easier to diagnose but no less urgent: she is febrile and tachycardic, her blood pressure is 85/50. You give her fluids and start her on antibiotics. Ultimately, despite your efforts, both mother and child die.

What went wrong? This chapter looks narrowly at these situations—the critical points after access and availability (including affordability) are already accomplished, when patients are in health care facilities that are staffed and equipped with appropriate technology. These are the situations in which the inputs are brought together and it is up to the provider to improve the health of the patient. Simply put, this chapter looks at the decisions and actions of the provider when seeing a patient. It is at this critical moment when we expect the doctor or nurse, or whoever is caring for the patient, to provide the best possible care by skillfully combining the available resources and technologies with the best clinical evidence and professional judgment.

Esmile and Vivej received poor-quality care at the time of delivery. Several clinical steps were not taken. The prolonged rupture of membranes was not diagnosed in a timely manner. Vivej needed either to have her labor induced or, failing that, to be referred for a cesarean section. Prophylactic antibiotics should have been administered. Just as important, the provider at the birthing center needed support and professional oversight, with guidelines, supervision, or default referral systems in place to provide a path to the best care possible. The multiple failures in this case led to puerperal and neonatal sepsis. At worst, these conditions have a fatality rate greater than one in four; at best, they lead to protracted care, recovery, and clinical expense that could have been avoided. It is possible, however, to imagine providers in a different setting, with the same physical resources, giving better care and avoiding this tragic scenario.

In the next section, we answer the questions raised in this scenario and in countless clinics and hospitals around the world. How much variation is there in the

Corresponding author: John Peabody, professor, University of California, San Francisco and University of California, Los Angeles; president, QURE Healthcare,
San Francisco, California, United States; jpeabody@qurehealthcare.com.

quality of care? How do we measure clinical practice? How and where has quality been systematically improved and practice variation reduced? What elements of care variation can be addressed by policy and what are the costs? Most important, what can be done to elevate the care given by providers in developing country settings? Our focus, therefore, is on the steps that can be taken to optimize the quality of care for patients like Esmile in pediatrics, Vivej in obstetrics, and other patients receiving care for the clinical conditions considered throughout the nine volumes of the third edition of *Disease Control Priorities* (*DCP3*).

PROBLEM OF VARIATIONS IN QUALITY OF CARE

Health policy makers, researchers, and clinicians recognize the wide variations in access to care (Peabody and others, forthcoming). However, once individuals and populations avail themselves of health care services, variations in health outcomes raise disturbing questions about the quality of care delivered, defined as "the degree to which health services for individuals and populations increase the likelihood of desired outcomes and are consistent with professional knowledge" (IOM 2013, 21). Variations in care entail policy challenges similar to those associated with variations in access, including equity and efficiency (Saleh, Alameddine, and Natafgi 2014). In studies comparing clinical practice with evidence-based standards, researchers found that high-quality care is provided inconsistently to large segments of the population (McGlynn and others 2003). For example, a landmark Institute of Medicine report found that, in the United States, medical errors kill more people than traffic accidents (Kohn, Corrigan, and Donaldson 2000).

Many subsequent studies have documented variations in quality of care in low- and middle-income countries (LMICs) (Barber, Bertozzi, and Gertler 2007; Barber, Gertler, and Harimurti 2007; Hansen and others 2008; Loevinsohn, Guerrero, and Gregorio 1995; National Academies of Sciences, Engineering, and Medicine 2015; Peabody, Nordyke, and others 2006; World Bank 2003). In India, studies have found alarmingly low rates of correct diagnosis, limited adherence to treatment guidelines, and frequent use of harmful or unnecessary drugs. In one study, only 31 percent of standardized patients who described symptoms of unstable angina and 48 percent who reported symptoms of asthma were given the correct drugs (Das and Hammer 2014). Even more worrying, providers prescribed an incorrect or harmful treatment to more than 60 percent of patients reporting asthma symptoms.

Clinicians failed to provide even the most basic care—only 12 percent of standardized patients who reported a child with symptoms of dysentery were told to give their child oral rehydration therapy (Das and others 2012). A study of 296 providers in India found that a mere 6 percent followed the six diagnostic standards of the International Standards for Tuberculosis Care (Achanta and others 2013).

Such deficits in quality of care can come from many sources, including gaps in knowledge, inappropriate application of available technology, and inability of organizations to monitor and support care standardization. This striking variation in quality within countries occurs across facilities, among providers, and between specialists and nonspecialists (Beracochea and others 1995; Das and Hammer 2007; Das and others 2012; Dumont and others 2002; Nolan and others 2001; Peabody, Gertler, and Leibowitz 1998; Weinberg 2001; Xu and others 2015).

Some cross-national comparisons have reached the same conclusion. A 2007 DCP-sponsored study that evaluated quality for three common clinical conditions in five countries simultaneously found that the average quality of care was low in every country (61 percent) and the difference in average score between countries was small (ranging from 60.2 to 62.6 percent). However, the quality scores within every country varied widely, ranging from 30 to 93 percent (Peabody and Liu 2007). This wide variation was constant across type of facility, medical condition, and domain of care.

Poor health outcomes are the result of many factors, ranging from the nature and severity of disease to patient behavior and structural elements of care (IOM and National Academy of Engineering 2011; Steinwachs and Hughes 2008; Xu and others 2015). Some factors are not amenable to change (genetic predisposition), while others are slow to affect outcomes (changes in payment incentives). Discouragingly, better access, more infrastructure, and structural measures of quality do not always translate into better health outcomes. Indeed, some structural indexes can be inversely related to health (for example, number of hospital beds versus health status) (Ng and others 2014). Thus, improving the quality of care may well provide the *greatest* sectoral opportunity to improve health outcomes (Peabody and others 2017). Care can be improved quickly and, if based on best evidence, improved care will improve outcomes and lower costs (Scott and Jha 2014). Reducing unwarranted variation and addressing poor-quality provider practices deserve the most urgent attention possible from policy makers (Kirkpatrick and Burkman 2010; Ransom, Pinsky, and Tropman 2000).

Providers, health care systems, governments, and payers are beginning to recognize this urgency and are seeking innovative, effective ways to improve the quality of care. Metrics and measurement, pathways, clinical checklists, educational interventions, and payment incentives all raise awareness and offer opportunities to provide accountability and improve care. These approaches have been tried in many LMICs, but their effectiveness varies. Changing practice at the system level is difficult and requires coordination, vision, planning, and consideration of how effective, high-impact interventions can be scaled up and applied across an entire system (Massoud and Abrampah 2015). At the level of individual providers, knowledge improvement and acquisition of new skills need to be motivated by both extrinsic and intrinsic factors, which are enabled through access to knowledge and measurement tools that change behavior and ideally are accompanied by peer support (Schuster, Terwoord, and Tasosa 2006; Woolf 2000). We have learned that improved clinical practice requires active participation (not passive learning), peer and leadership support, and communication of relevant feedback (Kantrowitz 2014; Mostofian and others 2015). Multifaceted interventions seem more successful than single interventions, underscoring the importance of practice-level change that focuses on supporting the individual provider (training) and creating a suitable environment for change (accountability).

Even more challenging than finding disease-level interventions for individual providers is identifying health care policies that improve the quality of care for populations. While clinical practice interventions, such as checklists, for acute and chronic diseases work at the provider-patient level, policies need to address group-level practice, for example, through incentives and indirect means. Preventing the deaths of Vivej and Esmile, for example, would have required the timely use of simple uterotonic commodities and prophylactic antibiotics, which might happen with better supervision. An effective policy, however, compels groups of providers to set up the supervision or the training that leads to the *use* of oxytocin or cephalosporins.

In the second edition of *DCP*, the chapter on quality of care largely summarized the emerging policy evidence that better quality could lead to better outcomes (Peabody, Taguiwalo, and others 2006). Just a decade later, every volume in this edition discusses quality of care. We consider in this chapter the different policy interventions that have been tried around the world. We begin with the quality infrastructure that is required for every policy intervention, then expand on the policy framework for changing clinical practice, and use this expanded framework to discuss the challenges, returns, and costs of improved quality.

QUALITY IMPROVEMENT INFRASTRUCTURE REQUIREMENTS

Clinical solutions are typically not generalizable because they are disease-specific, vary by clinical condition, and rely on the training of health care providers and the context of the health care system (Dayal and Hort 2015). Policy, however, is designed to work at the group level—that is, at scales larger than the individual level. Effective quality improvement policies that work at the group level have several common features, specifically the means to collect information and synthesize it and the means to encourage skills and technologies to be applied in a timely fashion. The following four common policy attributes, detailed below, improve quality:

- Measurement of the clinical activity (including measurement tied to feedback)
- Standards for those measurements (based on scientific evidence for standardizing care)
- Training of providers (including supervision)
- Incentives that align and motivate providers (including financial incentives, but also incentives of professionalism and reputation).

Measurement

Accurate, affordable, and valid measurements "are the basis for quality of care assessments" (Peabody and others 2004, 771). For too long, routine measures of quality in LMICs relied on structural elements (rosters, catalogs, and inventories of coverage and access), giving little thought to how these elements improve health. Such elements are relatively easy to count and measure, but are only remotely linked to better outcomes. Improving quality requires measurement of the care process—that is, what providers do when they see patients (Ansong-Tornui and others 2007; Peabody, Taguiwalo, and others 2006; Peabody and others 2011).

Measurement of the care process is critical, creating awareness of deficits in practice, gaps in care, and accountability at the individual and system levels, which improves focus and motivation. To serve as an instrument of change and accountability, provider-level measurement needs to be ongoing and cyclical. Transparency of results can increase knowledge and change intentions, but requires a supportive context to be effective (National Patient Safety Foundation 2015).

When coupled with useful feedback and done in a timely manner, measurement is the foundation for improving quality. If the measures are reliable, affordable, and anchored in valid, evidence-based criteria, quality of care can be followed over time and the impact of policy interventions can be assessed (Felt-Lisk and others 2012). Various quality measures have been developed, each with its own set of advantages and disadvantages. Although no measure is perfect, adequate measures exist, and every health system—from small clinics to national governments—can benefit from measurement. Feedback has the potential to promote improvement, but studies are limited, tending to focus on health care report cards (Baker and Cebul 2002; Dranove and others 2003; Kolstad 2013; Shaller and others 2003), which include public disclosure of quality scores that may not provide the same motivation to improve scores as when feedback is provided privately.

The available methods for measuring performance include provider self-reports, patient vignette simulations, patient self-reports, and reviews of medical records. These methods vary in their ability to capture improvement and account for differences in the type of patients treated (case-mix adjustment). They also vary in their economic feasibility (Epstein 2006; Spertus and others 2003), reliability (repeated measures), validity (against a gold standard), and ability to be "gamed" (Petersen and others 2006). The policy challenge is that performance-measurement methods may need to be developed and adapted to low-resource settings (Engelgau and others 2010). Table 10.1 lists available methods for measuring quality of the care process.

Table 10.1 Methods for Measuring Quality of the Care Process

Method	Advantage	Issues
Chart abstraction or review of medical record	• Nearly ubiquitous and theoretically could be obtained after the patient-provider encounter; in practice, record keeping in most LMICs is inadequate • Electronic medical record technology: improved uniformity, legibility, communication • Records of clinical events	• May lack relevant clinical details, especially when written for other purposes, such as legal protection • Poor record keeping and documentation lead to incomplete and inaccurate content • Illegibility of handwritten notes • Inaccuracies in the process of abstracting to produce data suitable for analysis • High costs involved in training medical abstractors • Variation in documentation practices across providers, facilities, and countries
Direct observation and recording of visits	• Records of clinical events • First-hand observation of actual encounters	• Ethical considerations • Need to inform providers and patients, which can induce the Hawthorne effect (bias when participant changes his or her behavior as a result of being evaluated) • High cost of training observers • Variations across observers
Administrative data	• Available in most facilities • Ubiquitous and inexpensive to collect when data collection system is in place	• Lack sufficient clinical detail • Inaccuracies in content • Poor data collection or management systems, especially in LMICs
Standardized patients	• The gold standard for process measurement • Captures technical and interpersonal elements of process • Reliable over a range of conditions, providing valid measurements that accurately capture variation in clinical practice among providers across patients	• Expensive • Not practical for routinely evaluating quality • Limited range of applicability (works best for adult conditions and conditions that can be simulated)
Clinical vignettes	• Can measure quality within a group of providers and evaluate quality at the population level • Responsive to variations in quality • Cases simulate actual patient visit and evaluate physician's knowledge • Validated against other methods and criteria for standard-of-quality measurement • Useful for comparison studies • Easy and inexpensive to administer • Ability to collect data independently	• Potential resistance of providers to complete the vignettes • Different methods for administering vignettes • Instrument validation • Link to patient-level data

Sources: Bertelsen 1981; Peabody and others 2004; Peabody and others 2011; Peabody, Nordyke, and others 2006.
Note: LMICs = low- and middle-income countries.

The usefulness of any method for measuring process depends on the completeness and accuracy of the data collected—a ubiquitous problem with charts, medical records, and administrative data. Another significant concern is patient case mix, given that different patient characteristics may affect quality (Zaslavsky 2001). Validity and comparability of results across measurement units (individual patients, providers, facilities, and countries) are questionable unless these differences are controlled for through complex instrument design and statistical techniques (Peabody and others 2004). Operational concerns, such as the need for highly trained staff, can increase the cost and complexity of implementing some methods.

Data Derived from Medical Charts

Chart abstraction, or review of the medical record, has long been used to measure quality of care. Clinical audits, physician report cards, and profiles are based on chart abstraction. Reliable health records can provide credible evidence of the health status of patients and assist policy makers with developing plans and making decisions to improve health care delivery (Haux 2006). The core strength of the medical record is that it is ubiquitous and could potentially be obtained after each encounter.

Chart reviews, however, suffer from many problems. First, the medical chart must be completed (and found) to proceed with an abstraction. Handwritten notes on paper charts may be illegible. Medical charts may be generated for reasons other than documenting the key clinical events of the visit (for legal protection or obtaining payment) and thus may lack crucial clinical details. Luck and others (2000) found that charts identified only 70 percent of activities performed during the clinical encounter. Even abstracting measures of quality from electronic medical records is challenging given the heterogeneity in record-keeping practices (Ali, Shah, and Tandon 2011; Parsons and others 2012). The costs and logistical challenges of securing medical records, training medical abstractors, and reviewing records can be significant. Throughout acquisition, verification, and abstraction, a process is needed to ensure that the data collected are reliable (Koh and Tan 2005). Beyond these costs and challenges, chart review also suffers from the inability to control for patient case mix and difficulty of comparing physicians caring for different patient populations.

Direct Observation and Recording of Visits

Direct observation and recording of visits are common practices in LMICs (Nolan and others 2001). Some of the most obvious challenges to using direct observation are the need to staff projects and train evaluators, which can be difficult to scale up. Ethical challenges must be addressed, and both providers and patients must be informed of the observation or recording. Although research performed in Tanzania showed that the Hawthorne effect can disappear after 10 to 15 observations, this notification introduces participation bias when providers change their behavior as a result of being evaluated (Leonard and Masatu 2006). Perhaps a more salient problem is that trained observers are costly, and variation between observers is difficult to remedy. These challenges have stimulated the search for other ways to measure and record what happens in clinical visits.

Administrative Data

Administrative data are available in all but the poorest settings. A data collection system, once established, can provide information on charges and many cost inputs. However, administrative data are assembled for purposes other than improving quality, such as documenting and processing medical claims (Calle and others 2000; Goeree and others 2009), and often lack sufficient clinical detail to be useful in evaluating clinical processes. In a 2004 study, an incorrect diagnosis was recorded 30 percent of the time (although the actual diagnosis was correct). The actual diagnosis was recorded only 57 percent of the time (Peabody and others 2004). As information systems advance, accuracy may improve, but the lack of adequate clinical detail will continue to limit the use of administrative data. Clinical databases such as registries may be helpful but are primarily available only in high-income countries (HICs) and for commercial interests.

Globally, both administrative and clinical health databases are of poor quality, and administrative databases are usually the only resource available in LMICs. Even when available, health information is underused for planning and decision making (Corrao and others 2009), especially in resource-constrained settings (Bosch-Capblanch and others 2009) and when data are paper based or decentralized to the district level (LaFond and Siddiqi 2003). District-level information systems often do not feed information back to the local level (Lippeveld, Sauerborn, and Bodart 2000). Paper-based information systems often generate poor-quality data (Lium, Tjora, and Faxvaag 2008), which weakens confidence in reported progress made toward health care system goals (Kerr and Fleming 2007) and toward the Sustainable Development Goals and the Millennium Development Goals (AbouZahr and Boerma 2005). In the absence of greater attention and resources from government or private

Standardized Patients

Using standardized patients, when unannounced, is the gold standard for measuring process (Luck and Peabody 2002). Trained to simulate patients with a given illness, standardized patients present themselves in a clinical setting to providers who have given their consent to participate in the study. After the visit, the standardized patient reports on the technical and interpersonal elements of the care process. Interest in using standardized patients has been growing in LMICs, with most studies done in China and India (Das and others 2012; Das and others 2015; Mohanan and others 2015; Sylvia and others 2015). Well-trained standardized patients are not susceptible to observation bias (Glassman and others 2000) and, when rigorously monitored, enable comparisons of quality within and between facilities.

However, this method also has major drawbacks, including high costs of training, significant difficulties in large-scale application (consistent training), and limited conditions that actors can reliably portray, for example, excluding surgical and pediatric cases (Felt-Lisk and others 2012).

Clinical Vignettes

The shortcomings of the previous methods have spurred development of more facile methods. One of these, developed in work starting in 1999, is the use of *validated* clinical performance vignettes (Peabody and others 2000). Clinical performance vignettes use a full set of clinical care elements to assess the patient-provider interaction (Glassman and others 2000).

There are many types of vignettes from which to choose—for example, multiple choice versus open-ended, or short case versus full clinical care delivery scenarios—producing variable results at predicting actual practice. Clinical performance and value vignettes have been validated in randomized evaluations against standardized patients in two large trials (Peabody and others 2000; Peabody and others 2004). In these studies, vignette scores for clinical performance and value consistently reflected quality as measured by standardized patients better than abstracted medical records and worked across different health care systems, clinical conditions, and levels of training among randomly sampled physicians.

Various types of vignettes have been used in diverse settings around the world (Canchihuaman and others 2011; Das and Hammer 2005a, 2005b; Holm and Burkhartzmeyer 2015; Jörg and others 2006; Kaptanoğlu and Aktas 2013; Li and others 2007; Tiemeier and others 2002; Veloski and others 2005). Vignettes are particularly effective in comparative evaluations because the same case or type of case can be presented to many providers simultaneously, and the results can be examined over time. Vignettes have been used in large cross-national studies, such as a six-country policy evaluation in Central Asia and Eastern Europe (Peabody and others, forthcoming). This study, involving 1,039 facilities and 3,121 providers, evaluated quality of care in obstetrics, newborns, and chronic disease. Because vignettes are inexpensive to administer, they are especially well suited for use in resource-poor settings (Peabody, Luck, and others 2014; Peabody, Shimkhada, and others 2014; Peabody, Taguiwalo, and others 2006).

Standards

Evidence-Based and Best-Practice Standards

Much of the early disagreement about what to measure has given way to a consensus that performance should be measured against evidence-based criteria. The scientific literature is replete with evidence-based quality metrics that describe processes as varied as whether a patient's blood pressure is under control, whether a patient is on the correct medication to slow down renal failure, whether the timing of a specific surgery is correct, or whether a diagnostic test is needed. Collectively, clinical care metrics are based on the evidence and the supposition that meeting these metrics results in better outcomes. Critics point out that evidence-based practice has only been established for a limited number of care elements (Contreras and others 2007; Karolinski and others 2009; Vogel and others 2014). However, clinicians routinely rely on best-practice standards, even as high-quality data from well-designed studies continue to emerge and evolve. In practical terms, there will never be a complete set of evidence-based standards, and quality of care will always rely on the best available evidence and local standards.

An important body of evidence-based, best-practice standards in LMICs comes from using surgical and childbirth safety checklists. Checklists have recently been rapidly introduced into LMIC settings, and the evidence indicates that using these evidence-based standards in checklist form improves health outcomes, primarily by setting a quality standard for treatment and facilitating communication within provider teams (Ergo and others 2012). An intervention in Michigan that used a surgical checklist to decrease catheter-related bloodstream infections in hospital intensive care units, for example, led the World Health Organization (WHO) to create the Surgical Safety

Checklist (Pronovost and others 2006). As of 2012, the WHO Surgical Safety Checklist has been adopted by 1,790 health care facilities worldwide (Treadwell, Lucas, and Tsou 2014), helping teams to manage crises, avoid clinical errors, and minimize health risks. However, successful uptake of checklists requires "constant supervision and instruction until it becomes self-evident and accepted" (Sendlhofer and others 2015).

Licensing, Certification, and Accreditation

Provider certification and hospital accreditation were introduced into health care in the early twentieth century and have been adopted globally as a cornerstone of health care quality assurance. The number of health care accreditation programs, including national accreditation systems, is doubling every few years, with as many as 70 programs around the world in 2013 (Saleh and others 2013). Accreditation has expanded beyond hospitals to include primary care, health systems, and laboratories. Additionally, many LMICs are replacing voluntary accreditation from independent organizations with national programs that, in some instances, link accreditation to licensing (Greenfield and Braithwaite 2008; Jovanovic 2005).

However, national licensing and accreditation programs require political commitment, human and financial resources, and planning. This issue is further complicated in LMICs by the complexity of the development of the accreditation process and the dearth of resources for implementing and maintaining a strong accreditation process. Evidence on the effectiveness of accreditation for enhancing clinical outcomes or defining when accreditation is most effective is limited and inconclusive: in a systematic review of the literature, health sector accreditation was consistently associated with professional development and promotion of change, but not consistently associated with quality improvement or other organizational and financial impacts (Greenfield and Braithwaite 2008). One study in the Philippines showed that licensing and accreditation independently and substantively improved clinical practice and health outcomes, but with modest impact (Quimbo and others 2008).

Training

Clinical training starts in medical or other professional schools and continues throughout a practitioner's professional career. Continuing medical education is often a requirement for licensing or certification and is part of almost every health care system. Continuing education has shown positive impacts on care. In Tanzania, training staff in the control of acute respiratory infections in young children reduced under-five mortality within two years (Mtango and Neuvians 1986). Physician-reported continuing medical education has been linked to better quality and health status when accountability is included using clinical performance vignettes (Luck and others 2014). A six-nation study linked continuing education to evidence-based practice as measured with simulated patients (Peabody and others, forthcoming). Using a systematic database of quality improvement studies, Rowe and colleagues at the U.S. Centers for Disease Control and Prevention (National Academies of Sciences, Engineering, and Medicine 2015) found that, in LMICs, training and supervision have modest positive effects on provider performance and that strategies may work better when used in combination than when used by themselves. Work by Das and others (2016) on providers in India suggests that better incentives can improve quality without any additional provider training.

Despite its ubiquity, continuing education will not greatly improve the quality of clinical practice or health outcomes (Davis and others 1999; Forsetlund and others 2009). An analysis of 62 studies and 20 systematic reviews found that the "continuing education 'system,' as it is structured today, is so deeply flawed that it cannot properly support the development of health professionals" (IOM, Committee on Planning a Continuing Health Professional Education Institute 2010, ix). Davis and others (2006) found that physicians cannot self-assess their skills accurately and suggested that external assessment, scoring, and feedback would drive more effective professional development. Moreover, physicians are often "not trained" to evaluate or use published guidelines and best practices. Passive dissemination of information (publishing guidelines, reading peer-reviewed articles) is generally ineffective at changing practice and is unlikely to change group-wide practice when used alone.

Newer educational techniques—targeted education, case-based learning, and interactive and multimodal teaching techniques—have had more success. Interventions that are multifaceted and include active participation and targeted feedback are much more likely to be effective than single interventions. Engaging clinicians is the key to translating training into improved quality (Mostofian and others 2015). Physicians engaged in hospital initiatives, for example, are much more likely to report successful experiences with quality improvement programs. Methods that require active physician learning (one-on-one meetings, small-group workshops, and programs tailored to a specific clinic) are effective at aligning patterns of physician practice with new clinical guidelines. In Guatemala, distance education that targeted diarrhea and cholera case management increased the accurate assessment and classification of diarrhea cases by 25 percent (Flores, Robles, and Burkhalter 2002).

Supervision

Supervision is an established method for assessing quality. The power and influence of peer review supervision, often conducted through professional societies, vary widely among countries (Heaton 2000). Large providers, such as hospitals or public health institutions, often have more resources for collecting information on provider practices and patient outcomes and for using those data to guide, educate, supervise, discipline, or recognize providers. Providers at clinics and primary care facilities also benefit from supervision (Loevinsohn, Guerrero, and Gregorio 1995). Other studies point to the benefits of quality review committees and standing groups that review all hospital deaths. However, oversight can also create an antagonistic relationship between workers and managers that may preclude cooperative problem solving and continuous improvement (Berwick 2002).

Incentives

Demand Incentives

Demand-side interventions, such as conditional cash transfer (CCT) and voucher programs, pay participants (not providers) a stipend for specific behaviors, for example, attending school, having up-to-date vaccinations, or visiting a health center for prenatal care (box 10.1). Although CCTs do not directly provide incentives to health care providers, they require quality health services, adding a supply- or provider-side component to demand-side interventions. There is also an indirect supply-side incentive when consumers use cash incentives to pay for services. A systematic review of the evidence suggests that CCTs improve the uptake of preventive services by children and pregnant women (Lagarde, Haines, and Palmer 2009).

However, in shorter time frames of months to a year, CCTs have difficulty driving lasting effects and affecting health (Beegle, Frankenberg, and Thomas 2001; World Bank 2003). From a policy perspective, it is also difficult to distinguish the effects of the CCT incentive from the impact of the cash itself, that is, it is unclear whether the behavioral change is associated with the conditional incentive or with an income effect (Fernald, Gertler, and Neufeld 2008). A systematic review of the impact of vouchers found modest evidence that the vouchers improved quality of care (Brody and others 2013). The question that remains is whether there are long-term effects because clinical practice was not improved.

Provider Payment

In the past two decades, health care administrators and policy makers in both LMICs and HICs have been using pay for performance (P4P) as a means to improve clinical practice. Although the details of programs vary, health care P4P programs link physician compensation to measures of clinical quality (Epstein, Lee, and Hamel 2004). P4P and other forms of results-based compensation have been used routinely in business settings. The challenge in health, however, is to identify suitable metrics that are under the control of the provider (Werner and Asch 2007). For example, care providers are hard pressed to reduce infant mortality rates that are driven primarily by poverty and nutrition, but they can readily change the frequency of unnecessary cesarean sections.

Even with suitable metrics, isolating and linking P4P changes in practice to better health has been challenging (Atkinson and others 2000; Derose and Petitti 2003). P4P might be linked, at best, to modest improvements in quality of care (Epstein 2007; Lindenauer and others 2007; Petersen and others 2006; Rosenthal and others 2005). However, most studies are not experimentally designed, and participation in P4P programs is voluntary, leading to selection bias. Although much of the literature on the equivocal benefit of provider incentive systems comes from HICs, the Quality Improvement Demonstration Study (QIDS), carried out in the Philippines as a social policy experiment, provides

---

Box 10.1

Progresa/Oportunidades

Progresa/Oportunidades is a major government initiative that used demand-side interventions (conditional cash transfers) to reduce long-standing poverty and develop human capital within poor households in Mexico (Fernald, Gertler, and Neufeld 2009). The demand incentives were payments to mothers for health behaviors, such as participation in programs like prenatal care, immunizations, and nutrition supplementation, as well as for children's school attendance. The intervention had a broad positive impact on many measures and improved patient outcomes such as stunting and anemia in preschool children (Fernald, Gertler, and Neufeld 2009; Rivera and others 2004). The implication of this work is that, for certain health outcomes, improving access was sufficient to improve outcomes. Although there are no data, this improvement occurred even though clinical practice was (certainly) varied.

strong experimental evidence that P4P can be effective in an LMIC (Quimbo and others 2008) (see box 10.2). Similar results were found in the work by Gertler and Vermeersch (2013).

The large QIDS randomized community-level experiment found greater improvement in health outcomes than previous P4P studies (Peabody and others 2017). This finding may have occurred because most other studies providing incentives to doctors have been conducted in wealthier countries and been nonrandomized, which introduces the possibility of selection bias wherein providers who adopt the incentives may be the most likely to respond and improve their clinical practice anyway (Petersen and others 2006). Three randomized P4P studies conducted in the United States found that rewarding physicians improved outpatient care, such as immunization rates (Fairbrother and others 1997; Fairbrother and others 2001; Kouides and others 1998). However, other randomized studies found that physician P4P had no effect on mammography, other cancer screening, or adherence to pediatric preventive guidelines (Grady and others 1997; Hillman and others 1998; Hillman and others 1999). Three hospital-based studies examining inpatient P4P programs in the United States also included control hospitals. These studies, which focused on adult care in cardiovascular disease, community-acquired pneumonia, and joint replacement, found modest improvements of 2 to 4 percentage points in outcomes beyond the performance seen in controls (Glickman, Boulding, and others 2007; Grossbart 2006; Lindenauer and others 2007). Although these studies had controls, the interventions were not randomly assigned.

Results- and Performance-Based Financing

Results-based financing (RBF) encompasses various types of interventions that provide demand-side incentives (for example, CCTs), refine provider payments (for example, P4P), and trigger government reforms.

The RBF lending projects financed by the Health Results Innovation Trust Fund and World Bank credits or loans (World Bank 2014) operationalized the concept of RBF at a large scale in many LMICs and intended to provide incentives to policy makers to build and leverage their quality infrastructure as a condition for financing. Since 2008, RBF projects like these have been widely adopted in more than 30 countries, with interventions at the national, subnational, district, facility, and community levels. Operationally, funds are provided to governments at the national and subnational level based on agreed-on disbursement-linked indicators and their established targets (often nation- and state-wide estimates). At the facility level, payments to individual facilities are based on their contracts with fund holders (often district or provincial health authorities). And, increasingly used at the community level, payments are

---

Box 10.2

Impact of P4P on Quality: Results of the Quality Improvement Demonstration Study

The Quality Improvement Demonstration Study (QIDS) is unique in that it was an explicit policy experiment that randomized communities into pay for performance (P4P) versus universal health coverage versus a true control. P4P improved both quality and outcomes.

QIDS was a large policy experiment conducted in the Philippines among 119 doctors, 3,162 children, and 30 communities, covering about one-third of the country. The communities were randomized into an incentives-based policy program rewarding physicians financially for providing higher-quality care to children than provided by universal health coverage and controls (Quimbo and others 2008). In the communities where doctors were eligible for the bonus payments, the number of children who were not wasted (underweight for height) increased 9 percentage points relative to control sites. The share of parents reporting at least good health for their children was 7 percentage points higher in P4P sites than in controls (Peabody, Shimkhada, and others 2014).

The introduction of P4P led to improvements in quality of care as measured by clinical case vignettes (Peabody and others 2011). Difference-in-differences model estimations indicated that P4P improved not only the measured quality of physician practice but also health outcomes. The impact of policy can be measured in a relatively short (two-year) time frame when evaluation is integrated into policy making and planning before implementation (Peabody and others 2017), making it possible to measure policy effectiveness and to identify ineffective polices early on.

provided to community organizations or community health workers based on RBF contracts with fund holders (often districts or facilities).

A flexible approach, RBF focuses on results:

- Payments linked to results (both demand and supply side) based on context-specific health priorities
- Contracts or agreements that clarify the responsibilities of all stakeholders
- Autonomy for those contracted to be able to use RBF funds to attain the agreed-on results most effectively
- Verification of results to ensure that they are accurate and reliable
- Data sharing to enhance the results, which can be used for planning, design, and implementation
- Community involvement to enhance accountability.

RBF operational data show improvement of quality (especially structural quality) in the RBF programs. Facilities' quarterly quality scores, calculated based on a supervisory checklist, improved in almost all of these programs. In Burundi, for example, quality scores improved significantly during the first two years following rollout of a national RBF program (figure 10.1). In Ethiopia, where RBF was implemented at the national government level, the Ministry of Health undertook Service Availability and Readiness Assessment (SARA) of its primary care facilities on an annual basis to achieve targets associated with disbursement-linked indicators and developed action plans to address weaknesses identified through SARA.

Impact evaluation studies show positive evidence about the impact of RBF programs on certain dimensions of quality. Several countries, including Argentina, Rwanda, and Zimbabwe, report improvement in quality of prenatal care (Basinga and others 2010; Gertler and Vermeersch 2013; World Bank 2014). Afghanistan demonstrated substantial improvements in quality of examinations and counseling, as well as time spent with patients (Engineer and others 2016). Under Argentina's Plan Nacer[1] incentives-based program, the estimated probability of low birthweight was reduced by 19 percent among beneficiaries, and in-hospital neonatal mortality for babies of enrolled mothers was reduced by 74 percent (Gertler, Giovagnoli, and Martinez 2014).

RBF programs exercise interventions beyond provider performance incentives, such as policy reform, system strengthening, transparency improvement, and management and accountability enhancement. Because of this, establishing the effectiveness of clinical interventions through randomized controlled trials becomes a challenge. How best to use operational data and experiences remains important in disentangling the effects of incentives and the key bottlenecks addressed by RBF.

LINKING POLICY AND PRACTICE AT THE PLATFORM LEVEL

How do quality infrastructure policies at the government level translate into improved clinical care at the patient level? At its heart, quality improves only when providers deliver the right care to the patient at the right time, do so efficiently, and focus on the patient. However, less variation among a group of providers depends on individual providers treating their patients and their diseases the same way. This section examines how policy and practice come together at the platform level. Specifically, we review the policy elements described above that would be implemented for 11 clinical conditions across four platforms.

We start by looking at where care services are delivered. Delivery occurs through various platforms, from community and public health settings to primary care clinics, first-level hospitals, and the most advanced facilities in every country.

The quality of care will vary in each setting, which means that the policy elements discussed above are relevant to each setting. These policy elements are categorized as quality measurement, practice standards, training management, and incentives.

Table 10.2 shows how each policy element might be implemented across the four delivery platforms.

Figure 10.1 Average Quality Score among All Health Centers in Burundi, 2010–12

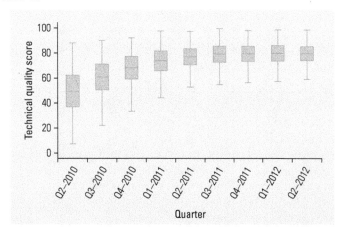

Source: Calculations based on operational data from the Burundi Health Sector Development Support Project.

Note: Quality score ("technical quality score") is measured based on a comprehensive supervisory checklist on a quarterly basis. Outlying values are not plotted on this graph.

Table 10.2 Infrastructure Elements for Improving Quality for 4 Delivery Platforms and 11 Representative Clinical Conditions

Infrastructure elements	Disease or condition	Delivery platforms							
		Community-based services		Primary health centers		First-level hospitals		Referral and specialized hospitals	
		Outcomes	Metrics	Outcomes	Metrics	Outcomes	Metrics	Outcomes	Metrics
Quality measurement									
Measurement	Reproductive health	Fertility management, contraception, family planning (information, condom availability, birth spacing)	Coverage rates or service use, provider knowledge, patient behavior (condom use); unintended pregnancy rate	Prenatal, perinatal care; recognition of high-risk pregnancies	Referral rates; folic acid coverage; ability to recognize high risk	Management of labor; vaginal delivery or cesarean section	Provider-level data on practice (vignettes, charts); patient-level data on outcomes (charts, patient reports)	Treatment of birth complications, such as sepsis	Provider-level data on use (vignettes, charts); patient-level data on outcomes (charts, registries, patient reports; mortality rates; readmission rates)
Feedback and accountability	Cardiovascular disease	Use of nutritional and exercise programs	Patient-level awareness of programs; availability of programs	Blood pressure, lipid, diabetes screening; management	Screening at the population level; screening with patient data on blood pressure, lipids	Triage of acute myocardial infarction and treatment of congestive heart failure	Provider-level data on practice; patient-level data on outcomes	Arrhythmias, endovascular procedures, valvular surgery	Provider-level data on use; patient-level data on outcomes
Practice standards									
Evidence-based practice	Sexually transmitted infections	Patient knowledge, safe sex practices	Patient surveys of knowledge, behaviors; provider surveys of clinical knowledge regarding sexually transmitted infections; cultural competency in communication	Syphilis screening, treatment of gonorrhea	Direct observation of successful management and treatment	Pelvic inflammatory disease	Provider-level data on practice; patient-level data on outcomes	Penile, cervical cancer	Provider-level data on use; patient-level data on outcomes

table continues next page

Table 10.2 Infrastructure Elements for Improving Quality for 4 Delivery Platforms and 11 Representative Clinical Conditions (continued)

Infrastructure elements	Disease or condition	Delivery platforms							
		Community-based services		Primary health centers		First-level hospitals		Referral and specialized hospitals	
		Outcomes	Metrics	Outcomes	Metrics	Outcomes	Metrics	Outcomes	Metrics
Checklists, clinical guidelines	Pediatric infectious diseases	Preventive, evidence-based measures to prevent disease	Immunization rates; incidence of disease	Diarrhea treatment, referral	Provider compliance with guidelines (charts, vignettes); provider's ability to diagnose, referral rates	Pneumonia (diagnosis, treatment of bacterial versus viral)	Provider-level data on use; patient-level data on outcomes	Cancer, bacterial meningitis, other serious infections	Provider-level data on use; patient-level data on outcomes
Licensing, certification, accreditation	Infectious disease	Provider hygiene, handwashing; proper disposal of needles	Direct observation of program implementation	Wound care with suturing; aseptic technique; instrument sterilization	Direct observation of explicit management or treatment criteria	Tuberculosis, HIV/AIDS diagnosis and treatment	Expert board review to determine if explicit criteria standards are met	Ebola, SARS, other outbreaks diagnosis and treatment	International body review to determine if explicit criteria are met; retransmission rates

Training, management

Infrastructure elements	Disease or condition	Community-based services		Primary health centers		First-level hospitals		Referral and specialized hospitals	
		Outcomes	Metrics	Outcomes	Metrics	Outcomes	Metrics	Outcomes	Metrics
Training	Mental health	Provider and community awareness of mental health; destigmatization of mental health illness	Provider and community attitudes, knowledge using surveys; incidence surveys of mental illness by socioeconomic status; destigmatization of mental health at community level	Acute mental health first aid and triage (suicide prevention, crisis intervention, disaster counseling); screening for ASD	Institutional training outcomes (provider knowledge) for diagnosis and counseling; provider's use of screening for ASD	Emergency care and hospitalization for acute psychosis; treatment and detoxification of substance abuse	Presence of care coordination and team practice with counseling and drug therapies available; provider's ability to diagnose; referral rates; treatment per institutional guidelines	Long-term care for dementia, chronic affective disorders, schizophrenia	Provider-level compliance according to evidence-based care; patient-level data: use of procedures, complications

table continues next page

Table 10.2 Infrastructure Elements for Improving Quality for 4 Delivery Platforms and 11 Representative Clinical Conditions (continued)

Infrastructure elements	Disease or condition	Delivery platforms							
		Community-based services		Primary health centers		First-level hospitals		Referral and specialized hospitals	
		Outcomes	Metrics	Outcomes	Metrics	Outcomes	Metrics	Outcomes	Metrics
Continuing medical education	Diabetes	Patient preventive behaviors: physical activity, healthy eating	Whether continuing medical education requirements are being met; provider knowledge regarding patient programs and ways to engage patient in behavioral change; patient knowledge	Diabetes management with behavioral interventions and medication	Knowledge-based testing	Treatment of renal failure, cardiovascular disease, and consumptive heart failure with medical therapies and medication	Knowledge-based testing; team-based practice measures	Transplant surgery	Provider use rates, provider's ability to identify transplant candidates; patient-level data on mortality, complications
Management	Accidents, injury, trauma	Provider's and patient's knowledge and use of preventive measures for injury (child safety, car seats, water safety, elder safety)	Provider and patient knowledge surveys	Provider's ability to recognize and assess severity of injury or complications	Provider-level data on ability to make correct diagnosis (vignettes), time to treatment, referral rates	Successful surgical treatment of trauma (minor surgery)	Mortality rates, wrong-site surgeries; proper use of surgery or surgical techniques; readmission	Successful surgical treatment of trauma (major surgery); treatment of burns	Mortality rates, wrong-site surgeries; proper use of surgery or surgical techniques; readmission rates
Professional oversight	Cancer	Smoking cessation, hepatitis B immunization rates, school-based human papillomavirus vaccination	Patient-level data on immunization rates, cancer incidence; hospital-based cancer registries	Screening for breast, colon, cervical, lung, and skin cancer	Assessment of provider's knowledge of risk and referral standards (set and disseminated); patient screening rates	Breast, skin cancer diagnosis; clinical staging	Provider's use of biopsies and compliance with treatment protocol	Colorectal cancer care screening (colonoscopy), colectomy, chemotherapy	Provider-level data on use, compliance with guidelines; patient-level data on outcomes

table continues next page

Table 10.2 Infrastructure Elements for Improving Quality for 4 Delivery Platforms and 11 Representative Clinical Conditions **(continued)**

Infrastructure elements	Disease or condition	Delivery platforms							
		Community-based services		Primary health centers		First-level hospitals		Referral and specialized hospitals	
		Outcomes	Metrics	Outcomes	Metrics	Outcomes	Metrics	Outcomes	Metrics
Incentives									
Performance-based remuneration	Orthopedics	Provider's knowledge and communication of preventive behaviors (healthy eating, immunization, healthy lifting); patient's behavior of the same	Provider's and patient's knowledge and behavior surveys; patient participation in preventive health programs; monitoring of physical activity of patients	Care for low-level trauma (simple broken bones), management of low-back pain	Provider's ability to diagnose low-back pain (vignettes); use of certain prescription drugs for pain management	Care for mid-level trauma and fractures	Proper use of surgery, drugs, antibiotics; mortality rate; bleeding during surgery; complications (thromboembolic disease)	Use and success of joint replacement	Proper use of surgery, drugs, antibiotics; mortality rate; bleeding during surgery; complications (thromboembolic disease)
Team-based, multidisciplinary care (global payment)	Malaria	Provider's knowledge and communication of vector control to patient (use of insecticides)	Provider's and patient's knowledge and behavior surveys; patient's participation in preventive health programs; community malaria rates	Provider's ability to recognize malaria rapidly; use of ACT	Provider's ability to diagnose malaria (vignettes); time to treat, proper use of ACT	Provider's ability to diagnose type of malaria (drug resistant or not); proper treatment, long-term follow-up, management	Provider's ability to diagnose malaria, recognize drug resistance; proper use of antimalarial drugs; proper management of relapse	Treatment and management of severe malaria-associated complications (cerebral malaria, renal dysfunction, hepatic dysfunction, acute respiratory distress, anemia, thrombocytopenia)	Patient-level data: mortality rate, complication rate; provider-level data: treatment of complications per evidence-based guidelines

Note: Quality interventions provided at lower-level platforms are also provided at higher-level facilities. ACT = artemisinin-based combination therapy. ASD = autism spectrum disorder; HIV/AIDS = human immunodeficiency virus/acquired immune deficiency syndrome; SARS = severe acute respiratory syndrome.

For each element, the table details how quality outcomes and metrics could be operationalized for a given disease or clinical condition. For example, community-based services in reproductive health (a condition) would focus on family planning and fertility management, which can be assessed by metrics of patient behavior (condom use); primary clinics would focus on high-risk pregnancies, which can be assessed using referral rates for women at risk. Outcomes and metrics tend to become more concrete as care progresses across platforms. Primary clinics and first-level hospitals, for example, might require chart-level data or provider-level assessments of skill, knowledge, and practice. Specialized hospitals, where care is more complex (treatment of birth complications) and outcome metrics are more serious (mortality rates), are likely to have more readily available data and better outcomes. A key element of quality improvement, whether at the specialized hospital or community clinic

level, is that the effectiveness of the improvement strategy must be assessed regularly. Recommendations published by the WHO and the International Association for Trauma Surgery and Intensive Care on quality improvement strategies are broadly applicable to all levels of care and types of settings and include strategies such as morbidity and mortality conferences to review errors occurring during the care of patients, panel reviews of preventable deaths, and tracking of complications, adverse events, sentinel events, and errors (WHO, Association for Trauma Surgery and Intensive Care, and International Society of Surgery 2009).

UPDATED QUALITY OF CARE FRAMEWORK

As shown in figure 10.2, health actions take place in the context of and are influenced by political (laws, governmental stability), cultural and social (societal norms,

Figure 10.2 DCP3 Approaches to Improving Quality of Care Framework

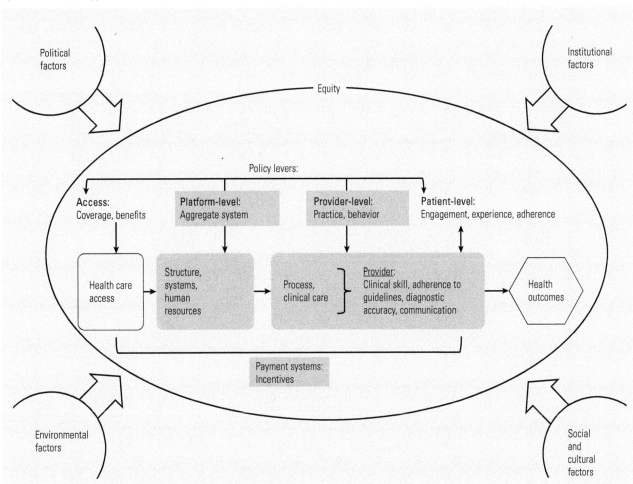

Note: Blue indicates items discussed in this chapter; DCP3 = Disease Control Priorities, third edition.

practices), environmental (natural disasters), and institutional (functioning health departments, corruption) factors. Demographic and socioeconomic makeup, including genetics and personal resources, also affect the health status of individuals seeking care.

The classic construct of structure, process, and outcome is at the core of the framework (Brook, McGlynn, and Cleary 1996; De Geyndt 1995; Donabedian 1980; McGlynn 1997). These three elements are described in table 10.3.

Structure refers to stable, material health care assets (infrastructure, tools, technology, implements), the resources of the organizations providing care, and the financing of that care (levels of funding, staffing, payment schemes, incentives). These factors can be measured inexpensively and data are typically readily available (De Geyndt 1995).

Process captures the interaction between caregivers and patients, including appropriateness of the care delivered, cognitive skill of the provider, and communication (Murray, Gakidou, and Frenk 1999). The private nature of the doctor-patient consultation, lack of measurement criteria, and absence of reliable measurement tools make it difficult to assess process, especially in LMICs (Peabody and others 2004). However, new approaches to measuring process have come a long way toward capturing process measures across settings.

Outcome includes direct measures of health status, death, or disability-adjusted life years as well as patient satisfaction or patient responsiveness to the health care system. Outcome measurement has matured in the past decade with the use of electronic medical records and data registries.

The updated framework in figure 10.2 adds policy levers for improving quality of care and showcases the provider's practice and behavior as well as the unique perspectives of policy makers, physicians, and patients, which are essential to establishing accountability. The early frameworks focused on the lack of structural inputs, whereas recent frameworks look at care processes (Kruk and others 2009). The Institute of Medicine was the first to include additional elements of care regarding safety and efficacy, patient focus, affordability and timeliness, and effectiveness (Berwick 2002; IOM, Committee on Quality Health Care in America 2001). The remainder of this section discusses these elements.

Safety and Efficacy

Patient safety has not received enough attention in LMICs. Globally, up to 1 in 10 patients is harmed by an adverse incident in a hospital not directly related to his or her clinical care, with approximately US$6 billion in costs per year (WHO 2008). Even procedures that are not considered high risk in HICs have the potential to lead to harm or poor outcomes in LMICs. For example, up to 1 in 4 cataract surgeries in India results in poor visual acuity (Lindfield and others 2012).

A study on patient safety practices in low-income countries suggests that improved staff-patient communication, use of protocols, control of infections, and standardization between providers can improve overall safety (Lindfield, Knight, and Bwonya 2015). Efficacy of care has an ascendant role in clinical practice as the practice of evidence-based medicine continues to expand. Many new and exciting studies of clinical efficacy are

Table 10.3 Quality-of-Care Framework

Elements of quality	Description	Subcomponents
Structure	Stable, material characteristics (infrastructure, tools, technology) and resources of the organizations that provide care and the financing of care (levels of funding, staffing, payment schemes, incentives)	• Physical characteristics • Management (executive leadership, board responsibilities) • Culture • Organizational design • Information management • Incentives
Process	The interaction between caregivers and patients during which structural inputs from the health care system are transformed into health outcomes	• Making the diagnosis • Providing evidence-based treatment
Outcomes	Measures of health status, deaths, or disability-adjusted life years (a measure that encompasses the morbidity and mortality of patients or groups of patients); outcomes such as patient satisfaction or patient responsiveness to the health care system	• Morbidity • Mortality • Patient satisfaction

Sources: Glickman, Boulding, and others 2007; Peabody, Taguiwalo, and others 2006.

driving better care, including the use of antibiotic prophylaxis before surgery and the elimination of antibiotics for otitis media.

Patient Focus

As with efficacy, focus on the patient and his or her perspective has become more prominent, leading evaluations of performance to include satisfaction as a necessary outcome. The availability and growing acceptance of patient satisfaction surveys are striking given that these tools were almost unheard of 20 years ago.

The focus on the patient is important because patients' or users' perspectives determine whether they seek care and where they obtain services (demand). This perspective is based on the individual's own opinions, previous experiences with the health system, and input received from others.

Perception of low quality has been reported as a major factor in the decision not to use or to bypass health services. For example, in a study in Tanzania, 42 percent of women who delivered children in a health care facility in rural parts of the country bypassed the local primary care clinic and delivered directly in a hospital or health center (Kruk and others 2014). This finding is striking because all of them lived near a functioning clinic with delivery services and the sample excluded women referred to a hospital. Primary care clinics tend to have poor infrastructure, lack equipment, and are understaffed, and women may choose care based on their perception of specific factors, such as a provider's attitude or competency and the availability of drugs and medical equipment.

Affordability and Timeliness

Determining affordability is challenging given that there is no recognized, consistent association between affordability and quality. High-quality care is often assumed to mean more expensive care (Starfield and others 1994). Indeed, early quality improvement efforts were often costly because the quality interventions themselves had to be paid for, and new measures of performance had to be introduced to calibrate the baseline quality and detect subsequent change (U.S. Congress, Office of Technology Assessment 1994).

However, high-quality care is potentially more affordable care because consistent, high-quality, standardized care entails fewer unnecessary tests, less time spent in the hospital, and fewer complications. In the United States, as much as one-third of health care costs are unnecessary, and as much as US$799 billion in costs is due to unexplained variation in practice and quality (Health

Affairs 2014). Estimates are not available for LMICs, but as much as one-third of health care costs may be due to unexplained variation in quality and unnecessary care in practice. A study in eight countries found that the introduction of surgical guidelines in hospitals led to less variation in quality, better health outcomes, and lower costs (Haynes and others 2009).

Effectiveness

Effectiveness refers to how well evidence-based practices are followed. Translating promising research findings and evidence, especially results that improve health or lower health care costs, into scalable interventions is challenging. The high stakes—and rare successes—have led to increasing calls for evidence-based policy making. Ideally, evidence-based policy making is based on evaluations of real-world economic effectiveness, allowing a determination to be made of value as well as efficacy.

With this effort has come interest in determining the comparative cost-effectiveness of clinical interventions. Few studies compare policy approaches to quality improvement. Peabody and others (2017) compared a demand-side intervention (universal health coverage for children under age five years) with a supply-side intervention (P4P scheme for physicians) and found that both interventions were effective, reducing wasting by about 9 percent (relative to controls). Costs were notably lower in the supply-side intervention than in the demand-side intervention, suggesting that increasing quality is more cost-effective than expanding insurance benefits in resource-constrained settings.

CHALLENGES FOR ASSESSMENT

The conversation on quality needs to include issues related to equity, misdiagnosis, perceptions, accountability, and learning from patients, all of which are challenging to assess.

Equity

Equity is an increasingly recognized part of the quality equation. Inequality—a situation in which poor-quality care is disproportionately provided to people from a particular disadvantaged group—is rampant worldwide (Barber, Bertozzi, and Gertler 2007; Barber, Gertler, and Harimurti 2007; Hansen and others 2008). Socioeconomically disadvantaged groups have poorer access to services and, once they have access, are less likely to receive effective treatment (Garrido-Cumbrera and others 2010; Health Affairs 2011; Rogers 2004).

If they are lucky enough to obtain treatment, they receive poorer-quality care than people from other groups. The impact of quality interventions on equity has not received enough attention in the literature.

Misdiagnosis

Misdiagnosis, also referred to as diagnostic error, is a significant shortcoming, with worrisome, albeit poorly understood, consequences (box 10.3). For example, a study reported that 5 percent of adults are misdiagnosed during outpatient visits, and about 50 percent of these errors could harm the patient (WHO 2000). Misdiagnosis in breast cancer is as high as 20 percent in some cases (Lozano and others 2006).

Misdiagnosis is likely to be especially high in LMICs (Galactionova and others 2015). A study in India found that only one-third of primary care providers articulated a diagnosis, either correct or incorrect, and when a diagnosis was given, close to 50 percent were wrong (Marchant and others 2015). In an observational study of primary care providers in rural China, the misdiagnosis rate was 74 percent, and clinicians provided medicine that was unnecessary or harmful to 64 percent of their patients (WHO and World Bank 2014). Diagnostic errors occur around the world and in all types of settings, suggesting a need to include misdiagnosis in conceptualizing quality-of-care deficiencies.

Real-world practicalities make investigating misdiagnoses a substantial challenge. Methodological problems include the difficulty of aggregating patients with the same diagnosis to overcome the unobserved (and unrecorded) case-mix variation, legitimate disagreements on reference standards for practice, reliance on recorded retrospective data, and challenges of measuring a clinician's cognitive thought processes. Perhaps the biggest methodological challenge is to reach some agreement regarding the correct diagnosis. Short of having a group of experts reexamine the patient, the correctness of diagnoses is difficult to evaluate.

Perceptions of Quality

Identifying a perspective—or multiple perspectives—from which to assess quality is difficult (Strauss and Corbin 1998; Tafreshi, Pazargadi, and Abed Saeedi 2007; Van der Bij, Vollmar, and Weggeman 1998; Wisniewski and Wisniewski 2005). Judging quality requires balancing the competing viewpoints of many players in the system. For example, payers and purchasers typically judge quality by how well insurance premium dollars are spent for each covered life; patients typically judge quality by how well their individual needs are addressed; and physicians assess quality by their own clinical judgment or training, patient demands, available resources, and cost-controlling mechanisms (Luck and others 2014).

Box 10.3

Misdiagnosis as a Core Element of Poor Quality

Diagnosis is a key determinant of a successful outcome (Freedman and Kruk 2014). Yet the extent of misdiagnosis has not been fully recognized (Jamison and others 2013; Ng and others 2014; OECD 2015; Rockers, Kruk, and Laugesen 2012; WHO 2000). A wrong diagnosis will lead, at best, to unnecessary evaluations and treatment and, at worst, to harmful tests and toxic treatment. Diagnostic errors result in potential delays in treatment, putting the patient at risk (WHO 2000) and leading to severe complications and overtreatment. They are an important cause of preventable morbidity and mortality (Freedman and Kruk 2014; Jamison and others 2013; Ng and others 2014; Rockers, Kruk, and Laugesen 2012).

The field of obstetrics provides a rich opportunity to study misdiagnosis in LMICs. A study examined the prevalence and consequences of misdiagnosis among 103 obstetrical providers in an urban area of the Philippines using identical vignettes and reviewing each provider's clinical records (Shimkhada and others 2016). The misdiagnosis of three common obstetric conditions—obstructed labor, postpartum hemorrhage, and preeclampsia—was almost 30 percent overall. Providers who misdiagnosed these conditions were more likely to have patients with a complication. Patients with a complication were significantly less likely to be referred to a hospital immediately and were more likely to be readmitted to a hospital after delivery, to have significantly higher medical costs, and to lose more income than patients without a complication.

When different perspectives collide—for example, when physician performance metrics (penalties for high surgical complication rates) are not in the best interest of the patient (a diabetic who is a higher surgical risk and may be turned down for surgery to keep complication rates low)—the patient's outcomes, including satisfaction, should be given the greatest weight.

Accountability

Establishing accountability is challenging. It can be difficult to determine which platform is responsible for achieving certain measurement goals and which individuals within each level should be held accountable for those measures (Emanuel and Emanuel 1996; Wachter 2013). The challenge of establishing accountability is tied to the larger challenge of convincing all players that poor quality should not be attributed to an individual clinician. Poor quality cuts across all types of care, facilities, providers, health insurance offerings, geographic areas, and patient populations. Accountability must be established at all levels (Brinkerhoff 2003). Holding physicians accountable may be especially difficult in a fee-for-service environment where individuals are used to being independent, and there are significant methodological, political, and legal obstacles to measuring accountability (Quimbo and others 2008).

A common trap is to let the availability of data determine which system-level metrics are tracked. System accountability is analogous to provider accountability, and metrics must be relevant, reliable, valid, comprehensive, and financially achievable; data availability should not drive the selection of metrics (Hsia 2003). Accountability also means that those who judge quality have the opportunity to go beyond explicit, evidence-based measures of practice or even structure. Recent work points to system- and platform-level accountability for collaboration, local ownership, and shared learning (Boucar and others 2014).

Learning from Patients

A final, neglected area of quality assessment is health system responsiveness to patients, specifically data on the patient's experience and satisfaction with care (Bernhart and others 1999). Therefore, improving the patient experience is a stand-alone goal of health systems in the updated framework (Rockers, Kruk, and Laugesen 2012; WHO 2000).

Initiatives such as the current push for universal health coverage assume that people will value and want to fund health benefits, whether through taxes or premiums. Public support, however, is shaped in important ways by an individual's health system experiences. For example, in addition to health outcome data, the Organisation for Economic Co-Operation and Development now measures the patient experience, including metrics on wait times, communication, and costs of care.

Methods of obtaining data on the patient experience include exit surveys (in person or anonymous), mailed or online questionnaires, and, increasingly, phone surveys. The large and growing penetration of mobile phones makes it more and more feasible to collect short telephone or mobile Web assessments of the patient experience in LMICs (Solon and others 2009).

IMPACT OF QUALITY IMPROVEMENT

Global health goals and projections are predicated on assumptions about achieving high coverage and improving the quality of care in high-mortality countries (Jamison and others 2013). Given the lack of high-quality data from LMICs, data from high-income settings are used to predict health gains from expanded coverage in LMICs. These extrapolations do not reflect the real-life impact of quality on use and eventual outcomes in LMICs. Diagnosis and treatment, for example, are often egregiously poor in understaffed, under-resourced and underregulated health systems. Yet it is critical to understand whether health care visits translate into quality health care—both for projecting better health and for estimating the health returns on initiatives such as universal health coverage.

Influence on Demand for Services and Outcomes

Quality of care is a major driver of use. Various studies have shown that perceived quality of care influences patterns of use—for example, perceptions of poor quality can motivate patients to stay at home or to choose far-away providers perceived to be more competent (Bohren and others 2014; Kruk and others 2009; Leonard 2014). Perceptions of poor quality are a strong factor pushing patients to bypass care, as are users' assessments of the complexity of their health needs (Akin and Hutchinson 1999; Kruk and others 2014; Leonard, Mliga, and Mariam 2002). In sum, patients in low-income settings increasingly behave like their rich-country counterparts: as active consumers making rational choices about their care rather than as passive beneficiaries of health care.

The demand for quality is likely to grow as coverage expands. Kruk and others (2015) found that, when childbirth at a health facility (that is, in-facility delivery) exceeds 80 percent of all births in a community, proximity to hospitals, not primary care clinics, matters in predicting delivery of care, potentially because of growing demand for high-quality care that is difficult for low-volume clinics to deliver.

How accurately do patients assess quality? Although patients are well positioned to report on interpersonal or nontechnical quality-of-care issues, such as clarity of communication, respect, confidentiality, and waiting times, they do not have full information with which to gauge the technical quality of care. Doyle, Lennox, and Bell (2013) found that the patient experience of care was positively associated with clinical effectiveness and safety in more than 75 percent of studies. For example, Glickman and others (2010) found that higher patient satisfaction was linked to lower mortality among patients with acute myocardial infarction. Similarly, more satisfied patients had lower 30-day hospital readmission rates and higher adherence to physician recommendations (Boulding and others 2011; Fenton and others 2012). Other research found little correlation between patient ratings of care and chart-measured adherence to standards of care, use of inpatient care, or mortality (Chang and others 2006).

Whether accurate or not, perceptions drive behavior. Patient ratings of quality and satisfaction are also associated with future care seeking, an important consideration given the rise of chronic diseases requiring ongoing contact with the health system (Bohren and others 2014; Groene 2011; Kruk and others 2014; Sun and others 2000). More work is needed to understand which patient assessments are most reliable and the best ways to collect these data.

Patient-reported quality and satisfaction are important indicators of the responsiveness and accountability of health systems (Thaddeus and Maine 1994). Responsiveness, defined as meeting patients' nonhealth expectations, should be a goal of every health system (WHO 2000). Yet recent research has documented disrespectful and abusive treatment of patients in health facilities. For example, nearly 20 percent of women in two districts of Tanzania reported harsh treatment by health workers, including yelling and slapping (Freedman and Kruk 2014). Such treatment leads to a loss of confidence (Kujawski and others 2015). Abusive treatment is distressingly common in other settings as well (Asefa and Bekele 2015; Gourlay and others 2014; Okafor, Ugwu, and Obi 2015; Sando and others 2014).

Fit between Services and Patient Needs

One promising strategy is to improve the fit between people's expectations and health needs and the health services available to them. This tailoring of care is an example of patient-centered reform (Groene 2011). For example, when the quality of obstetric care provided at first-level, low-volume facilities is of poor quality, referrals to higher levels of emergency care is inefficient, resulting in excessively high maternal and newborn mortality (Hsia and others 2012; Thorsen and others 2014). Women who deliver in the health system clearly prefer higher-volume, higher-quality facilities, as evidenced by choice of provider. Thus, the answer to improved quality and outcomes may be to establish high-volume maternity health centers or hospital units and provide support for travel to these facilities, rather than to invest more in primary care obstetrics or low-volume, first-level facilities. Focusing on customer service and respect requires paying attention to staffing, training, and supervision.

Health systems that can satisfy people's expectations may experience a double benefit: better health outcomes and greater support for the health system. For example, women who bypassed their first-level clinic and delivered in hospitals rated quality of care more highly than women who delivered in first-level clinics across a wide range of indicators (Kruk and others 2014). Experiencing responsive health services may enhance confidence in government. A multicountry study of LMICs found that a combination of high-quality care and financial risk protection raised the probability of having trust in government by 13 percent (Rockers, Kruk, and Laugesen 2012). More responsive, patient-centered health systems should be a health and political priority.

COSTS OF IMPROVING QUALITY

Almost all deficits in the quality of care can be addressed if enough resources are made available for the purpose. The question is not, "Can we improve the quality of health care services?" Instead, it is, "How can we use the resources available to achieve that improvement?" Thus, when resource constraints are considered, policy makers will have to choose from a range of interventions, and the question becomes, "What are the most efficient and feasible ways to improve health outcomes?" For example, nosocomial infections could be treated with costly antibiotics, new facilities, and equipment. However, it is likely to be far more efficient to introduce a handwashing protocol, to ensure that providers comply with it, and to develop a rapid response team that can be deployed when infections occur.

The costs of improving quality are different from the costs of the intervention itself. For example, the cost of delivering care to patients with closed fractures requiring internal fixation includes facility costs (patient room, equipment, sterile supplies), personnel costs (clinicians, support staff), and patient costs (transportation to the facility, time costs). If a high proportion of patients develop nosocomial infections, the cost of quality would be the costs incurred to reduce the risk of facility-associated infection through strategies such as providing training, supervising staff, procuring new cleaning and sterilization equipment, and developing care pathways or checklists.

Cost-effectiveness analysis (CEA) can be used to determine how cost-efficient a quality improvement intervention is. CEAs compare the resources consumed and the effects on the desired outcome of an intervention to improve the quality of care against a valid comparison, which is either business-as-usual or a different intervention. Three results are possible. First, the intervention may fail to improve the outcome of interest and is not cost-effective at any price. Second, the intervention may achieve the intended improvements, but require additional resources, in which case implementation is a matter of willingness to pay for the level of improvement achieved. Third, the intervention may improve health outcomes as a result of better quality while also reducing overall expenditure. Lower cost comes from spending a lesser amount on care or avoiding an expensive complication or an adverse event. Economically, it is best to implement all interventions matching the third result.

There is a dearth of literature on the cost-efficiency of quality of care interventions (IOM, Committee on Quality of Health Care in America 2001). Several difficulties are involved in determining efficiency:

- Inaccurate, incomplete, or unavailable routinely collected data
- Fidelity of the intervention to the outcome stated in research design
- The challenge of choosing comparison groups to isolate the variable of interest
- The difficulty of capturing all of the effects of the intervention to account for positive or negative spillover effects
- The challenge of calibrating the extent to which the quality improvement can be attributed to the intervention
- The perceived costs and economic consequences meaningful to different audiences
- The difficulty of valuing in-kind contributions
- The difficulty of capturing complexity of a system and the implications for economic evaluation.

Nevertheless, CEA can show substantive returns from better quality. In one study in Niger, high quality from a quality improvement collaborative conducted in childbirth facilities reduced the overall costs per birth an average of 20 percent (from US$35 to US$28); when accounting for the decrease in average clinical costs due to improved efficiency and the reductions in postpartum hemorrhage, the authors determined that the incremental cost of the improvement collaborative was US$2.43 (Broughton, Boucar, and Alagane 2012). The incremental cost-effectiveness was an impressive US$147 per disability-adjusted life year averted, compared with US$870 for the rotavirus vaccine, US$135 for hypertension treatment, and US$1,480 for a tobacco tax (Tran and others 2014). Interventions to improve health care quality can also save money as shown in the example of improving uptake of Kangaroo Mother Care for premature and low birthweight infants in Nicaragua (Broughton and others 2013). In this case, the cost of the improvement intervention was less than the cost savings realized from decreased treatment costs resulting from improved adherence to evidence-based standards of care.

Despite the many difficulties in determining efficient ways to address deficits in the quality of health care, it is important to include these cost analyses in every quality improvement intervention. Systematic accounting for the resources and rigorous evaluation of the effects on the outcomes of interest are essential for prioritizing decision making. Basic guidance on what costs to include in economic evaluations and how to analyze cost and effectiveness data is needed to move the field of health care quality forward.

CONCLUSIONS

In LMICs, quality of care is an emerging conversation. Mostly ignored a few decades ago, studies are now examining health system priorities once access to care has been addressed. Conversations over the past 10 years have largely acknowledged the importance of quality of care in resource-constrained LMICs. Quality of care is discussed in all volumes of *DCP3*.

Quality of care matters because it relates directly to outcomes and can be addressed in a shorter time frame than other policy interventions. The updated quality framework presented in this chapter describes the urgency, connections, and responsibilities for creating quality infrastructure that ties this responsibility to individual providers through the diseases they address and the patients who access care via various health care platforms. The framework is applicable across country settings, emphasizing the fundamental role that providers and patients play in determining quality. With the growing evidence base on quality improvement efforts around the globe, there is reason for renewed hope that quality can be improved and *done so rapidly*. Successful policies will always be linked to practice on a disease-by-disease basis and will only occur where access to health care is not in question.

NOTES

World Bank Income Classifications as of July 2014 are as follows, based on estimates of gross national income (GNI) per capita for 2013:

- Low-income countries (LICs) = US$1,045 or less
- Middle-income countries (MICs) are subdivided:
  (a) lower-middle-income = US$1,046 to US$4,125
  (b) upper-middle-income (UMICs) = US$4,126 to US$12,745
- High-income countries (HICs) = US$12,746 or more.

1. A program that delivers insurance for maternal and child health services to uninsured families.

REFERENCES

AbouZahr, C., and T. Boerma. 2005. "Health Information Systems: The Foundations of Public Health." *Bulletin of the World Health Organization* 83 (8): 578–83.

Achanta, S., J. Jaju, A. M. Kumar, S. B. Nagaraja, S. R. Shamrao, and others. 2013. "Tuberculosis Management Practices by Private Practitioners in Andhra Pradesh, India." *PLoS One* 8 (8): e71119.

Akin, J. S., and P. Hutchinson. 1999. "Health-Care Facility Choice and the Phenomenon of Bypassing." *Health Policy and Planning* 14 (2): 135–51.

Ali, M. K., S. Shah, and N. Tandon. 2011. "Review of Electronic Decision-Support Tools for Diabetes Care: A Viable Option for Low- and Middle-Income Countries?" *Journal of Diabetes Science and Technology* 5 (3): 553–70.

Ansong-Tornui, J., M. Armar-Klemesu, D. Arhinful, S. Penfold, and J. Hussein. 2007. "Hospital Based Maternity Care in Ghana: Findings of a Confidential Enquiry into Maternal Deaths." *Ghana Medical Journal* 41 (3): 125–32.

Asefa, A., and D. Bekele. 2015. "Status of Respectful and Non-Abusive Care during Facility-Based Childbirth in a Hospital and Health Centers in Addis Ababa, Ethiopia." *Reproductive Health* 12 (1): 33.

Atkinson, S., R. L. R. Medeiros, P. H. L. Oliveira, and R. D. Almeida. 2000. "Going Down to the Local: Incorporating Social Organisation and Political Culture into Assessments of Decentralised Health Care." *Social Science and Medicine* 51 (4): 619–36.

Baker, D. W., and R. D. Cebul. 2002. "Should Consumers Trust Hospital Quality Report Cards?" *Journal of the American Medical Association* 287 (24): 3206–07.

Barber, S. L., S. M. Bertozzi, and P. J. Gertler. 2007. "Variations in Prenatal Care Quality for the Rural Poor in Mexico." *Health Affairs (Millwood)* 26 (3): 310–23.

Barber, S. L., P. J. Gertler, and P. Harimurti. 2007. "Differences in Access to High-Quality Outpatient Care in Indonesia." *Health Affairs (Millwood)* 26 (3): 352–66.

Basinga, P., P. J. Gertler, A. Binagwaho, A. L. B. Soucat, J. R. Sturdy, and others. 2010. "Paying Primary Health Care Centers for Performance in Rwanda." Human Development Network Chief Economist's Office and Africa Region Health, Nutrition and Population Unit, World Bank, Washington, DC.

Beegle, K., E. Frankenberg, and D. Thomas. 2001. "Bargaining Power within Couples and Use of Prenatal and Delivery Care in Indonesia." *Studies in Family Planning* 32 (2): 130–46.

Beracochea, E., R. Dickson, P. Freeman, and J. Thomason. 1995. "Case Management Quality Assessment in Rural Areas of Papua New Guinea." *Tropical Doctor* 25 (2): 69–74.

Bernhart, M. H., I. G. Wiadnyana, H. Wihardjo, and I. Pohan. 1999. "Patient Satisfaction in Developing Countries." *Social Science and Medicine* 48 (8): 989–96.

Bertelsen, J. 1981. "Who Should Abstract Medical Records? A Study of Accuracy and Cost." *Evaluation and the Health Professions* 4 (1): 79–92.

Berwick, D. M. 2002. "A User's Manual for the IOM's 'Quality Chasm' Report." *Health Affairs (Millwood)* 21 (3): 80–90.

Bohren, M. A., E. C. Hunter, H. M. Munthe-Kaas, J. P. Souza, J. P. Vogel, and others. 2014. "Facilitators and Barriers to Facility-Based Delivery in Low- and Middle-Income Countries: A Qualitative Evidence Synthesis." *Reproductive Health* 11 (1): 71.

Bosch-Capblanch, X., O. Ronveaux, V. Doyle, V. Remedios, and A. Bchir. 2009. "Accuracy and Quality of Immunization Information Systems in Forty-One Low-Income Countries." *Tropical Medicine and International Health* 14 (1): 2–10.

Boucar, M. L., K. Hill, A. Coly, S. Djibrina, Z. Saley, and others. 2014. "Improving Postpartum Care for Mothers and Newborns in Niger and Mali: A Case Study of an Integrated Maternal and Newborn Improvement Programme." *British Journal of Obstetrics and Gynaecology* 121 (Suppl 4): 127–33.

Boulding, W., S. W. Glickman, M. P. Manary, K. A. Schulman, and R. Staelin. 2011. "Relationship between Patient Satisfaction with Inpatient Care and Hospital Readmission within 30 Days." *American Journal of Managed Care* 17 (1): 41–48.

Brinkerhoff, D. 2003. *Accountability and Health Systems: Overview, Framework, and Strategies*. Bethesda, MD: Partners for Health Reformplus Project, Abt Associates.

Brody, C. M., N. Bellows, M. Campbell, and M. Potts. 2013. "The Impact of Vouchers on the Use and Quality of Health Care in Developing Countries: A Systematic Review." *Global Public Health* 8 (4): 363–88.

Brook, R. H., E. A. McGlynn, and P. D. Cleary. 1996. "Measuring Quality of Care." *New England Journal of Medicine* 335 (13): 966–70.

Broughton, E. I., A. M. Boucar, and D. Alagane. 2012. "Cost-Effectiveness of a Quality Improvement Collaborative for Obstetric and Newborn Care in Niger." *International Journal of Health Care Quality Assurance* 26 (3): 250–61.

Broughton, E. I., I. Gomez, N. Sanchez, and C. Vindell. 2013. "The Cost-Savings of Implementing Kangaroo Mother Care in Nicaragua." *Revista Panamericana de Salud Publica* 34 (3): 176–82.

Calle, J. E., P. J. Saturno, P. Parra, J. Rodenas, M. J. Pérez, and others. 2000. "Quality of the Information Contained in the Minimum Basic Data Set: Results from an Evaluation in Eight Hospitals." *European Journal of Epidemiology* 16 (11): 1073–80.

Canchihuaman, F. A., P. J. Garcia, S. S. Gloyd, and K. K. Holmes. 2011. "An Interactive Internet-Based Continuing Education Course on Sexually Transmitted Diseases for Physicians and Midwives in Peru." *PLoS One* 6 (5): e19318.

Chang, J. T., R. D. Hays, P. G. Shekelle, C. H. Malean, D. H. Solomon, and others. 2006. "Patients' Global Ratings of Their Health Care Are Not Associated with the Technical Quality of Their Care." *Annals of Internal Medicine* 144 (9): 665–72.

Contreras, G. Y., B. S. Olavaria, S. M. Pérez, D. P. Haemmerli, M. L. Cafferata, and others. 2007. "Practices in the Care of the Low-Risk Delivery in Hospitals in Southern Chile." *Ginecología y Obstetricia de México* 75 (1): 24–30.

Corrao, S., V. Arcoraci, S. Arnone, L. Calvo, R. Scaglione, and others. 2009. "Evidence-Based Knowledge Management: An Approach to Effectively Promote Good Health-Care Decision-Making in the Information Era." *Internal and Emergency Medicine* 4 (2): 99–106.

Das, J., and J. Hammer. 2005a. "Which Doctor? Combining Vignettes and Item Response to Measure Clinical Competence." *Journal of Development Economics* 78 (2): 348–83.

———. 2005b. "Which Doctor? Combining Vignettes and Item Response to Measure Doctor Quality." Policy Research Working Paper 3301, World Bank, Washington, DC.

———. 2007. "Location, Location, Location: Residence, Wealth, and the Quality of Medical Care in Delhi, India." *Health Affairs (Millwood)* 26 (3): 338–51.

———. 2014. "Quality of Primary Care in Low-Income Countries: Facts and Economics." *Annual Review of Economics* 6 (1): 525–53.

Das, J., A. Holla, A. Das, M. Mohanan, D. Tabak, and others. 2012. "In Urban and Rural India, A Standardized Patient Study Showed Low Levels of Provider Training and Huge Quality Gaps." *Health Affairs (Millwood)* 31 (12): 2774–84.

Das, J., A. Holla, A. Mohpal, and K. Muralidharan. 2016. "Quality and Accountability in Healthcare Delivery: Audit-Study Evidence from Primary Care in India." *American Economic Review* 106 (12): 3765–99.

Das, J., A. Kwan, B. Daniels, S. Satyanarayana, R. Subbaraman, and others. 2015. "Use of Standardised Patients to Assess Quality of Tuberculosis Care: A Pilot, Cross-Sectional Study." *The Lancet Infectious Diseases* 15 (11): 1305–13.

Davis, D. A., P. E. Mazmanian, M. Fordis, R. Van Harrison, K. E. Thorpe, and others. 2006. "Accuracy of Physician Self-Assessment Compared with Observed Measures of Competence: A Systematic Review." *Journal of the American Medical Association* 296 (9): 1094–102.

Davis, D. A., M. A. O'Brien, N. Freemantle, F. M. Wolf, P. Mazmanian, and others. 1999. "Impact of Formal Continuing Medical Education: Do Conferences, Workshops, Rounds, and Other Traditional Continuing Education Activities Change Physician Behavior or Health Care Outcomes?" *Journal of the American Medical Association* 282 (9): 867–74.

Dayal, P., and K. Hort. 2015. "Quality of Care: What Are Effective Policy Options for Governments in Low- and Middle-Income Countries to Improve and Regulate the Quality of Ambulatory Care?" Policy Brief 4 (1), Asia Pacific Observatory on Health Systems and Policies, WHO, Geneva.

De Geyndt, W. 1995. "Managing the Quality of Health Care in Developing Countries." Technical Paper 258, World Bank, Washington, DC.

Derose, S. F., and D. B. Petitti. 2003. "Measuring Quality of Care and Performance from a Population Health Care Perspective." *Annual Review of Public Health* 24 (1): 363–84.

Donabedian, A. 1980. "Methods for Deriving Criteria for Assessing the Quality of Medical Care." *Medical Care Review* 37 (7): 653–98.

Doyle, C., L. Lennox, and D. Bell. 2013. "A Systematic Review of Evidence on the Links between Patient Experience and Clinical Safety and Effectiveness." *BMJ Open* 3 (1): e001570.

Dranove, D., D. Kessler, M. McClellan, and M. Satterthwaite. 2003. "Is More Information Better? The Effects of 'Report Cards' on Health Care Providers." *Journal of Political Economy* 111 (3): 555–88.

Dumont, A., L. De Bernis, D. Bouillin, A. Gueye, J. P. Dompnier, and others. 2002. "Maternal Morbidity and Qualification of Health-Care Workers: Comparison between Two Different Populations in Senegal." *Journal de Gynécologie, Obstétrique, et Biologie de la Reproduction (Paris)* 31 (1): 70–79.

Emanuel, E. J., and L. L. Emanuel. 1996. "What Is Accountability in Health Care?" *Annals of Internal Medicine* 124 (2): 229–39.

Engelgau, M., K. Okamoto, K. V. Navaratne, and S. Gopalan. 2010. "Prevention and Control of Selected Chronic NCDs in Sri Lanka: Policy Options and Action." HNP Discussion Paper 2010, World Bank, Washington, DC.

Engineer, C. Y., E. Dale, A. Agarwal, A. Agarwal, O. Alonge, and others. 2016. "Effectiveness of a Pay-for-Performance Intervention to Improve Maternal and Child Health Services in Afghanistan: A Cluster-Randomized Trial." *International Journal of Epidemiology* 45 (2): 451–59.

Epstein, A. M. 2006. "Pay for Performance in the United States and Abroad." *New England Journal of Medicine* 355 (4): 406–08.

———. 2007. "Pay for Performance at the Tipping Point." *New England Journal of Medicine* 356 (5): 515–17.

Epstein, A. M., T. H. Lee, and M. B. Hamel. 2004. "Paying Physicians for High-Quality Care." *New England Journal of Medicine* 350 (4): 406–10.

Ergo, A., L. Paina, L. Morgan, and R. Eichler. 2012. *Creating Stronger Incentives for High-Quality Health Care in Low- and Middle-Income Countries.* Report for the Maternal and Child Health Integrated Program (MCHIP). Washington, DC: U.S. Agency for International Development (USAID).

Fairbrother, G., S. Friedman, K. L. Hanson, and G. C. Butts. 1997. "Effect of the Vaccines for Children Program on Inner-City Neighborhood Physicians." *Archives of Pediatrics and Adolescent Medicine* 151 (12): 1229–35.

Fairbrother, G., M. J. Siegel, S. Friedman, P. D. Kory, and G. C. Butts. 2001. "Impact of Financial Incentives on Documented Immunization Rates in the Inner City: Results of a Randomized Controlled Trial." *Ambulatory Pediatrics* 1 (4): 206–12.

Felt-Lisk, S., G. Ferry, R. Roper, M. Au, J. Walker, and others. 2012. "Sustainability, Partnerships, and Teamwork in Health IT Implementation: Essential Findings from the Transforming Healthcare Quality through IT Grant." AHRQ Publication 12-0075-EF, Agency for Healthcare Research and Quality, Rockville, MD.

Fenton, J. J., A. F. Jerant, K. D. Bertakis, and P. Franks. 2012. "The Cost of Satisfaction: A National Study of Patient Satisfaction, Health Care Utilization, Expenditures, and Mortality." *Archives of Internal Medicine* 172 (5): 405–11.

Fernald, L. C., P. J. Gertler, and L. M. Neufeld. 2008. "Role of Cash in Conditional Cash Transfer Programmes for Child Health, Growth, and Development: An Analysis of Mexico's Oportunidades." *The Lancet* 371 (9615): 828–37.

————. 2009. "10-Year Effect of Oportunidades, Mexico's Conditional Cash Transfer Programme, on Child Growth, Cognition, Language, and Behaviour: A Longitudinal Follow-up Study." *The Lancet* 374 (9706): 1997–2005.

Flores, R., J. Robles, and B. R. Burkhalter. 2002. "Distance Education with Tutoring Improves Diarrhea Case Management in Guatemala." *International Journal of Quality Health Care* 14 (Suppl 1): 47–56.

Forsetlund, L., A. Bjorndal, A. Rashidian, G. Jamtvedt, M. A. O'Brien, and others. 2009. "Continuing Education Meetings and Workshops: Effects on Professional Practice and Health Care Outcomes." *Cochrane Database of Systematic Reviews* 2 (2): CD003030.

Freedman, L. P., and M. E. Kruk. 2014. "Disrespect and Abuse of Women in Childbirth: Challenging the Global Quality and Accountability Agendas." *The Lancet* 384 (9948): e42–44.

Galactionova, K., F. Tediosi, D. de Savigny, T. Smith, and M. Tanner. 2015. "Effective Coverage and Systems Effectiveness for Malaria Case Management in Sub-Saharan African Countries." *PLoS One* 10 (5): e0127818.

Garrido-Cumbrera, M., C. Borrell, L. Palència, A. Espelt, M. Rodríguez-Sanz, and others. 2010. "Social Class Inequalities in the Utilization of Health Care and Preventive Services in Spain, a Country with a National Health System." *International Journal of Health Services* 40 (3): 525–42.

Gertler, P., P. Giovagnoli, and S. Martinez. 2014. "Rewarding Provider Performance to Enable a Healthy Start to Life: Evidence from Argentina's Plan Nacer." Working Paper 6884, World Bank Group, Washington, DC.

Gertler, P., and C. Vermeersch. 2013. "Using Performance Initiatives to Improve Medical Care Productivity and Health Outcomes." Working Paper 19046, National Bureau of Economic Research, Cambridge, MA.

Glassman, P. A., J. Luck, E. M. O'Gara, and J. W. Peabody. 2000. "Using Standardized Patients to Measure Quality: Evidence from the Literature and a Prospective Study." *Joint Commission Journal on Quality Improvement* 26 (11): 644–53.

Glickman, S. W., W. Boulding, M. Manary, R. Staelin, M. T. Roe, and others. 2010. "Patient Satisfaction and Its Relationship with Clinical Quality and Inpatient Mortality in Acute Myocardial Infarction." *Circulation: Cardiovascular Quality and Outcomes* 3 (2): 188–95.

Glickman, S. W., W. Boulding, R. Staelin, J. Mulgund, M. T. Roe, and others. 2007. "A Framework for Quality Improvement: An Analysis of Factors Responsible for Improvement at Hospitals Participating in the Can Rapid Risk Stratification of Unstable Angina Patients Suppress Adverse Outcomes with Early Implementation of the ACC/AHA Guidelines (CRUSADE) Quality Improvement Initiative." *American Heart Journal* 154 (6): 1206–20.

Goeree, R., L. Levin, K. Chandra, J. M. Bowen, G. Blackhouse, and others. 2009. "Health Technology Assessment and Primary Data Collection for Reducing Uncertainty in Decision Making." *Journal of the American College of Radiologists* 6 (5): 332–42.

Gourlay, A., A. Wringe, I. Birdthistle, G. Mshana, D. Michael, and others. 2014. "'It Is Like That, We Didn't Understand Each Other': Exploring the Influence of Patient-Provider Interactions on Prevention of Mother-to-Child Transmission of HIV Service Use in Rural Tanzania." *PLoS One* 9 (9): e106325.

Grady, K. E., J. P. Lemkau, N. R. Lee, and C. Caddell. 1997. "Enhancing Mammography Referral in Primary Care." *Preventive Medicine* 26 (6): 791–800.

Greenfield, D., and J. Braithwaite. 2008. "Health Sector Accreditation Research: A Systematic Review." *International Journal for Quality in Health Care* 20 (3): 172–83.

Groene, O. 2011. "Patient Centredness and Quality Improvement Efforts in Hospitals: Rationale, Measurement, Implementation." *International Journal for Quality in Health Care* 23 (5): 531–37.

Grossbart, S. R. 2006. "What's the Return? Assessing the Effect of 'Pay for Performance' Initiatives on the Quality of Care Delivery." *Medical Care Research and Review* 63 (1): 29S–48S.

Hansen, P. M., D. H. Peters, A. Edward, S. Gupta, A. Arur, and others. 2008. "Determinants of Primary Care Service in Afghanistan." *International Journal for Quality in Health Care* 20 (6): 375–83.

Haux, R. 2006. "Individualization, Globalization, and Health: About Sustainable Information Technologies and the Aim of Medical Informatics." *International Journal of Medical Informatics* 75 (12): 795–808.

Haynes, A. B., T. G. Weiser, W. R. Berry, S. R. Lipsitz, A. H. Breizat, and others. 2009. "A Surgical Safety Checklist to Reduce Morbidity and Mortality in a Global Population." *New England Journal of Medicine* 360 (5): 491–99.

Health Affairs. 2011. "Achieving Equity in Health." Health Policy Brief, October 6.

———. 2014. "Geographic Variation in Medicare Spending." Health Policy Brief, March 6.

Heaton, C. 2000. "External Peer Review in Europe: An Overview from the ExPeRT Project. External Peer Review Techniques." *International Journal for Quality in Health Care* 12 (3): 177–82.

Hillman, A. L., K. Ripley, N. Goldfarb, I. Nuamah, J. Weiner, and others. 1998. "Physician Financial Incentives and Feedback: Failure to Increase Cancer Screening in Medicaid Managed Care." *American Journal of Public Health* 88 (11): 1699–701.

Hillman, A. L., K. Ripley, N. Goldfarb, J. Weiner, I. Nuamah, and others. 1999. "The Use of Physician Financial Incentives and Feedback to Improve Pediatric Preventive Care in Medicaid Managed Care." *Pediatrics* 104 (4, Pt 1): 931–35.

Holm, M., and H. Burkhartzmeyer. 2015. "Implementation of a Phased Medical Educational Approach in a Developing Country." *Global Health Action* 8 (November): 29882.

Hsia, D. C. 2003. "Medicare Quality Improvement: Bad Apples or Bad Systems?" *Journal of the American Medical Association* 289 (3): 354–56.

Hsia, R. Y., N. A. Mbembati, S. Macfarlane, and M. E. Kruk. 2012. "Access to Emergency and Surgical Care in Sub-Saharan Africa: The Infrastructure Gap." *Health Policy and Planning* 27 (3): 234–44.

IOM (Institute of Medicine). 2013. *Announcement. Crossing the Quality Chasm: The IOM Health Care Quality Initiative.* Washington, DC: Health and Medicine Division, National Academy of Sciences, Engineering, Medicine.

IOM, Committee on Planning a Continuing Health Professional Education Institute. 2010. *Redesigning Continuing Education in the Health Professions.* Washington, DC: National Academies Press.

IOM, Committee on Quality of Health Care in America. 2001. *Crossing the Quality Chasm: A New Health System for the 21st Century.* Washington, DC: National Academies Press.

IOM and National Academy of Engineering. 2011. "Healthcare System Complexities, Impediments, and Failures." In *Engineering a Learning Healthcare System: A Look at the Future, Workshop Summary,* edited by C. Grossmann, W. A. Goolsby, L. Olsen, and J. M. McGinnis, 117–70. Washington, DC: National Academies Press.

Jamison, D. T., L. H. Summers, G. Alleyne, K. J. Arrow, S. Berkley, and others. 2013. "Global Health 2035: A World Converging within a Generation." *The Lancet* 382 (9908): 1898–955.

Jörg, F., N. Borgers, A. J. Schrijvers, and J. J. Hox. 2006. "Variation in Long-Term Care Needs Assessors' Willingness to Support Clients' Requests for Admission to a Residential Home: A Vignette Study." *Journal of Aging and Health* 18 (6): 767–90.

Jovanovic, B. 2005. "Hospital Accreditation as Method for Assessing Quality in Healthcare." *Archive of Oncology* 13 (3–4): 156–57.

Kantrowitz, B. 2014. "The Science of Learning." *Scientific American* 311 (2): 68–73.

Kaptanoğlu, A. Y., and I. Aktas. 2013. "Measuring Quality of Care Using a Vignette-Based Survey in Turkish Hospitals." *Korean Journal of Critical Care Medicine* 1 (1): 5–7.

Karolinski, A., P. Micone, R. Mercer, L. Gibbons, F. Althabe, and others. 2009. "Evidence-Based Maternal and Perinatal Healthcare Practices in Public Hospitals in Argentina." *International Journal of Gynaecology and Obstetrics* 105 (2): 118–22.

Kerr, E. A., and B. Fleming. 2007. "Making Performance Indicators Work: Experiences of U.S. Veterans Health Administration." *British Medical Journal* 335 (7627): 971–73.

Kirkpatrick, D. H., and R. T. Burkman. 2010. "Does Standardization of Care through Clinical Guidelines Improve Outcomes and Reduce Medical Liability?" *Obstetrics and Gynecology* 116 (5): 1022–26.

Koh, H. C., and G. Tan. 2005. "Data Mining Applications in Healthcare." *Journal of Healthcare Information Management* 19 (2): 64–72.

Kohn, L. T., J. M. Corrigan, and M. S. Donaldson, eds. 2000. *To Err Is Human: Building a Safer Health System.* Washington, DC: National Academies Press.

Kolstad, J. T. 2013. "Information and Quality When Motivation Is Intrinsic: Evidence from Surgeon Report Cards." *American Economic Review* 103 (7): 2875–910.

Kouides, R. W., N. M. Bennett, B. Lewis, J. D. Cappuccio, W. H. Barker, and others. 1998. "Performance-Based Physician Reimbursement and Influenza Immunization Rates in the Elderly. The Primary-Care Physicians of Monroe County." *American Journal of Preventive Medicine* 14 (2): 89–95.

Kruk, M. E., S. Hermosilla, E. Larson, and G. M. Mbaruku. 2014. "Bypassing Primary Care Clinics for Childbirth: A Cross-Sectional Study in the Pwani Region, United Republic of Tanzania." *Bulletin of the World Health Organization* 92 (4): 246–53.

Kruk, M. E., S. Hermosilla, E. Larson, D. Vail, Q. Chen, and others. 2015. "Who Is Left Behind on the Road to Universal Facility Delivery? A Cross-Sectional Multilevel Analysis in Rural Tanzania." *Tropical Medicine and International Health* 20 (8): 1057–66.

Kruk, M. E., M. Paczkowski, G. Mbaruku, H. de Pinho, and S. Galea. 2009. "Women's Preferences for Place of Delivery in Rural Tanzania: A Population-Based Discrete Choice Experiment." *American Journal of Public Health* 99 (9): 1666–72.

Kujawski, S., G. Mbaruku, L. P. Freedman, K. Ramsey, W. Moyo, and others. 2015. "Association between Disrespect and Abuse during Childbirth and Women's Confidence in Health Facilities in Tanzania." *Maternal and Child Health Journal* 19 (10): 2243–50.

LaFond, A., and M. Siddiqi. 2003. "Second International RHINO Workshop on Enhancing the Data Quality and Use of Routine Health Information at District Level." RHINO (Routine Health Information Network), Mpekweni Sun, Eastern Cape, South Africa, September 29–October 4.

Lagarde, M., A. Haines, and N. Palmer. 2009. "The Impact of Conditional Cash Transfers on Health Outcomes and Use of Health Services in Low- and Middle-Income Countries." *Cochrane Database of Systematic Reviews* 4 (October): CD008137.

Leonard, K. L. 2014. "Active Patients in Rural African Health Care: Implications for Research and Policy." *Health Policy and Planning* 29 (1): 85–95.

Leonard, K. L., and M. C. Masatu. 2006. "Outpatient Process Quality Evaluation and the Hawthorne Effect." *Social Science and Medicine* 63 (9): 2330–40.

Leonard, K. L., G. R. Mliga, and D. H. Mariam. 2002. "Bypassing Health Centres in Tanzania: Revealed Preferences for Quality." *Journal of African Economics* 11 (4): 441–71.

Li, L., Z. Wu, Y. Zhao, C. Lin, D. Detels, and others. 2007. "Using Case Vignettes to Measure HIV-Related Stigma among Health Professionals in China." *International Journal of Epidemiology* 36 (1): 178–84.

Lindenauer, P. K., D. Remus, S. Roman, M. B. Rothberg, E. M. Benjamin, and others. 2007. "Public Reporting and Pay for Performance in Hospital Quality Improvement." *New England Journal of Medicine* 356 (5): 486–96.

Lindfield, R., A. Knight, and D. Bwonya. 2015. "An Approach to Assessing Patient Safety in Hospitals in Low-Income Countries." *PLoS One* 10 (3): e0121628.

Lindfield, R., K. Vishwanath, F. Ngounou, and R. C. Khanna. 2012. "The Challenges in Improving Outcome of Cataract Surgery in Low- and Middle-Income Countries." *Indian Journal of Ophthalmology* 60 (5): 464–69.

Lippeveld, T., R. Sauerborn, and C. Bodart. 2000. *Design and Implementation of Health Information Systems.* Geneva: WHO.

Lium, J. T., A. Tjora, and A. Faxvaag. 2008. "No Paper, but the Same Routines: A Qualitative Exploration of Experiences in Two Norwegian Hospitals Deprived of the Paper-Based Medical Record." *BMC Medical Informatics and Decision Making* 8 (2): PMC2245928.

Loevinsohn, B. P., E. T. Guerrero, and S. P. Gregorio. 1995. "Improving Primary Health Care through Systematic Supervision: A Controlled Field Trial." *Health Policy and Planning* 10 (2): 144–53.

Lozano, R., P. Soliz, E. Gakidou, J. Abbott-Klafter, D. M. Freehan, and others. 2006. "Benchmarking of Performance of Mexican States with Effective Coverage." *The Lancet* 368 (9548): 1729–41.

Luck, J., and J. W. Peabody. 2002. "Using Standardised Patients to Measure Physicians' Practice: Validation Study Using Audio Recordings." *British Medical Journal* 325 (7366): 679.

Luck, J., J. W. Peabody, L. M. DeMaria, C. S. Alvarado, and R. Menon. 2014. "Patient and Provider Perspectives on Quality and Health System Effectiveness in a Transition Economy: Evidence from Ukraine." *Social Science and Medicine* 114 (August): 57–65.

Luck, J., J. W. Peabody, T. R. Dresselhaus, M. Lee, and P. Glassman. 2000. "How Well Does Chart Abstraction Measure Quality? A Prospective Comparison of Standardized Patients with the Medical Record." *American Journal of Medicine* 108 (8): 642–49.

Marchant, T., R. D. Tilley-Gyado, T. Tessema, K. Singh, M. Gautham, and others. 2015. "Adding Content to Contacts: Measurement of High-Quality Contacts for Maternal and Newborn Health in Ethiopia, North East Nigeria, and Uttar Pradesh, India." *PLoS One* 10 (5): e0126840.

Massoud, R., and N. Abrampah. 2015. "Scaling-Up of High-Impact Interventions." In *Improving Aid Effectiveness in Global Health*, edited by E. Beracochea, 139–47. New York: SpringerVerlag.

McGlynn, E. A. 1997. "Six Challenges in Measuring the Quality of Health Care." *Health Affairs (Millwood)* 16 (3): 7–21.

McGlynn, E. A., S. M. Asch, J. Adams, J. Keesey, J. Hicks, and others. 2003. "The Quality of Health Care Delivered to Adults in the United States." *New England Journal of Medicine* 384 (26): 2635–45.

Mohanan, M., M. Vera-Hernandez, V. Das, S. Giardili, J. D. Goldhaber-Fiebert, and others. 2015. "The Know-Do Gap in Quality of Health Care for Childhood Diarrhea and Pneumonia in Rural India." *Journal of the American Medical Association Pediatrics* 169 (4): 349–57.

Mostofian, F., C. Ruban, N. Simunovic, and M. Bhandari. 2015. "Changing Physician Behavior: What Works?" *American Journal of Managed Care* 21 (1): 75–84.

Mtango, F. D., and D. Neuvians. 1986. "Acute Respiratory Infections in Children under Five Years: Control Project in Bagamoyo District, Tanzania." *Transactions of the Royal Society of Tropical Medicine and Hygiene* 80 (6): 851–58.

Murray, C. J., E. E. Gakidou, and J. Frenk. 1999. "Health Inequalities and Social Group Differences: What Should We Measure?" *Bulletin of the World Health Organization* 77 (7): 537–43.

National Academies of Sciences, Engineering, and Medicine. 2015. *Improving Quality of Care in Low- and Middle-Income Countries.* Washington, DC: National Academies Press.

National Patient Safety Foundation. 2015. *Shining a Light: Safer Health Care through Transparency; Report of the Roundtable on Transparency.* Boston, MA: National Patient Safety Foundation.

Ng, M., N. Fullman, J. L. Dieleman, A. D. Flaxman, C. J. Murray, and others. 2014. "Effective Coverage: A Metric for Monitoring Universal Health Coverage." *PLoS Medicine* 11 (9): e1001730.

Nolan, T., P. Angos, A. J. Cunha, L. Muhe, S. Qazi, and others. 2001. "Quality of Hospital Care for Seriously Ill Children in Less-Developed Countries." *The Lancet* 357 (9250): 106–10.

OECD (Organisation for Economic Co-Operation and Development). 2015. *Health Care Quality Indicators.* Paris: OECD.

Okafor, I. I., E. O. Ugwu, and S. N. Obi. 2015. "Disrespect and Abuse during Facility-Based Childbirth in a

Low-Income Country." *International Journal of Gynecology and Obstetrics* 128 (2): 110–13.

Parsons, A., C. McCullough, J. Wang, and S. Shih. 2012. "Validity of Electronic Health Record–Derived Quality Measurement for Performance Monitoring." *Journal of the American Medical Informatics Association* 19 (4): 604–9.

Peabody, J. W., L. DeMaria, S. N. Nguyen, O. Smith, A. Hoth, and others. Forthcoming. "Quality of Care in Six Eastern European Countries Using Clinical Performance and Value Vignettes: A Cross-Sectional Study." *Bulletin of the World Health Organization.*

Peabody, J. W., P. J. Gertler, and A. Leibowitz. 1998. "The Policy Implications of Better Structure and Process on Birth Outcomes in Jamaica." *Health Policy* 43 (1): 1–13.

Peabody, J. W., and A. Liu. 2007. "A Cross-National Comparison of the Quality of Clinical Care Using Vignettes." *Health Policy and Planning* 22 (5): 294–302.

Peabody, J. W., J. Luck, L. M. DeMaria, and R. Menon. 2014. "Quality of Care and Health Status in Ukraine." *BMC Health Services Research* 14: 446.

Peabody, J. W., J. Luck, P. A. Glassman, T. R. Dresselhaus, and M. Lee. 2000. "Comparison of Vignettes, Standardized Patients, and Chart Abstraction: A Prospective Validation Study of 3 Methods for Measuring Quality." *Journal of the American Medical Association* 283 (13): 1715–22.

Peabody, J. W., J. Luck, P. Glassman, S. Jain, M. Spell, and others. 2004. "Measuring the Quality of Physician Practice by Using Clinical Vignettes: A Prospective Validation Study." *Annals of Internal Medicine* 141 (10): 771–80.

Peabody, J. W., R. J. Nordyke, F. Tozija, J. Luck, J. A. Munoz, and others. 2006. "Quality of Care and Its Impact on Population Health: A Cross-Sectional Study from Macedonia." *Social Science and Medicine* 62 (9): 2216–24.

Peabody, J. W., S. Quimbo, J. Florentino, R. Shimkhada, X. Javier, and others. 2017. "Comparative Effectiveness of Two Disparate Policies on Child Health: Experimental Evidence from the Philippines." *Health Policy and Planning* czw179. doi:http://dx.doi.org/10.1093/heapol/czw179.

Peabody, J. W., R. Shimkhada, S. Quimbo, J. Florentino, M. Bacate, and others. 2011. "Financial Incentives and Measurement Improved Physicians' Quality of Care in the Philippines." *Health Affairs (Millwood)* 30 (4): 773–81.

Peabody, J. W., S. Shimkhada, S. Quimbo, O. Solon, X. Javier, and others. 2014. "The Impact of Performance Incentives on Health Outcomes: Results from a Cluster Randomized Controlled Trial in the Philippines." *Health Policy and Planning* 29 (5): 615–21.

Peabody, J. W., M. M. Taguiwalo, D. A. Robalino, and J. Frenk. 2006. "Improving the Quality of Care in Developing Countries." In *Disease Control Priorities in Developing Countries*, second edition, edited by D. T. Jamison, J. G. Breman, A. R. Measham, G. Alleyne, M. Claeson, D. B. Evans, P. Jha, A. Mills, and P. Musgrove. Washington, DC: World Bank.

Petersen, L. A., L. D. Woodard, T. Urech, C. Daw, and S. Sookanan. 2006. "Does Pay-for-Performance Improve the Quality of Health Care?" *Annals of Internal Medicine* 145 (4): 265–72.

Pronovost, P., D. Needham, S. Berenholtz, D. Sinopoli, H. Chu, and others. 2006. "An Intervention to Decrease Catheter-Related Bloodstream Infections in the ICU." *New England Journal of Medicine* 355 (26): 2725–32.

Quimbo, S. A., J. W. Peabody, R. Shimkhada, K. Woo, and O. Solon. 2008. "Should We Have Confidence If a Physician Is Accredited? A Study of the Relative Impacts of Accreditation and Insurance Payments on Quality of Care in the Philippines." *Social Science and Medicine* 67 (4): 505–10.

Ransom, S. B., W. W. Pinsky, and J. E. Tropman, eds. 2000. *Enhancing Physician Performance: Advanced Principles of Medical Management.* Tampa, FL: American College of Physician Executives.

Rivera, J. A., D. Sotres-Alvarez, J. P. Habicht, T. Shamah, and S. Villalpando. 2004. "Impact of the Mexican Program for Education, Health, and Nutrition (Progresa) on Rates of Growth and Anemia in Infants and Young Children: A Randomized Effectiveness Study." *Journal of the American Medical Association* 291 (21): 2563–70.

Rockers, P. C., M. E. Kruk, and M. J. Laugesen. 2012. "Perceptions of the Health System and Public Trust in Government in Low- and Middle-Income Countries: Evidence from the World Health Surveys." *Journal of Health Politics, Policy, and Law* 37 (3): 405–37.

Rogers, W. A. 2004. "Evidence-Based Medicine and Justice: A Framework for Looking at the Impact of EBM upon Vulnerable or Disadvantaged Groups." *Journal of Medical Ethics* 30 (2): 141–45.

Rosenthal, M. B., R. G. Frank, Z. Li, and A. M. Epstein. 2005. "Early Experience with Pay-for-Performance: From Concept to Practice." *Journal of the American Medical Association* 294 (14): 1788–93.

Saleh, S. S., M. S. Alameddine, and N. M. Natafgi. 2014. "Beyond Accreditation: A Multi-Track Quality-Enhancing Strategy for Primary Health Care in Low- and Middle-Income Countries." *International Journal of Health Services* 44 (2): 355–72.

Saleh, S. S., J. Bou Sleiman, D. Dagher, H. Sbeit, and N. Natafgi. 2013. "Accreditation of Hospitals in Lebanon: Is It a Worthy Investment?" *International Journal for Quality in Health Care* 25 (3): 284–90.

Sando, D., T. Kendall, G. Lyatuu, H. Ratcliffe, K. McDonald, and others. 2014. "Disrespect and Abuse during Childbirth in Tanzania: Are Women Living with HIV More Vulnerable?" *Journal of Acquired Immune Deficiency Syndromes* 67 (Suppl 4): S228–34.

Schuster, R. J., N. A. Terwoord, and J. Tasosa. 2006. "Changing Physician Practice Behavior to Measure and Improve Clinical Outcomes." *American Journal of Medical Quality* 21 (6): 394–400.

Scott, K. W., and A. K. Jha. 2014. "Putting Quality on the Global Health Agenda." *New England Journal of Medicine* 371 (1): 3–5.

Sendlhofer, G., N. Mosbacher, L. Karina, B. Kober, L. Jantscher, and others. 2015. "Implementation of a Surgical Safety Checklist: Interventions to Optimize the Process and Hints to Increase Compliance." *PLoS One* 10 (2): e0116926.

Shaller, D., S. Sofaer, S. Findlay, J. Hibbard, D. Lansky, and others. 2003. "Consumers and Quality-Driven Health Care: A Call to Action." *Health Affairs (Millwood)* 22 (2): 95–101.

Shimkhada, R., O. Solon, D. Tamondong-Lachica, J. W. Peabody. 2016. "Misdiagnosis of Obstetrical Cases and the Clinical Cost and Consequences to Patients: A Cross-Sectional Study of Urban Providers in the Philippines." *Global Health Action* 9 (1): 32672.

Solon, O., K. Woo, S. A. Quimbo, R. Shimkhada, J. Florentino, and others. 2009. "A Novel Method for Measuring Health Care System Performance: Experience from QIDS in the Philippines." *Health Policy and Planning* 24 (3): 167–74.

Spertus, J. A., M. J. Radford, N. R. Every, E. F. Ellerbeck, E. D. Peterson, and others. 2003. "Challenges and Opportunities in Quantifying the Quality of Care for Acute Myocardial Infarction: Summary from the Acute Myocardial Infarction Working Group of the American Heart Association/American College of Cardiology First Scientific Forum on Quality of Care and Outcomes Research in Cardiovascular Disease and Stroke." *Circulation* 107 (12): 1681–91.

Starfield, B., N. R. Powe, J. R. Weiner, M. Stuart, D. Steinwachs, and others. 1994. "Costs vs. Quality in Different Types of Primary Care Settings." *Journal of the American Medical Association* 272 (24): 1903–08.

Steinwachs, D. M., and R. G. Hughes. 2008. "Health Services Research: Scope and Significance." In *Patient Safety and Quality: An Evidence-Based Handbook for Nurses*, edited by R. G. Hughes, 8–43. Rockville, MD: Agency for Healthcare Research and Quality.

Strauss, A., and J. Corbin. 1998. *Basics of Qualitative Research: Techniques and Procedures for Developing Grounded Theory.* 2nd ed. Newbury Park, CA: Sage.

Sun, B. C., J. Adams, E. J. Orav, D. W. Rucker, T. A. Brennan, and others. 2000. "Determinants of Patient Satisfaction and Willingness to Return with Emergency Care." *Annals of Emergency Medicine* 35 (5): 426–34.

Sylvia, S., Y. Shi, H. Xue, X. Tian, H. Wang, and others. 2015. "Survey Using Incognito Standardized Patients Shows Poor Quality Care in China's Rural Clinics." *Health Policy and Planning* 30 (3): 322–33.

Tafreshi, M. Z., M. Pazargadi, and Z. Abed Saeedi. 2007. "Nurses' Perspectives on Quality of Nursing Care: A Qualitative Study in Iran." *International Journal of Health Care Quality Assurance* 20 (4): 320–28.

Thaddeus, S., and D. Maine. 1994. "Too Far to Walk: Maternal Mortality in Context." *Social Science and Medicine* 38 (8): 1091–110.

Thorsen, V. C., T. Meguid, J. Sundby, and A. Malata. 2014. "Components of Maternal Healthcare Delivery System Contributing to Maternal Deaths in Malawi: A Descriptive Cross-Sectional Study." *African Journal of Reproductive Health* 18 (1): 16–26.

Tiemeier, H., W. J. de Vries, M. van Het Loo, J. P. Kahan, N. Klazinga, and others. 2002. "Guideline Adherence Rates and Interprofessional Variation in a Vignette Study of Depression." *Quality and Safety in Health Care* 11 (3): 214–18.

Tran, B. X., V. M. Nong, R. M. Maher, P. K. Nguyen, and H. N. Luu. 2014. "A Systematic Review of Scope and Quality of Health Economic Evaluation Studies in Vietnam." *PLoS One* 9 (8): e103825.

Treadwell, J. R., S. Lucas, and A. Y. Tsou. 2014. "Surgical Checklists: A Systematic Review of Impacts and Implementation." *BMJ Quality and Safety* 23 (4): 299–318.

U.S. Congress, Office of Technology Assessment. 1994. *Identifying Health Technologies that Work: Searching for Evidence.* OTA-H-608. Washington, DC: U.S. Government Printing Office.

Van der Bij, J. D., T. Vollmar, and M. C. Weggeman. 1998. "Quality Systems in Health Care: A Situational Approach." *International Journal of Health Care Quality Assurance* 11 (2): 65–70.

Veloski, J., S. Tai, A. S. Evans, and D. B. Nash. 2005. "Clinical Vignette-Based Surveys: A Tool for Assessing Physician Practice Variation." *American Journal of Medical Quality* 20 (3): 151–57.

Vogel, J. P., A. M. Gülmezoglu, G. J. Hofmeyr, and M. Temmerman. 2014. "Perspectives on Elective Induction of Labor." *Clinical Obstetrics and Gynecology* 7 (2): 331–42.

Wachter, R. 2013. "Personal Accountability in Healthcare: Searching for the Right Balance." *BMJ Quality and Safety* 22 (2): 176–80.

Weinberg, N. 2001. "Using Performance Measures to Identify Plans of Action to Improve Care." *Joint Commission Journal on Quality and Patient Safety* 27 (12): 683–88.

Werner, R. M., and D. A. Asch. 2007. "Clinical Concerns about Clinical Performance Measurement." *Annals of Family Medicine* 5 (2): 159–63.

WHO (World Health Organization). 2000. *World Health Report 2000: Health Systems, Improving Performance.* Geneva: WHO.

———. 2008. *Summary of the Evidence on Patient Safety: Implications for Research.* Geneva: WHO.

WHO, Association for Trauma Surgery and Intensive Care, and International Society of Surgery. 2009. *Guidelines for Trauma Quality Improvement Programmes.* Geneva: WHO.

WHO and World Bank. 2014. *Monitoring Progress towards Universal Health Coverage at Country and Global Levels: Framework, Measures, Targets.* Geneva: WHO; Washington, DC: World Bank.

Wisniewski, M., and H. Wisniewski. 2005. "Measuring Service Quality in a Hospital Colposcopy Clinic." *International Journal of Health Care Quality Assurance* 18 (2–3): 217–29.

Woolf, S. H. 2000. "Changing Physician Practice Behavior." *Journal of Family Practice* 49 (2): 126–29.

World Bank. 2003. *World Development Report 2004: Making Services Work for Poor People.* Washington, DC: World Bank.

———. 2014. *Health Results Innovation Trust Fund Annual Report 2014.* Washington, DC: World Bank.

Xu, Y., Y. Liu, T. Shu, W. Yang, and M. Liang. 2015. "Variations in the Quality of Care at Large Public Hospitals in Beijing, China: A Condition-Based Outcome Approach." *PLoS One* 10 (10): e0138948.

Zaslavsky, A. M. 2001. "Statistical Issues in Reporting Quality Data: Small Samples and Casemix Variation." *International Journal for Quality in Health Care* 13 (6): 481–88.

High-Quality Diagnosis: An Essential Pathology Package

Kenneth A. Fleming, Mahendra Naidoo, Michael Wilson,
John Flanigan, Susan Horton, Modupe Kuti, Lai Meng Looi,
Christopher P. Price, Kun Ru, Abdul Ghafur, Jinaxiang Wang,
and Nestor Lago

INTRODUCTION

A young child living in Sub-Saharan Africa presents to a rural health care clinic with a one-week history of fevers, night sweats, chills, and malaise. The child's mother does not know if the child has lost weight in the recent past; when weighed, the child is significantly below the expected weight for her age. No other family members, including other young siblings, report similar symptoms. Physical examination reveals a fever, mild increase in heart and respiratory rates, and enlarged lymph nodes along both sides of her neck. The clinic does not have access to imaging studies, and the only available pathology laboratory tests show that the patient does not have serologic evidence of human immunodeficiency virus/acquired immune deficiency syndrome (HIV/AIDS) infection or malaria. She is mildly anemic as measured by a manual spun hematocrit. The physician wants to refer the patient to a hospital in a nearby city, but the family does not have sufficient resources.

The physician offers to collect blood for pathology testing and send it to that hospital for testing, but because the hospital requires advance payment for pathology tests, the family again does not have the resources. The physician completes the notes, indicating that the differential diagnosis is broad—including tuberculosis, nontuberculous mycobacterial infection, disseminated fungal infection, Epstein-Barr virus infection (infectious mononucleosis), and malignant lymphoma—and that accurate diagnosis requires pathology investigations, including both microbiology and anatomic pathology. The family leaves the clinic, and the patient is lost to follow-up.

This scenario is played out daily in many countries across the world and illustrates one aspect of the crucial role that pathology has in ensuring effective health care, namely, diagnosis. Despite recent progress in controlling communicable disease, the need for pathology is growing as the burden of noncommunicable diseases increases. There were approximately 14 million new cases of cancer and 8.2 million cancer-related deaths in 2012 (Stewart and Wild 2014), but treating these cases accurately is impossible unless the pathological diagnosis is known. Cancer is predicted to increase by 70 percent by 2032, with more than 60 percent of these new cases in Asia, Central and South America, and Sub-Saharan Africa. Similarly, diagnosing and treating patients with diabetes mellitus—another developing epidemic in low- and middle-income countries (LMICs)—is impossible without the ability to measure the levels of glucose in the blood. The diagnosis and risk stratification of cardiovascular disease requires pathology, for example, to check levels of serum lipids such as cholesterol.

Corresponding author: Kenneth A. Fleming, Center for Global Health, National Cancer Institute, Washington, DC, United States; Green Templeton College, University of Oxford, United Kingdom; kenneth.fleming@medsci.ox.ac.uk.

This chapter specifies an essential minimal package of services that should be available in LMICs to provide access to pathology services that are of acceptable quality, affordable, and timely to a majority of the population, especially outside of major cities.

RANGE OF PATHOLOGY SERVICES

The term *pathology* means the *study of disease*. The knowledge gained from this study has led to development of the many diagnostic tests used in clinical practice. These tests are performed on body fluids, including blood, urine, sweat, saliva, and sputum; on tissue biopsies; and on cells obtained from needle-aspirated specimens.

The diagnostic role is a key aspect of what pathology laboratories do and is fundamental to the effective working of any health care system. An interview-based study of cardiologists and oncologists in Germany and the United States indicated that 66 percent of clinical decisions are based on results of in vitro diagnostic tests (Rohr and others 2016).

Pathology also supports clinical care by assessing disease severity and prognosis, for example, determining the staging and grading of a cancer by histopathology; this information is fundamental to deciding and managing treatment plans for patients. Equally important is the role of the pathology laboratory in monitoring clinical response to treatment, for example, analyzing blood levels of markers of renal function in patients with renal failure.

Pathology plays a number of other key roles. One is quality assurance within the health care system. In 2013, autopsies showed an estimated 20 percent major discrepancy between the pre-mortem clinical diagnosis and the autopsy diagnosis (Kuijpers and others 2014). Similarly, through the examination of surgical specimens, surgeons can learn whether they are fully excising tumors; through the use of microbiological culturing, physicians can correctly identify the cause of a fever. Pathology contributes to disease surveillance by helping identify new and emerging diseases such as the Zika virus; pathology facilitates the maintenance of disease registries that help inform national health policy and allocation of resources. Finally, forensic pathology is integral to legal systems around the world.

In all of these roles, pathology services encompass a number of disciplines and subspecialties; table 11.1 describes the main ones. In the United States and most other regions, these pathology disciplines are divided into two main groups:

- **Clinical pathology**, also called *laboratory medicine*, which is largely concerned with analysis of blood and

other fluids and involves, for instance, clinical biochemistry, microbiology, and hematology
- **Anatomic pathology**, which is concerned with cell and tissue analysis and involves cytology, histology, and autopsy.

In high-income countries (HICs), pathology services typically are provided in one of three ways:

- **Central laboratories that deliver most of their services in hospital settings.** Central laboratories have a common infrastructure that supports their various components, including specimen collection services, transport and reception, and a mechanism for transmitting the results of tests and accompanying reports to the ordering clinicians and patients. They have laboratory information systems (LIS) that are ideally connected to electronic patient records.
- **Smaller laboratories in more rural environments** that offer a more limited repertoire of tests, as well as point-of-care testing (POCT) in community settings.
- **A small number of laboratories, often in conjunction with university departments, that provide the most specialized tests.** These laboratories also undertake research, both in the field of pathology itself and with other disciplines as part of multidisciplinary teams. They also organize and provide education and training in pathology and related disciplines.

Although the core of laboratory activities may be considered the performance of tests and the analysis of the results (the analytical phase), it is important to recognize that the pre- and postanalytical phases are equally important for generating accurate laboratory test results (box 11.1). These phases range from the selection of the most appropriate tests or investigations to the interpretation of their results and the provision of clinical advice across the spectrum of medical specialties. In practice, this involvement may require a review of medical records and discussions with ordering clinicians. An example is the multidisciplinary meeting (tumor boards in the United States), in which pathologists, surgeons, and chemotherapy and radiation oncologists, radiologists, nurses, and others involved in cancer care of a patient meet to review all relevant information and decide on the best approach for treatment and management.

Pathologists may also provide leadership for hospital-wide quality assurance efforts. Increasingly, pathologists are assuming additional clinical roles in many health systems, for example, serving as infectious disease doctors, managing patients with metabolic disorders, and providing specialized oncology services.

Table 11.1 Major Pathology Disciplines and Roles

Clinical biochemistry	Study of the biochemical basis of disease
Cytopathology	Study of disease in individual cells
Forensic pathology	Determination of cause and manner of death for legal purposes
Hematology	Study of blood disorders
Histopathology[a]	Study of disease in human tissue
Immunopathology	Study of the immunologic basis of disease
Medical microbiology	Study of infection
Molecular pathology and genetics	Study of the molecular and genetic basis of diseases and heritable conditions
Pediatric and perinatal pathology	Study of the diseases of pregnancy, childbirth, and children
Transfusion medicine	Study of the collection, preparation, storage, and clinical use of blood products

Note: A selection of the major disciplines was derived, in part, from https://www.rcpath.org.
a. Histopathology includes a number of subdisciplines, such as dermatopathology, neuropathology, and others that focus on diseases of a single organ or organ system.

Box 11.1

Three Phases of Laboratory Testing

- *Preanalytical phase.* Selecting the appropriate test, obtaining the specimen, labeling it with the patient's name, providing timely transport to the laboratory, registering receipt in the laboratory, and processing before testing.
- *Analytical phase.* Performing the test and interpreting the result.
- *Postanalytical phase.* Preparing a report detailing the result and its interpretation, authorizing the report, and transmitting the report to the clinician so that the clinician can institute appropriate action.

In HICs, the largest proportion of errors in pathology occurs in the pre- and postanalytical phases (Plebani 2009). In the preanalytical phase, these errors include failing to ensure that the specimen is collected from the right patient, that the correct specimen type is collected, and that the specimen is collected at the right time. In the postanalytical phase, errors include reporting the wrong result and failing to read the report, making the wrong or no decision, or taking the wrong or no action.

Clearly, pathology is not a stand-alone service. Its value is as a crucial and integral part of the system of care in which the outcomes for patients and the operational and economic benefits for the system depend on all of the parts working effectively together. Without accurate diagnosis, everything else is compromised.

CHALLENGES TO PATHOLOGY SERVICES IN LMICs

The child described in the clinical vignette at the beginning of this chapter needed access to microbiology, hematology, and immunology services, and she almost certainly would have needed access to the expertise of a histopathologist. Yet access to diagnostic pathology services is not available in many countries and regions.

Ideally, the public sectors of LMICs should have three tiers of laboratories—with a small additional number of national or regional research or reference laboratories (WHO AFRO and U.S. CDC 2010). The tier 1 laboratories are widely distributed in the community and typically perform a small number of simple clinical pathology tests. Tier 2 and tier 3 laboratories are progressively fewer in number, provide tests of increasing complexity and capacity, and are found in progressively larger population centers. In many countries, however, especially poorer ones, such structures do not exist. Their absence has several causes, the most important of which is lack of human capacity, resulting in far too few trained personnel to staff the laboratories to provide adequate population coverage at all levels.

Inadequate Staffing

Data on staffing are lacking for much of the world, but the available data illustrate the problem. In Sub-Saharan Africa, at least five countries have no anatomic pathologist. Surveys of the other countries in the region have shown that the number of anatomic pathologists per patient population is approximately 1:1,000,000, or about one-fiftieth the ratio in the United Kingdom and the United States (Adesina and others 2013; African Strategies for Advancing Pathology Group Members 2015). In China, there were approximately 10,300 pathologists in all disciplines in 2015 (unpublished data from Chinese Society of Pathology 2015), constituting an estimated shortfall of 60,000–120,000. In 2014, there were only eight pathologists in a population of 14 million in Cambodia (Vathana and Stauch 2014); the ratio of pathologists per patient population in Vietnam was estimated to be 1:254,000 (Van Dang 2014). In upper-middle-income countries, the situation is somewhat better; for example, in Malaysia the ratio is 1:75,000 (Looi 2008).

Variable Standards

In addition to staff shortages, widely variable standards are an issue. Although the quality of services, particularly those provided in large cities in middle-income countries, can be good, frequently it is seriously inadequate in both urban and rural areas (Daramola and others 2016; Orem and others 2012).

A characteristic of many LMICs is that private laboratories—most staffed by pathologists from the public sector—are often run in parallel to the public sector and provide services to the population. The facilities in some of these laboratories can be as good as any internationally, but many are much less satisfactory. In India, where 70 percent of the laboratories are private, only 1 percent are accredited (Singh 2013). In Kampala, Uganda, which had more than 900 laboratories in 2011—96 percent of which were private—only 45 laboratories achieved the first step of the five-step process for international accreditation (Elbireer and others 2013).

The result of these challenges is that much of the population in LMICs does not have access to quality pathology services. As noncommunicable diseases that are particularly reliant on pathology for diagnosis and management become more prevalent, the level of misdiagnosis is likely to rise. This increase will result in unnecessary deaths and avoidable prolonged illness and distress, with attendant social disruption and negative impacts on productivity. The deficiencies also mean that data needed for disease surveillance and registries, and other types of population data needed to guide public policy and resource allocation, are not available. In addition, good quality pathology is necessary for the achievement of 11 of the 13 goals of the United Nation's health-related Sustainable Development Goals (table 11.2); the deficiencies will impede attainment of these goals.

Table 11.2 Health-Related Sustainable Development Goals and Pathology

Sustainable Development Goals	Is pathology relevant?	Specific pathology examples
3.1: By 2030, reduce the global maternal mortality ratio to less than 70 per 100,000 live births	Yes	Testing for most common causes of maternal mortality, for example, infections; also blood transfusion for hemorrhage and autopsy to establish cause of death
3.2: By 2030, end preventable deaths of newborns and children under age five years, with all countries aiming to reduce neonatal mortality to at least as low as 12 per 1,000 live births and under-five mortality to at least as low as 25 per 1,000 live births	Yes	Testing and monitoring for most common causes of infant mortality, for example, infections, autopsy
3.3: By 2030, end the epidemics of HIV/AIDS, tuberculosis, malaria, and neglected tropical diseases, and combat hepatitis, water-borne diseases, and other communicable diseases	Yes	Testing for communicable diseases, for example, blood tests for HIV/AIDS and malaria, antiretroviral resistance
3.4: By 2030, reduce by one-third premature mortality from noncommunicable diseases through prevention and treatment and promote mental health and well-being	Yes	Histo- and cytopathology for cancer diagnosis; hematology and biochemistry for diabetes diagnosis and management; pathology support for surveillance and other data platforms, for example, cancer registries
3.5: Strengthen the prevention and treatment of substance abuse	Yes	Toxicology tests
3.6: By 2020, halve the number of global deaths and injuries from road traffic accidents	Yes	Autopsy reports, blood banks for transfusion support

table continues next page

Table 11.2 Health-Related Sustainable Development Goals and Pathology (continued)

Sustainable Development Goals	Is pathology relevant?	Specific pathology examples
3.7: By 2030, ensure universal access to sexual and reproductive health care services, including family planning, information, and education; and the integration of reproductive health into national strategies and programs	Yes	Blood and urine testing for pregnancy and for sexually transmitted diseases
3.8: Achieve universal health coverage, including financial risk protection; access to quality essential health care services; and access to safe, effective, quality, and affordable essential medicines and vaccines	No	—
3.9: By 2030, substantially reduce the number of deaths and illnesses from hazardous chemicals, and air, water, and soil pollution and contamination	Yes	Toxicology testing and diagnosis of related diseases
3a: Strengthen the implementation of the World Health Organization Framework Convention on Tobacco Control in all countries, as appropriate	Yes	Testing for smoking cessation in urine
3b: Support the research and development of vaccines and medicines for the communicable and noncommunicable diseases that primarily affect LMICs; provide access to affordable essential medicines and vaccines, in accordance with the Doha Declaration on the Trade-Related Aspects of Intellectual Property Rights (TRIPS) Agreement and Public Health	Yes	Pathology systems provide data, for example, surveillance, and research platforms
3c: Substantially increase health financing and the recruitment, development, training, and retention of the health workforce in LMICs, particularly in LICs and small island LMICs	No	—
3d: Strengthen the capacity of all countries, particularly LMICs, for early warning, risk reduction, and risk management of national and global health risks	Yes	Surveillance for emerging disease and through cancer registries

Note: HIV/AIDS = human immunodeficiency virus/acquired immune deficiency syndrome; LICs = low-income countries; LMICs = low- and middle-income countries; — = not applicable.

THE ESSENTIAL PATHOLOGY PACKAGE

The essential pathology package consists of a minimal suite of services that should be available in LMICs to provide access to pathology that is of reasonable quality, affordable, and timely to a majority of the population, especially that outside the main cities. The key concept is an integrated network of tiered laboratories (box 11.2, table 11.3), the tiers being similar to that described in the previous section. Thus, tier 1 is widely distributed in the community (both rural and urban). It has limited pathology capacity and staffing but can perform some basic tests and can refer patients and specimens to the next tier. The next tier has many fewer laboratories, probably located in sizable towns. It has greater capacity, performing most routine tests and when necessary, can refer more specialized tests to the to the next tier. These next-tier laboratories will probably be based in the largest towns and are capable of performing all routine tests and many specialized ones. Finally, depending on the country and its pathology capacity, there may be a highly specialized laboratory performing complex testing that can act as a referral center for the country or even a region. These last two levels will often have educational and research capacity and be part of a university medical school.

This model is similar to the three-tier model in many LMICs (WHO AFRO and U.S. CDC 2010); the crucial aspect is that the model must be an integrated network of laboratories for more efficient and effective referral of patients across networks than would be the case with independent laboratories. This approach provides economies of scale, such as sharing use and costs of staff, equipment, and reagents. Other benefits include better communication, exchange of staff and knowledge, provision of education and training, and opportunities for research. This integrated approach would result in development of a critical mass of expertise and the optimal use of scarce resources.

Definition of Laboratory Tiers

- *Tier 1.* Primary care and health center laboratories primarily serving outpatients in community settings, performing point-of-care tests and single-use tests, and referring more complex work to tier 2 or tier 3. These laboratories are staffed at the technician level.
- *Tier 2.* Laboratories in first-level hospitals that receive specimens from their own patients and receive referrals from tier 1 facilities. Usually, they have a pathologist and perform a selected number of routine tests.
- *Tier 3.* Laboratories in second-level hospitals that receive specimens from their own patients and receive referrals from tier 1 and 2 facilities. These laboratories have significant numbers of pathology staff and cover all routine testing in the major pathology disciplines.

- *Tier 4.* Laboratories in national or teaching hospitals that receive specimens from their own patients and receive referrals from tier 1, 2, and 3 facilities. They provide routine tests and highly specialized tests. In small countries, these facilities may be regional and shared by more than one country.

Each country and region has a different burden of disease and availability of staff, and some shifting of capacity may occur across the tier boundaries. For example, if a tier 2 pathologist makes regular visits, then fine needle aspiration cytology could be performed and reported in a tier 1 laboratory. In many countries, shortages of staff require that one laboratory fulfill the functions of both tier 3 and 4.

Table 11.3 Pathology Tiers

Laboratory features	Tier 1	Tier 2 (includes tier 1 capabilities)	Tier 3 (includes tier 2 capabilities)	Tier 4 (includes tier 3 capabilities)
Tests and test categories	POCT and single-use tests: malaria, tuberculosis, urinalysis, pregnancy, blood glucose, hemoglobin/hematocrit, ESR, blood typing Slide microscopy: malaria, wet preparation, stool parasites Preparation of FNAC and tissue specimens to send to tier 2 facilities	Many routine diagnostic and prognostic tests **Clinical biochemistry** urea and electrolytes, HBA1c for diabetes, liver, renal, bone, and lipid profiles **Hematology** complete blood counts, CD4 count, simple coagulation studies and thalassemia tests, support for whole blood transfusion **Microbiology culture** blood, urine, cerebrospinal fluid, sputum; simple antimicrobial susceptibility testing; serology for hepatitis A, B, or C and common infections	All routine and some specialized tests **Clinical chemistry** Endocrine tests: thyroid; cardiac markers, troponin, BNP; dynamic function tests, GTT; tumor markers: AFP, Ca-125, blood gases; therapeutic drug monitoring; serum and urine electrophoresis **Microbiology** Additional antimicrobial susceptibility testing, fungal cultures, mycobacterial cultures, viral load **Hematology** More advanced blood analysis, for example, component therapy, hemolysis, bone marrow studies, hematological malignancies, immunological studies	Specialized services as appropriate, surveillance, toxicology studies, support for transplantation, rare tumors, nutritional studies, support for clinical trials, mutational studies (cytogenetics, molecular analysis), gene analysis

table continues next page

Table 11.3 Pathology Tiers (continued)

Laboratory features	Tier 1	Tier 2 (includes tier 1 capabilities)	Tier 3 (includes tier 2 capabilities)	Tier 4 (includes tier 3 capabilities)
		Anatomic pathology	**Anatomic pathology**	
		FNAC, tissue biopsies and surgical excisions—processing, H&E stain and interpretation	Same as for tier 2, but with special stains including immunohistochemistry: ER, PR for breast cancer	
		Hospital autopsy	Specialized autopsy	
Staffing	Laboratory technicians supervised by general pathologist from distance	General pathologist, laboratory technicians, laboratory assistants; one of technicians manages laboratory	Mono-specialty pathologists, clinical scientists, specialized laboratory technicians, laboratory assistants, dedicated laboratory manager, possibly laboratory information systems coordinator, quality care manager	Same as for tier 3 plus clinical trial specialists, data specialist
				Additional specialist educational capacity
			Facilities and responsibilities for education and training of all levels of medical and nonmedical staff	
Communication infrastructure	Paper or electronic, mobile	Paper or electronic or laboratory information system	Electronic or laboratory information system; telepathology (optional)	Same as tier 3 but more data linkages to trials and registries
Equipment	Simple microscope	Automated blood and biochemistry analyzers; microbiology analyzers and incubators; blood typing including refrigerators; tissue processor and microtome for anatomic pathology	Automated tissue processor, equipment for full autopsy, immunohistochemistry station	Molecular biology and cytogenetics
	Rapid diagnostic tests			Immunofluorescence
	POCT and single-use tests			Electron microscopy for renal disease
	Specimen and patient identification			Possible biobanking for research
	FNAC and biopsy fixation			
Turnaround time	Rapid, POCT, and single-use tests: 0–3 hours	An hour to several days	Routine: 1 hour to several days	Same as tier 3
	Send-outs, several days		Complex: 7 days	
			Autopsy: 30–60 days	
Networks and surveillance	Accumulates and forwards incidence data to higher tier	Report to emerging disease, AST, cancer, and other NCD registries	Links to emerging disease, AST, cancer, and other NCD registries	Research on disease incidence trends, including AST and emerging diseases

Note: AFP = alpha-fetoprotein; AST = antimicrobial susceptibility testing; BNP = brain natriuretic peptide; Ca-125 = cancer antigen 125; ER and PR = receptor tests for breast cancer; ESR = erythrocyte sedimentation rate; FNAC = fine needle aspiration cytology; GTT = glucose tolerance test; H&E = hematoxylin and eosin stain (basic histopathology test); HBA1c = glycated hemoglobin test; NCD = noncommunicable disease; POCT = point-of-care tests.
Assumptions
1. Tiers may be adjusted as necessary to reflect the local burden of disease or local practice patterns and availability of trained staff.
2. Changes in technologies over time can shift tests and workloads across tiers.
3. Tests are examples (as applied to broad groups of infectious disease, cancer, and other NCD) and are not an exhaustive list.

In 2008, such national integrated laboratory systems were proposed as a key development for pathology services in Sub-Saharan Africa in the Maputo Declaration on Strengthening of Laboratory Systems (WHO AFRO 2008). Ethiopia was one of the first countries to successfully develop such a model; the model was subsequently endorsed in the Freetown Declaration of 2015 (ASLM and WHO AFRO 2015) as the cornerstone of effective health care. Although infectious diseases were the focus of the original model, the principles are equally applicable to noncommunicable diseases.

A key component in ensuring the sustainability of such a model is the tier 4 laboratory. These centers would offer specialized services as well as develop and provide research, education, and training, especially to the linked tier 1 and 2 facilities. Furthermore, these centers are most likely to develop innovations appropriate to the country's needs. Without these fostering and supporting roles, the long-term sustainability of the lower-tier laboratories will not be feasible. Linking such facilities to other centers of excellence (North-South, South-South) to provide access to further expertise and resources is important for continuing long-term development.

The model outlined in box 11.2 is intended to represent the minimum that a lower-middle-income country would provide. Countries at higher levels of development can build on this model to deliver increased provision appropriate to their needs. Conversely, the model serves as a goal for LICs to achieve as resources become available and are invested.

To ensure this network is sustainable, effective, and of good quality, five components are vital:

- Leadership
- Education, training, and continuing professional development
- Emerging technologies
- Quality management and accreditation
- Reimbursement policies for pathology services.

Leadership

The effective and efficient operation of a pathology laboratory is a multidisciplinary effort. Pathology services are primarily delivered by three groups of professionally qualified staff—pathologists, clinical scientists, and technicians (also referred to as *technologists*)—supported by assistants, managers and administrators, and technology specialists. In most places, clinical scientists or technicians undertake the role of administrator or manager. Pathologists provide leadership and serve as the interface between laboratory and clinical services; in some countries and specialties, pathologists share these roles with clinical scientists. Pathologists and clinical scientists also oversee quality improvement and service development as well as pathology-led research and development. Laboratory technologists are responsible for delivering the technical aspects of the service.

The goal of this joint effort is to provide a service that is patient oriented and meets clinical needs. These clinical needs are defined by standards of care, expectations of individual physicians, and patients. Accordingly, laboratory leadership needs to monitor the activities of staff to ensure that clinically relevant services are being provided.

This administrative oversight is a key leadership responsibility required by International Organization for Standardization (ISO) 15189:2012, the international reference document for best laboratory practice (ISO 2012).

Laboratories produce information that result from their processes, personnel, and equipment. This information is also influenced by the clinical settings in which the laboratories operate and from which they receive specimens. Patient-specific, disease-specific, and therapy-specific factors may influence the information that the laboratories produce. Those in leadership positions need to understand the interactions between these factors, especially as those interactions affect how the information will be used for patient care. The Joint Commission International's accreditation standards for hospitals state that for the purpose of clinical consultation and rendering of medical opinion, the laboratory should be led by physicians, preferably pathologists (JCI 2014). Pathologists, as clinicians, have insights into the thought processes behind requests for laboratory tests and the decisions that may be made with the information received. These insights are not only invaluable in determining how to most effectively organize and direct laboratory services, but they are also crucial to provision of clinical advice on the further investigation and management of individual patients. Clinical scientists, who have had training significantly similar to that received by clinical pathologists, may also provide this level of leadership.

Reflecting the integral role that pathology plays in the wider heath care system, laboratory leadership also needs to be involved in the development of national strategic plans for laboratories. These plans detail the long-term vision and mission of the nation's laboratory services. To be effective, development of this national blueprint needs to recognize the local disease burden, available clinical skills and services, clinical requirements for diagnosis and monitoring, and technical realities. The primary involvement of clinical laboratory leadership, in conjunction with other clinicians, is to provide guidance for the definition of policy that delineates the organization, scope, and nature of the laboratory service according to the tiers providing health care in the respective countries (WHO AFRO and U.S. CDC 2010).

Pathologists provide leadership at the operational level. Doing so entails the ability to read about and understand scientific and technological advances in the field of medicine as well as improvements in laboratory technology. Changing clinical demands for patient care, as documented in new and revised versions of locally applicable clinical care guidelines, require a laboratory director's involvement and informed response. Similarly, advances in the technical capacity of laboratories, including the introduction of new tests and the withdrawal of obsolete ones, need to be assessed in relation to their ability to improve the clinical effectiveness of the laboratory, as well as the clinical effectiveness and cost-effectiveness of the whole care pathway. To effectively lead the response to such changes, pathologists need the authority to alter aspects of the operations to ensure that laboratories remain true to their goal of enhancing the quality of patient care.

Education, Training, and Continuing Professional Development

Educating and training larger numbers of qualified personnel is clearly of paramount importance in developing a sustainable pathology network. There are three major categories of staff: pathologists, clinical scientists and technologists, and technicians. Their education consists largely of a combination of formal courses for degrees and diplomas and hands-on training and experience under the supervision of qualified individuals.

Pathologists

Historically, pathologists in LMICs were educated in Australia, Europe, and North America; the individuals often resided in the HICs for the duration of their training programs. Although those funded by governments or charities were expected or required to return home when the training was completed, large numbers stayed in HICs. In contrast, clinical scientists and technicians predominantly received their education locally.

Pathologists are medically qualified practitioners who have undergone postgraduate education and training in pathology. There are three main models of training; the first two are common in LMICs:

- In the first training model, pathologists are trained as generalists dealing with all aspects of pathology, both clinical and anatomic; this is also called *general pathology*. This postgraduate training period is usually two to four years. In some countries, the course entails a university degree.
- In the second model, pathologists are trained only as either clinical or anatomic pathologists. The postgraduate training period is two to three years.
- In the third model, pathologists are trained as monospecialists, for example, as hematologists, microbiologists, or clinical biochemists. Such individuals tend to be employed in academic centers. This model reflects countries with more-developed health care systems, such as South Africa. The postgraduate training period is usually a minimum of four years. In much of South America, pathologists are only trained as mono-specialty anatomic pathologists; the other disciplines of pathology are staffed by clinical scientists, such as clinical biochemists.

These training courses are largely experiential in nature, with considerable hands-on involvement in pathology service delivery supplemented by small group teaching and formal lectures.

Clinical Scientists and Technologists

In some countries, clinical scientists perform functions similar to those of pathologists. They follow a similar pathway of education and training to achieve the required competence, for example, in clinical biochemistry, immunology, microbiology, or virology. Clinical scientists may also be responsible for the performance of specialized services, such as molecular genetics, toxicology investigations, and electron microscopy. These individuals generally have degrees in chemistry, biological science, or biomedical science, usually followed by a master's or doctoral degree in such areas as microbiology or clinical biochemistry. The training period is four to eight years. There may be subsequent subspecialization in such fields as virology.

Technologists are also sometimes referred to as *medical laboratory scientists* or *biomedical scientists*. Their education and training in some places involves the acquisition of a university degree, while in others it is similar to that of technicians.

Technicians

Technical staff are usually educated and trained through college courses, often part-time over several years. The education may encompass all of the specialities of pathology or it may be restricted to one of the major specialities, such as anatomic pathology or microbiology; such specialization is a feature of more developed laboratory services. In some countries, technical staff do not have formal qualifications and only receive hands-on training in the laboratory.

In most countries, in addition to the professional qualification or appropriate university degree, individuals need to be registered with the national registration body as an indication of required competence before being allowed to practice.

LMICs have increasingly developed their own pathologist postgraduate educational and training systems. In Sub-Saharan Africa, 21 countries have developed training programs in the past 25 years. In the 14 countries for which comparative data are available, the number of pathologists increased from 70 in 1990 to 370 in 2015 (Nelson and others 2016). Similarly, in Malaysia, the number of pathologists increased from approximately 50 in the 1980s (Jegathesan and de Witt 1982) to more than 500 in 2016 (Looi 2008).

However, in many countries, especially low-income countries (LICs), the shortage is such that training enough pathologists to fully staff all relevant sections of health care systems is not possible, even in the medium term. Accordingly, the expansion of the training of scientists and technicians and the exploration of task-shifting and task-sharing are needed, with parallel development of shorter training programs focused on specific tasks, such as cytology screening.

A program of continuing professional development (CPD) is necessary to maintain the standards and long-term sustainability of the pathology network. Many individuals and institutions provide CPD events, often delivered by visiting individuals and organizations, on an informal basis; systematic institutional and national programs are rare in LMICs. One of the most common support requests from pathologists in LMICs is for provision of and access to CPD. Without such programs, the knowledge and skills of individuals can become out of date, especially as the pace of advances accelerates.

Emerging Technologies

Diagnostics
In all health care systems, the need for medical tests at any point in the care pathway requires that specimens be collected and sent to laboratories for analysis and interpretation. Laboratory testing can be centralized, provided at the point of care, or more typically a combination of the two. The selection of which approach to take is partly driven by the availability of a given test at the point of care, the level of test volumes, and the need to have test results available at the time of the patient

encounter. These considerations need to be balanced against the generally higher cost of providing POCT, albeit resulting in savings elsewhere in the care pathway, and the technical challenges of generating accurate test results at that level.

A tiered system of laboratory testing that focuses on the type of care provided within each tier, as well as the number of tests performed within each tier, can be used to design approaches to testing. For example, tier 1 facilities would most benefit from POCT; tier 3 facilities would benefit most from centralized laboratory testing. Test devices used for disease surveillance purposes can be designed for centralized use only.

Device manufacturers and public-private partnerships have developed new technologies for laboratory testing to provide both POCT and centralized testing within a tiered system of health care delivery, increase and improve access to laboratory testing in general, and bring new diagnostic tests to the public. Key challenges for the development and use of emerging tests are shown in box 11.3. In particular, simplicity of specimen collection, device use, and interpretation and communication of test results are critically important because new devices will be used in many LMICs by persons with widely varying languages, backgrounds, training, and expertise.

Many of today's laboratory analyzers require a reliable external power supply, and because electricity supply can be intermittent in many LMICs, even with back-up facilities such as diesel generators, there is increasing focus on developing devices that require no

---

Box 11.3

Effectiveness Criteria for Emerging Tests

- Any new tests should provide results for a specified clinical problem to guide clinical decisions, for monitoring disease status or response to therapy, or for data collection for disease surveillance.
- Results of tests designed to be used in clinical care should be available in a time frame that will guide clinical decision making.
- Tests should be easy to perform, and results must be easy to interpret and communicate.
- Target performance characteristics—such as sensitivity, specificity, predictive values, precision, and accuracy—for the intended uses should be specified before test development.

- Manufacturers' claims regarding test performance characteristics should be independently verified.
- Test platforms should be usable and stable in locations of intended use.
- Test platforms should meet procurement requirements for supply chain, maintenance, availability of quality control standards, durability, and stability in variable climatic conditions.
- Test costs should be affordable in locations of intended use.

Source: Based on Wu and Zaman 2012.

power or have built-in power generation (Pollock and others 2013; Whitesides and Wilding 2012; Yetisen, Akram, and Lowe 2013). In addition, because of the challenges of supply chains and storage in many LMICs, interest is growing in developing POCT devices that require minimal or no reagents other than the devices and that can be stored for long periods in hot and humid climates with no performance degradation. For larger analyzers used in central laboratories, one goal is to develop test platforms that can support a number of different assays rather than platforms that are unique to one set of tests. The development of flexible platforms would minimize the number of devices needed, with associated reductions in acquisition and maintenance costs; it would also allow for rapid introduction of new assays, a particularly important consideration in light of emerging diseases in LMICs.

Molecular diagnostic techniques have historically been substantially more expensive and required technical expertise and laboratory infrastructure unavailable in most LMICs. This field of diagnostics is rapidly evolving to the point where some tests are becoming practicable for use in LMICs (St. John and Price 2014), and this trend is likely to accelerate. Access to these tests is becoming a routine part of health care delivery because a number of diseases and conditions are only detectable using these methods. For example, many cancers are now classified using molecular tests, and the use of some drugs requires molecular testing to determine whether specific biomarkers are present.

Point-of-Care Testing

POCT is usually performed by medical staff, nurses, or medical assistants using small, mobile testing devices. It can be used anywhere on the care pathway—first-level, second-level, or third-level care—as well as in patients' homes. This approach differs from centralized laboratory testing, which is performed by specialized technicians using large-capacity (high-throughput) analyzers.

Although POCT technologies are broadly based on the same techniques used in centralized laboratory analyzers, they have reduced reagent and sample volume requirements, rely upon stabilization of reagents, and typically use single-use cassettes for testing.

In LMICs, POCT has been used extensively to help guide the treatment of several diseases and conditions. Expanded access to POCT is cost-effective in extending life expectancy in patients with HIV/AIDS (Cassim and others 2014; Hyle and others 2014; Wu and Zaman 2012). Access to smear microscopy, rapid malaria diagnostic testing, or both has played an important role in decreasing malaria-related morbidity and mortality (WHO 2015b). Access to rapid detection of infection

and limited antimicrobial susceptibility testing for tuberculosis has significantly enhanced global efforts in diagnosis and treatment (WHO 2015a).

However, the use of small specimen volumes causes substantial challenges in the design of systems that can yield consistent test results (Bond and Richards-Kortum 2015). As a result, POCT may not produce test results that agree with those generated by larger laboratory analyzers. The results from POCTs need to be harmonized with those from a central laboratory analyzer so that health care providers are familiar with any variations in the results.

Data Handling

Clinical laboratories generate large volumes of data for patient care as well as for quality control and other laboratory-management operations. As access to laboratory services increases in LMICs, paper reporting systems will not support the high volumes of data. An integrated, tier-based laboratory system requires the ability to transmit data to and from multiple testing sites as well as to forward results to clinicians and selected test results to patients for self-monitoring, to public health authorities, and to disease registries. These data-handling needs will only be achieved by the use of LIS (NPP 2014). Although many commercial systems are not affordable in LMICs, open-source systems are available that may provide opportunities for local use. Development of robust, reliable LIS that can be integrated with other parts of health care data systems needs to be a priority in all regions. Mobile phones may facilitate the process.

Part of the data used in diagnostic testing consists of images, including for surgical pathology (histopathology) and cytopathology, hematology (blood smear examinations), microbiology (identification of parasites based on morphologic examination), microscopic examination of urine specimens, and malaria smears. One approach to diagnostic testing, consultation, and quality control is the use of telepathology—the transmission of images via Internet connections to and from remote sites. Previously, this technology was expensive and required access to bandwidth not available in most of the world. More recently, costs have decreased, and improved Internet connectivity is available in many regions.

Quality Management and Accreditation

Although access to quality pathology laboratory testing is an essential part of modern medical practice, in some settings most laboratories are not accredited and do not meet minimal standards for good laboratory practice. These laboratories are unlikely to consistently generate accurate or reliable test results. The absence of accurate and reliable results can lead to incorrect diagnoses, inappropriate treatment, wasted resources, and even lost lives. Such situations give credence to the saying that "no test is better than a bad test."

Causes of Suboptimal Testing

Laboratory testing is a complex process with preanalytical, analytical, and postanalytical phase variables (box 11.1). Considering analytical influences alone, test methodologies affect the magnitude of false positive and false negative results. Sensitivity and specificity profiles influence choices for screening and confirmatory tests. The competence of personnel, regular quality control, state of equipment and laboratory infrastructure, and access to reagents affect the accuracy of test results. A lapse in any step in the long chain of processes can result in incorrect and potentially harmful test results. Ethics and accountability are as important in laboratories as in any other component of health care.

Quality Management

To control these variables, it is essential that laboratories make the commitment to a quality management system and organization structure that ensures that tests are fit-for-purpose, standard operating procedures are documented and followed, personnel are suitably qualified and trained, and regular audits are conducted. The practice of interlaboratory comparisons, such as external quality assurance (EQA) and proficiency testing (PT) programs, has evolved to encourage laboratories to meet validated performance benchmarks. Many comprehensive EQA and PT programs are available regionally and globally (box 11.4). These programs vary in strength; some are educational, while others have a validation focus.

Audit practices have extended beyond internal activities to assessments by third parties using national and international peer-determined standards. The formal assessment of laboratories by independent external agencies against such standards, known as *accreditation*, is the norm in HICs, where requirements for laboratory practices are often mandated by law. Apart from ensuring quality, accreditation status affects the profitability and marketability of laboratories; only accredited tests are reimbursed by health insurance. Through mutual recognition agreements, such as the Asia-Pacific Laboratory Accreditation Cooperation, the Inter-American Accreditation Cooperation, and the International Laboratory Accreditation Cooperation, the tests performed by accredited laboratories are recognized by signatories across country boundaries.

In LMICs, the culture of interlaboratory comparison, audit, and accreditation has yet to become firmly established. In India, it is estimated that fewer than 1 percent of the approximately 100,000 pathology laboratories are accredited (Singh 2013). A 2013 survey reported that more than 90 percent of countries in Sub-Saharan Africa had no laboratories accredited to international quality standards; of the laboratories that were accredited, more than 90 percent were in South Africa (Schroeder and Amukele 2014). Laboratory accreditation has not been established in many LMICs in Southeast Asia, partly because most LMICs do not have national health insurance plans, and the incentive of reimbursement for tests conducted by accredited laboratories does not apply. In addition, most LMICs lack strong regulatory oversight of laboratory practice. Laboratory tests performed by public laboratories, which are frequently resource constrained, are heavily subsidized by governments,

---

Box 11.4

Examples of External Quality Assessment Programs

International Programs

- Royal College of Pathologists of Australasia Quality Assurance Programs, Australia
- National External Quality Assessment Services, United Kingdom
- College of American Pathologists, United States
- Randox International Quality Assessment Scheme, international
- International Academy of Pathology, international with regional and national divisions.

National and Local Programs

- Bureau of Laboratory Quality Standards, Thailand
- External Quality Assessment schemes of Faculty of Medical Technology, Mahidol University, Thailand
- Laboratory Quality Assurance Scheme, Malaysia
- National Center for Clinical Laboratories, China
- Indian Association of Medical Microbiologists, India
- National Health Laboratory Service, South Africa (this program extends to other Sub-Saharan African countries).

while private laboratories benefit from out-of-pocket payments. EQA and PT are not mandatory. The situation pits profit against quality, and many LMICs struggle with the mushrooming of corner shop–type private laboratories with substandard practices and questionable accountability.

However, practices in many emerging economies are rapidly changing, and laboratory accreditation is now actively sought. Although most laboratories started by seeking accreditation from foreign agencies (for example, Australia's National Association of Testing Agencies and the College of American Pathologists), this approach has proved unsustainable because of the high expense. Today, government-backed national accreditation agencies adopting international standards, especially ISO 15189 for medical testing laboratories, provide assessments at a more reasonable cost. Examples of accreditation agencies are listed in box 11.5.

However, legislation-backed regulation of laboratories in LMICs remains the exception (Looi 2008; Wattanasri, Manoroma, and Viriyayudhagorn 2010), and participation in EQA or PT programs and accreditation is entirely voluntary. For these emerging economies, the impetus to gain accreditation has been competition and market driven, especially in light of trade agreements such as the ASEAN (Association of Southeast Asian Nations) Free Trade Area, the World Trade Organization, and the imminent Trans-Pacific Partnership Agreement.

In Sub-Saharan Africa, because public laboratories are the main providers of services, the WHO Regional Office for Africa in 2009 introduced the Stepwise Laboratory Improvement Process Towards Accreditation checklist and the Strengthening Laboratory Management Toward Accreditation training curriculum. These programs were jointly developed with the U.S. Centers for Disease Control and Prevention, the Clinton Health Access Initiative, and the American Society for Clinical Pathology to assist laboratories to move toward accreditation status (Gershy-Damet and others 2010). Although much remains to be done, these tools have transformed the laboratory mindset and practice landscape in Sub-Saharan Africa (Alemnji and others 2014; Yao and others 2014).

The cooperation of the WHO, governments, and national professional bodies has been crucial in the global paradigm shift in laboratory testing to quality and international standardization. However, many challenges remain for LMICs; the most important are resource constraints; establishment of national EQA, PT, and accreditation programs; and legislation-backed regulation of laboratories. Ensuring the long-term, good quality of the services provided by the essential pathology package requires the adoption of an appropriate form of accreditation, within which EQA is embedded.

Reimbursement Policies for Pathology Services

Pathology tests are almost universally costed according to the complexity and the volume of tests performed, often referred to as the *cost-per-test* or *activity-based costing*. Who pays for the tests varies and is closely related to overall health reimbursement policies.

Box 11.5

Examples of Accreditation Bodies

- College of American Pathologists, Laboratory Accreditation Program, United States
- Joint Commission International, United States
- National Association of Testing Authorities, Australia
- South African National Accreditation System, South Africa
- United Kingdom Accreditation Service, United Kingdom
- International Accreditation New Zealand, New Zealand
- Comité Français d'Accréditation, France
- Standards Council of Canada, Canada

- China National Accreditation Service for Conformity Assessment, China
- Hong Kong Accreditation Service, Hong Kong SAR, China
- National Accreditation Board for Testing and Calibration Laboratories, India
- Bureau of Laboratory Quality Standards, Thailand
- Medical Technology Council, Thailand
- Department of Standards Malaysia, Malaysia
- General Coordination for Accreditation, Brazil
- Bureau of Accreditation, Vietnam
- Komite Akreditasi Nasional, Indonesia.

China has a complex reimbursement system for pathology services. The national health care system accounts for the majority of medical reimbursement, but individual provinces and cities have their own differing reimbursement policies. This variation is reflected in the big gap in health care benefits between wealthy and poor regions in China (Chen, Zhao, and Si 2014; Pan and others 2016). In Tianjin, a large city with a population in excess of 13 million people, the health care policy states that public medical insurance covers approximately 70 percent of laboratory testing provided in local hospitals. The remaining laboratory tests are paid on an out-of-pocket basis. In practice, however, the government usually only reimburses basic laboratory tests; because complex tests carry high price tags, only 40 percent of the actual cost of pathology testing is covered (Lei, Chen, and Lu 2014; Mao 2012; Pan and others 2014). In addition, the circumstances under which pathology tests can be used are restricted. The result is that most of the burden of the costs of laboratory tests falls on patients. In some rural areas, especially the more rural regions of western China, coverage of medical costs, including pathology services, is even less generous.

In India—with more than 40,000 hospitals and 100,000 diagnostic laboratories—the private sector delivers 70 percent of health care, including laboratory services. Public financing for health care is less than 1 percent of gross domestic product; only 17 percent of the population is covered by any kind of health insurance. Accordingly, more than 70 percent of health expenditures, including for pathology services, is borne by families as out-of-pocket payments (*The Hindu* 2014).

In Sub-Saharan Africa, the picture is mixed. In South Africa 80 percent of the population has health care, including pathology, paid for by the government. Patients only make a payment if they can afford to. About 7 percent have personal insurance, while the remainder pay out of pocket. A similar situation exists in Zimbabwe and Botswana. In East Africa, there is a mixture of government, insurance, and self-payment. In other countries, self-payment is more common. Payment for testing is made in advance, with patients and families purchasing the necessary supplies to perform the tests in addition to paying the fee required for testing.

Some LMICs have community-based health insurance programs that households can join, but the coverage provided varies. Ghana's program covers only hospital-based services. In Bangladesh, nongovernmental organizations operate insurance programs and cover services in their own clinics. Whether laboratory tests are covered in these programs depends on the details of the particular programs (Robyn, Sauerborn, and Bärnighausen 2013; Soors and others 2010; Wang 2012).

The key factor that applies to all programs is that both patients and clinicians worldwide have a tendency to prefer to use their limited financial resources for treatment rather than diagnosis. If payment is out of pocket, the tendency is for fewer, less complex, and lower-quality tests; the opposite is the case when reimbursement is provided by national or private programs. Invariably, this bias reduces the eventual quality of the outcome. Moreover, it adversely affects the ability of health care systems and governments to standardize health care delivery, collect epidemiological data, and assess the effectiveness of policies and interventions.

To optimize the benefits of pathology provision, as little as possible of the costs should be on an out-of-pocket basis. Where countries adopt a model of universal health coverage, we propose that pathology reimbursement be an integral component of the reimbursement system. Clearly, it will be important to ensure that in such a model, pathology costs are kept in check, for example, by the institution of guidelines on the use of tests.

Economics of Pathology in Different Countries

This section analyzes the costs of pathology laboratories using data from countries with different income levels and with varied health systems (table 11.4). These analyses provide some interesting insights, although data are

Table 11.4 Approximate Annual Salary of Pathology Staff, by Country Income Category, 2010 U.S. Dollars

WHO employee category and corresponding pathology staff	Low-income country	Lower-middle-income country
2: laboratory assistant (secondary education or diploma)	2,220	4,800
3: laboratory technician (bachelor's degree)	2,870	6,170
4: scientific officer (master's degree)	4,550	9,800
Pathologist (physician with additional training)	13,650	29,400

Source: Based on ongoing estimates from Serje 2015.
Note: WHO = World Health Organization. The WHO data are from International Labour Organization salary databases. Equivalencies for technicians, and construction of the top category at three times the salary of category 4 by authors, also is based on unpublished data for Tata Memorial Hospital, Mumbai, as a guideline.

limited and not always readily comparable. These variations on unit costs of tests help explain why estimating the costs of an essential pathology package is challenging.

Pathology's Share of Health Costs

One study for the United States suggested that laboratory tests account for 4.5 percent to 10 percent of total health expenditures (Avivar 2012), compared with 5 percent for Spain (Avivar 2012), 3.3 percent for the United Kingdom (Department of Health, United Kingdom 2006), and 3 percent for Australia (CIE 2016). The payment system in the United States, in which doctors receive payment on a per test basis (and are particularly conscious of potential litigation) means that the United States is likely to be an outlier among HICs. In South Africa, the costs of pathology are about 3.5 percent of total health care expenditure (Pillay 2012). We have no data on the share of pathology costs in overall health expenditure in other LMICs.

Cost per Laboratory Test

Cost per laboratory test undertaken varies considerably. Important factors include the type of test (the diagnostic area), the volume of tests undertaken in the laboratory (the scale), the level of national income and salaries of technical personnel, whether the test is undertaken in the normal workflow or on an urgent or rapid-turnaround basis, and a hard-to-measure efficiency factor. Since the level of the laboratory (tiers 1 through 4) affects the mix of tests undertaken, the cost per test also varies with the level of the laboratory.

Some diagnostic areas are more standardized and more automated than others. Data from the United Kingdom (Department of Health, United Kingdom 2008) found that the median direct cost—excluding equipment costs, costs of space, and overhead costs—of a specific routine test in biochemistry across a sample of laboratories was £1.00 compared with £2.40 in hematology, £6.90 in microbiology, and £48.10 in histopathology (2006/07 costs) (the corresponding costs in 2012 U.S. dollars are US$1.94, US$9.03, US$13.39, and US$93.31). In some disciplines, it has been possible to use equipment, such as large analyzers, to lower the costs per test. In these areas, staff costs are a smaller proportion of the test cost (68 percent to 87 percent for biochemistry tests across different sites and 74 percent to 89 percent for hematology, with one outlier). In other disciplines in which automation is not as extensive, the unit costs are higher, and staff costs are a higher proportion of test costs at 72 percent to 92 percent for microbiology and 93 percent to 97 percent for histopathology (Department of Health, United Kingdom 2008). As science and technology progress, areas such as microbiology may become more automated and less costly; however, newer and less automated tests will continue to be developed.

There are strong economies of scale in laboratory testing (for example, Department of Health, United Kingdom 2008; Cunnama and others 2016 for tuberculosis tests in South Africa). However, the tradeoff is that increased centralization of tests is also associated with increased turnaround time and potential loss of patients to follow-up. In table 11.5 the smallest laboratory performs

Table 11.5 Estimated Ingredients for General Pathology Laboratories at Different Levels, Lower-Middle-Income Countries

Assumptions	Tier 1 laboratory	Tier 2 laboratory	Tier 3 laboratory
Facility description	5 health workers; no inpatients	100 beds	200–400 beds
		5 surgeries per day	15–20 surgeries per day
		500 outpatients per week	1,500 outpatients per week
Population served	30,000	50,000–200,000	3 million to 6 million
Approximate annual hospital budget	US$150,000	US$6 million	US$18 million
Laboratory staff, excluding administrative support	1 laboratory technician	1 general pathologist	4 pathologists
		4 laboratory technicians	2 clinical scientists
		2 laboratory assistants	12 laboratory technicians
			8 laboratory assistants
			1 medical officer
Laboratory test volume per week	100 malaria slides plus point-of-care tests	850	2,500

table continues next page

Table 11.5 Estimated Ingredients for General Pathology Laboratories at Different Levels, Lower-Middle-Income Countries **(continued)**

Assumptions	Tier 1 laboratory	Tier 2 laboratory	Tier 3 laboratory
Equipment needs	US$2,000–US$5,000 (microscope; small devices)	US$150,000–US$200,000	Varies according to functions
Annual salary cost, (using table 11.4)	US$4,800	US$63,680	US$259,440
Overall annual laboratory budget, assuming consumables: salaries are 4:1 in hospitals	n.a.	US$318,400 (5.3 percent of hospital budget)	US$1.3 million (7.2 percent of hospital budget)

Sources: Based on economic ratios from table 11.6, salaries from table 11.4, and expert judgment. Published data were for hospitals; insufficient data were available to make complete estimates for a tier 1 facility.
Note: n.a. = not applicable.

about one test per employee per day, compared with 24 in the medium-sized laboratory in India, and 43 billable tests in the largest laboratory in the United States. We used 300 days worked per person per year as a rough guide for this calculation. No data on staff were available for Thailand.

The level of national income affects the technology used in conducting tests, and hence the relative shares of different cost components. In LMICs, salary costs are lower relative to the cost of reagents and test kits, so tests tend to be less automated; however, staff costs form a smaller proportion of overall costs. In HICs, salary costs are higher relative to the cost of consumables, and there is more automation; but salary costs form a higher proportion of overall costs (see table 11.6; some caution in interpretation is needed because the four laboratories in the table do not serve identical functions). In the United States, the ratio of staff to consumables in total costs has increased. The ratio was 40:60 in 1980 for one clinical biochemistry laboratory in a university hospital, but rose to 60:40 by 1990 (Benge, Csako, and Parl 1993). It is likely that LMICs will follow a similar trend as salaries increase and drive increased automation.

Estimated Costs for the Essential Pathology Package

Although the variations in the unit costs of tests make estimating laboratory costs challenging, systematic factors are involved as well. We first estimate salary costs for technical staff using the WHO-CHOICE data (table 11.4) for the average LMIC. We then construct stylized laboratories using expert judgment combined with published data summarized in table 11.6. We combine these stylized data with the salary data and with the estimate that consumables in the laboratory cost approximately four times as much as salaries in Asia (which is slightly lower than the

ratio for the two big hospital laboratories in India and Thailand, summarized in table 11.6). In Sub-Saharan Africa, the current ratio is closer to 1:1 (Kuti, personal communication); this ratio is likely not to be optimal given that too few tests are undertaken in Sub-Saharan Africa.

These inputs yield estimates of recurrent laboratory costs as a proportion of hospital budget of slightly more than 5 percent for a first-level hospital, and slightly more than 7 percent for a second-level hospital. Our estimates can be compared with data for Ghana, where the share of laboratories in total hospital costs was 2.3 percent for a first-level hospital with 117 beds and one doctor, and 4.1 percent for a second-level hospital with 100 beds and three doctors (Aboagye, Degboe, and Obuobi 2010). In India, the corresponding shares were 7.3 percent for a first-level hospital of 400 beds and 24 doctors, and 9.2 percent for a second-level hospital of 778 beds and 237 doctors (Chatterjee, Levin, and Laxminarayanan 2013).

We do not have enough data to estimate laboratory costs for primary health centers. One study of 12 government primary health centers in Ghana (Dalaba and others 2013) estimated that the costs of laboratory supplies amounted to less than 1 percent of the overall cost of the center. This figure excludes the cost of consumables for POCT that do not enter the laboratory.

Because of too little published data, our confidence that these numbers apply in LICs is low. Professional salaries in LICs are about half the level of those in lower-middle-income countries (table 11.4). However, it is unlikely that the costs of laboratories would be half as well. The volume of tests is likely to be lower, and unit costs are likely to be higher by an unknown amount. The data from Malawi (Gopal, personal communication) show that salaries of laboratory personnel are closer to the levels of lower-middle-income countries than the

Table 11.6 Structure and Annual Cost of Tier 3 and 4 Laboratories in Four Settings

	Lilongwe, Malawi	Tata Memorial Hospital, India Hemopathology lab	King Chulalongkorn Memorial Hospital, Thailand	Major teaching hospital, United States
Types of test	91% histology, 9% cytology	Primarily hematological malignancies	85% biochemistry; 15% hematology	Full service
Staff	2 pathologists 2 laboratory technicians 1 laboratory assistant	2 physicians 2 senior residents 6 scientists (2 PhDs) 2 technical officers (MSc) 13 technicians (BSc) 6 assistants Total 31	n.a.	7 pathologists 7 technical supervisors 19 phlebotomists 4 blood banks 18 molecular and microbiology labs 26 clinical biochemistry and hematology labs 11 processors 25 outpatient laboratory technicians 117 total, excluding administration
Approximate population coverage	1 of only 2 such laboratories, country of 15 million	City of 21 million, state of 112 million, diagnostic center for region	City of 6.3 million	City of 650,000 State of 5.3 million
Annual number of tests	1,680	227,000	2.16 million	1.5 million billable (7 million total)
Annual budget US$ (year)	243,000 (2012)	976,270 (2012)	25.3 million in 2002 ($ 2012)	18 million (2015) (2.7% of hospital budget)
Budget shares (%)				—c
• Space, utilities	n.a.	2.8	1.9 (equipment + space)	
• Equipment	22.6	11.2	13.2	
• Staff	61.7	13.9	84.9	
• Consumables	14.4	71.1	0	
• Miscellaneous	1.2a	1.1b	n.a.	

Sources: Gopal (personal communication) and Gopal and others 2013; Gujral and others 2010 for India; budget shares calculated by chapter author from published data; Charuruks, Chamnanpai, and Seublinvog 2004 for Thailand.

Note: n.a. = not available.

a. Communications costs, telepathology link with University of North Carolina.

b. Quality control, usually additional tests.

c. Data (Christopher Price, personal communication) from a hospital trust in the United Kingdom suggest that the split is 72 percent staff, 26 percent equipment rental, 1 percent equipment maintenance, and 1 percent other.

WHO data predict, likely because technically qualified staff are sufficiently scarce that if they were paid less, they would not remain in public laboratories in LICs.

In summary, our rough estimates (table 11.5) are that recurrent laboratory costs for a first-level hospital should be slightly more than 5 percent of the hospital budget; for a second- or third-level hospital, they should be slightly more than 7 percent of the budget. Of this share, about 16 percent consists of staff costs, and the balance consists of consumables. Costs for a tier 1 laboratory are

more modest, but most of the testing at this level is point of care, and we do not have data on the cost of POCT. What is known from HICs is that POCT is generally more expensive on a cost-per-test basis compared with centralized testing, primarily because POCT is based on single-use technology.

The cost of setting up a laboratory is estimated to be US$2,000–US$5,000 for a tier 1 laboratory; US$150,000–US$200,000 for a tier 2 laboratory at a second-level hospital; and a considerably larger amount at a third-level hospital, but no estimates were made because of the wide variety of equipment choices available. In comparison, the equipment for a specialized (primarily histopathology) laboratory in Malawi cost US$150,000 to set up; about half of this cost is in addition to the cost of training two technicians in other countries (Gopal, personal communication). The cost of training two technicians in other countries was a further US$74,000.

CONCLUSIONS

The differential diagnosis of the child in the vignette at the beginning of this chapter, ranging from tuberculosis to lymph node cancer, was wide, and each diagnosis would have required completely different treatments and management. Most of the possible diagnoses were life threatening; without the appropriate treatment, the prognosis was poor. Conversely, with the right diagnosis and resultant treatment, the prognosis would have been good. The widespread availability of and timely access to good quality pathology, as described in the essential pathology package, would have provided that accurate diagnosis.

Key Messages

Pathology is a cross-cutting discipline upon which the other health disciplines depend and a crucial component in the care pathway. Pathologists are diagnosticians who, as part of the clinical team, play a key role in linking clinical services with laboratory services, providing leadership, and capitalizing on the opportunities arising from rapidly emerging new technologies. Pathology contributes to research in both communicable and noncommunicable diseases, and it plays a central role in national policy planning.

Recommendations

Implementation of the essential pathology package is needed to address the lack of timely, accurate pathology in many LMICs; the rapidly increasing burden of noncommunicable diseases makes such implementation a priority. Our economic analysis shows that provision of the essential pathology package is affordable at approximately 6 percent of a hospital's budget. An integrated network is crucial to achieving the benefits of shared knowledge, expertise, communication, and economies of scale.

The sustainability and quality of the essential pathology package depends on investment in education and training and in appropriate emerging technologies, including LIS. Standards of practice need to be assessed across the network by an ongoing system of internal and external (accreditation) audits. Reimbursement systems, especially for universal health coverage, need to include pathology to minimize out-of-pocket expenses and disincentives to appropriate use. Finally, ongoing research is important to obtain more accurate data on the economic benefits of pathology and on the most cost-effective solutions.

NOTE

World Bank Income Classifications as of July 2014 are as follows, based on estimates of gross national income (GNI) per capita for 2013:

- Low-income countries (LICs) = US$1,045 or less
- Middle-income countries (MICs) are subdivided:
  (a) lower-middle-income = US$1,046–US$4,125
  (b) upper-middle-income(UMICs)=US$4,126–US$12,745
- High-income countries (HICs) = US$12,746 or more.

REFERENCES

Aboagye A. Q. Q., A. K. B. Degboe, and A. A. D. Obuobi. 2010. "Estimating the Cost of Healthcare Delivery in Three Hospitals in Southern Ghana." *Ghana Medical Journal* 44 (3): 83–92.

Adesina, A., D. Chumba, A. M. Nelson, J. Orem, D. J. Roberts, and others. 2013. "Improvement of Pathology in Sub-Saharan Africa." *The Lancet Oncology* 14 (4): e152–57. doi:10.1016 /S1470-2045(12)70598-3.

African Strategies for Advancing Pathology Group Members. 2015."Quality Pathology and Laboratory Diagnostic Services Are Key to Improving Global Health Outcomes: Improving Global Health Outcomes Is Not Possible without Accurate Disease Diagnosis." *American Journal of Clinical Pathology* 143 (3): 325–28. doi:10.1309/AJCP6K0DZCNVCSCI.

Alemnji, G. A., C. Zeh, K. Yao, and P. N. Fonjungo. 2014. "Strengthening National Health Laboratories in Sub-Saharan Africa: A Decade of Remarkable Progress." *Tropical Medicine and International Health* 19 (4): 450–58.

ASLM (African Society for Laboratory Medicine) and WHO AFRO (World Health Organization Regional Office for Africa). 2015. "The Freetown Declaration." Statement at Regional Global Health Security Consultation on Laboratory Strengthening, Freetown, Sierra Leone, October 15–16. http://new.aslm.org/programmes/global-health-security /freetown-declaration.

Avivar, C. 2012. "Strategies for the Successful Implementation of Viral Laboratory Automation." *Open Virology Journal* 6 (S1): 151–21.

Benge, H., G. Csako, and F. F. Parl. 1993. "A 10-Year Analysis of Revenues, Costs, Staffing and Workload in an Academic Medical Centre Clinical Chemistry Laboratory." *Clinical Chemistry* 39: 1780–87.

Bond, M. M., and R. R. Richards-Kortum. 2015. "Drop-to-Drop Variation in the Cellular Components of Fingerprick Blood:

Implications for Point-of-Care Diagnostic Development." *American Journal of Clinical Pathology* 144 (6): 885–94. doi:10.1309/AJCP1L7DKMPCHPEH.

Cassim, N., L. M. Coetzee, K. Schnippel, and D. K. Glencross. 2014. "Estimating Implementation and Operational Costs of an Integrated Tiered CD4 Service Including Laboratory and Point of Care Testing in a Remote Health District in South Africa." *PLoS One* 9 (12): e115420.

Charuruks, N., S. Chamnanpai, and T. Seublinvog. 2004. "Cost Analysis of Laboratory Tests: A Study of the Central Laboratory of King Chulalongkorn Memorial Hospital." *Journal of the Medical Association of Thailand* 87: 955–63.

Chatterjee, S., C. Levin, and R. Laxminarayanan. 2013. "Unit Cost of Medical Services at Different Hospitals in India." *PLoS One* 8 (7): e69728. doi:10.1371/journalpone 0069728.

Chen, M., Y. Zhao, and L. Si. 2014. "Who Pays for Health Care in China? The Case of Heilongjiang Province." *PLoS One* 9 (10): e108867. doi:10.1371/journal.pone.0108867.

CIE (Centre for International Economics). 2016. *The Economic Value of Pathology: Achieving Better Health, and a Better Use of Health Resources.* Canberra: CIE. http://www.thecie .com.au/wp-content/uploads/2016/04/Economic-value-of -pathology_-Final-Report-April-2016.pdf.

Cunnama, L., E. Sinanovic, L. Ramma, N. Foster, L. Berrie, and others. 2016. "Using Top-Down and Bottom-Up Costing Approaches in LMICS: The Case for Using Both to Assess the Incremental Costs of New Technologies at Scale." *Health Economics* 25: 53–66.

Dalaba, M. A., P. Akweongo, G. Savadogo, H. Saronga, J. Williams, and others. 2013. "Cost of Maternal Health Services in Selected Primary Health Centres in Ghana: A Step-down Allocation Approach." *BMC Health Services Research* 13 (1): 287–95.

Daramola, A. O., A. A. Banjo, A. Bennett, F. Abdulkareem, and A. M. Shaaban. 2016. "Breast Cancer Reporting in Lagos, Nigeria: Implications for Training and Education in Africa." *Journal of Global Oncology* 2 (2). doi:10.1200/JGO.2015.003079.

Department of Health, United Kingdom. 2006. *Report of the Review of NHS Pathology Services in England.* London. http://collection.europarchive.org/tna/20070706124823 /http://dh.gov.uk/en/Publicationsandstatistics/Publications /PublicationsPolicyAndGuidance/DH_4137606.

———. 2008. *Report of the Second Phase of the Review of NHS Pathology Services in England.* London. http://webarchive .nationalarchives.gov.uk/20130107105354/http://www.dh .gov.uk/prod_consum_dh/groups/dh_digitalassets/@dh /@en/documents/digitalasset/dh_091984.pdf.

Elbireer, A. M., J. B. Jackson, H. Sendagire, A. Opio, D. Bagenda, and others. 2013. "The Good, the Bad, and the Unknown: Quality of Clinical Laboratories in Kampala, Uganda." *PLoS One* 8 (5): e64661. doi:10.1371/journal.pone.0064661.

Gershy-Damet, G. M., P. Rotz, D. Cross, F. Cham, J. B. Ndihokubwayo, and others. 2010. "The World Health Organization African Region Laboratory Accreditation Process." *American Journal of Clinical Pathology* 134 (3): 393–400.

Gopal, S., R. Krysiak, N. G. Liomba, M.-J. Horner, C. G. Shores, and others. 2013. "Early Experience after Developing a Pathology Laboratory in Malawi, with Emphasis on

Cancer Diagnoses." *PLoS One* 8 (8): e70361. doi:10.1371 /journal.pone.0070361.

Gujral, S., K. Dongre, S. Bhindare, P. G. Subramanian, H. K. V. Narayan, and others. 2010. "Activity-Based Costing Methodology as Tool for Costing in Haematopathology Laboratory." *Indian Journal of Pathology and Microbiology* 53 (1): 68–74.

The Hindu. 2014. "Only 17% have Health Insurance Cover." December 22. http://www.thehindu.com/news/national/only -17-have-health-insurance-cover/article6713952.ece.

Hyle, E. P. L., K. Meye, K. Kelly, S. Christensen, K. Daskilewicz, and others. 2014. "The Clinical and Economic Impact of Point-of-Care CD4 Testing in Mozambique and Other Resource-Limited Settings: A Cost-Effectiveness Analysis." *PLoS Medicine* 11 (9): e1001725.

ISO (International Organization for Standardization). 2012. *Medical Laboratories: Requirements for Quality and Competence.* ISO 15189:2012. Geneva: ISO.

JCI (Joint Commission International). 2014. *Accreditation Standards for Hospitals,* fifth edition. Oak Brook, IL: JCI. http:// www.jointcommissioninternational.org/jci-accreditation -standards-for-hospitals-5th-edition/.

Jegathesan, M., and G. F. de Witt. 1982. "Organisation of Laboratory Services in Malaysia." *Malaysian Journal of Pathology* 5: 1–5.

Kuijpers, C. C., J. Fronczek, F. R. van de Goot, H. W. Niessen, P. J. van Diest, and others. 2014. "The Value of Autopsies in the Era of High-Tech Medicine: Discrepant Findings Persist." *Journal of Clinical Pathology* 67 (6): 512–19. doi:10.1136/jclinpath-2013-202122.

Lei, H. D., J. B. Chen, and X. S. Lu. 2014. "Analysis of the Personal Burden of Inpatients in a Hospital in Tianjin." *Foreign Medical Sciences* 31 (1): 38–40.

Looi, L. M. 2008. "The Pathology Act Explained." *Malaysian Journal of Pathology* 30 (1): 1–10.

Mao, A. Y. 2012. "Study on the Impact of Public Health Insurance System Reform over 20 Years in China, How Patients' Actual Reimbursement Rate Changed." *Chinese Health Economics* 31 (10): 19–22.

Nelson, A. M., D. A. Milner, T. R. Rebbeck, Y. Iliyasu, and K. A. Fleming. 2016. "Africa: Pathology in the Sub-Sahara." In *The State of Oncology in Africa 2015,* edited by P. Boyle, T. Ngoma, R. Sullivan, N. Ndlovu, P. Autier, and others. Lyon, France: iPRI Scientific Publication 4, iPRI.

NPP (National Pathology Programme). 2014. *Digital First: Clinical Transformation through Pathology Innovation.* London: NPP. https://www.england.nhs.uk/wp-content/uploads/2014/02 /pathol-dig-first.pdf.

Orem, J., S. Sandin, C. E. Weibull, M. Odida, H. Wabinga, and others. 2012. "Agreement between Diagnoses of Childhood Lymphoma Assigned in Uganda and by an International Reference Laboratory." *Clinical Epidemiology* 4: 339–47. doi:10.2147/CLEP.S35671.

Pan, L., P. He, H. F. Wu, Y. Den, W. B. Zhang, and others. 2014. "Investigation and Analysis of City Public Hospital Outpatient and Inpatient Medical Expenses of Inpatients and Payment." *Chinese General Practice* 17 (34): 4127–32.

Pan, J., S. Tian, Q. Zhou, and W. Han. 2016. "Benefit Distribution of Social Health Insurance: Evidence from China's Urban Resident Basic Medical Insurance." *Health Policy and Planning* 1–7. doi:10.1093/heapol/czv141.

Pillay, T. S. 2012. "Containing Costs in the Era of National Health Insurance—The Need for and Importance of Demand Management in Laboratory Medicine." *South African Medical Journal* 103 (1): 24. doi: 10.7196/samj.6383.

Plebani, M. 2009. "Exploring the Iceberg of Errors in Laboratory Medicine." *Clinica Chimica Acta* 404: 16–23.

Pollock, N. R., S. McGray, D. J. Colby, F. Noubary, H. Nguyen, and others. 2013. "Field Evaluation of a Paper-Based Point-of-Care Fingerstick Transaminase Test." *PLoS One* 8 (9): e75616. doi:10.1371/journal.pone.0075616. eCollection 2013.

Robyn, P. J., R. Sauerborn, and T. Bärnighausen. 2013. "Provider Payment in Community-Based Health Insurance Schemes in Developing Countries: A Systematic Review." *Health Policy and Planning* 28 (2): 111–22.

Rohr U.-P., C. Binder, T. Dieterle, F. Giusti, C. G. M. Messina, and others. 2016. "The Value of In-Vitro Diagnostic Testing in Medical Practice: A Status Report." *PLoS One* 11: e0149856. doi:10.1371.journal.pone.0149856.

Schroeder, L. F., and T. Amukele. 2014. "Medical Laboratories in Sub-Saharan Africa that Meet International Quality Standards." *American Journal of Clinical Pathology* 141 (6): 791–95.

Serje, J. 2015. "Estimates of Health Sector Salaries across Four Occupational Levels for UN Member States." Unpublished, WHO, Geneva.

Singh, T. D. 2013. "Accreditation of Diagnostic Laboratories." *The Sangai Express*, September 28.

Soors, W., N. Devadasan, V. Durairaj, and Criel B. 2010. "Community Health Insurance and Universal Coverage: Multiple Paths, Many Rivers to Cross." World Health Report Background Paper 48, WHO, Geneva.

Stewart, B., and C. P. Wild, eds. 2014. *World Cancer Report.* Lyon: International Agency for Research on Cancer.

St. John, A., and C. P. Price. 2014. "Existing and Emerging Technologies for Point-of-Care Testing." *Clinical Biochemistry Review* 35: 155–67.

Van Dang, D. 2104. "Pathology and Telepathology in Vietnam." *Pathology* 46 (Suppl 2): S8.

Vathana, C. S., and G. Stauch. 2014. "Pathology and Telepathology in Cambodia." *Pathology* 46 (Suppl 2): S8.

Wang, L. 2012. "Study on the Healthcare Benefit in Sub-Saharan African Countries." *Foreign Medical Sciences (Health Economics)* 29 (4).

Wattanasri, N., W. Manoroma, and S. Viriyayudhagorn. 2010. "Laboratory Accreditation in Thailand: A Systemic Approach." *American Journal of Clinical Pathology* 134 (4): 534–40.

Whitesides, G. M., and P. Wilding. 2012. "Laboratory on a Stamp: Paper-Based Diagnostic Tools." Interview by Molly Webster and Vikram Sheel Kumar. *Clinical Chemistry* 58: 956–58.

WHO (World Health Organization) 2008. *Consultation on Technical and Operational Recommendations for Clinical Laboratory Testing Harmonization and Standardization.* WHO: Geneva. http://www.who.int/healthsystems/round9_9.pdf.

———. 2015a. *Global Tuberculosis Report.* 20th edition. Geneva: WHO.

———. 2015b. *World Malaria Report 2015.* Geneva: WHO.

WHO AFRO (World Health Organization Regional Office for Africa). 2008. *The Maputo Declaration on Strengthening of Laboratory Systems.* Statement issued at Consensus Meeting on Clinical Laboratory Testing Harmonization and Standardization, Maputo, Mozambique, January 22–24. http://www.who.int/diagnostics_laboratory/Maputo -Declaration_2008.pdf.

———, and US CDC (United States Centers for Disease Control and Prevention). 2010. *Guidance for Development of National Laboratory Strategic Plans.* Atlanta: CDC. http://www.who.int/hiv/amds/amds_guide_dev_nat_lab _strat.pdf.

Wu, G., and M. H. Zaman. 2012. "Low-Cost Tools for Diagnosing and Monitoring HIV Infection in Low-Resource Settings." *Bulletin of the World Health Organization* 90 (12): 914–20.

Yao, K., M. Talkmore, E. T. Luman, and J. N. Nkengasong. 2014. "The SLMTA Programme: Transforming the Laboratory Landscape in Developing Countries." *African Journal of Laboratory Medicine* 3 (2). doi:10.4102/ajlm.v3i2.194.

Yetisen, A. K., M. S. Akram, and C. R. Lowe. 2013. "Paper-Based Microfluidic Point-of-Care Diagnostic Devices." *Laboratory on a Chip* 13: 2210–51.

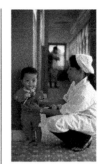

Chapter 12

Palliative Care and Pain Control

Eric L. Krakauer, Xiaoxiao Kwete, Stéphane Verguet,
Hector Arreola-Ornelas, Afsan Bhadelia, Oscar Mendez,
Natalia M. Rodriguez, Zipporah Ali, Silvia Allende,
James F. Cleary, Stephen Connor, Kristen Danforth,
Liliana de Lima, Liz Gwyther, Ednin Hamzah, Dean T. Jamison,
Quach Thanh Khanh, Suresh Kumar, Emmanuel Luyirika,
Anne Merriman, Egide Mpanumusingo, Diana Nevzorova,
Christian Ntizimira, Hibah Osman, Pedro Perez-Cruz,
M. R. Rajagopal, Lukas Radbruch, Dingle Spence,
Mark Stoltenberg, Neo Tapela, David A. Watkins,
and Felicia Knaul

INTRODUCTION

Palliative care has been shown to provide significant and diverse benefits for patients with serious, complex, or life-limiting health problems. Such benefits include the following:

- Reduced physical, psychological, and spiritual suffering (Abernethy and others 2003; Gwyther and Krakauer 2011; Higginson and others 2014; Krakauer 2008; Singer and others 2016; Temel and others 2010; WHO 2008; Zimmerman and others 2014)
- Improved quality of life (Singer and others 2016; Zimmerman and others 2014)
- Prolonged survival in some situations (Connor and others 2007; Temel and others 2010).

Palliative care also can lower costs to health care systems (Chalkidou and others 2014; DesRosiers and others 2014; Gomez-Batiste and others 2012; Jamison and others 2013; Knaul and others 2017; Summers 2016). For these reasons, it is recognized globally as an ethical responsibility of all health care systems and a necessary component of universal health coverage (World Health Assembly 2014). Yet palliative care is rarely accessible in low- and middle-income countries (LMICs). This chapter describes an essential package (EP) of palliative care services and treatments that could and should be accessible to everyone everywhere, as well as the sites or platforms where those services and treatments could be offered. Thus, it was necessary to make a preliminary estimate of the burden of health-related suffering requiring palliative care.

To roughly estimate the need for palliative care, we identified the serious, complex, or life-limiting conditions listed in the *International Classification of Diseases* (ICD)-10 that most commonly result in physical, psychological, social, or spiritual suffering (WHO 2015a). We then estimated the types, prevalence, and duration of suffering resulting from each condition. On the basis

Felicia Knaul is senior author.

Corresponding author: Eric L. Krakauer, Harvard Medical School, Boston, Massachusetts, United States; eric_krakauer@hms.harvard.edu.

of this characterization of the burden of suffering, we propose an EP of palliative care and pain control designed to do the following:

- Prevent or relieve the most common and severe suffering related to illness or injury.
- Be affordable, even in LMICs.
- Provide financial risk protection for patients and families by providing a realistic alternative to expensive, low-value treatment.

We costed the EP in one low-income country (Rwanda), one lower-middle-income country (Vietnam), and one upper-middle-income country (Mexico) and projected these costs for LMICs in general (Knaul and others 2017). At the conclusion of this chapter, we provide guidance on how to integrate the EP into health systems as an essential element of universal health coverage (UHC) in LMICs. We also discuss how to augment the EP as soon as is feasible to further prevent and relieve suffering.

This chapter draws directly on the work of the *Lancet* Commission on Global Access to Palliative Care and Pain Control (the *Lancet* Commission) (Knaul and others 2017).

THE NEED FOR PALLIATIVE CARE

In 2015, there were 56 million deaths, including nearly 9 million from malignant neoplasms, more than 1 million from human immunodeficiency virus/aquired immune deficiency syndrome (HIV/AIDS), more than 17 million from cardiovascular diseases, and more than 3 million from chronic obstructive pulmonary disease (COPD) (WHO 2016). These and other serious, complex, or life-limiting health problems generate multiple kinds of suffering, typically categorized in the palliative care literature as follows (WHO 2002):

- Pain and other physical distress
- Psychological distress
- Social distress
- Spiritual distress.

Existing data, mostly from high-income countries (HICs), indicate that well over 50 percent of patients who die of malignant neoplasms and HIV/AIDS experience pain (Foley and others 2006). Pain is also common among those who die of heart disease, COPD, renal failure, neurologic disease, and dementia (Moens, Higginson, and Harding 2014; Solano, Gomes, and Higginson 2006). A recent meta-analysis of pain prevalence studies,

almost all from HICs, revealed that 75 percent of patients receiving anti-cancer treatment or with advanced, metastatic disease had pain, most of which was moderate or severe (Doyle and others 2017; Van den Beuken-van Everdingen, Hochstenbach, and Joosten 2016). Dyspnea—shortness of breath—is especially common among people who die of COPD and heart failure and only slightly less common among those who die of malignant neoplasms and HIV/AIDS (Moens, Higginson, and Harding 2014).

Depressed mood and anxiety are quite common among patients with a variety of advanced life-threatening illnesses. Data on prevalence of social and spiritual distress among these patients are scant. A study in the United States found that 44 percent of patients with advanced cancer experienced spiritual pain. In an impoverished rural district in Malawi, 76 percent of patients receiving palliative care needed social supports. In Germany, approximately 50 percent of patients receiving palliative care needed such supports (Herce and others 2014; Ostgathe and others 2011).

The *Lancet* Commission on Global Access to Palliative Care and Pain Relief (Knaul and others 2017) identified (a) the 20 ICD-10 conditions that most commonly result in a need for palliative care and (b) the specific categories of suffering typically caused by each condition (table 12.1). Almost all of the identified conditions can cause any of the four categories of suffering. In addition, psychological and social distress can be a cause of at least some of the ICD-10 conditions (Farmer and others 2006). To determine the number of deaths per year from each condition, and hence gain insight into the need for palliative care, the Commission used mortality data from the WHO Global Health Estimates (GHE) for 2015 (Mathers and others 2018, chapter 4 of this volume) and aligned these data with the ICD-10 conditions using a conversion document from the WHO (2017). The Commission then estimated the percentage of people who die from each condition ("decedents") who have health-related suffering that requires palliative care.

The Commission also identified the conditions that often lead to physical, psychological, social, or spiritual suffering, even among nondecedents, defined as people who do not die in a given year. These conditions include some that may be curable (drug-resistant tuberculosis and some malignancies), others that may be well controlled for long periods (HIV/AIDS and musculoskeletal disorders), and others from which patients may recover (serious injuries). It also was necessary to identify the specific types of suffering within each category (for example, pain, dyspnea, and nausea are types of physical suffering) and to estimate the prevalence and duration of each type.

Table 12.1 Conditions Responsible for the Need for Palliative Care

Condition/disease	Patients		Decedents					
			Symptoms (%)					
			Total		Physical		Psychological	
			All symptoms		All symptoms		All symptoms	
	Rank	%	Total days	At least days	Total days	At least days	Total days	At least days
a. LMICs								
Malignant neoplasms	1	26	47	45	50	46	36	36
CVD	2	17	11	12	12	12	7	9
Lung disease	3	11	9	11	8	11	12	12
Injuries	4	6	0	1	0	1	1	1
TB	5	6	6	6	4	4	10	9
Premature birth and trauma	6	5	0	0	0	0	0	0
HIV	7	5	12	8	11	8	12	12
Liver disease	8	5	3	3	3	3	2	1
NI heart disease	9	4	3	3	3	3	4	4
Dementia	10	3	4	4	3	3	10	10
All other		11	5	8	5	8	6	6
All (millions)		20.6	9,143	2,473	7,191	2,378	1,952	1,054
b. Global								
Malignant neoplasms	1	30	51	49	54	51	39	39
CVD	2	16	10	10	11	11	6	8
Lung disease	3	11	8	10	7	10	11	11
Injuries	4	6	0	1	0	1	1	1
TB	5	5	4	5	3	3	8	7
Dementia	6	5	6	6	4	4	13	13
Liver disease	7	5	2	3	3	3	2	1
Premature birth and trauma	8	4	0	0	0	0	0	0
HIV	9	4	9	6	9	6	10	9
NI heart disease	10	4	3	3	3	3	3	4
All other		11	6	8	6	9	7	7
All (millions)		25.6	11,900	3,231	9,347	3,105	2,553	1,376

Source: Adapted with permission from Knaul and others 2017.
Note: CVD = cardiovascular disease; HIV = human immunodeficiency virus; LMICs = low- and middle-income countries; NI = non-ischemic; TB = tuberculosis.
a. The other illness conditions that commonly result in a need for palliative care are hemorrhagic fever, leukemia, dementia, inflammatory disease of the central nervous system, degeneration of the central nervous system; chronic ischemic heart disease, renal failure, congenital malformations, atherosclerosis, chronic musculoskeletal disorders, and malnutrition.

The Commission identified 20 conditions that account for 81 percent of global deaths and 80 percent of deaths in LMICs. Based on mortality figures for 2015 and our estimates, at least 50.5 million people each year with these conditions in LMICs, including decedents and nondecedents, require palliative care. Approximately 60 percent of these patients are nondecedents. More than 46 million

deaths occurred in LMICs in 2015; of these, about 20 million or 45 percent experienced health-related suffering that required palliative care. Patients in LMICs account for 17 billion days per year of need for palliative care—80 percent of the annual global total. Among decedents in LMICs, 10 conditions account for approximately 90 percent of patients and 95 percent of total days of health-related suffering. The other 10 conditions each account for less than 3 percent of decedents and days with health-related suffering.

THE GLOBAL SUFFERING DIVIDE: DISPARATE ACCESS TO PALLIATIVE CARE AND PAIN CONTROL

Despite compelling evidence of a huge burden of remediable health-related suffering and of the efficacy of palliative care and pain treatment, these essential health services are rarely accessible in LMICs. Data from the International Narcotics Control Board show that 91 percent of the morphine consumed worldwide in 2013 was consumed in HICs, which have only 19 percent of the world's population; people in LMICs, which account for 81 percent of the world's population, only consumed 9 percent (Pain and Policy Studies Group 2017). Given that morphine is essential to relieve moderate and severe pain (WHO 1996, 2012) and that morphine consumption is the most common—although imperfect—measure of palliative care accessibility, the data reveal an enormous disparity between rich and poor in meeting the need for palliative care.

Available data indicate that 74 percent of countries—virtually all of them LMICs—had at best isolated palliative care provision as of 2013 (Connor and Sepulveda Bermedo 2014). Among the 9 percent of countries where palliative care is "at a stage of advanced integration into mainstream service provision," only Romania and Uganda are LMICs, and most people in need lack access to palliative care even in these two countries (Connor and Sepulveda Bermedo 2014, 39–40). The global suffering divide appears to be one of the world's largest health care inequities. The EP of palliative care that we propose is designed specifically to be the minimum acceptable package for the lowest income settings. Accordingly, although necessary for all countries, the EP is not exhaustive; palliative care can be improved by expanding the package to include additional medicines, equipment, and human resources.

AN ESSENTIAL PACKAGE OF PALLIATIVE CARE AND PAIN CONTROL

Patients with life-threatening illnesses are the sole focus of palliative care according to the current WHO definition, and there are calls for it to be revised and expanded (Gwyther and Krakauer 2011; WHO 2002). There is large-scale, unrelieved health-related suffering among other groups as well. In particular, patients in LMICs

typically lack access to relief of pain and other types of suffering that result from common health problems that may be cured (drug-resistant tuberculosis and some malignancies) or controlled for a long period (HIV/AIDS and musculoskeletal disorders) or from which patients are likely to recover (serious injuries). The need for palliative care in low-resource settings is often determined by the magnitude of suffering, the inadequacy of existing capacity to respond, and the resultant need for relief. Therefore, the EP of palliative care and pain control that we propose should be as follows:

- Accessible at all levels of health care systems and in patients' homes.
- Adapted to local cultures, as well as clinical and social situations. For example, in resource-poor settings, the social circumstances of the patient and family members may be a major source of the patient's suffering and may need to be a focus for palliative care (Gwyther and Krakauer 2011).
- Integrated with disease prevention and treatment programs, although not considered a substitute for these, and assist patients in accessing and adhering to optimum disease treatment—if they desire such treatment and if it may be more beneficial than harmful according to patients' values, balanced with scientific evidence. Further, palliative care workers have a responsibility to advocate for access to comprehensive health care including, but not restricted to, disease-modifying treatments, such as cancer chemotherapy, antiretroviral treatment, or effective medicines for multidrug resistant tuberculosis (Gwyther and Krakauer 2011; Shulman and others 2014).
- Applied not only to persons who are dying but also to those living with long-term physical, psychological, social, or spiritual sequelae of serious, complex, or life-limiting illnesses or of their treatment. The EP should be applied to relieve acute pain and other acute symptoms when medically indicated.
- With adequate levels of palliative care training and skill, applied by health care workers of various kinds, including primary care providers, generalists, and specialists in many disciplines and from basic to intermediate to specialist.

Design of the Essential Package

The EP that we propose is a key component of health systems and is designed to relieve the most common and severe suffering related to illness or injury, to be low cost and feasible to deliver in LMICs, and to protect patients and their families from catastrophic health expenditures (table 12.2). It consists of a list of

Table 12.2 Delivery Platforms for the Essential Palliative Care Interventions

Intervention	Delivery platform			
	Intersectoral	Mobile outreach or home care	Health center (PHC)	First-, second-, and third-level hospitals
Control of chronic pain related to serious, complex, or life-limiting health problems	• Routine social assessment • Income and in-kind support[a]	• Surveillance and emotional support by community health workers as often as needed (sometimes daily) • Visits by PHC nurse or doctor as needed	• Oral immediate-release morphine and other essential medicines and simple equipment for prevention and relief of chronic pain	—
Control of other types of physical and psychological suffering[b] related to serious, complex, or life-limiting health problems	• Routine social assessment • Income and in-kind support[a]	• Emotional support and suffering surveillance by community health workers as often as needed (sometimes daily) • Visits by PHC nurse or doctor as needed	• Essential medicines and simple equipment for prevention and relief of other types of physical and psychological suffering • Psychological counseling	—
Control of refractory suffering (chronic pain, other types of physical and psychological suffering[b] that have not or cannot be controlled at lower level)	• Routine social assessment • Income and in-kind support[a]	—	—	• Oral immediate-release morphine and injectable morphine and other essential medicines and simple equipment for prevention and relief of chronic pain and other types of physical and psychological suffering[c] • Psychological counseling[c]
Acute pain related to surgery or serious injury	—	—	—	• Essential medicines and simple equipment for prevention and relief of acute pain[c]

Note: PHC = public health care. — = this type of care not provided in this setting.

a. Support provided only for patients living in extreme poverty and for one caregiver per patient.

b. Physical suffering includes breathlessness, fatigue, weakness, nausea, vomiting, diarrhea, constipation, pruritus, bleeding, and wounds. Psychological suffering includes anxiety or worry, depressed mood, confusion or delirium, and dementia.

c. Care devolves to lower level once effective treatment is established.

medicines, based on the WHO Model List of Essential Medicines for Palliative Care (WHO 2015b, 2015c). Centrally important in this list is immediate-release morphine. The EP includes equipment (lock boxes) and procedures to assure against misuse of opioids. The package also includes some small and inexpensive equipment. In addition, the package specifies several types of palliative care interventions and the platform or health care system level at which each intervention and each item in the package should be available. Finally, the package includes intersectoral inputs in the form of income and in-kind support required by any patient or family caregiver living in extreme poverty. (See annex table 12A.1 for an exhaustive list of medicines and other inputs required for the EP.)

Medicines

Morphine, in oral immediate-release and injectable preparations, is the most **clinically important** of the essential palliative care medicines (WHO 2011). It must be accessible in the proper form and dose by any patient with terminal dyspnea or with moderate or severe pain that is either acute, chronic and associated with malignancy, or chronic in a patient with a terminal prognosis. We do not recommend the use of opioids for chronic pain outside of cancer, palliative, and end-of-life care, except under special circumstances and with strict monitoring (Dowell, Haegerich, and Chou 2016). All physicians who ever care for patients with moderate or severe pain of the types described, or for patients with terminal dyspnea, should be able to prescribe oral and injectable morphine for inpatients and outpatients in any dose necessary to provide adequate relief as determined by the patients. Physicians should be able to prescribe an adequate supply of morphine so that obtaining refills is feasible for patients or families without requiring unreasonably frequent, expensive, or arduous travel.

Although ensuring access to morphine for anyone in need is imperative, it also is necessary to take reasonable precautions to prevent diversion and nonmedical use. Model guidelines for this purpose are available (Joranson, Maurer, and Mwangi-Powell 2010). Oral immediate release and injectable morphine should be accessible at all third-, second, and first-level hospitals. Personnel at health centers also should be trained in opioid analgesia and safe storage so that morphine may be safely dispensed by prescription in these settings as well.

Among the other essential palliative medicines are oral and injectable haloperidol and oral fluoxetine or another selective serotonin reuptake inhibitor (SSRI). Although these medicines are considered psychiatric or psychotropic medicines, they have multiple essential uses in palliative care and are safe and easy to prescribe. For example, haloperidol is the first-line medicine in many cases for relief of nausea, vomiting, agitation, delirium, and anxiety. An SSRI, such as fluoxetine, is the first-line pharmacotherapy for depressed mood or persistent anxiety, both of which are common among patients with serious, complex, or life-limiting health problems. All physicians at any level of the health care system and who care for patients with these symptoms should be trained and permitted to prescribe these medicines—not solely psychiatrists or neurologists.

Equipment

The EP includes equipment that often is needed for palliative care yet may not be available in all health centers and hospitals in LMICs. Such equipment includes pressure-reducing mattresses, adult diapers, opioid lock boxes nasogastric tubes, and urinary catheters (annex table 12A.1). For the sake of efficiency, the EP does not include materials needed for palliative care that should be standard equipment for any health center or hospital, such as gauze and tape for dressing wounds, nonsterile examination gloves, syringes, and angiocatheters.

Psychological and Spiritual Counseling

Interventions to relieve psychological distress may be provided not only by psychologists but also by adequately trained and supervised physicians, nurses, or social workers at any level of the health care system (Belkin and others 2011; Patel 2014; Rahman and others 2016). For patients or family members with complicated psychological problems, such as suicidality, psychotic disorders, or bipolar disorder, referral should be made to psychiatrists, if possible. In addition, hospital-based staff members should routinely ask patients with serious, complex, or life-limiting health problems if they desire spiritual counseling, and hospitals should allow local volunteer spiritual counselors to visit inpatients upon request by the patient or family.

Social Supports

Social supports should be accessible both for any patient in need of palliative care and for their main caregiver in instances of extreme poverty. Given that extreme poverty is both a cause and an effect of serious, complex, or life-limiting health problems, it is crucial that meaningful social supports are accessible (Bamberger 2016). Such social supports include transportation vouchers, cash payments, food packages, and other types of in-kind support (annex table 12A.1) (Carrillo and others 2011; Syed, Gerber, and Sharp 2013). In most cases, funding for these social supports should come not from health care budgets but from antipoverty or social welfare programs. Thus, to be able to implement all aspects of the full EP, there must be intersectoral coordination.

Human Resources

The EP should include adequate time for trained personnel at each level of the health care system to provide palliative care consisting of the interventions, medicines, equipment, counseling, and social supports described earlier. These personnel include doctors, nurses, counselors such as social workers or psychologists, pharmacists, community health workers, and family caregivers (annex table 12A.1). Community health workers require a minimum of several hours of training to prepare them to recognize and report any uncontrolled suffering to a supervisor. Capable family caregivers should be trained, equipped, and encouraged by staff at health centers to provide basic nursing care such as wound and mouth care and medicine administration. Nurses and doctors at health centers who provide palliative care or who instruct family caregivers need basic training and all doctors who care for patients with serious, complex, or life-limiting health problems at hospitals require intermediate training. Ideally, all countries should have palliative care specialist physicians to lead training and service implementation and to advise governments on palliative care policy (World Health Assembly 2014).

Augmenting the Essential Package

After the EP of palliative care and pain control is universally accessible, additional palliative medicines, equipment, and services should be made accessible by all countries to further prevent and relieve health-related suffering as soon as resources permit (Lutz, Jones, and Chow 2014; Miner 2005; Shulman and others 2015). This augmentation would consist of the following:

- Generic slow-release oral morphine or generic transdermal fentanyl patches
- Palliative surgery
- Palliative radiotherapy
- Palliative cancer chemotherapy
- Canes and wheelchairs.

In many LMICs, rehabilitation and long-term care services are either inadequate or inaccessible by the poor. As a result, community-based palliative care teams often assume responsibility for these tasks (Ratcliff and others 2017). However, all countries should develop policies and allocate funding specifically for the implementation of these much-needed services (World Health Assembly 2016).

COSTS OF THE ESSENTIAL PACKAGE OF PALLIATIVE CARE AND PAIN CONTROL

In most LMICs, the cost of caring for patients with serious, complex, or life-limiting health problems is borne primarily not by governments but out-of-pocket by patients and their families. Serious, complex, or life-limiting health problems put patients' families at risk of financial ruin and caregivers at risk of exhaustion and health problems of their own (Emanuel and others 2008; Emanuel and others 2010). Data on the obvious and hidden costs of palliative care and any cost savings are important to inform governmental decisions about including palliative care among public health care services and about covering palliative care with government health insurance.

Data on Costs and Cost Savings

Multiple studies from HICs indicate that palliative care can reduce costs for patients and families, as well as for health systems (Chalkidou and others 2014; DesRosiers and others 2014; Gomez-Batiste and others 2012; Jamison and others 2013; Summers 2016). Not only can palliative care improve patient outcomes, it also can reduce health care costs by reducing length of stay in the hospital, hospital admissions, and demand for expensive disease-modifying treatments of dubious benefit near the end of life. Patients who receive palliative care, especially early in their disease course, incur lower health care costs (Albanese and others 2013; May 2016; Morrison and others 2008), have shorter hospitalization (Morrison and others 2008; Postier and others 2014), enjoy equal or higher quality of life (Zimmerman and others 2008), and live equally long or longer (Elsayem and others 2004) than patients who do not receive palliative care. Palliative care also has been shown to increase satisfaction of family caregivers (Zimmerman and others 2008). Thus, evidence indicates that palliative care can generate positive externalities and can lower indirect costs to society, but data on costs and cost savings of palliative care in LMICs are limited (Emanuel and others 2010; Hongoro and Dinat 2011; Mosoiu, Dumitrescu, and Connor 2014).

Method for Costing an Essential Package of Palliative Care and Pain Control in LMICs

To estimate the cost of delivering high-quality palliative care and pain control in LMICs, we used a method developed by the *Lancet* Commission (Knaul and others 2017). We obtained input from palliative care clinicians and global health experts with extensive experience in LMICs to devise a method of costing the EP of palliative care and pain control described in this chapter.

After creating the package of interventions, inexpensive essential medicines, simple equipment, human resources, and intersectoral social supports, as well as the sites or platforms where each part of the package should be accessible (table 12.2 and annex table 12A.1), we then estimated amounts of each item that would be required by patients with each ICD-10 health condition that generates a need for palliative care or pain control. We also estimated the staffing needs in full-time equivalents (FTEs) to apply the package at each site. Using WHO GHE mortality data (WHO 2016), we were able to estimate the total amount of medicines, equipment, and personnel FTEs, as well as the intersectoral social supports needed to provide palliative care and pain control to all patients in need in any country.

To determine the cost of delivering the EP in a specific country, we then identified the reported unit price of all medicines, equipment, social supports, and monthly FTE salaries of the palliative care providers in that country (De Lima and others 2014; McCoy and others 2008). The total cost of the EP was the total cost of all components. To cost human resources, we used monthly total pretax (including mandatory benefits), public sector, FTE-reported salaries. We also considered the most basic operational inputs required to support the provision of the EP at every level of care and added, on average, 8 percent to our overall figures.

Application of the Method in Specific Countries

To provide examples for policy makers of the expected cost of the health care components of the EP per patient in need of palliative care in one low-income country, one lower-middle-income country, and one upper-middle-income country, we applied our method in Rwanda, Vietnam, and Mexico (table 12.3) using the prices reported in each.

Not surprisingly, the cost of achieving universal access to the EP would require a much higher share of total government expenditure on health in Rwanda (between 7.0 and 10.0 percent) than in Mexico (less than 1.0 percent) or Vietnam (between 1.0 and 1.7 percent). As a proportion of gross domestic product, there would be an almost tenfold difference in cost of the EP between Rwanda (0.25 percent) and Mexico (0.03 percent) or Vietnam (0.04 percent).

We also produced preliminary estimates of the costs of the intersectoral social supports previously mentioned, considering only patients living in extreme poverty (daily income below US$1.9) and a patient's one main caregiver living in extreme poverty (World Bank 2017). (These illustrative estimates assume that a stringent means test (screening process) can be implemented to identify those living in extreme poverty. However, experience with means tests in many places suggests that they may be costly to administer and subject to abuse.) Our assumption is that intersectoral social supports are both financed and provided by sectors of government working on poverty alleviation, and not by ministries of health. On the basis of data on subsidies provided to families by existing anti-poverty programs in Mexico, and given the small proportion of families below the poverty line (3 percent), the social supports would represent a very

Table 12.3 Per Patient Cost of the Health Care Components of the Essential Package of Palliative Care and Pain Control in Mexico, Rwanda, and Vietnam, US$, 2015 Current Value

	Rwanda[d]	Vietnam[e]	Mexico
Medicines	52	27	122
Morphine (oral or injectable)	*20*	*14*	*90*
Equipment	31	5	31
Palliative care team (HR)	121	78	584
Operational Costs (8% of total)	16	9	59
Total	**219**	**119**	**796**
% GDP[a]	0.25	0.04	0.03
% health expenditure[b]	3.35	0.56	0.50
% public health expenditure[c]	8.79	1.04	0.97

Note: GDP = gross domestic product; HR = human resources.

a. GDP, World Development Indicators, World Bank, http://data.worldbank.org/indicator/NY.GDP.MKTP.CD.

b. Health expenditure, total (% of GDP), World Development Indicators, World Bank, http://data.worldbank.org/indicator/SH.XPD.TOTL.ZS.

c. Health expenditure, public (% of total health expenditure), World Development Indicators, World Bank, http://data.worldbank.org/indicator/SH.XPD.PUBL.

d. For costing in Rwanda, the following substitutions were made: Fluoxetine was substituted with SSRI and reusable cloth diapers instead of disposable.

e. Costing in Vietnam does not include *Parenteral Fluconazole* as pricing for this medicine was unavailable in the country.

small additional cost, about 1 percent, compared to the health components of the EP. For Rwanda, as would be the case for other low-income countries, the total cost would be quite high, largely because more than 60 percent of families live in extreme poverty. Thus, the EP would have an anti-poverty function for the most financially vulnerable patients with palliative care needs and caregivers.

Limitations of the Method

This costing method has several limitations. First, it does not include the costs of initial palliative care capacity building, including secure supply-chain building for controlled substances, human resource training and policy changes to officially integrate palliative care into the health care system and to ensure essential medicine accessibility. Second, our calculations are based on a particular model of palliative care delivery. For example, our model assumes that inpatient care is available at health centers for one patient at a time whose family is unable to provide adequate care in the home but who does not require higher-level care. Where inpatient care at health centers is not available, costs may differ. Our model includes estimated FTEs of all palliative care team members. Where larger or smaller FTEs are devoted to palliative care, costs will differ.

CONCLUSIONS

A universally accessible EP of palliative care and pain control can prevent and relieve suffering for chronically or terminally ill patients. It is indispensable for achieving universal health coverage and for realizing Sustainable Development Goal 3: "ensure healthy lives and promote well-being for all at all ages" (United Nations General Assembly 2015, 16). It therefore is a medical and moral imperative to include such a package in publicly financed universal health coverage. In addition, the EP of palliative care and pain control that we propose may reduce costs for health care systems and national economies and provide financial risk protection for patients and their families.

To ensure that the EP of palliative care and pain control is universally accessible, governments should enact appropriate policies and ensure that health care providers have the necessary competencies by including training in palliative care and pain control in standard undergraduate and postgraduate curricula in medicine, nursing, and other clinical fields (Stjernswärd, Foley, and Ferris 2007; World Health Assembly 2014).

ANNEX

The annex to this chapter is available at http://www .dcp-3.org/DCP.

- Annex 12A. The Essential Package of Palliative Care: Interventions, Medicines, Equipment, Human Resources, and Intersectoral Supports

NOTES

This chapter was adapted from Knaul, F. M., P. E. Farmer, E. L. Krakauer, L. de Lima, A. Bhadelia, and others. 2017. "Alleviating the Access Abyss in Palliative Care and Pain Relief: An Imperative of Universal Health Coverage. Report of the *Lancet* Commission on Global Access to Palliative Care and Pain Control." *The Lancet*. doi:10.1016/S0140-6736(17)32513-8.

World Bank Income Classifications as of July 2015 are as follows, based on estimates of gross national income (GNI) per capita for 2014:

- Low-income countries (LICs) = US$1,045 or less
- Middle-income countries (MICs) are subdivided:
  (a) lower-middle-income = US$1,046 to US$4,125
  (b) upper-middle-income (UMICs) = US$4,126 to US$12,735
- High-income countries (HICs) = US$12,736 or more.

REFERENCES

Abernethy, A. P., D. C. Currow, P. Frith, B. S. Fazekas, A. McHugh, and others. 2003. "Randomised, Double Blind, Placebo Controlled Crossover Trial of Sustained Release Morphine for the Management of Refractory Dyspnea." *BMJ* 327: 523–29.

Albanese, T. H., S. M. Radwany, H. Mason, C. Gayomali, and K. Dieter. 2013. "Assessing the Financial Impact of an Inpatient Acute Palliative Care Unit in a Tertiary Care Teaching Hospital." *Journal of Palliative Medicine* 16 (3): 289–94.

Bamberger, J. 2016. "Reducing Homelessness by Embracing Housing as a Medicaid Benefit." *JAMA Internal Medicine* 176 (8): 1051–52.

Belkin, G. S., J. Unutzer, R. C. Kessler, H. Verdell, G. J. Raviola, and others. 2011. "Scaling Up for the 'Bottom Billion'; '5×5' Implementation of Community Mental Health Care in Low-Income Regions." *Psychiatric Services* 62 (12): 1494–1502.

Carrillo, J. E., V. A. Carrillo, H. R. Perez, D. Salas-Lopez, A. Natale-Pereira, and others. 2011. "Defining and Targeting Health Care Access Barriers." *Journal of Health Care for the Poor and Underserved* 22 (2): 562–75.

Cassell, E. J. 1982. "The Nature of Suffering and the Goals of Medicine." *New England Journal of Medicine* 306 (11): 639–45.

Chalkidou, K., P. Marquez, P. K. Dhillon, Y. Teerawattananon, T. Anothaisintawee, and others. 2014. "Evidence-Informed

Frameworks for Cost-Effective Cancer Care and Prevention in Low, Middle, and High-Income Countries." *The Lancet Oncology* 15 (3): e119–31. http://dx.doi.org/10.1016/S1470 -2045(13)70547-3.

Connor, S., B. Pyenson, K. Fitch, C. Spence, and K. Iwasaki. 2007. "Comparing Hospice and Non-Hospice Patient Survival among Patients Who Die within a Three-Year Window." *Journal of Pain and Symptom Management* 33 (3): 238–46.

Connor, S., and M. C. Sepulveda Bermedo, eds. 2014. *Global Atlas of Palliative Care at the End of Life*. London: Worldwide Palliative Care Alliance. http://www.who.int/nmh/Global _Atlas_of_Palliative_Care.pdf.

De Lima, L., T. Pastrana, L. Radbruch, and R. Wenk. 2014. "Cross-Sectional Pilot Study to Monitor the Availability, Dispensed Prices, and Affordability of Opioids around the Globe." *Journal of Pain and Symptom Management* 48 (4): 649–59.

DesRosiers, T., C. Cupido, E. Pitout, L. van Niekerk, M. Badri, and others. 2014. "A Hospital-Based Palliative Care Service for Patients with Advanced Organ Failure in Sub-Saharan Africa Reduces Admissions and Increases Home Death Rates." *Journal of Pain and Symptom Management* 47 (4): 786–92.

Dowell, D., T. M. Haegerich, and R. Chou. 2016. "CDC Guideline for Prescribing Opioids for Chronic Pain—United States." *MMWR* 65 (1): 1–48.

Doyle, K. E., S. K. El Nakib, M. R. Rajagopal, S. Babu, G. Joshi, and others. 2017. "Predictors and Prevalence of Pain and Its Management in Four Regional Cancer Hospitals in India." *Journal of Global Oncology*. http://ascopubs.org/doi /pdf/10.1200/JGO.2016.006783.

Elsayem, A., K. Swint, M. J. Fisch, J. L. Palmer, S. Reddy, and others. 2004. "Palliative Care Inpatient Service in a Comprehensive Cancer Center: Clinical and Financial Outcomes." *Journal of Clinical Oncology* 22 (10): 2008–14.

Emanuel, N., M. A. Simon, M. Burt, A. Joseph, N. Sreekumar, and others. 2010. "Economic Impact of Terminal Illness and the Willingness to Change It." *Journal of Palliative Medicine* 13 (8): 941–44.

Emanuel, R. H., G. A. Emanuel, E. B. Reitschuler, A. J. Lee, E. Kikule, and others. 2008. "Challenges Faced by Informal Caregivers of Hospice Patients in Uganda." *Journal of Palliative Medicine* 11 (5): 746–53.

Farmer, P. E., B. Nizeye, S. Stulac, and S. Keshavjee. 2006. "Structural Violence and Clinical Medicine." *PLoS* 3 (10): e449. http://journals.plos.org/plosmedicine/article ?id=10.1371/journal.pmed.0030449.

Foley, K. M., J. L. Wagner, D. E. Joranson, and H. Gelband. 2006. "Pain Control for People with Cancer and AIDS." In *Disease Control Priorities in Developing Countries* (second edition), edited by D. T. Jamison, J. G. Breman, A. R. Measham, G. Alleyne, M. Claeson, D. B. Evans, P. Jha, A. Mills, and P. Musgrove. Washington, DC: World Bank.

Gaskin, D. J., and P. Richard. 2011. "Appendix C: The Economic Costs of Pain in the United States." In *Institute of Medicine. Relieving Pain in America: A Blueprint for Transforming Prevention, Care, Education, and Research*, 301–37. Washington DC: National Academies Press. https://www .ncbi.nlm.nih.gov/books/NBK92521/.

Gomez-Batiste, X., C. Caja, J. Espinosa, I. Bullich, M. Martinez-Muñoz, and others. 2012. "The Catalonia World Health Organization Demonstration Project for Palliative Care Implementation: Quantitative and Qualitative Results at 20 Years." *Journal of Pain Symptom Management* 43 (4): 783–94.

Gwyther, L., and E. L. Krakauer. 2011. "WPCA Policy Statement on Defining Palliative Care." Worldwide Palliative Care Alliance, London. http://www.thewhpca.org/resources /item/definging-palliative-care.

Herce, M. E., S. N. Elmore, N. Kalanga, J. W. Keck, E. B. Wroe, and others. 2014. "Assessing and Responding to Palliative Care Needs in Rural Sub-Saharan Africa: Results from a Model Intervention and Situation Analysis in Malawi." *PLoS One* 9 (10): e110457. http://www.plosone.org/article /info%3Adoi%2F10.1371%2Fjournal.pone.0110457.

Higginson, J., C. Bausewein, C. C. Reilly, W. Gao, M. Gysels, and others. 2014. "An Integrated Palliative and Respiratory Care Service for Patients with Advanced Disease and Refractory Breathlessness: A Randomised Controlled Trial." *The Lancet Respiratory Medicine* 2 (12): 979–87.

Hongoro, C., and N. Dinat. 2011. "A Cost Analysis of a Hospital-Based Palliative Care Outreach Program: Implications for Expanding Public Sector Palliative Care in South Africa." *Journal of Pain and Symptom Management* 41 (6): 1015–24.

Jamison, D. T., L. H. Summers, G. Alleyne, K. J. Arrow, S. Berkley, and others. 2013. "Global Health 2035: A World Converging within a Generation." *The Lancet* 382 (9908): 1898–955.

Joranson, D., M. Maurer, and F. Mwangi-Powell, eds. 2010. "Guidelines for Ensuring Patient Access to, and Safe Management of, Controlled Medicines." Kampala: African Palliative Care Association. http://integratepc.org/wp -content/uploads/2013/05/patient_access1.pdf.

Knaul, F. M., P. E. Farmer, E. L. Krakauer, L. de Lima, A. Bhadelia, and others. 2017. "Alleviating the Access Abyss in Palliative Care and Pain Relief: An Imperative of Universal Health Coverage. Report of the *Lancet* Commission on Global Access to Palliative Care and Pain Control." *The Lancet*. doi:10.1016/S0140-6736(17)32513-8.

Krakauer, E. L. 2008. "Just Palliative Care: Responding Responsibly to the Suffering of the Poor." *Journal of Pain and Symptom Management* 36 (5): 505–12.

Lutz, S. T., J. Jones, and E. Chow. 2014. "Role of Radiation Therapy in Palliative Care of the Patient with Cancer." *Journal of Clinical Oncology* 32 (26): 2913–19.

Mathers, C., G. Stevens, D. Hogan, A. Mahanani, and J. Ho. 2018. "Global and Regional Causes of Death: Patterns and Trends, 2000–15." In *Disease Control Priorities* (third edition): Volume 9, *Improving Health and Reducing Poverty*, edited by D. T. Jamison, H. Gelband, S. Horton, P. Jha, R. Laxminarayan, C. N. Mock, and R. Nugent. Washington, DC: World Bank.

May, P., M. M. Garrido, J. B. Cassel, A. S. Kelley, D. E. Meier, and others. 2016. "Palliative Care Teams' Cost-Saving Effect Is Larger for Cancer Patients with Higher Numbers of Comorbidities." *Health Affairs* 35 (1): 44–53.

McCoy, D., S. Bennett, S. Witter, B. Pond, B. Baker, and others. 2008. "Salaries and Incomes of Health Workers in Sub-Saharan Africa." *The Lancet* 371 (9613): 675–81.

Miner, T. J. 2005. "Palliative Surgery for Advanced Cancer: Lessons Learned in Patient Selection and Outcome Assessment." *American Journal of Clinical Oncology* 28 (4): 411–14.

Moens, K., I. J. Higginson, and R. Harding. 2014. "Are There Differences in the Prevalence of Palliative Care-Related Problems in People Living with Advanced Cancer and Eight Non-Cancer Conditions? A Systematic Review." *Journal of Pain and Symptom Management* 48 (4): 660–77.

Morrison, R. S., J. D. Penrod, J. B. Cassel, M. Caust-Ellenbogen, A. Litke, and others. 2008. "Cost Savings Associated with U.S. Hospital Palliative Care Consultation Programs." *Archives of Internal Medicine* 168 (16): 1783–90.

Mosoiu, D., M. Dumitrescu, and S. R. Connor. 2014. "Developing a Costing Framework for Palliative Care Services." *Journal of Pain and Symptom Management* 48 (4): 719–29.

Ostgathe, C., B. Alt-Epping, H. Golla, J. Gaertner, G. Lindena, and others. 2011. "Non-Cancer Patients in Specialized Palliative Care in Germany: What Are the Problems?" *Palliative Medicine* 25 (2): 148–52.

Pain and Policy Studies Group. 2017. Opioid Consumption Data. Madison, University of Wisconsin. http://www.painpolicy.wisc.edu/opioid-consumption-data.

Patel, V. 2014. *Where There Is No Psychiatrist*. London: Gaskell.

Postier, A., J. Chrastek, S. Nugent, K. Osenga, and S. J. Friedrichsdorf. 2014. "Exposure to Home-Based Pediatric Palliative and Hospice Care and Its Impact on Hospital and Emergency Care Charges at a Single Institution." *Journal of Palliative Medicine* 17 (2): 183–88.

Rahman, A., S. U. Hamdani, N. R. Awan, R. A. Bryant, K. S. Dawson, and others. 2016. "Effect of a Multicomponent Behavioral Intervention in Adults Impaired by Psychological Distress in a Conflict-Affected Area of Pakistan: A Randomized Clinical Trial." *Journal of the American Medical Association* 316 (24): 2609–17.

Ratcliff, C., A. Thyle, S. Duomai, and M. Manak. 2017. "Poverty Reduction in India through Palliative Care: A Pilot Project." *Indian Journal of Palliative Care* 23 (1): 41–45.

Shulman, L. N., T. Mpunga, N. Tapela, C. M. Wagner, T. Fadelu, and others. 2014. "Bringing Cancer Care to the Poor: Experiences from Rwanda." *Nature Reviews Cancer* 14 (12): 815–21.

Shulman, L. N., C. M. Wagner, R. Barr, G. Lopes, G. Longo, and others. 2015. "Proposing Essential Medicines to Treat Cancer: Methodologies, Processes, and Outcomes." *Journal of Clinical Oncology* 34 (1): 69–75.

Singer, A. E., J. R. Goebel, Y. S. Kim, S. M. Dy, S. C. Ahluwalia, and others. 2016. "Populations and Interventions for Palliative and End-of-Life Care: A Systematic Review." *Journal of Palliative Medicine* 19 (9): 995–1008. doi:10.1089/jpm.2015.0367.

Solano, J. P., B. Gomes, and I. J. Higginson. 2006. "A Comparison of Symptom Prevalence in Far Advanced Cancer, AIDS, Heart Disease, Chronic Obstructive Pulmonary Disease and Renal Disease." *Journal of Pain and Symptom Management* 31 (1): 58–69.

Stjernswärd, J., K. M. Foley, and F. D. Ferris. 2007. "The Public Health Strategy for Palliative Care." *Journal of Pain and Symptom Management* 33 (5): 486–93.

Summers, L. H. 2016. "No Free Lunches but Plenty of Cheap Ones." *Larry Summers's Blog*, February 7. http://larrysummers.com/2016/02/08/no-free-lunches-but-plenty-of-cheap-ones/.

Syed, S. T., B. S. Gerber, and L. K. Sharp. 2013. "Traveling towards Disease: Transportation Barriers to Health Care Access." *Journal of Community Health* 38 (5): 976–93.

Temel, J. S., J. A. Greer, A. Muzikansky, E. R. Gallagher, S. Admane, and others. 2010. "Early Palliative Care for Patients with Metastatic Non–Small-Cell Lung Cancer." *New England Journal of Medicine* 363 (8): 733–742.

United Nations General Assembly. 2015. "Transforming Our World: The 2030 Agenda for Sustainable Development." UNGA A/RES/70/1. http://www.un.org/ga/search/view_doc.asp?symbol=A/RES/70/1&Lang=E.

Van den Beuken-van Everdingen, M. H. J., L. J. Hochstenbach, and E. A. J. Joosten. 2016. "Update on Prevalence of Pain in Patients with Cancer: Systematic Review and Meta-Analysis." *Journal of Pain and Symptom Management* 51 (6): 1070–90.

WHO (World Health Organization). 1996. *Cancer Pain Relief, with a Guide to Opioid Availability* (second edition). Geneva: WHO. http://apps.who.int/iris/bitstream/10665/37896/1/9241544821.pdf.

———. 2002. "Definition of Palliative Care." WHO, Geneva. http://www.who.int/cancer/palliative/definition/en/.

———. 2006. "Amended Constitution of the World Health Organization." http://www.who.int/governance/eb/who_constitution_en.pdf.

———. 2011. *Ensuring Balance in National Policies on Controlled Substances: Guidance for Availability and Accessibility of Controlled Medicines*. Geneva: WHO. http://www.who.int/medicines/areas/quality_safety/GLs_Ens_Balance_NOCP_Col_EN_sanend.pdf.

———. 2012. *WHO Guidelines on the Pharmacological Treatment of Persisting Pain in Children with Medical Illnesses*. Geneva: WHO. http://apps.who.int/iris/bitstream/10665/44540/1/9789241548120_Guidelines.pdf.

———. 2015a. WHO International Classification of Diseases (ICD)-10. Geneva: WHO. http://apps.who.int/classifications/icd10/browse/2015/en.

———. 2015b. "WHO Model List of Essential Medicines, 19th list." Geneva, WHO. http://www.who.int/medicines/publications/essentialmedicines/en/index.html.

———. 2015c. "WHO Model List of Essential Medicines for Children, 5th list." WHO, Geneva. http://www.who.int/medicines/publications/essentialmedicines/en/index.html.

———. 2016. "Cause-Specific Mortality." WHO, Geneva. http://www.who.int/healthinfo/global_burden_disease/estimates/en/index1.html.

———. 2017. "WHO Methods and Data Sources for Country-Level Causes of Death 2000–2015." Geneva: WHO. http://www.who.int/healthinfo/global_burden_disease/GlobalCOD_method_2000_2015.pdf.

World Bank. 2017. "Poverty Headcount Ratio at $1.90 a Day (2011 PPP) (% of Population)." World Bank, Washington, DC. http://data.worldbank.org/indicator/SI.POV.DDAY.

World Health Assembly. 2014. "Strengthening of Palliative Care as a Component of Comprehensive Care throughout the Life Course." WHA 67.19. http://apps.who.int/gb/ebwha/pdf_files/WHA67/A67_R19-en.pdf.

———. 2016. "Multisectoral Action for a Life Course Approach to Healthy Ageing: Draft Global Strategy and Plan of Action on Ageing and Health." WHA A69/17. http://apps.who.int/gb/ebwha/pdf_files/WHA69/A69_17-en.pdf.

Zimmerman, C., R. Riechelmann, M. Krzyzanowska, G. Rodin, and I. Tannock. 2008. "Effectiveness of Specialized Palliative Care: A Systematic Review." *Journal of the American Medical Association* 299 (14): 1698–709.

Zimmerman, C., N. Swami, M. Krzyzanowska, B, Hannon, N. Leighl, and others. 2014. "Early Palliative Care for Patients with Advanced Cancer: A Cluster-Randomised Controlled Trial." *The Lancet* 383 (9930): 1721–30. http://dx.doi.org/10.1016/S0140-6736(13)62416-2.

Strengthening Health Systems to Provide Emergency Care

Teri A. Reynolds, Hendry Sawe, Andrés M. Rubiano,
Sang Do Shin, Lee Wallis, and Charles N. Mock

INTRODUCTION

All around the world, acutely ill and injured people of all ages seek care every day. They will call neighbors, the police, or universal emergency numbers for help. They will be assisted by family members, community members with first-aid training, or professional prehospital providers. They may travel to a health care facility by foot, motorcycle, taxi, or ambulance. On arrival, they may or may not find a designated emergency area and providers capable of delivering the care they need.

Emergency care systems (ECSs) address a wide range of acute conditions, including injuries, communicable and noncommunicable diseases, and complications of pregnancy. Especially when there are barriers to health care access, people may seek care *only* when acutely ill or injured. Emergency care is an essential component of universal health coverage—a critical mechanism for ensuring accessible, affordable, high-quality care—and for many people around the world, it is the primary point of access to the health system.

The World Health Organization (WHO) has defined a series of essential functions for an ECS that span from prehospital care and transport through facility-based emergency unit care to early operative and critical care (figure 13.1). Each of these functions can be achieved in

many ways, depending on available resources, and each is essential to the delivery of effective emergency care.

Each of the previous eight volumes of this edition of *Disease Control Priorities* (third edition) (*DCP3*) presents a package of essential services and highlights urgent services for conditions likely to result in morbidity or mortality if not addressed rapidly. An ECS is an integrated mechanism to address these time-sensitive conditions, and this chapter integrates the urgent interventions from all the *Disease Control Priorities* packages with the WHO ECS framework to derive a package of essential emergency care services, including key policy strategies for system development. This effort is intended to identify ways in which national health care systems globally can be strengthened to provide emergency care more effectively.

WHAT IS EMERGENCY CARE?

Emergency care has been defined by various attributes, such as time-to-care provision and acuity of the condition addressed. Common definitions include care delivered within minutes or hours (Kobusingye and others 2006) and care for conditions that require rapid intervention to avoid death or disability (Hirshon and others 2013).

Corresponding author: Teri Reynolds, Department for Management of Noncommunicable Diseases, Disability, Violence, and Injury Prevention, World Health Organization, Geneva, Switzerland; reynoldst@who.int.

Figure 13.1 WHO Emergency Care System Infographic

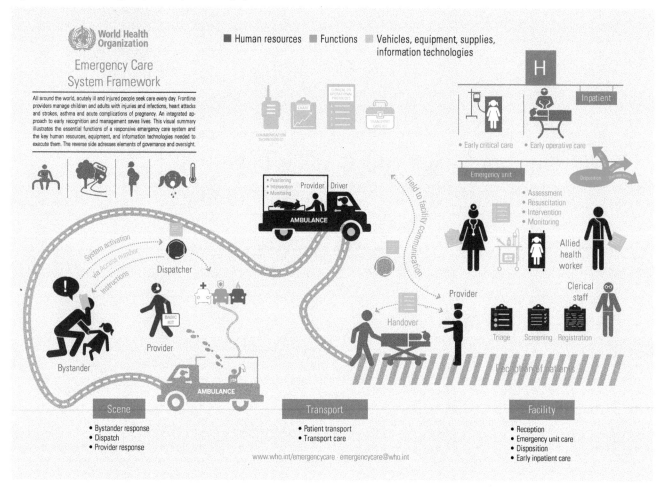

Source: WHO, http://www.who.int/emergencycare/emergencycare_infographic/en/.
Note: H = hospital; WHO = World Health Organization.

Definitions of emergency care that focus on the acuity of the condition itself have the advantage of being independent of the rapidity or level of care that can be achieved by the system and, instead, encompass all rapidly progressive conditions. This approach is preferable to definitions grounded in a specific period for care delivery, since much emergency care would fall outside of a time-bound definition in regions where long transport times are the norm and referrals may take days.

To facilitate consistent understanding across systems at varying levels of development, emergency care is considered here to encompass health services for conditions that require rapid intervention to avert death and disability (such as shock or respiratory failure) or for which delays of hours can worsen prognosis or render care less effective (such as treatment of infections, management of asthma exacerbations, or suturing of wounds).

However, users of the health care system may not themselves be able to judge whether a condition is life-threatening; the belief that an emergency condition exists requires at least urgent preliminary assessment by health care professionals.

People in need of care may access the system at many points, including by activating the prehospital system, by visiting a primary health center, or by presenting directly to a hospital-based emergency unit (figure 13.2); providers at every level of the health system deliver emergency care, whether or not they have the dedicated training and resources to do so effectively. Frontline emergency care may involve early recognition and initial resuscitation for dangerous conditions followed by transfer for definitive care (for example, chest drain placement, volume resuscitation, and transfusion performed before transfer for surgery) or may encompass

Figure 13.2 Access to Emergency Care

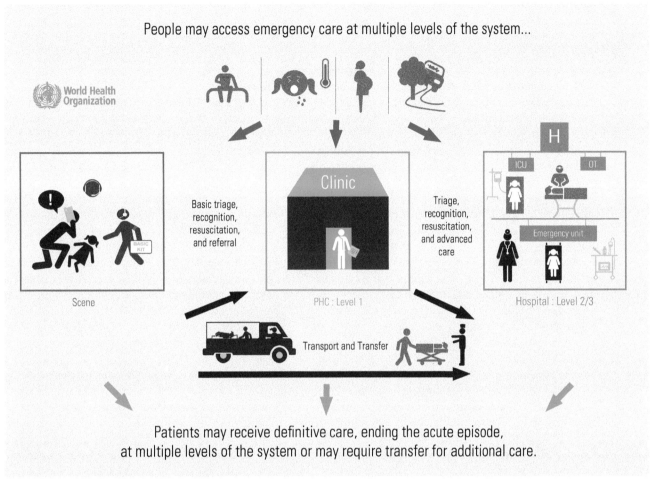

People may access emergency care at multiple levels of the system...

Scene

Basic triage, recognition, resuscitation, and referral

Clinic
PHC : Level 1

Triage, recognition, resuscitation, and advanced care

H
ICU OT
Emergency unit
Hospital : Level 2/3

Transport and Transfer

Patients may receive definitive care, ending the acute episode, at multiple levels of the system or may require transfer for additional care.

Source: World Health Organization, http://www.who.int/emergencycare.
Note: H = hospital; ICU = intensive care unit; OT = operating theatre; PHC = primary health clinic.

definitive therapy (such as administration of antibiotics for pneumonia, wound repair, or nonoperative fracture management).

In keeping with the WHO ECS framework, the use of the term *emergency care* in this chapter encompasses care that occurs both before and beyond the emergency unit itself (figure 13.1), including prehospital care and the early operative care and critical care that may occur in an operating room or an inpatient intensive care unit (ICU). Although the focus of this chapter's package is on facility-based emergency care, many of these services can be mapped onto prehospital systems at increasing levels of development. In general, depending on the level of development of a prehospital system, the services may be very basic, similar to those available at a community-based health center, or may include sophisticated critical care approaching that available in an ICU.

Further details on emergency care specific to the prehospital setting are covered in chapter 14 of volume 1 of *DCP3* (Thind and others 2015).

WHY FOCUS ON EMERGENCY CARE?

Expanding the availability of disease-specific treatments and procedures is essential. The effectiveness of these interventions is compromised, however, without the initial emergency care interface that links undifferentiated patient presentations to appropriate definitive care. For the most part, people seeking care for acute illness or injury do not know if they have a condition requiring oxygen, antibiotics, pericardiocentesis, or surgery. They generally present complaining of fever, pain, or difficulty breathing rather than pneumonia, appendicitis, or tamponade. They do not necessarily know when they are critically ill and cannot go directly to ICUs or operating rooms. In most parts of the world, initial emergency care is delivered by frontline providers (often cadres other than doctors) acting with limited diagnostic resources. Emergency care includes both the early assessment that helps narrow a chief complaint toward a diagnosis, as well as the initial management that allows survival until a diagnosis-oriented therapy can be identified and accessed. The failure (a) to designate and staff emergency care areas, (b) to train frontline providers in recognition of and resuscitation for dangerous conditions, and (c) to create organized ECSs to match people rapidly with the care they need, will cost lives, even where life-saving resources are already available somewhere in the system (Dare and others, 2015; Grimes and others 2011; Hsiao and others 2013; Irfan, Irfan, and Spiegel 2012).

A systematic approach to emergency care—centered on acuity-based triage, early recognition and resuscitation, and simple initial management and referral—has been shown to decrease the mortality associated with a range of medical and surgical conditions. Implementation of a systematic emergency unit approach to early recognition and treatment has been shown to reduce significantly mortality from both pneumonia and sepsis (Gaieski and others 2010; Hortmann and others 2014; Rivers 2001). Better-organized trauma systems have been shown to decrease preventable deaths among the severely injured by 50 percent and to improve functional outcomes among survivors (Siman-Tov, Radomislensky, and Peleg 2013; Tallon and others 2012). Recognition and emergency treatment for myocardial infarction delivered within 60 minutes rather than hours has been shown to reduce mortality twofold (Terkelsen and others 2010); early noninvasive positive pressure ventilation reduces in-hospital mortality (RR [95% CI]: 0.66 [0.48, 0.89]) in patients with heart failure (Vital, Ladeira, and Atallah 2013). Early treatment with aspirin (within 48 hours) for ischemic stroke has been shown to reduce both morbidity and mortality (Sandercock and others 2014), and early intensive blood-pressure lowering (within six hours) has been shown to improve functional outcomes in hemorrhagic stroke (Anderson and others 2013). Three obstetric emergencies—hemorrhage, hypertensive disorders, and sepsis—are responsible for more than half of the maternal deaths worldwide (Say and others 2014) and are highly treatable with simple emergency care interventions (Holmer and others 2015).

Despite the substantial positive impact emergency care can have, however, many low- and middle-income countries (LMICs) lack the fundamentals of organized emergency care: basic prehospital care and transport,

a dedicated area and standards for hospital-based emergency care, and a core of nonrotating providers trained in the care of emergencies and assigned to the emergency unit. These gaps are reflected in wide global discrepancies in outcomes across the range of emergency conditions:

- Overall mortality rates from diabetic ketoacidosis are less than 1 percent in high-income countries (HICs) (Nyenwe and Kitabchi 2011) but are as high as 30 percent in LMICs (Mbugua and others 2005).
- The estimated lifetime risk of maternal mortality in HICs is 1 in 3,300, compared to 1 in 41 in LMICs (Alkema and others 2016).
- Although available data are limited and range widely, mortality from sepsis in LMICs is likely to be more than twice that in HICs (Silva and others 2004; Stevenson and others 2014; Tanriover and others 2006).
- Even within a single country, the discrepancy in outcomes associated with limited access to emergency care can be dramatic: in one Indian study, being poor was associated with reduced access to timely emergency treatments for acute myocardial infarction and with a 50 percent relative increase in mortality (Xavier and others 2008).
- Finally, modeling studies estimate that between 20 and 38 percent of the global injury burden (between 1 million and 2 million fatalities each year and around 52 million disability-adjusted life years, or DALYs) could be averted if severe injury outcomes in LMICs were similar to those in HICs (Higashi and others 2015; Mock and others 2012).

Overall, the global burden of disease that potentially can be addressed by prehospital and facility-based emergency care is estimated at a staggering 54 percent of the annual deaths in LMICs (Thind and others 2015) (figure 13.3).

Although severe global discrepancies exist in outcomes from emergency conditions, both these modeling estimates and direct evidence suggest that emergency care has the potential to narrow this gap dramatically. Powerful examples of feasible life-saving emergency care interventions in LMICs include the following:

- Organizing low-cost prehospital systems was associated with a dramatic decrease in all-condition mortality in Cambodia and Iraq (Husum and others 2003), in road-traffic mortality in Iraq (Murad and others 2012), and in snakebite mortality in Nepal (Sharma and others 2013). A recent review and meta-analysis estimated that simple prehospital systems can reduce injured patients' risk of death by 25 percent (Henry and Reingold 2012).

Figure 13.3 Burden of Disease That Can Potentially Be Addressed by Prehospital and Emergency Care in Low- and Middle-Income Countries

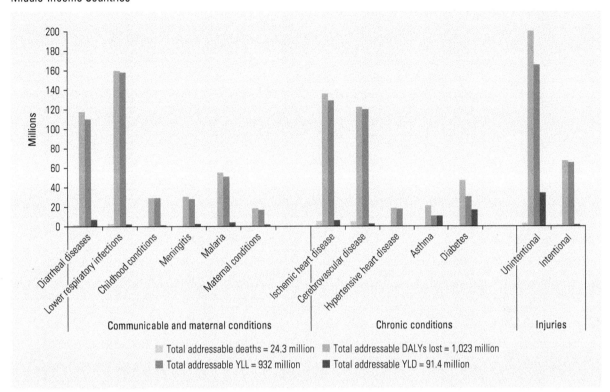

Total addressable deaths = 24.3 million   Total addressable DALYs lost = 1,023 million
Total addressable YLL = 932 million   Total addressable YLD = 91.4 million

Source: Thind and others 2015 (data from WHO 2013).
Note: DALYs = disability-adjusted life years; LMICs = low- and middle-income countries; YLD = years lived with disability; YLL = years of life lost.

- Designating an area for emergency care of all critical patients at a third-level hospital in Romania transformed care and halved mortality.[1]
- In Malawi, restructuring a hospital intake area to create a dedicated emergency care area and initiating formal triage were associated with halved inpatient mortality and a reduction in the proportion of deaths occurring within 24 hours from 36 to 12.6 percent (Molyneux, Ahmad, and Robertson 2006).
- Timely simple interventions (fluids, antibiotics, and clinical monitoring) within the first six hours of hospitalization in Ugandan adults with serious infection reduced mortality from 46 to 33 percent (Jacob and others 2012).
- In rural Mali, improved access to emergency obstetric care halved the risk of maternal mortality and reduced the risk nearly threefold among women with hemorrhage (Fournier and others 2009). Growing evidence indicates that a range of simple nonsurgical interventions for complications of childbirth can dramatically improve maternal mortality in LMICs (Kausar and others 2012; Miller, Lester, and Hensleigh 2004; Paxton and others 2005).

- The introduction of standardized resuscitation protocols in Colombia reduced hospital length of stay and all-cause mortality among injured patients by a quarter (Kesinger, Puyana, and Rubiano 2014).
- Short course trainings in trauma management were associated with reduced mortality in injured patients from 19.9 to 15.1 percent in China (Wang and others 2010) and from 8.8 to 6.3 percent in Rwanda with no significant increase in resource usage (Petroze and others 2015).
- Finally, one modeling study, although dependent on the assumption of available oxygen, predicted that the use of pulse oximetry, combined with current WHO guidelines for recognition of severe illness, has the potential to avert up to 148,000 deaths per year in the 15 countries across Africa and Asia with the highest global burden of childhood pneumonia (Floyd and others 2015).

Evidence from around the world shows that emergency care is an effective means of saving lives, and evidence from LMICs suggests that feasible and simple steps to improve emergency care could rapidly improve outcomes and reduce global disparities in outcomes. More broadly, the recently adopted United Nations Sustainable Development Goals (SDGs)[2] and their associated targets provide guidance for coordinated action to end poverty, protect the planet, and promote health on a global level. ECSs directly address nearly all the health-related SDG targets, as well as those on disasters and violence (table 13.1), and the SDG targets are unlikely to be met without strengthening ECSs globally.

THE WHO EMERGENCY CARE SYSTEM FRAMEWORK

To facilitate systematic assessment and targeted development of integrated ECSs, the WHO ECS framework (annex 13A) was designed with input from more than 30 LMICs. This consensus-based document defines essential emergency care functions at the scene of injury or illness, during transport, and through emergency unit

Table 13.1 Sustainable Development Goals Directly Addressed by Emergency Care

Sustainable Development Goal targets	Emergency care interventions
3.1: By 2030, reduce the global maternal mortality ratio to less than 70 per 100,000 live births	Interventions include treatment for obstetric emergencies such as hemorrhage, hypertensive disorders, and sepsis.
3.2: By 2030, end preventable deaths of newborns and children under age five years, with all countries aiming to reduce neonatal mortality to at least as low as 12 per 1,000 live births and under-five mortality to at least as low as 25 per 1,000 live births	Interventions include treatment of acute pediatric diarrhea, pneumonia, and sepsis.
3.3: By 2030, end the epidemics of HIV/AIDS, tuberculosis, malaria, and neglected tropical diseases, and combat hepatitis, water-borne diseases, and other communicable diseases	Interventions include recognition and treatment of acute infections.
3.4: By 2030, reduce by one-third premature mortality from noncommunicable diseases through prevention and treatment and promote mental health and well-being	Interventions include treatment of acute exacerbations of noncommunicable diseases such as heart attack, stroke, and asthma.
3.5: Strengthen the prevention and treatment of substance abuse	Interventions include treatment of overdose and emergency-unit harm-reduction interventions.
3.6: By 2020, halve the number of global deaths and injuries from road-traffic accidents	Interventions include postcrash emergency care for injury.
3.7: By 2030, ensure universal access to sexual and reproductive health care services, including family planning, information, and education; and the integration of reproductive health into national strategies and programs	Interventions include time-sensitive postexposure treatments.
3.8: Achieve universal health coverage, including financial risk protection; access to quality essential health care services; and access to safe, effective, quality, and affordable essential medicines and vaccines	Interventions include continuous access to timely essential services for acute illness and injury. Emergency care is the primary point of access to the health system for many, especially among vulnerable populations.
3.9: By 2030, substantially reduce the number of deaths and illnesses from hazardous chemicals and air, water, and soil pollution and contamination	Interventions include management of acute exposures.
3d: Strengthen the capacity of all countries, particularly LMICs, for early warning, risk reduction, and risk management of national and global health risks	The ECS is a critical site for syndromic surveillance and for preparedness to mitigate the risk of health system collapse in the face of mass events.
11.5: By 2030, significantly reduce the number of deaths and the number of people affected and substantially decrease the direct economic losses relative to global gross domestic product caused by disasters, including water-related disasters, with a focus on protecting the poor and people in vulnerable situations	The ECS is an essential substrate for emergency response and health system resilience.
16.1 Significantly reduce all forms of violence and related death rates everywhere	Interventions include treatment for victims of violence and early recognition of vulnerable individuals.

Source: Sustainable Development Goal targets, http://www.un.org/sustainabledevelopment/sustainable-development-goals/.
Note: ECS = emergency care system; HIV/AIDS = human immunodeficiency virus/acquired immune deficiency syndrome.

and early inpatient care. The functions are mapped across the WHO Health System Building Blocks (WHO 2010), and each function is associated with general categories of human and material resources as well as information and governance elements. The framework—intended to facilitate system planning and development activities—identifies the components of each essential function to allow policy makers and planners to coordinate system development activities and identify and use existing processes and resources more effectively.

Different systems may achieve each function in different ways, based on available resources. For example, system activation may occur in a high-resource setting with a universal access number linked to a central, computerized dispatch and global positioning system. In other settings, system activation may involve the use of simple mobile phone–based protocols that guide dispatchers to provide advice on first aid and use landmark maps to identify patient location.

At the same time, the framework is designed to account for all the basic functions of emergency care. Each function corresponds to specific human, material, and governance requirements. In the case of patient transfer, for example, it is impossible for one person to drive and care for a patient simultaneously, so essential human resources include both the driver and provider. The authority responsible for medical equipment is not likely to be the same as that responsible for vehicle maintenance, and distinct governance components are required. The framework identifies minimum resource categories and ensures that all essential functions are addressed.

Since few countries will have the available resources to implement all components of a fully developed ECS at once, the WHO ECS framework is designed to allow policy makers to identify gaps in care delivery and to create context-relevant priority action plans for system development. The framework is linked with the WHO Emergency Care System Assessment (ECSA) tool, a survey-based tool designed to help policy makers and planners assess a national or regional ECS and set priorities for system development (WHO, n.d.). The ECSA allows users to rate the level of development of components of an ECS on a progressive scale. By providing specific descriptions of each progressive stage, the tool provides a road map, allowing users to generate action priorities rapidly from identified gaps (figure 13.4). For example, for a given component rated at the lowest level (level one), the next most appropriate and feasible targets would likely be the elements described in levels two and three.

WHO ECSAs and associated priority development meetings have been conducted in more than 25 countries across multiple regions. Although each country's assessment differs, shared challenges have been identified across many low- and low-middle-income countries, including the following:

- The need for better coordination of prehospital and facility-based care
- Limited or no coverage of prehospital systems, especially in rural areas
- Critical emergency care service gaps at first-level hospitals (some countries report gaps in both equipment and skills, whereas several middle-income countries report limited emergency care due to first-level hospital provider knowledge gaps, even when equipment is available)
- Lack of nonrotating staff assigned to the emergency unit, which limits coordinated action to improve care and processes
- Limited data on emergency care delivery and poor links for existing data to system planning and quality-improvement efforts
- Lack of standard clinical management and documentation in prehospital and facility settings
- Gaps in dedicated emergency care training across the system, especially regarding integration into formal curricula and ongoing certification requirements
- Insufficient funding and lack of dedicated funding streams
- Lack of security for prehospital and facility-based emergency care staff.

Areas targeted for priority action by multiple countries include the following:

- Designating or strengthening the authority of a government agency to ensure better coordination
- Creating policies to improve access to emergency care, including legislation mandating access without requirement for prior payment and explicit integration of emergency care services into national insurance plans
- Coordinating development of dedicated emergency units with fixed staff at first-level hospitals
- Establishing dedicated emergency care training programs for diverse cadres, including (depending on the system) lay people; undergraduate health professions students; and a range of providers, such as clinical officers, nurses, and generalist and specialist doctors
- Implementing standardized clinical charts based on WHO data sets to facilitate systematic clinical approaches, as well as standardized data collection to inform quality improvement and system planning
- Developing and disseminating formal triage and condition-specific management protocols.

Figure 13.4 Example of Progressive Ratings in the WHO Emergency Care System Assessment Tool

* 8.3 Emergency unit staffing in facilities:

> An **emergency unit** is any dedicated intake area for acutely ill and injured patients. This may be referred to as the emergency department/room/ward, accident and emergency, casualty, etc.
>
> **First-level hospitals** are the lowest level of hospital that receives referrals. In many countries these are district hospitals.
>
> **Third-level hospitals** are the highest level of facility.
>
> **Note** that in some countries there may be other facility levels in between first-level and third-level that are not addressed here.

	First-level hospitals	Third-level hospitals
[1] There are no dedicated emergency units or no providers with specific responsibility for emergency unit patients until they are admitted.	○	○
[2] There are staff that register and direct patients in the emergency unit to inpatient areas (the unit has a sorting function, but minimal care is provided).	○	○
[3] Providers from inpatient services have on-call responsibility to cover emergency unit patients, but are not assigned to be in the emergency unit.	○	○
[4] Providers from inpatient services are assigned to be in the emergency unit, rotating through for limited intervals (for example, one-month blocks).	○	○
[5] There are a core of nonrotating providers that permanently staff the emergency unit.	○	○
I don't know.	○	○
Cannot answer for another reason (explain):	○	○

Source: WHO, http://who.int/emergencycare/activities/en.

In addition to guiding in-country system development efforts, these shared priorities and country-identified needs also serve to guide WHO technical resource development and program agendas.

ESSENTIAL PACKAGE OF EMERGENCY CARE

Each volume of this edition of *Disease Control Priorities* highlights a set of urgent time-dependent elements from among its essential package. Although these elements do not in themselves form a comprehensive package of basic emergency care services, they identify a range of services that an effective ECS must be able to provide. As such, they serve as a foundation for the package described here.

Each essential package defines a set of services, including the capacity to recognize or manage specific conditions and to perform specific procedures or other interventions. Although many of the urgent elements specify a diagnosis (pneumonia or meningitis) or diagnosis-specific intervention (appendectomy), most emergency care is by its nature syndrome-based (addressing shortness of breath, shock, or altered mental status). Even in a fully resourced system, the entire arc of emergency unit assessment and management may occur before establishing a diagnosis. This scenario is especially true where diagnostic resources are limited. In this chapter, the essential urgent services identified in other packages from *DCP3* are integrated with the components necessary to the practice of frontline care for the undifferentiated acutely ill patient, creating a comprehensive package of basic emergency care services (table 13.2).

The emergency care package includes nearly all the urgent elements identified in other packages from this edition, except where these do not fall in the scope of emergency care (for example, electroconvulsive therapy for depression or hepatitis B vaccination). In addition, the critical presenting *syndromes* in emergency care—difficulty breathing, shock, altered mental status—and their commonly associated diagnoses are used to identify additional elements (table 13.3). As with the other packages in this edition, the essential

Table 13.2 Essential Package of Emergency Care

Protocols with Training and Capacity to Perform			
Primary health center	**First-level hospital**	**Referral and specialized hospitals**	**Crosscutting policy interventions**
Recognition of danger signs in children and adults	Acuity-based triage of children and adults		• Ensure that the National Ministry of Health has a directorate dedicated to emergency care (not limited to disaster response).
Vital signs measurement			• Conduct a standardized national assessment of the emergency care system (using the WHO ECSA or a similar tool) to identify gaps and inform system development.
BLS	ALS		• Ensure that emergency care is explicitly incorporated into the National Health Plan.
Neonatal resuscitation (including kangaroo care and thermal care for preterm newborns)	Full supportive care for preterm newborns		• Establish national legislation ensuring access to emergency care without regard to ability to pay.
Basic approach to difficulty in breathing, shock, altered mental status, trauma	Advanced approach to difficulty in breathing, shock, altered mental status, trauma	Advanced condition-specific algorithms for life-threatening conditions	• Ensure that hospitals at all levels include dedicated emergency units—areas dedicated to the provision of emergency care and staffed with at least a core of nonrotating personnel who are specifically trained in the care of emergency conditions. • Disseminate dedicated training for emergency care across cadres, including training in basic emergency care for all prehospital providers, basic emergency care training for all cadres of facility-based providers who treat patients with emergency conditions, dedicated emergency care training integrated into undergraduate medical and nursing curricula, and residency or specialist training programs in emergency medicine.
Detection of sepsis	Emergency management of sepsis		• Establish acuity-based triage systems at all facilities that regularly receive acutely ill and injured patients. • Establish prehospital care systems based on WHO or other international standards, including a dedicated certification pathway for prehospital care providers and a toll-free, universal access number for emergency care.

table continues next page

Table 13.2 Essential Package of Emergency Care **(continued)**

Protocols with Training and Capacity to Perform			
Primary health center	**First-level hospital**	**Referral and specialized hospitals**	**Crosscutting policy interventions**
			• Develop critical process and clinical protocols as identified in the WHO ECS framework (including transport and referral protocols, prehospital and facility-based clinical treatment protocols, disaster and mass casualty).
Detect and initiate treatment of severe malnutrition	Advanced treatment of severe malnutrition		• Implement standardized clinical charts and registries incorporating essential data points, such as those based on WHO standards, to facilitate quality improvement efforts.
Post exposure prevention of STI/ HIV, emergency contraception, counseling			
	Basic case-based syndromic surveillance and reporting		
	Basic communicable disease isolation	Advanced communicable disease isolation	
	Disaster and mass casualty protocols	Advanced regional response protocols for disaster and mass casualty	

Emergency Unit Procedures		
Primary health center	**First-level hospital**	**Referral and specialized hospitals**
Cervical spine immobilization	Endotracheal intubation	
Oral and nasal airway placement	Surgical airway	
Bedside swallow evaluation		
	BVM ventillation	Mechanical Ventilation
		Noninvasive positive pressure ventilation
	Oxygen administration	
	Needle decompression for tension pneumothorax	
	Placement of chest drain	
	IV fluid infusion (peripheral) for neonates, children, adults	IV infusion (central)
		Pericardiocentesis
	Defibrillation	Pacing
		Cardioversion (including synchronized)
Safe physical restraint		
	NGT placement	

table continues next page

Table 13.2 Essential Package of Emergency Care (continued)

	Emergency Unit Procedures	
Primary health center	**First-level hospital**	**Referral and specialized hospitals**
	Lumbar puncture	
	Passive rewarming techniques	Active invasive rewarming techniques
Drainage of superficial abscess		
Basic wound care	Suturing laceration	
	Escharotomy/fasciotomy	
Splinting for extremity injury	Nonoperative fracture management (closed reduction and casting)	
	Reduction of simple dislocated joint	
	Placement of external fixator; use of traction	
	Relief of urinary obstruction: catheterization or suprapubic cystostomy	
Management of labor and delivery in low risk women (BEMNOC)	(See operative services below)	
	Procedural sedation	
	Regional block	

	Operating Theatre Services	
Primary health center	**First-level hospital**	**Referral and specialized hospitals**
	Spinal anesthesia	
	General anesthesia	
	Repair of perforations: for example, perforated peptic ulcer, typhoid ileal perforation	Surgical intervention for gastrointestinal bleeding
	Appendectomy	
	Colostomy	
	Gallbladder removal	
	Hernia, including incarceration	
	Trauma laparotomy	
	Open reduction and internal fixation for fractures	
	Irrigation and debridement of open fractures	
	Emergency surgery for obstruction	
	Trauma-related amputations	

table continues next page

Table 13.2 Essential Package of Emergency Care (continued)

Operating Theatre Services		
Primary health center	**First-level hospital**	**Referral and specialized hospitals**
	Burr hole	
	Drainage of septic arthritis	
	Surgery for ectopic pregnancy	
	Cesarean section	
	Hysterectomy for uterine rupture or intractable postpartum hemorrhage	
	Dilation and curretage	

Radiology Services		
Primary health center	**First-level hospital**	**Referral and specialized hospitals**
	Comprehensive X-ray services	CT services
	Radiology performed ultrasound	
	Point of care ultrasound	

Laboratory Services		
Primary health center	**First-level hospital**	**Referral and specialized hospitals**
Point of care testing: glucose, malaria, urinalysis and urine pregnancy test, hemoglobin.	Point of care HIV testing. Laboratory complete blood counts, simple coagulation studies, urea, and electrolytes. Slide microscopy for cell counts, malaria, and wet preparation. STI testing. Capcity to collect blood culture in emergency unit prior to antibiotic administration.	Comprehensive laboratory services for emergency diagnoses, including troponin and cardiac markers, blood gas, thyroid studies, therapeutic drug levels

Medications		
ABCDEs		
Primary health center	**First-level hospital**	**Referral and specialized hospitals**
	IV paralytic (depolarizing and nondepolarizing agent)	
Oral steroids	IV steroids (for airway, CNS, and antenatal)	
Inhaled bronchodilator	Nebulized bronchodilator	
IM adrenaline	IV adrenaline	
Oral rehydration solution	IV fluids for rehydration	
	Transfusion (whole blood, FFP, packed red blood cells)	
Oral aspirin		Systemic anticoagulation

table continues next page

Table 13.2 Essential Package of Emergency Care **(continued)**

Medications		
ABCDEs		
Primary health center	First-level hospital	Referral and specialized hospitals
		Thrombolytic (streptokinase for STEMI)
	Insulin	
Oral (buccal) glucose	IV glucose	

Antidotes		
Primary health center	First-level hospital	Referral and specialized hospitals
Activated charcoal		
	Naloxone	Antithyroid agents
	Bicarbonate infusion	
	Atropine	
	Antivenin[a]	
	Pyridoxine	
Oral Vitamin K	IV Vitamin K	

Cardiac		
Primary health center	First-level hospital	Referral and specialized hospitals
Oral diuretics	IV diuretics	
		Adenosine
		Advanced vasopressor support
		Amiodarone
	Nitroglycerin SL	IV Nitroglycerin
	IV antihypertensive agent	IV Betablockers or CCB
		IV Calcium
	Oral potassium	IV Potassium

CNS		
Primary health center	First-level hospital	Referral and specialized hospitals
Oral antipsychotic	IM & IV antipsychotic	
Oral and rectal benzodiazepine	IM & IV benzodiazepine	
Oral and IM analgesia	IV analgesia	
	Local anesthesia for injection	

table continues next page

Table 13.2 Essential Package of Emergency Care **(continued)**

Obstetrics and Gynecology		
Primary health center	**First-level hospital**	**Referral and specialized hospitals**
Initiate antenatal steroids		
IM magnesium sulphate (loading dose)	Magnesium sulphate infusion[a]	
	Oxytocin for IV infusion	
	Second-line agent for PPH	
	Anti-D immunoglobulin	
	Oral agents for management of ectopic pregnancy, emergency contraception	

Vaccines		
Primary health center	**First-level hospital**	**Referral and specialized hospitals**
Tetanus vaccine		
Rabies vaccine	Antirabies immunoglobulin[a]	

Antimicrobials		
Primary health center	**First-level hospital**	**Referral and specialized hospitals**
Oral antibiotics for lung, skin, GI, or GU source (including syndromic STI treatment); PPROM)	IV antibiotics (for lung, skin, GI, GU, or CNS source; PPROM)	
Topical antifungals		
Oral antifungal		IV antifungal
Oral antimalarials	IV antimalarials	
Oral antihelminthics		
	Oral antiviral (acyclovir or equivalent)	IV antiviral (acyclovir or equivalent)
Opthalmic topical antibacterial		
Topical antidermatoparasitic agent		

Other		
Primary health center	**First-level hospital**	**Referral and specialized hospitals**
Oral paracetamol		
Oral antiemetic	IV antiemetic	
Oral zinc		
Topical agents for burn dressing		

table continues next page

Table 13.2 Essential Package of Emergency Care (continued)

		Other
Primary health center	**First-level hospital**	**Referral and specialized hospitals**
Topical steroid	Mannitol	
		Agents for acute glaucoma (IV acetazolamide, opthalmic topical steroid, opthalmic topical beta-blocker)
Surface and skin disinfectants		

Note: All resources mapped to lower levels are expected to be available at higher levels. ABCDEs = airway, breathing, circulation, disability, exposure; ALS = advanced life support; BEMNOC = basic emergency newborn and obstetric care; BLS = basic life support; BVM = bag valve mask; CCB = calcium channel blocker; CNS = central nervous system; CT = computed tomography scan; ECS = emergency care system; ECSA = emergency care system assessment; FFP = fresh frozen plasma; GI = gastrointestinal; GU = genitourinary infection; HIV = human immunodeficiency virus; IM = intramuscular; IV = intravenous; NGT = nasogastric tube; PPH = postpartum hemorrhage; PPROM = preterm premature rupture of the membranes; SL = sublingual; STEMI = ST-elevated myocardial infarction; STI = sexually transmitted infections; WHO = World Health Organization.
a. In many regions, antivenin will be kept centrally by public health authorities. Ensure timely availability to first-level hospitals.

Table 13.3 Key Diagnoses Associated with Critical Syndromes

Difficulty breathing	**Shock**	**Altered mental status**
Airway injury and inflammation	Sepsis	Coma
Foreign body	Gastroenteritis and diarrhea	Delirium
Pneumohemothorax	Bradycardia	Hypo- and hyperglycemia
Pneumonia	Hemorrhage	Hypoxia
Pleural effusion	Cardiac valvular disease	Hypo- and hyperthermia
Asthma	Abnormal cardiac rhythm or cardiac failure	Electrolyte or thyroid abnormality
Chronic obstructive pulmonary disease	Gastrointestinal bleeding	Liver disease
Anemia	Tension pneumothorax	Kidney disease
Myocardial ischemia	Anaphylaxis	Poisoning and envenomation
Cardiac failure	Spinal cord injury	Psychosis
Pericardial effusion		Seizure
Pulmonary embolism		Stroke
Drug overdose		Tumor
Chest wall injury		Traumatic brain injury
Paralysis		Central nervous system infections, including HIV-related

Note: HIV = human immunodeficiency virus.

package for emergency care highlights interventions that should be considered part of universal health coverage (Jamison and others 2013).

The following general assumptions were used as a guide in assigning components to levels of the system. It is not assumed that primary health centers have the capacity to deliver intravenous infusions or that emergency units in first-level hospitals have electrocardiogram and cardiac monitoring available. Hence, intravenous therapies are only included at the first-level hospital and above, and therapies dependent on a diagnosis of cardiac rhythm are included only at the second- or third-level hospitals. Practice conditions will vary among countries and regions, and so this constitutes a minimum package. Countries and regions with greater capacity at lower levels of the health system may want to map package components from higher levels to lower-level facilities.

COST-EFFECTIVENESS OF EMERGENCY CARE SERVICES IN LMICS

Many examples of individual emergency care services are highly cost-effective in LMICs, including the following:[3]

- *Dedicated emergency unit with formal triage.* The creation of the dedicated emergency unit in Malawi described earlier (associated with halved inpatient mortality and a reduction in the proportion of early deaths from 36 to 12.6 percent) had a cost of US$1.95 per patient (Molyneux, Ahmad, and Robertson 2006).
- *Oxygen for pneumonia.* In Papua New Guinea, introduction of an improved oxygen system (oxygen concentrators and pulse oximeters) decreased mortality risk for children with pneumonia by 35 percent. The estimated cost of this system was US$118 per patient treated, US$3,868 per life saved, and US$116 per DALY averted (Duke and others 2008).
- *Pulse oximetry for childhood pneumonia.* The modeling study that described the impact of implementing pulse oximetry combined with WHO guidelines showed that the intervention was extremely cost-effective, with estimates ranging from US$3.26 to US$72.01 per DALY averted, in the 15 countries across Africa and Asia with the highest global burden of childhood pneumonia (Floyd and others 2015).
- *Treatment of acute myocardial infarction.* In India, the incremental cost of treating, with either aspirin to a 95 percent coverage level or aspirin plus streptokinase to an 80 percent coverage level, treatment-eligible patients with acute myocardial infarction who were not yet being treated was US$0.56 and US$701 per DALY averted, respectively (Megiddo and others 2014). Early electrocardiogram diagnosis to facilitate triage and referral was shown to be cost-effective in India at US$17 per quality-adjusted life year (QALY) (Gaziano and others 2017).
- *Emergency obstetric care.* In rural India, an emergency obstetric hospital provided services at an estimated cost of US$0.43 per capita per year for the community (or US$1.50 per woman of childbearing age) (McCord and others 2001).
- *Trauma surgery.* In a Cambodian hospital dealing almost exclusively with injury (about 90 percent of cases), surgical interventions (though not all were emergency surgeries) cost approximately US$133 per DALY averted (Gosselin and Heitto 2008).
- *Emergency obstetric services.* A small hospital in rural Bangladesh demonstrated substantial DALYs averted primarily through the institution of emergency obstetric services (McCord and Chowdhury 2003).

PRIORITIES FOR ACTION

The following key priorities for policy makers and planners were derived from the WHO ECS framework (annex 13A) and represent key policy components to support delivery of the essential package of care:

- Ensure that the national ministry of health has a directorate dedicated to emergency care (not limited to disaster response).
- Conduct a standardized national assessment of the ECS (using the WHO ECSA or a similar tool) to identify gaps and inform system development.
- Ensure that emergency care is explicitly incorporated into the national health plan.
- Establish national legislation ensuring access to emergency care without regard to ability to pay.
- Ensure that hospitals at all levels include dedicated emergency units—areas dedicated to the provision of emergency care and staffed with at least a core of nonrotating personnel who are specifically trained in the care of emergency conditions.
- Disseminate dedicated training for emergency care across cadres, including training in basic emergency care for all prehospital providers, basic emergency care training for all cadres of facility-based providers who treat patients with emergency conditions, dedicated emergency care training integrated into undergraduate medical and nursing curricula, and residency or specialist training programs in emergency medicine.
- Establish acuity-based triage systems at all facilities that regularly receive acutely ill and injured patients.
- Establish prehospital care systems based on WHO or other international standards, including a dedicated certification pathway for prehospital care providers and a toll-free, universal access number for emergency care.
- Develop critical process and clinical protocols as identified in the WHO ECS framework (including transport and referral protocols, prehospital and facility-based clinical treatment protocols, and disaster and mass casualty protocols.
- Implement standardized clinical charts and registries incorporating essential data points, such as those based on WHO standards, to facilitate quality improvement efforts.

CONCLUSIONS

Conditions that can be addressed by emergency care (such as injuries, infections, obstetrical complications, stroke, myocardial infarction, and respiratory failure) account for a substantial health burden. The interventions needed to address these conditions are very cost-effective, even in limited-resource settings, but critical gaps remain in emergency care governance and delivery in LMICs. Improving the organization of and planning for emergency care services substantially improves the outcomes of patients with emergency conditions. Most of the evidence for such improvements comes from HICs, but there is growing evidence that such improvements can also be made—affordably, sustainably, and with dramatic impact—in LMICs. The WHO ECS framework and the complementary essential package of emergency care services represent a mechanism by which emergency care can be scaled up globally, accelerating progress toward universal health coverage and a range of other SDG targets.

ACKNOWLEDGMENT

The authors acknowledge with thanks the contributions of Stas Salerno Amato, Morgan Broccoli, and Jennifer Nash to the tables and figures in the chapter.

ANNEX

The annex to this chapter is as follows. It is available at http://www.dcp-3.org/DCP.

- Annex 13A: WHO Emergency Care Systems Framework.

NOTES

World Bank Income Classifications as of July 2014 are as follows, based on estimates of gross national income (GNI) per capita for 2013:

- Low-income countries (LICs) = US$1,045 or less
- Middle-income countries (MICs) are subdivided:
  (a) lower-middle-income = US$1,046 to US$4,125
  (b) upper-middle-income (UMICs) = US$4,126 to US$12,745
- High-income countries (HICs) = US$12,746 or more.

1. R. Arafat, Ministry of the Interior, Department for Emergency Situations, Government of Romania, personal communication with the author based on internal facility data, March 2016.

2. For more information on the SDGs, see http://www.un.org /sustainabledevelopment/sustainable-development-goals/.
3. All costs are adjusted to 2012 US$.

REFERENCES

Alkema, L., D. Chou, D. Hogan, S. Zhang, A. B. Moller, and others. 2016. "Global, Regional, and National Levels and Trends in Maternal Mortality between 1990 and 2015, with Scenario-Based Projections to 2030: A Systematic Analysis by the UN Maternal Mortality Estimation Inter-Agency Group." *The Lancet* 387 (10017): 462–74.

Anderson, C. S., E. Heeley, Y. Huang, J. Wang, C. Stapf, and others. 2013. "Rapid Blood-Pressure Lowering in Patients with Acute Intracerebral Hemorrhage." *New England Journal of Medicine* 368 (25): 2355–65.

Dare, A. J., J. S. Ng-Kamstra, J. Patra, S.H. Fu, P. S. Rodriguez, and others. 2015. "Deaths from Acute Abdominal Conditions and Geographical Access to Surgical Care in India: A Nationally Representative Spatial Analysis." *The Lancet Global Health* 3 (10): e646–e653.

Duke, T., F. Wandi, M. Jonathan, S. Matai, M. Kaupa, and others. 2008. "Improved Oxygen Systems for Childhood Pneumonia: A Multihospital Effectiveness Study in Papua New Guinea." *The Lancet* 372 (9646): 1328–33.

Floyd, J., L. Wu, D. Hay Burgess, R. Izadnegahdar, D. Mukanga, and others. 2015. "Evaluating the Impact of Pulse Oximetry on Childhood Pneumonia Mortality in Resource-Poor Settings." *Nature* 528 (7580): S53–S59.

Fournier, P., A. Dumont, C. Tourigny, G. Dunkley, and S. Dramé. 2009. "Improved Access to Comprehensive Emergency Obstetric Care and Its Effect on Institutional Maternal Mortality in Rural Mali." *Bulletin of the World Health Organization* 87 (1): 30–38.

Gaieski, D. F., M. E. Mikkelsen, R. A. Band, J. M. Pines, R. Massone, and others. 2010. "Impact of Time to Antibiotics on Survival in Patients with Severe Sepsis or Septic Shock in Whom Early Goal-Directed Therapy Was Initiated in the Emergency Department." *Critical Care Medicine* 38 (4): 1045–53.

Gaziano, T., M. Suhrcke, E. Brouwer, C. Levin, I. Nikolic, and others. 2017. "Costs and Cost-Effectiveness of Interventions and Policies to Prevent and Treat Cardiovascular and Respiratory Diseases." In *Disease Control Priorities* (third edition): Volume 5, *Cardiovascular, Respiratory, and Related Disorders*, edited by D. Prabhakaran, S. Anand, T. Gaziano, J.-C. Mbanya, Y. Wu, and R. Nugent. Washington, DC: World Bank.

Gosselin, R. A., and M. Heitto. 2008. "Cost-Effectiveness of a District Trauma Hospital in Battambang, Cambodia." *World Journal of Surgery* 32 (11): 2450–53.

Grimes, C. E., K. G. Bowman, C. M. Dodgion, and C. B. Lavy. 2011. "Systematic Review of Barriers to Surgical Care in Low-Income and Middle-Income Countries." *World Journal of Surgery* 35 (5): 941–50.

Henry, J., and A. Reingold. 2012. "Prehospital Trauma Systems Reduce Mortality in Developing Countries: A Systematic

Review and Meta-Analysis." *Journal of Trauma Acute Care Surgery* 73 (1): 261–68.

Higashi, H., J. J. Barendregt, N. J. Kassebaum, T. G. Weiser, S. W. Bickler, and others. 2015. "Burden of Injuries Avertable by a Basic Surgical Package in Low- and Middle-Income Regions: A Systematic Analysis from the Global Burden of Disease 2010 Study." *World Journal of Surgery* 39 (1): 1–9.

Hirshon, J., N. Risko, E. J. Calvello, S. Stewart de Ramirez, M. Narayan, and others. 2013. "Health Systems and Services: The Role of Acute Care." *Bulletin of the World Health Organization* 91 (5): 386–88.

Holmer, H., K. Oyerinde, J. G. Meara, R. Gillies, J. Liljestrand, and others. 2015. "The Global Met Need for Emergency Obstetric Care: A Systematic Review." *British Journal of Obstetrics and Gynaecology* 122 (2): 183–89.

Hortmann, M., H. J. Heppner, S. Popp, T. Lad, and M. Christ. 2014. "Reduction of Mortality in Community-Acquired Pneumonia after Implementing Standardized Care Bundles in the Emergency Department." *European Journal of Emergency Medicine* 21 (6): 429–35.

Hsiao, M., S. K. Morris, A. Malhotra, W. Suraweera, and P. Jha. 2013. "Time-Critical Mortality Conditions in Low-Income and Middle-Income Countries." *The Lancet* 381 (9871): 998–94.

Husum, H., M. Gilbert, T. Wisborg, Y. Van Heng, and M. Murad. 2003. "Rural Prehospital Trauma Systems Improve Trauma Outcome in Low-Income Countries: A Prospective Study from North Iraq and Cambodia." *Journal of Trauma* 54 (6): 1188–96.

Irfan, F. B., B. B. Irfan, and D. A. Spiegel. 2012. "Barriers to Accessing Surgical Care in Pakistan: Healthcare Barrier Model and Quantitative Systematic Review." *Journal of Surgical Research* 176 (1): 84–94.

Jacob, S. T., P. Banura, J. M. Baeten, C. C. Moore, D. Meya, and others. 2012. "The Impact of Early Monitored Management on Survival in Hospitalized Adult Ugandan Patients with Severe Sepsis: A Prospective Intervention Study." *Critical Care Medicine* 40 (7): 2050–58.

Jamison, D. T., L. H. Summers, G. Alleyne, K. J. Arrow, S. Berkley, and others. 2013. "Global Health 2035: A World Converging within a Generation." *The Lancet* 382 (9908): 1898–955.

Kausar, F., J. L. Morris, M. Fathalla, O. Ojengbede, A. Fabamwo, and others. 2012. "Nurses in Low Resource Settings Save Mothers' Lives with Non-Pneumatic Anti-Shock Garment." *Maternal Child Nursing: The American Journal of Maternal/Child Nursing* 37 (5): 308–16.

Kesinger, M. R., J. C. Puyana, and A. M. Rubiano. 2014. "Improving Trauma Care in Low- and Middle-Income Countries by Implementing a Standardized Trauma Protocol." *World Journal of Surgery* 38 (8): 1869–74.

Kobusingye, O., A. A. Hyder, D. Bishai, M. Joshipura, E. R. Hicks, and others. 2006. "Emergency Medical Services." In *Disease Control Priorities in Developing Countries*, second edition, edited by D. T. Jamison, J. G. Breman, A. R. Measham, G. Alleyne, M. Claeson, D. Evans, P. Jha, A. Mills, and P. Musgrove, 1261–80. Washington, DC: World Bank and Oxford University Press.

Mbugua, P. K., C. F. Otieno, J. K. Kayima, A. A. Amayo, and S. O. McLigeyo. 2005. "Diabetic Ketoacidosis: Clinical Presentation and Precipitating Factors at Kenyatta National Hospital, Nairobi." *East African Medical Journal* 82 (Suppl 12): S191–S196.

McCord, C., and Q. Chowdhury. 2003. "A Cost-Effective Small Hospital in Bangladesh: What It Can Mean for Emergency Obstetric Care." *International Journal of Gynecology and Obstetrics* 81 (1): 83–92.

McCord, C., R. Premkumar, S. Arole, and R. Arole. 2001. "Efficient and Effective Emergency Obstetric Care in Rural Indian Community Where Most Deliveries Are at Home." *International Journal of Gynaecology and Obstetrics* 75 (3): 297–307.

Megiddo, I., S. Chatterjee, A. Nandi, and R. Laxminarayan. 2014. "Cost-Effectiveness of Treatment and Secondary Prevention of Acute Myocardial Infarction in India: A Modeling Study." *Global Heart* 9 (4): 391–98.

Miller, S., F. Lester, and P. Hensleigh. 2004. "Prevention and Treatment of Postpartum Hemorrhage: New Advances for Low-Resource Settings." *Journal of Midwifery and Women's Health* 49 (4): 283–92.

Mock, C., M. Joshipura, C. Arreola-Risa, and R. Quansah. 2012. "An Estimate of the Number of Lives That Could Be Saved through Improvements in Trauma Care Globally." *World Journal of Surgery* 36 (5): 959–63.

Molyneux, E., S. Ahmad, and A. Robertson. 2006. "Improved Triage and Emergency Care for Children Reduces Inpatient Mortality in a Resource-Constrained Setting." *Bulletin of the World Health Organization* 84 (4): 314–19.

Murad, M. K., D. B. Issa, F. M. Mustafa, H. O. Hassan, and H. Husum. 2012. "Prehospital Trauma System Reduces Mortality in Severe Trauma: A Controlled Study of Road Traffic Casualties in Iraq." *Prehospital Disaster Medicine* 27 (1): 36–41.

Nyenwe, E. A., and A. E. Kitabchi. 2011. "Evidence-Based Management of Hyperglycemic Emergencies in Diabetes Mellitus." *Diabetes Research and Clinical Practice* 94 (3): 340–51.

Paxton, A., D. Maine, L. Freedman, D. Fry, and S. Lobis. 2005. "The Evidence for Emergency Obstetric Care." *International Journal of Gynecology and Obstetrics* 88 (2): 181–93.

Petroze, R. T., J. C. Byiringiro, G. Ntakiyiruta, S. M. Briggs, D. L. Deckelbaum, and others. 2015. "Can Focused Trauma Education Initiatives Reduce Mortality or Improve Resource Utilization in a Low-Resource Setting?" *World Journal of Surgery* 39 (4): 926–33.

Rivers, E., B. Nguyen, S. Havstad, J. Ressler, A. Muzzin, and others. 2001. "Early Goal-Directed Therapy in the Treatment of Severe Sepsis and Septic Shock," *New England Journal of Medicine* 8, no. 345 (19): 1368–77.

Sandercock, P. A., C. Counsell, M. C. Tseng, and E. Cecconi. 2014. "Oral Antiplatelet Therapy for Acute Ischaemic Stroke." *Cochrane Database of Systematic Reviews* 26 (3): CD000029.pub3.

Say, L., D. Chou, A. Gemmill, Ö. Tunçalp, A. B. Moller, and others. 2014. "Global Causes of Maternal Death: A WHO

Systematic Analysis." *The Lancet Global Health* 2 (6): e323–e333.

Sharma, S. K., P. Bovier, N. Jha, E. Alirol, L. Loutan, and others. 2013. "Effectiveness of Rapid Transport of Victims and Community Health Education on Snake Bite Fatalities in Rural Nepal." *American Journal of Tropical Medicine and Hygiene* 89 (1): 145–50.

Silva, E, P. M. de Almeida, A. C. B. Sogayar, T. Mohovic, C. L. Silva, and others. 2004. "Brazilian Sepsis Epidemiological Study (BASES Study)." *Critical Care Medicine* 8 (4): R251–R261.

Siman-Tov, M., I. Radomislensky, and K. Peleg. 2013. "Reduction in Trauma Mortality in Israel during the Last Decade (2000–2010): The Impact of Changes in the Trauma System." *Injury* 44 (11): 1448–52.

Stevenson, E. K., A. R. Rubenstein, G. T. Radin, R. S. Wiener, and A. J. Walkey. 2014. "Two Decades of Mortality Trends among Patients with Severe Sepsis: A Comparative Meta-Analysis." *Critical Care Medicine* 42 (3): 625–31.

Tallon, J. M., D. B. Fell, S. A. Karim, S. Ackroyd-Stolarz, and D. Petrie. 2012. "Influence of a Province-Wide Trauma System on Motor Vehicle Collision Process of Trauma Care and Mortality: A 10-Year Follow-Up Evaluation." *Canadian Journal of Surgery* 55 (1): 8.

Tanriover, M. D., G. S. Guven, D. Sen, S. Unal, and O. Uzun. 2006. "Epidemiology and Outcome of Sepsis in a Tertiary-Care Hospital in a Developing Country." *Epidemiology and Infection* 134 (2): 315–22.

Terkelsen, C. J., J. T. Sørensen, M. Maeng, L. O. Jensen, H. H. Tilsted, and others. 2010. "System Delay and Mortality among Patients with STEMI Treated with Primary Percutaneous Coronary Intervention." *Journal of the American Medical Association* 304 (7): 763–71.

Thind, A., R. Hsia, J. Mabweijano, E. Romero Hicks, A. Zakariah, and others. 2015. "Prehospital and Emergency Care." In *Disease Control Priorities* (third edition): Volume 1, *Essential Surgery*, edited by H. T. Debas, P. Donkor, A. Gawande, D. T. Jamison, M. Kruk, and C. N. Mock. Washington, DC: World Bank.

Vital, F. M. R., M. T. Ladeira, and A. N. Atallah. 2013. "Non-Invasive Positive Pressure Ventilation (CPAP or Bilevel NPPV) for Cardiogenic Pulmonary Oedema." *Cochrane Database of Systematic Reviews* 5: CD005351.

Wang, P., N. P. Li, Y. F. Gu, X. B. Lu, J. N. Cong, and others. 2010. "Comparison of Severe Trauma Care Effect before and after Advanced Trauma Life Support Training." *Chinese Journal of Traumatology* 13 (6): 341–44.

WHO (World Health Organization). 2010. *Monitoring the Building Blocks of Health Systems: A Handbook of Indicators and Their Measurement Strategies.* WHO: Geneva. http://www.who.int/healthinfo/systems/WHO_MBHSS_2010_full_web.pdf.

———. 2013. "Global Health Estimates for Deaths by Cause, Age, and Sex for Years 2000–2011." WHO, Geneva. http://www.who.int/healthinfo/global_burden_disease/en/.

———. n.d. "Emergency and Trauma Care," WHO, Geneva. http://www.who.int/emergencycare/activities/en.

Xavier, D., P. Pais, P. J. Devereaux, C. Xie, D. Prabhakaran, and others. 2008. "Treatment and Outcomes of Acute Coronary Syndromes in India (CREATE): A Prospective Analysis of Registry Data." *The Lancet* 371 (9622): 1435–42.

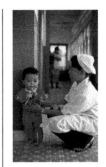

14

Community Platforms for Public Health Interventions

Melissa Sherry, Abdul Ghaffar, and David Bishai

INTRODUCTION

Community health platforms are the partnerships formed to assess and ensure public health. They provide the context in which outside interventions should be implemented and sustained, and they offer a way to develop and maintain community-centered solutions. Although local boards of health and health departments are the official bodies with the mandate to sustain strong community health platforms, they do not always achieve their full potential (Bellagio District Public Health Workshop Participants 2016). In the absence of an effective government presence, nongovernmental organizations (NGOs) can build community health platforms.

Well-functioning community health platforms can serve as vehicles for health information and advocacy and can convene local resources to support successful public health interventions. Well-designed and well-implemented community health platforms can function as the engine in the public health cycle of convening communities to monitor, review, and act (figure 14.1). These are functional tasks that are best conducted in a partnership among public health professionals, politicians, and community members. Effective partnerships among these parties ensure that health data are collected to answer questions posed by the community, that local health data are shared with the community to guide actions, and that actions marshal all of a community's human and capital resources as well as public revenue.

Then the cycle repeats. A community that has the ability to engage successfully in the cycle shown in figure 14.1 has a platform that can support all types of community health initiatives.

The provision of legal authority for community health platforms can be traced to England's first health law, the Public Health Act of 1848, which gave cities the option to create local health boards (Rosen 1958; Szreter 1988). In the mid-nineteenth century, functional health departments were established throughout Canada, Europe, and the United States before the development of effective medical care and drove the dramatic decline in mortality in the twentieth century (McKeown, Record, and Turner 1975). However, western governments had largely omitted the creation of functioning local health departments when they formed colonies in the Americas, Africa, and Asia; countries that gained independence in the mid-1900s faced an urgent need to catch up. By the late 20th century, the growing recognition that public health and primary care were lagging became the topic of international concern. In 1978, an International Conference on Primary Health Care in Alma-Ata, USSR, attended by nearly all member nations of the World Health Organization and the United Nations Children's Fund, demonstrated the degree of concern about access to primary health care (Lawn and others 2008). It resulted in the Declaration of Alma-Ata.

Corresponding author: Melissa Sherry, Johns Hopkins Bloomberg School of Public Health, Baltimore, Maryland, United States; msherry4@jhu.edu.

Figure 14.1 Public Health Cycle: Monitor, Review, and Act

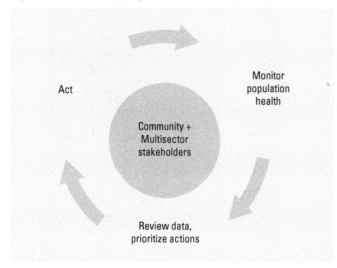

Chapter Overview

The Declaration of Alma-Ata asserted that health is a fundamental human right and that community consultation and participation in health care are essential elements of successful programs (Lawn and others 2008; Rohde and others 2008). Following the declaration, global health indicators improved despite inadequate adherence to the principles laid out in the declaration. The recent transition from the Millennium Development Goals to the Sustainable Development Goals of the United Nations has renewed attention to strategies that build on local capacity to strengthen community health platforms (Open Working Group of the General Assembly 2014).

This chapter presents a brief review of how the public health cycle supports the sustained success of any of the interventions discussed in the *Disease Control Priorities* volumes. It offers a typology of the stages of development of community health platforms, as well as a framework for assessing their success. We illustrate four stages of development of community health platforms with four case studies that range from a most developed case in Indonesia to a primitive case of near-paralysis of the state's efforts in public health. The chapter closes with a discussion of investment opportunities for policy makers who are interested in strengthening community health platforms.

Background and Historical Context

The lack of a clear roadmap to implement community involvement, combined with changes in the global economy, slowed the progress of low- and middle-income countries in achieving the primary health care goals set by Alma-Ata (Lawn and others 2008; Rohde and others 2008). The Cold War fostered a culture of development planning that emphasized interventions that were rapidly deployed and easily measured. Health commodities, such as vaccines, oral rehydration solutions, micronutrients, contraceptives, and antibiotics, became the focus of health care systems (Lawn and others 2008; Perry 2013). The emphasis of global health donors on results and short project cycles made the focus on commodities rather than systems more expedient.

The urgency of saving lives in the moment and the truth that the commodities really did save lives perpetuated a stronger emphasis on delivery of medical services and health care goods and a lighter emphasis on communities' development of Alma-Ata—style platforms. The term *vertical* was used to define projects focused on getting a selected health commodity or service to households in the most expedient way, typically using a stand-alone organization of staff, vehicles, and capital. The term *horizontal* was used to define initiatives to build more comprehensive institutions of primary care services and for population-level public health. A short-term focus on vertical programs delivering good health at low cost crowded out attention to building long-term horizontal platforms. The *World Development Report 1993: Investing in Health* (World Bank 1993) offered an excellent listing of population-level public health interventions that could be implemented, but it neglected any discussion of how to make them happen, other than by raising money. This report was novel in that it demonstrated for the first time that international health investments could be justified on the basis of having measureable outcomes and effects.

Volume 1 of the first edition of *Disease Control Priorities in Developing Countries (DCP1)* also offered a comprehensive list of public health policies, with recommendations for developing and financing state capacity in data collection and data analysis (Mosley, Bobadilla, and Jamison 1993). The authors shared aspirations for better policy environments that would be conducive to structural approaches to public health. Volume 2 of the second edition of *Disease Control Priorities in Developing Countries (DCP2)* explicitly recognized the need for community-driven global health efforts to strengthen health systems and infrastructure and suggested the need to strengthen platforms that would allow communities to hold health systems accountable for improved quality and access to services (Mills, Rasheed, and Tollman 2006). *DCP2* also emphasized that a lack of intersectoral action through cross-sector partnerships and the failure of health systems to address community-level barriers to accessing the health system were key constraints for health system strengthening (Mills, Rasheed, and Tollman 2006).

However, *DCP1, DCP2,* and the *World Development Report 1993* did not offer specific recommendations about how to create conducive policy environments that could enable and sustain public health interventions, cross-sectoral partnerships, and community engagement with local health departments (Macinko, Starfield, and Erinosho 2009; Mosley, Bobadilla, and Jamison 1993; Rohde and others 2008).

The lack of a roadmap for creating community health platforms and cross-sectoral action made room for vertical programming to dominate the policy landscape (Lawn and others 2008; Macinko, Starfield, and Erinosho 2009; Rohde and others 2008). These vertical programs saved lives, but they left populations vulnerable by failing to create resilient systems in situ that would marshal local political will and local resources to address the root causes of poor population health.

Actions that improve public health are often met with resistance about who will pay for them, because results are often less tangible and urgent than medical interventions. Further, public health actions often threaten the livelihoods of industries and occupations whose harmful aspects are regulated. Resistance is to be expected. Examples of public health actions range from the need to pay for sewers and waterworks to the need to enact and enforce restrictions on tobacco, food labeling, and road safety. Solving these problems is fundamental to public health. Solutions are often political, and vertical approaches are only partial responses.

The inability to sustain a local consensus and to mobilize community buy-in regarding the health risks leads to difficulty in imposing the measures needed to control health threats. Poorly performing public health departments are part of the reason that HIV/AIDS (human immunodeficiency virus/acquired immune deficiency syndrome) and the Ebola virus arose and overwhelmed many health systems.

Essential Public Health Functions

To improve public health functioning, between 1989 and 1994, groups at the Centers for Disease Control and Prevention and the U.S. Public Health Service developed a list of 10 essential public health functions to benchmark the quality of practice in public health agencies (Dyal 1995). The consensus was that country health ministries and regional offices needed to define national-level lists of functions and items deemed essential and that the lists should be country specific (Bettcher, Sapirie, and Goon 1998). Countries and regions have adapted their own priority lists of essential public health functions on the basis of local stakeholder input

(Bishai and others 2016). For example, the Pan American Health Organization's (PAHO) list of Essential Public Health Functions (EPHFs) is as follows (PAHO 2001):

1. Monitor health status to identify community health problems.
2. Diagnose and investigate health problems and health hazards in the community.
3. Inform, educate, and empower people about health issues.
4. Mobilize community partnerships to identify and solve health problems.
5. Develop policies and plans that support individual and community health efforts.
6. Enforce laws and regulations that protect health and ensure safety.
7. Link people to needed personal health services and assure the provision of health care when otherwise unavailable.
8. Assure a competent public and personal health care workforce.
9. Evaluate effectiveness, accessibility, and quality of personal and population-based health services.
10. Research for new insights and innovative solutions to health problems.
11. Engage in disaster preparedness to reduce the impact of emergencies and disasters on health.

PAHO's 11 items fall into the same basic cycle of monitor, review, and act shown in figure 14.1. EPHFs 1 and 2 are for monitoring; EPHFs 3–5 are for reviewing, typically through participatory multistakeholder community engagement; and EPHFs 6–11 are for acting. The best community health platforms successfully make their populations healthy by understanding what constitutes health threats and by sharing this information with community members from multiple sectors. Community health platforms mobilize parts of a coherent solution using the strengths and resources present in the community.

Health Care and Health Facilities

The care of the sick and the delivery of health commodities are integral parts of public health practice and are parts of the work plan of community health platforms. Community health workers can play multiple roles in generating health data (PAHO 2001, EPHFs 1–2), informing and mobilizing communities (PAHO 2001, EPHFs 3–5), and helping to provide primary care services (PAHO 2001, EPHFs 7–9). Many of the interventions discussed in Volume 4 of the third edition of *Disease Control Priorities* (*DCP3*) rely on facilities and community health workers (Patel and others 2015). When community health platforms fulfill their mandate to provide essential public health functions like those mentioned earlier, interventions based in facilities and involving community health workers become integrated and sustained by local support and action.

MEASURING SUCCESS IN COMMUNITY HEALTH PLATFORMS

The literature shows that community health platforms that enable participation and engagement lead to improved health outcomes (Edmunds and Albritton 2015; George and others 2015; Kenny and others 2013; McCoy, Hall, and Ridge 2012; O'Mara-Eves and others 2015; Rifkin 1996, 2014). Measuring health outcomes associated with community participation can be difficult, but community participation in public health generally leads to improvements in health knowledge, service quality, and health-related outcomes (Kenny and others 2013; Russell and others 2008).

The degree to which a community health platform is high functioning lies along a continuum. At one end is development that extends from mere delivery of services. At the other end is facilitation of an active community through an engagement platform whereby communities are informed and enabled to take shared responsibility for addressing their changing health risks and concerns (Beracochea 2015; Cyril and others 2015; Dooris and Heritage 2013; Draper, Hewitt, and Rifkin 2010; George and others 2015; McCoy, Hall, and Ridge 2012; Raeburn and others 2006; Rosato and others 2008; Russell and others 2008).

The breadth of the literature on community health platforms demonstrates the range of ways that the concept can be applied. Types of platforms described in published and gray literature generally fall into the following categories:

- Health committees
- Community health worker interventions
- Community-based participatory research and health scorecards
- NGOs or academic community partnerships for specific community interventions (Beracochea 2015; Draper, Hewitt, and Rifkin 2010; George and others 2015; Kenny and others 2013; Marmot and others 2008; Meier, Pardue, and London 2012; Rifkin 1996; Tiwari, Lommerse, and Smith 2014; UK Aid and DFID/HDRC 2011).

The literature also covers concepts of community engagement, participation, and mobilization as they relate to multiple types of community platforms (Cyril and others 2015; Draper, Hewitt, and Rifkin 2010; Frumence and others 2014; Meier, Pardue, and London 2012; Rifkin 1996, 2014; Rosato and others 2008; Russell and others 2008; UK Aid and DFID/HDRC 2011).

The likelihood that community engagement will result in improved health outcomes depends on many factors. Cyril and others (2015) identified the following components of success: engaging in real power sharing, building collaborative partnerships, providing bidirectional learning, incorporating the voice and agency of beneficiary communities in research protocol, and using multicultural health care workers for intervention delivery. Draper, Hewitt, and Rifkin (2010) suggested a continuum of process measures for use in evaluating community participation in a health system context (table 14.1).

Table 14.1 Example of Process Indicators for Participation

Indicators of participation	Continuum of community participation		
	Values for mobilization	Values for collaboration	Values for empowering
Leadership: Professionals introducing interventions, or by community of intended beneficiaries	Health professionals assume leadership. Local leadership does not necessarily try to widen the decision-making base in the community.	Collaborative decision making occurs between health professionals and community leaders. Local leadership tries to present the interests of different groups.	Program is led by community members who are selected through a representative process. Health professionals give leadership training, if necessary.
Planning and management: The way partnerships between leadership and the community are forged	Health professionals tell the community how it may participate. They decide the program's focus, goals, and activities and provide the necessary resources.	Health professionals initiate collaboration. Communities are invited to participate within a predetermined remit. Activities reflect community priorities and involve local people and existing community organizations.	Partnerships between communities and health professionals are created and institutionalized. Professionals facilitate, and the community defines priorities and manages the program. Local people learn skills they need for management and evaluation.

table continues next page

Table 14.1 Example of Process Indicators for Participation (continued)

Indicators of participation	Continuum of community participation		
	Values for mobilization	Values for collaboration	Values for empowering
Women's involvement	The inclusion of women is not specifically sought outside their traditional roles.	Women actively participate in some aspects of the program, but they have minor decision-making roles.	The active participation of women in positions of decision making and responsibility is a program objective.
External support for program development: In terms of finance and program design	Funding comes from outside the community and is controlled by health professionals. Program components are designed by health professionals.	The majority of funding comes from outside the community, but local people are asked to contribute time, money, and materials. Health professionals allocate resources, although they may consult community members. The program is designed by health professionals in discussion with community representatives. Each role in the program, including those for women and minority groups, is negotiated.	Community members work to find ways of mobilizing resources, including through external funding and their own resources (for example, microfinancing). The program is designed by community members with technical advice from health professionals on request. The design is flexible and incorporates wide community participation, including that of women and minority groups.
Monitoring and evaluation: The way intended beneficiaries are involved in these activities	Health professionals design monitoring and evaluation protocols, choose outcomes, and analyze data in ways to suit their information needs. The approach is mainly one of hypothesis testing and statistical analyses of health-related outcomes. Communities might not be made aware of the findings.	Health professionals design mixed method monitoring and evaluation protocols and perform analyses, but community members are involved in data collection. A broad definition of "success" is used. Responses to monitoring findings are jointly decided, and community feedback is both sought and given.	Communities do a participatory evaluation that produces locally meaningful findings. A variety of data collection methods is used, and the community chooses the indicators for success. Health professionals assist at the request of the community. Communities are actively involved in participatory monitoring and decide how to respond to monitoring findings. Communities contribute to wider external evaluations.
Score given	1–2	3–4	5

Source: Draper, Hewitt, and Rifkin 2010.
Note: Scores range from a low of 1 (lowest level of community participation) to 5 (highest level of community participation).

Figure 14.2 From Passive to Active Community Participation

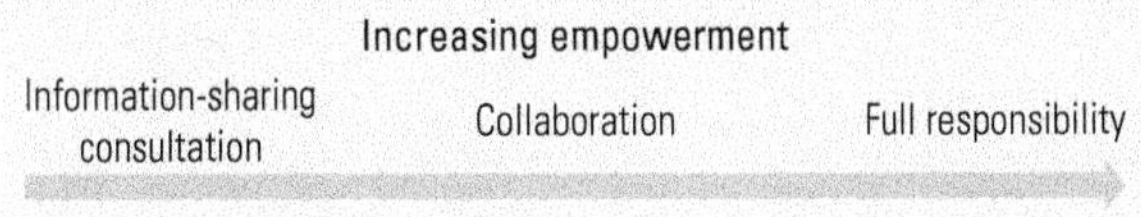

Source: Rosato and others 2008.

Figure 14.2 summarizes a process of increasing empowerment in the development of community participation.

INTERVENTIONS, POLICIES, AND EFFECTIVENESS

Community Health Platform Case Studies

We describe the continuum of developmental stages that low- and middle-income countries move through in their health systems as they improve in their ability to empower communities to take on health challenges. Using themes that emerged from the literature, we identified broad domains of function in the development of community health platforms:

- **Level of community engagement:** To what extent was the community empowered to engage with the health care system?
- **Health-system context and role of the government:** Was the health system decentralized? Did local health departments have power to innovate and to work with communities? Was the government a support or a hindrance to community health platforms?
- **Breadth of intersectoral partnerships:** Was the community able to work with NGOs, community-based

organizations, local governments, and other sectors in addition to the health sector? Did this ability predict the comprehensiveness of improvements? Was the community able to influence action across sectors?

- **Sustainability:** Was the community health platform's ability to be both scalable and sustainable a key factor in its success and longevity? This category includes the financing strategies and the ability to create lasting change while reducing inefficiencies across the system. Is the community health platform legally recognized?

- **Leadership and platform structure that promotes integration across all partners:** Who initiated the community's involvement with the health system? Did the platform create opportunities for shared vision, shared leadership and decision making, and shared financing across sectors?

Identifying Case Studies Demonstrating Community Health Platform Development

Among the countries with recent rapid reductions in mortality under age 5 years, Indonesia and Peru offer informative examples of community health platforms that have been sustainable and high achieving (Altobelli 2008; Blas, Sommerfeld, and Kurup 2011; Kowitt and others 2015; Rasanathan and others 2012; Siswanto 2009; Tanvatanakul and others 2007; Tiwari, Lommerse, and Smith 2014; Westphal and others 2011). Table 14.2 shows a staged typology of community health platforms as countries move from low-functioning platforms with little accountability (level 1) to high-functioning platforms that promote intersectoral action (level 4).

Factors That Support Successful Community Health Platforms

Supportive factors that emerged from the case study review and that contribute to sustainability include government participation, advocacy, cross-sectoral partnerships, and community-owned vetting mechanisms.

Successful community health platforms were developed to fit in the political and cultural context of the local area they served, but they were strengthened by advocacy from NGOs or universities, which also

Table 14.2 Continuum of Functioning, from High to Low, across Functional Domains of Community Health Platforms

Features	Level 1-> Poor functioning, not accountable	Level 2-> Contractor and donor driven, uncoordinated across sectors	Level 3-> Sectorwide partnerships, working to address burden of disease, but unsuccessful in improving health outcomes	Level 4 Frontier of intersectoral collaboration where all sectors and community are involved in creating health aspects in all policies, intersectoral action, existence of a global budget, and successful health outcomes
Community engagement	No platform exists for community engagement or priority setting.	Limited community engagement is through select organizations or contractors working with community for specific purposes.	Community is engaged and able to voice needs to government and other sectors.	Community works closely with government sectors, NGOs, and other community organizations to ensure needs are met.
Role of government	Government is centralized. Health system is fragmented and lacks resources to support intersectoral action for health. No accountability exists.	Contractors and donors guide government decisions. Government does not work to integrate sectors or address community needs.	Government participates in cross-sectoral partnerships.	Government is decentralized, focuses on partnerships with community and other sectors, has high accountability and transparency, has sufficient funding to support the public health and medical system, has legislation that enables public health and community integration, and uses global budgeting.
Partnerships across community	No substantial partnerships exist across sectors.	Partnerships exist between sectors, but they are limited to a few partners working together at a time, not sectorwide.	Multiple partnerships exist across sectors; integrating entity brings together government sectors, community, NGOs, and others.	Action across sectors is fully realized.

table continues next page

Table 14.2 Continuum of Functioning, from High to Low, across Functional Domains of Community Health Platforms (continued)

Features	Level 1-> Poor functioning, not accountable	Level 2-> Contractor and donor driven, uncoordinated across sectors	Level 3-> Sectorwide partnerships, working to address burden of disease, but unsuccessful in improving health outcomes	Level 4 Frontier of intersectoral collaboration where all sectors and community are involved in creating health aspects in all policies, intersectoral action, existence of a global budget, and successful health outcomes
Sustainability	Spending is wasteful, and duplication of efforts occurs; platform is not sustainable without continuous donor funding.	Sustainability is low, and platform is reliant on outside assistance to maintain health system.	Sustainability is moderate: intersectoral action improves efficiency and reduces duplication of efforts. However, continued reliance on outside funding remains necessary	Partnerships across sectors are used to fill gaps in funding across government. Improved social determinants result in improved health and less medical spending, with minimal reliance on outside funding sources.
Health outcomes	Health MDGs are not met.	Few MDGs are met.	Improvements are achieved in reaching MDGs, but substantial improvements are still needed.	Majority of MDGs are met, and social determinants are being addressed.
Type of integrator	There is no integrator.	Contractor or NGO integrates with one or two other sectors at a time.	Government or community board integrates with multiple sectors.	Government brings together all sectors in partnership to improve health.

Source: Authors.

Note: MDGs = Millennium Development Goals; NGOs = nongovernmental organizations.

provided technical support for emerging platforms. Support from the government was essential for longer-term sustainability, but strong internal and external advocates from nongovernment sectors helped communities engage with governments and health systems, which led to more formal structures.

Successful community health platforms relied on coordination across sectors to meet health goals, which resulted in reduced duplication of efforts and more efficient use of government funding. Successful platforms also provided a mechanism to vet new projects or accept funding from external donors or NGOs based on the priorities of communities. The ability of platforms to set their own health agenda further reduced duplication of efforts and empowered communities to establish control over their own health priorities.

Case Study: Gerbangmas Movement as a Community Health Platform, Lumajang District, Indonesia, Level 4

Among lower-middle-income countries, Indonesia has achieved the highest reduction in the rate of mortality under age 5 years in recent decades (Rohde and others 2008; Siswanto 2009). One component in this success was a network of community health posts (*posyandus*)

that involved communities in primary health care. In the 1980s and 1990s, these posts offered limited services, and quality and performance varied (Blas, Sommerfeld, and Kurup 2011; Siswanto 2009). After Indonesia decentralized in 2001, district governments were empowered to run district-level health systems.

The experience of Lumajang district in East Java is notable as an example of a health-in-all-policies approach driven by public health and community participation, as well as for its ability to adapt and sustain itself despite political and environmental changes over time. The district health office originally created enriched health posts with three key functions: community education, community empowerment, and community services. The enriched health post hosted activities such as clinical maternal and child health, family planning, nutrition, immunization, diarrhea control, under-five growth stimulation, and early childhood education. Other sectors outside of health care, such as education, became involved (Blas, Sommerfeld, and Kurup 2011; Siswanto 2009).

Starting in 2005, with encouragement from the governor, the district health office led subsequent efforts to create the Gerbangmas movement, a platform for communities, the public health sector, and other government sectors to work collaboratively to achieve 21 indicators of concern (Blas, Sommerfeld, and Kurup 2011; Siswanto 2009). The more specific objectives were to achieve 14 indicators for human development, 1 indicator for the economy, and 6 indicators for the household environment that together represented the priorities of the government and the community, as well as the religious, education, industry and trade, health, family planning, agriculture, and public works sectors (Blas, Sommerfeld, and Kurup 2011; Siswanto 2009). The sectors worked together with support from the district governor, leadership from a local NGO to address family welfare issues, and a funding stream that allowed all sectors to contribute to progress on the chosen indicators.

This movement for community development resulted in improvements in all indicators (Marmot and others 2008). The multisectoral Gerbangmas movement was sustainable and successful, even in the context of a changing economic and government landscape. Although the Gerbangmas movement has experienced numerous changes over time, its central tenants of building a community health platform to lead cross-sector partnerships has remained relevant in Indonesia for the past 15 years. Lessons learned from this case study illustrate important roles for local government, cross-sector partnerships, and leadership.

Heath Systems and Role of Local Government

The development of the Gerbangmas movement stemmed from decentralization of the Indonesian health system, allowing peripheral innovation. The local government offered support and leadership for the initiative, as well as a mechanism for funding. Once the movement was planned and funded, the district health office created a single vehicle through which the communities, the health system, and other sectors could collaborate around common goals without competing for volunteers or resources. The district health office did not dominate the partnership; it included itself as a stakeholder, with leadership provided by a neutral entity.

Partnerships across Sectors

The partnership structure provided clear roles for each sector to develop programs to help achieve the shared indicators. The district PKK (a family welfare semigovernmental NGO consisting of spouses of government officials and community members) helped coordinate and support the partnership across organizations. The funding structure created a common pool of funds from which communities were able to draw for investment in interventions in multiple sectors. Some sectors also contributed funds to achieve action plans. Essentially, the partnership structure of this movement allowed sectors to compete for community dollars in their respective programs, while preventing duplication of efforts and competition across sectors (Blas, Sommerfeld, and Kurup 2011; Siswanto 2009).

The district governor mandated that all community empowerment programs use the Gerbangmas movement as an entry point, thereby reducing competition and keeping outside interests (such as those from NGOs) from affecting the success of the partnerships across sectors (Blas, Sommerfeld, and Kurup 2011; Siswanto 2009). With the community at the center of the partnership structure, a hierarchy that placed all sectors on equal footing, and a common set of indicators to work toward, the Gerbangmas movement helped sectors work together effectively.

Leadership and Integration

The district health office was the initial champion for the Gerbangmas movement, which eventually assumed the role of the integrated health platform. During the initial scale-up from health posts to enriched health posts, the district health office garnered support from local government and encouraged involvement of other sectors (such as education) while demonstrating the importance of involving other sectors in achieving common health goals. As the health posts evolved into enriched posts, or Gerbangmas health posts (figure 14.3), the district health office took a step back to participate as a member of a team engaging other sectors; an NGO took on a more significant role as an integrator and coordinator of the movement. Part of the significance of an NGO's heading an integrated platform is that such an organization can be sector neutral, allowing each sector equal weight in achieving agreed-upon goals. Notably, the community itself held power over the management of the programs and the priorities of the Gerbangmas movement.

Role of Communities

Community volunteers conducted needs surveys in their respective villages, and maps of community needs were developed on the basis of the data gathered. The community problems in each village were discussed in open forums where members created action plans. Final proposals were drawn up that became the community action plans. Community members had input on the allocation of funds. Financing came from government funding allocation and from financial contributions from the community. Community volunteers also participated in the monitoring and evaluation of activities that had been carried out each year.

District Gerbangmas teams trained subdistrict teams. A training-of-trainers approach helped educate

Figure 14.3 Evolution of Conventional Health Posts to Gerbangmas Health Posts in Lumajang District

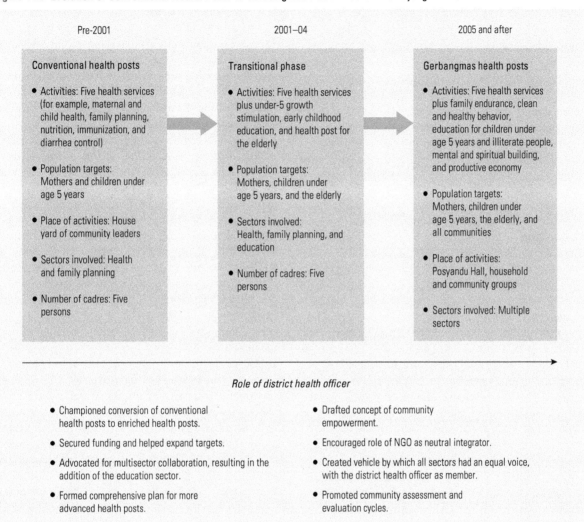

Pre-2001

Conventional health posts

- Activities: Five health services (for example, maternal and child health, family planning, nutrition, immunization, and diarrhea control)

- Population targets: Mothers and children under age 5 years

- Place of activities: House yard of community leaders

- Sectors involved: Health and family planning

- Number of cadres: Five persons

2001–04

Transitional phase

- Activities: Five health services plus under-5 growth stimulation, early childhood education, and health post for the elderly

- Population targets: Mothers, children under age 5 years, and the elderly

- Sectors involved: Health, family planning, and education

- Number of cadres: Five persons

2005 and after

Gerbangmas health posts

- Activities: Five health services plus family endurance, clean and healthy behavior, education for children under age 5 years and illiterate people, mental and spiritual building, and productive economy

- Population targets: Mothers, children under age 5 years, the elderly, and all communities

- Place of activities: Posyandu Hall, household and community groups

- Sectors involved: Multiple sectors

Role of district health officer

- Championed conversion of conventional health posts to enriched health posts.

- Secured funding and helped expand targets.

- Advocated for multisector collaboration, resulting in the addition of the education sector.

- Formed comprehensive plan for more advanced health posts.

- Drafted concept of community empowerment.

- Encouraged role of NGO as neutral integrator.

- Created vehicle by which all sectors had an equal voice, with the district health officer as member.

- Promoted community assessment and evaluation cycles.

Source: Adapted from Siswanto 2009.
Note: NGO = nongovernmental organization.

many community volunteers and village staff members on the way to assess community health, facilitate community dialogue about the findings to lead to community involvement in proposing and implementing action plans, and evaluate the results of those plans (Blas, Sommerfeld, and Kurup 2011; Siswanto 2009).

Sustainability

Sustainability was supported by an overall structure that included resources, funding, and training from partnering organizations and did not rely on grant funds or external donor dollars (Blas, Sommerfeld, and Kurup 2011; Siswanto 2009). In addition, the partnership structure did not depend on the success of any single organization or leader. The largest hurdle to sustainability was the turnover of government officials. Sustainability relied on the new district governor's approval of the Gerbangmas movement in the subsequent five-year plan. In response, the district government created an official book on the Gerbangmas movement, including write-ups of the success of the movement in the governor's accountability report. The report covered a summary of the governor's achievements during his term and included the movement as policy in the district regulation, which was ratified by the district legislative body (Blas, Sommerfeld, and Kurup 2011; Siswanto 2009).

Case Study: Local Health Administration Committees, Peru, Level 3

The Peruvian government has legalized, regulated, and institutionalized community participation as a means of ensuring its role in primary health care (Altobelli 2008; Beracochea 2015; Blas, Sommerfeld, and Kurup 2011; Iwami and Petchey 2002). Local health administration communities (comunidades locales de administración en salud, or CLAS) are private, nonprofit civil associations that have agreements with the government to receive and administer public funding for the purpose of implementing primary health care services responsive to community needs.

Evolution of Local Health Administration Committees

The path to development of the CLAS movement was a complicated one. The CLAS movement emerged in 1994, following the collapse of the health sector in Peru. Terrorism and hyperinflation were major national challenges, and decentralization was beginning (Altobelli 2008; Beracochea 2015; Blas, Sommerfeld, and Kurup 2011; Iwami and Petchey 2002). Rural areas had a strong mistrust of the government; initial efforts to expand primary health care in these areas resulted in further mistrust, because community members often felt mistreated by physicians (Altobelli 2008; Beracochea 2015; Blas, Sommerfeld, and Kurup 2011; Iwami and Petchey 2002). When Jaime Freundt became the minister of health in the mid-1990s, he sought reform through a process that involved convening technical experts and community members. As a result, a new form of CLAS was proposed (Altobelli 2008; Beracochea 2015; Blas, Sommerfeld, and Kurup 2011; Iwami and Petchey 2002).

Role of Communities

In the new CLAS, community members were part of a civil association under the authority of the Peruvian Civil Code. Community members had a formal relationship with the government by electing community representatives to a general assembly that worked with the regional health directorates (Altobelli 2008; Beracochea 2015; Blas, Sommerfeld, and Kurup 2011; Iwami and Petchey 2002).

The elected assembly provided a way to demand accountability from health personnel (Altobelli 2008; Beracochea 2015; Blas, Sommerfeld, and Kurup 2011; Iwami and Petchey 2002). The CLAS became a platform through which community representatives and volunteers could perform public health roles of community assessment, identifying health priorities across local

areas, guiding interventions, and choosing where resources should be allocated. The CLAS structure also allowed communities to control the quality of care and distribution of services. Unlike a community advisory board in which participation is often based on board members' advising those with the power to make decisions and allocate funding, each CLAS had the power and resources to act as the local health department for its respective community.

The CLAS's financing came from direct government transfers from general revenue, reimbursements from the government health insurance program for the poor, and in-kind stocks of medicines and supplies from the regional health directorates. Control over allocation of these funds resided in the hands of the CLAS (Altobelli 2008; Beracochea 2015; Blas, Sommerfeld, and Kurup 2011; Iwami and Petchey 2002). The CLAS assemblies conducted community assessments for health needs and helped identify unmet health needs to determine how best to tailor primary health care services to local contexts (Iwami and Petchey 2002).

Sustainability

The CLAS movement began as a pilot with 250 health facilities incorporated into the program. Early evaluations showed improved equity, quality, and coverage of health services in CLAS facilities, compared to non-CLAS facilities (Beracochea 2015). Advocates helped demonstrate the positive effects of the model, and in 2007, the Peruvian Congress approved a statute for citizen participation in primary health care at local levels. The passage of this law ensured the sustainability of the CLAS movement and confirmed Peru's commitment to empowering communities to have some control over their own health care (Altobelli 2008).

CLAS Achievements

The CLAS movement increased the availability of physicians in rural areas; improved access to care for the poor; improved usage rates, especially for children; improved quality in health facilities; and improved connections among people in Peruvian communities (Altobelli 2008; Beracochea 2015; Blas, Sommerfeld, and Kurup 2011; Iwami and Petchey 2002). These achievements were the result of the communities' ability to allocate budgets to attract higher numbers of physicians to areas where they were needed and to provide full or partial fee exemptions based on financial need. In addition, the number of women members of the CLAS general assembly grew substantially (Altobelli 2008; Beracochea 2015; Blas, Sommerfeld, and Kurup 2011; Iwami and Petchey 2002).

Heath Systems and Role of Government

One interesting lesson learned from the CLAS movement is that public mistrust of the government can be counteracted through structures for communities to take ownership and oversight of public programs (Altobelli 2008; Beracochea 2015; Blas, Sommerfeld, and Kurup 2011; Iwami and Petchey 2002). The CLAS movement was a key driver in creating transparency, participation, and social control over the health system that built community trust and improved relations between communities and the government (Altobelli 2008). The Ministry of Health, with internal and external champions, was instrumental in helping the CLAS expansion to continue and become law (Altobelli 2008).

Partnerships across Sectors

In addition to primary health care needs, CLAS began to focus on the development needs of communities through community work plans that used discretionary funds and partnerships with local municipalities to allocate dollars to community-identified development projects (Beracochea 2015). CLAS appears to be well on its way to transitioning from level 3 to level 4 in the typology of table 14.2; CLAS is already a community platform for addressing health needs and is broadening its intersectoral reach to partner with additional sectors. The CLAS movement has been spreading through the SEED-SCALE model of sustainability (Taylor and Taylor 2002). Successful models in each region served as training centers and hubs for lateral diffusion of innovations.

Case Study: Community Scorecards in Nine Districts, Uganda, Level 2

Examples of contractor- and donor-driven platforms (level 2 in table 14.2) are fairly common in practice, and extensive literature documents this approach. We present a district scorecard program conducted in Uganda in 2004 to promote community oversight of health services at the primary care level.

The goal of the intervention was to strengthen provider accountability through a process that used community organizations as facilitators of village-level meetings to inform communities about the status of health service delivery in their area relative to the standards held in surrounding areas (Abdul Latif Jameel Poverty Action Lab 2015; Björkman and Svensson 2009, 2010). Facilitators encouraged community members to identify areas for improvement in health service provision and to develop action plans that could lead to improvements (Abdul Latif Jameel

Poverty Action Lab 2015; Björkman and Svensson 2009, 2010). The intervention sought to create a community-led process of monitoring to ensure that health care workers were performing their assigned tasks (Abdul Latif Jameel Poverty Action Lab 2015; Björkman and Svensson 2009, 2010). The results of the study indicated that, compared to control communities, community-based monitoring improved the quality and quantity of primary care delivered, reduced the number of deaths among children under age 5 years, improved outpatient service use, and improved quality measures such as wait time in primary care (Abdul Latif Jameel Poverty Action Lab 2015; Björkman and Svensson 2009, 2010).

Analysis of Uganda District Scorecards

The example of the district scorecard study in Uganda represented a limited intervention that was driven by outside agencies for the purposes of involving the community in health service improvement. Despite positive outcomes, ongoing success was reliant on ongoing collection of scores from scorecards by third-party entities (Abdul Latif Jameel Poverty Action Lab 2015; Björkman and Svensson 2009, 2010).

Health Systems and Role of Government

In Uganda's decentralized system, local health unit management committees monitored the day-to-day health service activities of the public dispensaries. The government was not the driver of the interventions and did not have a large role in the improvements to community health, other than through its role in running the committees (Abdul Latif Jameel Poverty Action Lab 2015; Björkman and Svensson 2009, 2010).

Partnerships across Sectors

Partnerships across sectors were limited in this example. NGOs and community organizations participated in community meetings, but there were few other partnerships across sectors or across government agencies (Abdul Latif Jameel Poverty Action Lab 2015; Björkman and Svensson 2009, 2010).

Leadership and Integration

The community health platform was originally developed by researchers at the University of Stockholm and the World Bank, and the researchers generated the report cards that served as the basis for the program. Local NGOs facilitated program meetings and served as community leaders for the intervention. There was no means for integration across sectors (Björkman and Svensson 2009, 2010).

Role of Communities

The role of communities was to attend meetings where health care provider performance and quality were examined, discuss health care delivery problems that could be improved, and develop action plans for needed changes (Abdul Latif Jameel Poverty Action Lab 2015; Björkman and Svensson 2009, 2010). Although the communities' ability to hold health care providers accountable was limited, they were able to participate in the improvement process and were given a voice for addressing their concerns.

Sustainability

Because the scorecards—determined to be a crucial piece of this intervention—were not developed by communities or the government, this intervention was scalable and sustainable only as long as researchers continued to provide data, or until a cheaper and more direct way of creating the scorecards was established (Abdul Latif Jameel Poverty Action Lab 2015; Björkman and Svensson 2009, 2010). Without further government and community buy-in to allocate resources to these activities, the district scorecard intervention faced many challenges in scalability and sustainability.

Case Study: Weak Government Platforms for Community Empowerment, Haiti, Level 1

Challenges to Development of Community Health Platforms

Haiti faces many challenges in developing local government engagement of community health platforms. It provides a case study where important lessons can be learned about the role of NGOs and donor agencies in helping promote or hinder development of community health platforms.

Haiti has long suffered from natural disasters, disease outbreaks, poverty and social divisions, political instability, and other social and political inequalities that have led to instability (Fatton 2006; James 2010). Numerous NGOs arrived with varying agendas; before the 2010 earthquake, an estimated 8,000–9,000 were working in the country (Batley and McLoughlin 2010; Zanotti 2010). Nearly all of the interventions in the education, health, and development sectors were led by NGOs, which provided 70 percent of health care services and 85 percent of education support (Vaux and Visman 2005; Zanotti 2010). The flow of funds through NGOs rather than the government weakened the elected government, created instability, and further undermined the accountability and sustainability of the state (Zanotti 2010). After the earthquake, the negligible state capacity

that did exist was destroyed, and the vulnerability of the state and subsequent reliance on NGOs, faith-based organizations, and formal providers for care was further exposed (Hill and others 2014).

Given the diversity of NGOs working throughout Haiti, health care delivery was largely inconsistent in quality, quantity, and coordination across the country (Hill and others 2014). The role of the Ministry of Public Health and Population was marginal, and external resources were often allocated according to the priorities of NGOs or donors (Hill and others 2014; Zanotti 2010). Ultimately, many of these NGOs did not have local origins, did not understand local context, and did not focus on creating sustainable, responsive platforms where communities could be empowered to address their own health needs (Zanotti 2010).

Analysis of Haiti's Challenges with Development of Successful Community Health Platforms

Unreliable health services and access to those services promoted health inequities and created a reliance on external entities that created difficulties for communities to voice their own needs (Hill and others 2014). Lack of service integration and coordination led to further fragmentation and duplication of efforts, and Haitians often relied on traditional medicine that was widely available (Hill and others 2014).

Despite the challenges, Haiti's structure also provides the opportunity for NGOs to develop community health platforms that are responsive and engage local communities. Several NGOs engaged the needs of communities and helped build community capacity in the areas of development, health, and education. Successful NGOs had several factors in common:

- They had local origins in Haiti.
- They had a diverse international network of donors and were not accountable to a single funder or government agency.
- They focused on addressing local needs and the needs of the poorest individuals.
- They shared a vision that tied economy, politics, and human rights (Zanotti 2010).

Health Systems and Role of Government

The weakness of the state and the reliance on NGOs created an environment in which external entities often influenced resource allocation and priority setting. The lack of a focus on Haitian governance and the subsequent lack of health system structure and community input created difficulties for the community to engage meaningfully in the public health process and hampered the creation of sustainable and responsive health care systems.

The ability of communities to hold the government accountable for health service access and quality was nearly absent.

Partnership across Sectors

Coordination among health and other sectors has been slow owing to lack of government leadership. However, successful NGOs acknowledged the importance of other sectors in improving health outcomes and worked on issues of sanitation, economic development, and education, in addition to health (Zanotti 2010). NGOs served as providers of services, as well as social advocates pursuing reforms to address poverty and social injustice (Zanotti 2010).

Leadership and Integration

One of the key difficulties that Haiti faces in creating community health platforms is that the country's leaders are highly influenced by external funding sources. The ability of an NGO to make decisions on the basis of community needs would be much greater if it did not depend on external agencies with specific agendas. Addressing community needs requires flexibility in setting agendas that not all NGOs possess.

Role of Communities

Successful NGOs were those that were able to engage communities, to set priorities for community input, and to include communities in identifying problems and developing and delivering solutions. These included, for example, community health workers and health care providers (Zanotti 2010).

Sustainability

One of Haiti's most significant challenges is creating sustainable solutions in the presence of NGOs that provide the majority of the health-related services in the country. NGOs that can create a platform through which communities can carry out basic public health functions and partner with other sectors to address the social determinants of health represent a way forward. NGOs that can empower communities and provide them with the necessary skills are setting the stage for the sustainability and effectiveness of a future health system.

STRENGTHENING COMMUNITY HEALTH PLATFORMS

Benefits of Strengthening Community Health Platforms

The reviewed literature and the focal case studies highlight the benefits of and provide a framework for strengthening community health platforms. The benefits arise whether the priority is (a) implementing or scaling up delivery of commodities, services, and programs or (b) building the capacity of communities to identify and address long-standing and emerging public health problems.

The benefits of stronger platforms arise because the more health platforms develop along the continuum in table 14.2, the better they can carry out the essential public health functions and the cycle of monitoring, reviewing, and acting to achieve solutions. Strength means the capability of health data collection through local surveillance and outbreak investigation. Strength means that public health personnel can find ways to share the data with their communities and to engage communities in developing local solutions that mobilize external resources as well as untapped resources in communities. Strength also means that local public health personnel can facilitate implementation of existing programs and develop modifications in response to emerging issues.

Because only some communities have community health platforms that can effectively carry out essential public health functions, outsiders often develop action plans that can succeed in the absence of these platforms. The unintended consequence of neglecting core strength in community health platforms is the continued building of partial substitutes for what community health platforms ought to be doing. The partial substitutes crowd out the necessary business of building indigenous strength.

Factors That Strengthen Community Health Platforms

Our review found the following identifiable factors that strengthen community health platforms:

- Access to data about health problems and health threats
- The means and will to share data and control with community members
- Achievement of a balance between delivering clinical services and preventing disease in whole populations
- Advocacy to maintain community engagement against pressure to consolidate control.

In some cases, these factors were present fortuitously. However, evidence suggests that the success factors can be present as the result of intention and effort. A commitment to engage community stakeholders cannot be maintained for long simply because of circumstances. However, a widespread political movement toward openness and grassroots engagement can make maintaining a community orientation easier.

Priorities for Investment in Strengthening Community Health Platforms

Effective strategies must come from taking stock of the current position of a community on the development continuum shown in table 14.2. Tools to measure a community's performance of essential public health functions have been used extensively in the Americas (Corso and others 2000; PAHO 2001; Upshaw 2000). Measurement of current strength in public health care services through a performance and quality improvement tool that targets the essential public health functions can help identify areas of emphasis within a district if the measures are provided to the public health staff to help create a performance improvement plan (Bishai and others 2016).

A strategy to develop community health platforms requires a modest investment in a central unit devoted to the quality of public health practice. Quality units are a growing feature in public health departments (Gunzenhauser and others 2010). The best practice for a quality unit is to use measurement of practice as a conversation starter rather than a disciplinary bludgeon. A public health practice quality unit for a central or regional health ministry requires a small investment. The budget should allow a team of district supervisors to make quarterly supervisory visits to specified districts and remain in regular electronic communication. Checklists and protocols for supervisory visits have been developed and are available from several sources. (The library of these resources can be found at http://www.ianphi.org/documents/pdfs/evaluationtool and https://sites.google.com/site/ephfjhu/.)

CONCLUSIONS

Communities vary in their level of sophistication in conducting a cycle of monitoring, reviewing, and acting on the basis of local data and local multisector community-engaged partnerships. Helping communities do this well is a concept that goes back to the foundations of the field of public health. Because good health can exist at low cost with vertical programs that rescue people regardless of their community's functional level, making the case for investing in community resilience can be challenging. The situation does not need to be an "either-or" option; the way forward ought to be a "both-and" option. Rescuing and building resilience are complementary. Especially where budgets are finite, strong community health platforms can marshal new resources to the service of public health.

Valuing Community Health Platforms

Given the common misinterpretation that cost-effectiveness (as dollars per disability-adjusted life year averted) is the key to understanding an intervention's value, one might be lulled into thinking that any investment that cannot show its disability-adjusted life years averted is wasteful—perhaps even unethical, given that people are dying of preventable causes every day.

Without initiatives to help community health platforms flourish around the world, the health gains promised by interventions will cost more and deliver less. Communities will miss opportunities to activate partners and resources that can shift health determinants in schools and workplaces and the commerce, transport, and culture sectors. Political will to make changes in public health law enforcement and regulation and to hold governments accountable is a precious resource that community health platforms can nurture and maintain. With the availability of local data, local forums for sharing data, and local multisectoral stakeholder engagement, the solutions will work better and deliver more. This human infrastructure has been neglected for far too long.

A Way Forward for Health Systems

With the Sustainable Development Goals and calls for health system resilience, we are entering a new era in which this neglect of community engagement and capacity is ending (Bellagio District Public Health Workshop Participants 2016). Community health platforms require a respectful trust that people being presented with data about their health problems and evidence about what works to solve the problems will choose wisely. Community health platforms require a recognition that health is too big for the health care sector alone; we need a decision-making forum that includes the education sector, commercial interests, transportation, law enforcement, and media. These partnerships are essential if we are to address upstream social determinants.

Our model of community health platforms is explicitly drawn at the local level. The national and global policy makers have important roles in setting up expectations and tools to support local communities. Fundamentally, human bodies are small objects; most of the time, what makes a body sick (or worse) is a microbe from across the street or a cigarette from the local store or a speeding car with a drunk driver behind the wheel. Protecting a body requires a protector that is close to that body. The emerging burden of noncommunicable diseases caused by health behavior choices, lifestyles, mental health trauma, and injuries underscores the need for local approaches. High-income country data show that noncommunicable disease burdens differ intensely at the scale of a census tract. Modern cities are seeing life-expectancy differentials of 20 years across neighborhoods.

The other advantage of local communities is their sheer number. For a failed state, efforts to work at the national level can remain frustrating for decades. At the local level, one can find failed communities, but one can also find successful communities. One can even find successful communities inside failed states and accomplish at subnational levels what cannot be done when a central government is not prioritizing health.

The model of community health platforms asks local government health officials to play a prominent role as conveners and integrators. Government presence does not suggest that government workers perform all of the roles in the public health cycle. The decisions about who does what emerge from the community, on the basis of its own stock of possible actors and doers. Community health platforms can mobilize resources through volunteers and voluntary activities independent of the budgets of governments and donors.

A Chinese proverb says that the best time to plant a tree was 20 years ago, and the second-best time is today. High-functioning community health platforms are the trees that we wish our ancestors had planted in every community many years ago. Future generations cannot afford to have us spend the next 20 years attending to local epidemics and global pandemics that could have been snuffed out and quickly controlled if all local communities had been performing all of the essential public health functions and engaging their communities in building a culture of health.

ACKNOWLEDGMENTS

The authors gratefully acknowledge helpful comments from Henry Mosley, MD, Johns Hopkins Bloomberg School of Public Health, Johns Hopkins University, Baltimore, MD, United States.

NOTE

World Bank Income Classifications as of July 2014 are as follows, based on estimates of gross national income (GNI) per capita for 2013:

- Low-income countries (LICs) = US$1,045 or less
- Middle-income countries (MICs) are subdivided:
  (a) lower-middle-income = US$1,046 to US$4,125
  (b) upper-middle-income (UMICs) = US$4,126 to US$12,745
- High-income countries (HICs) = US$12,746 or more.

REFERENCES

Abdul Latif Jameel Poverty Action Lab. 2015. "The Power of Information in Community Monitoring." *J-PAL Policy Briefcase*, July. https://www.povertyactionlab.org/sites/default/files/publications/Community%20Monitoring_2.pdf.

Altobelli, L. 2008. "Case Study of CLAS in Peru: Opportunity and Empowerment for Health Equity." Prepared for Case Studies of Programmes Addressing Social Determinants of Health and Equity, Priority Public Health Conditions–Knowledge Network, World Health Organization (WHO) Commission on Social Determinants of Health, with support from the Alliance for Health Policy and Systems Research, WHO, Geneva.

Batley, R., and C. McLoughlin. 2010. "Engagement with Non-State Service Providers in Fragile States: Reconciling State Building and Service Delivery." *Development Policy Review* 28 (10): 131–54.

Bellagio District Public Health Workshop Participants. 2016. "Public Health Performance Strengthening at Districts: Rationale and Blueprint for Action." White paper prepared after the Bellagio Conference, New York City, November 21–25. www.who.int/alliance-hpsr/bellagiowhitepaper.pdf.

Beracochea, E. 2015. *Improving Aid in Global Health*. New York: Springer.

Bettcher, D. W., S. Sapirie, and E. H. Goon. 1998. "Essential Public Health Functions: Results of the International Delphi Study." *World Health Statistics Quarterly* 51 (1): 44–54.

Bishai, D., M. K. Sherry, C. Pereira, S. Chicumbe, F. Mbofana, and others. 2016. "Development and Usefulness of a District Health Systems Tool for Performance Improvement in Essential Public Health Functions in Botswana and Mozambique." *Journal of Public Health Management and Practice* 22 (6): 586–96.

Björkman, M., and J. Svensson. 2009. "Power to the People: Evidence from a Randomized Field Experiment on Community-Based Monitoring in Uganda." *Quarterly Journal of Economics* 124 (2): 735–69.

———. 2010. "When Is Community-Based Monitoring Effective? Evidence from a Randomized Experiment in Primary Health in Uganda." *Journal of European Economic Association* 8 (2–3): 571–81.

Blas, E., J. Sommerfeld, and A. S. Kurup. 2011. *Social Determinants Approaches to Public Health: From Concept to Practice.* Geneva: World Health Organization.

Corso, L. C., P. J. Wiesner, P. K. Halverson, and C. K. Brown. 2000. "Using the Essential Services as a Foundation for Performance Measurement and Assessment of Local Public Health Systems." *Journal of Public Health Management and Practice* 6 (5): 1–18.

Cyril, S., B. J. Smith, A. Possamai-Inesedy, and A. M. Renzaho. 2015. "Exploring the Role of Community Engagement in Improving the Health of Disadvantaged Populations: A Systematic Review." *Global Health Action* 8: 29842.

Dooris, M., and Z. Heritage. 2013. "Healthy Cities: Facilitating the Active Participation and Empowerment of Local People." *Journal of Urban Health* 90 (Suppl 1): 74–91.

Draper, A. K., G. Hewitt, and S. Rifkin. 2010. "Chasing the Dragon: Developing Indicators for the Assessment of Community Participation in Health Programmes." *Social Science and Medicine* 71 (6): 1102–09.

Dyal, W. W. 1995. "Ten Organizational Practices of Public Health: A Historical Perspective." *American Journal of Preventive Medicine* 11 (Suppl 6): 6–8.

Edmunds, M., and E. Albritton. 2015. "Global Public Health Systems Innovations: A Scan of Promising Practices." AcademyHealth, Washington, DC, and Robert Wood Johnson Foundation, Princeton, NJ.

Fatton, R. 2006. "Haiti: The Saturnalia of Emancipation and the Vicissitudes of Predatory Rule." *Third World Quarterly* 27 (1): 115–33.

Frumence, G., T. Nyamhanga, M. Mwangu, and A. K. Hurtig. 2014. "Participation in Health Planning in a Decentralised Health System: Experiences from Facility Governing Committees in the Kongwa District of Tanzania." *Global Public Health* 9 (10): 1125–38.

George, A., K. Scott, S. Garimella, S. Mondal, R. Ved, and K. Sheikh. 2015. "Anchoring Contextual Analysis in Health Policy and Systems Research: A Narrative Review of Contextual Factors Influencing Health Committees in Low and Middle Income Countries." *Social Science and Medicine* 133: 159–67.

Gunzenhauser, J., Z. Eggena, J. Fielding, K. Smith, D. Jacobson, and N. Bazini-Barakat. 2010. "The Quality Improvement Experience in a High-Performing Local Health Department: Los Angeles County." *Journal of Public Health Management and Practice* 16 (1): 39–48.

Hill, P. S., E. Pavignani, M. Michael, M. Murru, and M. Beesley. 2014. "The 'Empty Void' Is a Crowded Space: Health Service Provision at the Margins of Fragile and Conflict Affected States." *Conflict and Health* 8 (20).

Iwami, M., and R. Petchey. 2002. "A CLAS Act? Community-Based Organizations, Health Service Decentralization and Primary Care Development in Peru." *Journal of Public Health Medicine* 26 (4): 246–51.

James, E. C. 2010. "Ruptures, Rights, and Repair: The Political Economy of Trauma in Haiti." *Social Science and Medicine* 70 (1): 106–13.

Kenny, A., N. Hyett, J. Sawtell, V. Dickson-Swift, J. Farmer, and P. O'Meara. 2013. "Community Participation in Rural Health: A Scoping Review." *BMC Health Services Research* 13: 64–72.

Kowitt, S. D., D. Emmerling, E. B. Fisher, and C. Tanasugarn. 2015. "Community Health Workers as Agents of Health Promotion: Analyzing Thailand's Village Health Volunteer Program." *Journal of Community Health* 40 (4): 780–88.

Lawn, J. E., J. Rohde, S. Rifkin, M. Were, V. K. Paul, and M. Chopra. 2008. "Alma-Ata 30 Years On: Revolutionary, Relevant, and Time to Revitalise." *The Lancet* 372 (9642): 917–27.

Macinko, J. S., B. Starfield, and T. Erinosho. 2009. "The Impact of Primary Healthcare on Population Health in Low- and Middle-Income Countries." *Journal of Ambulatory Care Management* 32 (2): 150–71.

Marmot, M., S. Friel, R. Bell, T. A. J. Houweling, and S. Taylor, for the Commission on Social Determinants of Health. 2008. "Closing the Gap in a Generation: Health Equity through Action on the Social Determinants of Health." *The Lancet* 372 (9650): 1661–69.

McCoy, D. C., J. A. Hall, and M. Ridge. 2012. "A Systematic Review of the Literature for Evidence on Health Facility Committees in Low- and Middle-Income Countries." *Health Policy Plan* 27 (6): 449–66.

McKeown, T., R. G. Record, and R. D. Turner. 1975. "An Interpretation of the Decline of Mortality in England and Wales during the Twentieth Century." *Population Studies* 29: 391–422.

Meier, B. M., C. Pardue, and L. London. 2012. "Implementing Community Participation through Legislative Reform: A Study of the Policy Framework for Community Participation in Western Cape Province of South Africa." *BMC International Health and Human Rights* 12: 15–29.

Mills, A., F. Rasheed, and S. Tollman. 2006. "Strengthening Health Systems." In *Disease Control Priorities in Developing Countries,* second edition, edited by D. T. Jamison, J. G. Bremen, A. R. Measham, G. Alleyne, M. Claeson, D. B. Evans, P. Jha, A. Mills, and P. Musgrove. Washington, DC: World Bank and Oxford University Press.

Mosley, W. H., J. L. Bobadilla, and D. T. Jamison. 1993. "The Health Transition: Implications for Health Policy in Developing Countries." In *Disease Control Priorities in Developing Countries,* edited by D. T. Jamison, W. H. Mosley, A. R. Measham, and J. L. Bobadilla. Washington, DC: World Bank; New York: Oxford University Press.

O'Mara-Eves, A., G. Brunton, S. Oliver, J. Kavanagh, F. Jamal, and J. Thomas. 2015. "The Effectiveness of Community Engagement in Public Health Interventions for Disadvantaged Groups: A Meta-Analysis." *BMC Public Health* 15: 129.

Open Working Group of the General Assembly. 2014. "Open Working Group Proposal for Sustainable Development Goals." A/68/970, United Nations, New York. http://undocs.org/A/68/970.

PAHO (Pan American Health Organization). 2001. *Public Health in the Americas.* Washington, DC: PAHO.

Patel, V., D. Chisholm, T. Dua, R. Laxminarayan, and M. E. Medina-Mora, eds. 2015. *Disease Control Priorities* (third edition): Volume 4, *Mental, Neurological, and Substance Use Disorders*. Washington, DC: World Bank.

Perry, H. B. 2013. "Primary Health Care: A Redefinition, History, Trends, Controversies and Challenges." White paper, Unpublished.

Raeburn, J., M. Akerman, K. Chuengsatiansup, F. Mejia, and O. Oladepo. 2006. "Community Capacity Building and Health Promotion in a Globalized World." *Health Promotion International* 21 (Suppl 1): 84–90.

Rasanathan, K., T. Posayanonda, M. Birmingham, and V. Tangcharoensathien. 2012. "Innovation and Participation for Healthy Public Policy: The First National Health Assembly in Thailand." *Health Expectations* 15 (1): 87–96.

Rifkin, S. B. 1996. "Paradigms Lost: Toward a New Understanding of Community Participation in Health Programmes." *Acta Tropica* 61 (2): 79–92.

———. 2014. "Examining the Links between Community Participation and Health Outcomes: A Review of the Literature." *Health Policy and Planning* 29 (Suppl 2): ii98–106.

Rohde, J., S. Cousens, M. Chopra, V. Tangcharoensathien, R. Black, and others. 2008. "30 Years after Alma-Ata: Has Primary Health Care Worked in Countries?" *The Lancet* 372 (9642): 950–61.

Rosato, M., G. Laverack, L. H. Grabman, P. Tripathy, N. Nair, and others. 2008. "Community Participation: Lessons for Maternal, Newborn, and Child Health." *The Lancet* 372 (9642): 962–71.

Rosen, G. 1958. *A History of Public Health*. Baltimore, MD: Johns Hopkins University Press.

Russell, N., S. Ingras, N. Johri, H. Kuoh, M. Pavin, and J. Wickstrom. 2008. "The Active Community Engagement Continuum." Project Working Paper, July, ACQUIRE Project, New York, and United States Agency for International Development, Washington, DC. http://www.acquireproject.org/fileadmin/user_upload/ACQUIRE/Publications/ACE-Working-Paper-final.pdf.

Siswanto, E. S. 2009. "Community Empowerment through Intersectoral Action: A Case Study of Gerbangmas in Lumajang District." *Jurnal Managemen Pelayanan Keshehatan* 12 (1).

Szreter, S. 1988. "The Importance of Social Intervention in Britain's Mortality Decline c. 1850–1914: A Reinterpretation of the Role of Public Health." *Social History of Medicine* 1 (1): 1–38.

Tanvatanakul, V., C. Vicente, J. Amado, and S. Saowakontha. 2007. "Strengthening Health Development at the Community Level in Thailand: What Events Should Be Managed?" *World Health and Population* 9 (1): 65–73.

Taylor, D. C., and C. E. Taylor. 2002. *A Just and Lasting Change: When Communities Own Their Own Futures*. Baltimore, MD: Johns Hopkins University Press.

Tiwari, R., M. Lommerse, and D. Smith. 2014. M^2 *Models and Methodologies for Community Engagement*. Singapore: Springer.

UK Aid and DFID/HDRC (Department for International Development, United Kingdom/Human Development Resource Centre). 2011. "Helpdesk Report: Community Engagement in Health Service Delivery." November 16, DFID, London.

Upshaw, V. 2000. "The National Public Health Performance Standards Program: Will It Strengthen Governance of Local Public Health?" *Journal of Public Health Management and Practice* 6 (5): 88–92.

Vaux, T., and E. Visman. 2005. *Service Delivery in Countries Emerging from Conflict*. Report, Centre for International Co-operation and Security, University of Bradford, Bradford, U.K.

Westphal, M. F., F. Zioni, M. F. Almeida, and P. R. Nascimento. 2011. "Monitoring Millennium Development Goals in Brazilian Municipalities: Challenges to Be Met in Facing Up to Iniquities." *Cadernos de saude publica* 27 (Suppl 2): S155–63.

World Bank. *World Development Report 1993: Investing in Health*. Washington, DC: World Bank.

Zanotti, L. 2010. "Cacophonies of Aid, Failed State Building and NGOs in Haiti: Setting the Stage for Disaster, Envisioning the Future." *Third World Quarterly* 31 (5): 755–71.

Chapter 15

Rehabilitation: Essential along the Continuum of Care

Jody-Anne Mills, Elanie Marks, Teri Reynolds, and Alarcos Cieza

INTRODUCTION

The World Health Organization (WHO) has defined rehabilitation as "a set of interventions designed to optimize functioning and reduce disability in individuals with health conditions, in interaction with their environment" (Nas and others 2015, 1). Rehabilitation interventions optimize well-being by addressing impairments, limitations, and restrictions in many areas (areas as disparate as mobility, vision, and cognition), as well as by considering personal and environmental factors (Nas and others 2015).

Individuals with health conditions or injuries may require rehabilitation across the course of their lifespan. The timing and type of intervention that a rehabilitation provider selects depend greatly on several factors. These include the etiology and severity of the person's health condition, the prognosis, the way in which the person's condition affects the person's ability to function in the environment, as well as the individual's identified personal goals.

Rehabilitation services may be delivered in any setting (including in hospitals and in communities), depending on individuals' needs and situation. In hospitals, acute rehabilitation is particularly important in facilitating recovery, maximizing the effect of emergency and

surgical services, preventing complications, and ensuring that the optimal functional outcome is achieved. Rehabilitation in the community similarly aims to optimize functioning in those who are not in the hospital system, to identify needs, and to provide services in a person's typical environment. Community rehabilitation services frequently are accessed by those with chronic health conditions or sensory impairment, as well as by children with developmental conditions.

The demand for community- and hospital-based rehabilitation services will continue to grow as the result of several factors. First is the significant epidemiological transition and demographic shift underway globally (Dalal and others 2015; Dias and others 2013; GBD 2015 Disease and Injury Incidence and Prevalence Collaborators 2016). Second, as access to care expands to universal health coverage, rehabilitation is essential for maximizing the effectiveness of a range of medical and surgical interventions. Finally, injuries (which remain an escalating public health concern in some countries) also contribute substantially to the demand for rehabilitation services (WHO 2014). These factors suggest that the positive health, social, and economic effects of rehabilitation will have a more profound influence on population health in coming years (WHO 2016a).

Corresponding author: Alarcos Cieza, Department for Management of Noncommunicable Diseases, Disability, Violence, and Injury Prevention, World Health Organization, Geneva, Switzerland; ciezaa@who.int.

GROWING DEMAND FOR REHABILITATION SERVICES

Health and Population Trends

The prevalence of noncommunicable diseases has increased by 13.7 percent in the past 10 years (GBD 2015 Disease and Injury Incidence and Prevalence Collaborators 2016). Noncommunicable diseases and associated health complications can have a profound effect across functioning domains, such as mobility, respiration, vision, cognition, and communication. Studies have shown that rehabilitation can effectively assist in prevention of and recovery from various health conditions. Stroke and cardiac rehabilitation have been shown to be effective in increasing independence, reducing mortality, and reducing hospital readmissions (Jolliffe and others 2000; Stroke Unit Trialists' Collaboration 2013; Taylor and others 2010). Similarly, rehabilitation following amputation improves physical functioning and improves the likelihood of home discharge from the hospital (Fleury, Salih, and Peel 2013; Kurichi and others 2009).

Demand for rehabilitation services directly corresponds to the incidence of injuries (such as those caused by road traffic crashes, burns, near drownings, falls, and poisonings). For every one of the more than 5 million people who die as the result of injuries every year, 10 to 15 more people are estimated to survive, many with ensuing impairment. A significant portion of injuries are caused by road traffic injuries (WHO 2014), which are predicted to become the seventh leading cause of death by 2030. The number of road traffic injuries is anticipated to increase, especially in low-income countries as economies develop and more people use vehicles (Gosselin and others 2009). Along with surgical and medical interventions, rehabilitation helps to mitigate the profound socioeconomic impact of nonfatal injuries.

The consequences of the demographic shift currently underway globally are substantial; the number of individuals older than age 60 years is projected to increase 56 percent globally by 2030 (UN 2015). Aging is associated with natural decrements in intrinsic capacity (such as declines in musculoskeletal strength and cognitive function) that increase vulnerability to health conditions and injuries (WHO 2015). Widespread availability of rehabilitation services is essential for health systems to be able to respond effectively to the needs of older populations. Numerous studies have concluded that community-based rehabilitation increases the safety and independence of older people, reduces the risk of falls, and decreases the need for hospital and nursing home admissions (Beswick and others 2008; Gillespie and others 2012). Ensuring that the disabilities associated with aging are minimized is a major priority for policy development (UN 2015); health systems need to take concerted action to ensure that they can provide older populations with the requisite services.

The potential benefits of rehabilitation services are not restricted to aging and adult populations. Children constitute a significant and important portion of users of rehabilitation services. Although fertility rates are slowly declining in many low- and lower-middle-income countries, populations continue to expand. For example, 48 percent of the population of Chad and 42 percent of the population of Timor-Leste are between ages 0–14 years (World Bank 2016). Furthermore, while child mortality rates are declining, not all who survive actually thrive (Grantham-McGregor and others 2007; WHO 2016b). Early interventions that optimize developmental outcomes for children with various health conditions (including neurological, congenital, and intellectual impairments), as well as injuries, can positively affect participation rates in education, community activities, and future capacity to work.

Expanded Access to Health Care

As access to more advanced emergency, trauma, and medical care expands, rehabilitation becomes proportionally more important. It constitutes an essential aspect of care for many of those who experience, or are at risk of experiencing, short-term or long-term residual impairment and functioning limitations following injuries or illnesses. These include the following:

- Individuals with injuries or medical conditions requiring lower-limb amputation. Amputations may effectively save lives, but mobility will decline substantially without proper postoperative stump management, strengthening, and training in the use of a mobility device such as a prosthesis (Fleury, Salih, and Peel 2013; Godlwana, Stewart, and Musenge 2015).
- Children with spastic cerebral palsy. Antispasmodic medication may be effective, but children's independence may be largely unchanged without adequate supported seating, splinting, and functional retraining (Aisen and others 2011; Novak and others 2013).
- People with burn injuries. Such individuals may benefit from skin grafting, but rehabilitation is required from the acute to long-term phase of recovery to prevent or minimize skin contractures, to regain strength

and dexterity, and to maximize functional outcomes (Proctor 2010).

- Those with spinal cord injuries (particularly complete and high-level injuries) who have received optimal care in the acute phase. Without access to appropriate rehabilitation and long-term care, such individuals may experience potentially fatal complications, such as pressure sores and urinary tract infections (Nas and others 2015).

Integrating rehabilitation into health care systems and providing early access to services can benefit both individuals and health systems. Such integration can help to ensure optimal outcomes from medical and surgical interventions, and it can mitigate the risks of ongoing complications that may burden the health system. Furthermore, the benefits of rehabilitation are realized beyond the health system. By restoring functioning, rehabilitation can enable people to take up or resume family and work roles and can enable them to participate in education and community life, with potentially substantial economic and social implications (WHO 2017).

UNMET REHABILITATION NEEDS AND PROMISING PROGRAMS IN MIDDLE-INCOME COUNTRIES

In many parts of the world, the capacity to provide rehabilitation is limited or nonexistent, and the needs of the population remain largely unmet (Anchique Santos and others 2014; Atijosan and others 2009). Analysis suggests that 92 percent of the burden of disease in the world is related to an etiology for which rehabilitation may be required; it further suggests that a strong negative relationship exists between countries with the highest rehabilitation need and the availability of rehabilitation professionals (Gupta, Castillo-Laborde, and Landry 2011).

The true effect of this unmet need is difficult to capture, partly because the benefits of rehabilitation are realized longitudinally and in outcomes that are more challenging to measure (such as participation in work and education). Moreover, few studies have assessed the long-term and comprehensive effects of rehabilitation; these effects may be made manifest in the ability to return to or engage in meaningful occupation and gainful employment, to participate in education, and to achieve a degree of independence with self-care tasks. Deductive inference suggests, however, that the health and social impacts of failing to receive necessary rehabilitation services will fall most heavily on those who are the most economically disadvantaged. The lack of robust impact studies notwithstanding, substantial evidence on the effectiveness of rehabilitation on health, economic, and quality of life outcomes provides ample impetus to adopt a systematic approach to building and strengthening rehabilitation services. Several examples from upper-middle-income countries demonstrate the feasibility of implementing rehabilitation interventions in health systems with limited resources for health and a diversity of approaches to doing so.

Expanding the Availability of Rehabilitation in Mexico

Mexico responded to its population's growing rehabilitation needs by developing 46 first-level rehabilitation units that provide evaluation, therapy, and referral; these units are staffed by physiatrists, physiotherapists, social workers, and nurses. The development of these units has increased Mexico's rehabilitation services capacity by 60 percent. In addition to these services, Mexico also has 1,444 community-based basic rehabilitation units distributed across the country, and rehabilitation services are integrated in general and specialized hospitals and institutions (Guzman and Salazar 2014).

Speeding Access to Acute Rehabilitation in Brazil

The Orthopaedic and Traumatology Institute at a hospital in São Paulo, Brazil, has created a simplified rehabilitation program to address the rehabilitation needs of those in its care. Before the program's development, people who sustained spinal cord injuries, amputations following limb injuries, and severe musculoskeletal injuries had to wait to receive therapy for up to one year following their injuries. For many people, this delay resulted in devastating secondary complications that easily could have been prevented, such as pressure sores, joint deformities, and chronic pain. The program has had a profound effect on the prevention of complications and resulting functional outcomes, and it demonstrates how facilities with limited resources can benefit from basic rehabilitation strategies (Mock and others 2006).

ECONOMIC CASE FOR INVESTMENT

The diversity in the scope of rehabilitation interventions and the settings in which they are provided create a challenge for cost-effectiveness assessments. This limitation notwithstanding, several examples of the application of rehabilitation in the context of specific conditions demonstrate cost savings. These tend to capture cost benefits in the acute phase of care for health systems and not the economic advantages for service users, which may be more profound.

Cost savings associated with rehabilitation are not always fully accrued by the health sector. They may be realized through reduction in ongoing care costs provided by social services, the persons themselves, or their family members. A multicenter cohort analysis from 62 rehabilitation services in third-level hospitals in the United Kingdom (Turner-Stokes and others 2016) found specialized rehabilitation for complex neurological conditions to be highly cost-efficient. The weekly care costs for a person with a spinal cord injury who was highly dependent were reduced by £847; approximately 22.7 months were needed to offset the cost of the rehabilitation episode.

Rehabilitation also has been found to be cost-effective in the context of preoperative and postoperative care. Provision of rehabilitation before and after lumbar spine fusion surgery in a hospital in Denmark resulted in lower costs for both the hospital and patients. In addition to the benefit of reduced hospital length of stay, costs were 1,625€ lower per patient once direct (hospital fees) and indirect fees (financial burden for patients before returning to work) were considered (Nielsen and others 2008).

Whereas large, high-quality methodical studies of rehabilitation cost-effectiveness originate predominately from high-income countries, studies from low- and middle-income countries (LMICs) suggest that the same is true in these settings. Cardiac rehabilitation in LMICs, for example, has been found to save costs, compared with routine management based on provider judgment. In Brazil, cardiac rehabilitation leads to mean monthly savings per patient of US$190. In Colombia, the economic benefit was calculated as significantly higher; the cost-effectiveness of a typical cardiac rehabilitation program for patients with heart failure is estimated to be US$998 per quality-adjusted life year, compared with usual care with five-year follow-up (Oldridge, Pakosh, and Thomas 2016).

Although the literature is limited to high-income countries, promising evidence of the cost-effectiveness of rehabilitation programs for reintegration into the workplace exists (European Agency for Safety and Health at Work 2016; Franche and others 2005). Studies suggest that although there is an initial investment in return-to-work programs (typically incurred by the employer), there can be a substantial return for society. Cost savings are almost entirely due to foregone benefit payments (Bardos, Burak, and Ben-Shalom 2015). One study found that return-to-work rehabilitation programs resulted in a 25 to 30 percent reduction in lost workdays

and a 40 percent reduction in health care costs (for individuals with short-term disabilities) (Beal 2007). Another study found that that for every dollar invested in return-to-work rehabilitation, $2.35 is returned to society (Na 2016). The magnitude of return on investment to taxpayers is dependent on the disability scheme in the country; regardless, without return-to-work programs, employees affected by injury or illness may face substantial reductions in standard of living. Depending on the availability of resources, such programs could be adjusted for most settings.

ESSENTIAL PACKAGE OF REHABILITATION INTERVENTIONS

The essential package of interventions presented in table 15.1 is an initial attempt to compile rehabilitation interventions in a minimum essential set of services. The interventions are based on the *International Classification of Functioning, Disability, and Health* (WHO 2001) and the *International Classification of Health Interventions* (WHO 2016c). As such, the interventions are not mapped to specific diagnoses and may be performed in the context of many health conditions. The rehabilitation interventions included in the essential package are targeted at resource-constrained settings, such as a district hospital in Sub-Saharan Africa. However, countries are not restricted to this level; when the package is applied in settings with greater resource availability, countries are encouraged to expand the scope, quality, and availability of interventions.

Certain important adjuncts to rehabilitation have not been included in this package of interventions. Prescription of medication (for example, analgesia to assist with pain management or antispasmodic medication to assist with tone or spasticity) also may be considered if it is in the scope of practice of the provider. Use of medication during selected interventions, or as an intervention in its own right, can assist with patient comfort and ability to participate in functional activities. Psychological interventions also are an important component of rehabilitation, not only in the context of mental health, but also for people experiencing different impairments (such as physical or sensory). Mental health interventions for adults and children are exclusively covered in the third edition of *Disease Control Priorities (DCP3)*, volume 4, *Mental, Neurological, and Substance Use Disorders* (chapters 4 [Hyman and others 2015] and 8 [Scott and others 2015]).

The rehabilitation workforce is potentially the most important mechanism for delivering the package

Table 15.1 Essential Package of Rehabilitation Interventions

Intervention area	Platform for delivery		
	Community[a]	Primary health center	Hospital[b]
Musculoskeletal system			
	Transfer training		Prescription[c] of mobility techniques customized to the condition and individual
	Mobility training (including gait training)		
			Acute mobilization—inpatients and outpatients
	Basic lower limb, upper limb, and trunk/spine exercise and symptom management programs according to standard protocols based on presentation	Simple lower limb, upper limb, and trunk/spine exercise and symptom management programs based on diagnosis (condition specific)	Prescription[c] of lower limb, upper limb, and trunk/spine exercise and symptom management programs customized to the condition and individual
	• Joint mobilization		
	• Stretches/range of movement		
	• Strengthening		
			Postamputation management
			• Stump care
			• Limb positioning
		Ponseti clubfoot treatment	
	Body repositioning for		
	• Pressure area care		
	• Supportive seating, in wheelchairs		
	Upper limb functional retraining		Prescription[c] of upper limb functional retraining techniques customized to the condition and individual
	• Functional gross and fine motor movement patterns		
	• Compensatory strategies		Prescription[c] of scar and contracture management techniques to optimize range of movement
Cardiorespiratory system	Cardiac rehabilitation (such as recommendations for physical activity, nutrition, and risk factor management)		Prescription[c] of a cardiac rehabilitation program customized to the condition and individual
	Breathing exercises to improve respiratory function, including sputum clearance techniques		Chest function interventions, including sputum clearance techniques

table continues next page

Table 15.1 Essential Package of Rehabilitation Interventions (continued)

	Platform for delivery		
Intervention area	Community[a]	Primary health center	Hospital[b]
Neurological systems and communication	Basic swallow retraining/interventions		Prescription[c] of swallow retraining techniques customized to the condition and individual
			Acute swallow management for inpatients
	Speech and communication interventions		Prescription[c] of speech and communication techniques customized to the condition and individual
	• Interventions for aphasia and ataxia		
	• Sign language		
	• Other alternative mechanisms of communication		
	Cognitive interventions		Prescription[c] of cognitive interventions customized to the condition and individual
	• Training in basic-level cognitive functions		
	• Cognitive compensatory strategies (techniques and provision of assistive products)		
	• Early stimulation for children		
Mechanical stabilization and assistive products		Prosthesis review and referral to hospital if indicated	Fabrication, fitting, and training in the use of a prosthesis[d]
		Splinting and orthosis review and referral to hospital if indicated	Splinting and orthosis[e] for upper limb, lower limb, and spine immobilization and stability
			Postoperative splinting and orthosis[e]
		Upper limb positioning	
		• Slings	
		• Casting	
			Compression therapy[f] for postamputation management, burns, and vascular and lymphatic conditions
	Provision and training in the use of assistive products, assistive technology, and compensatory strategies for		Provision and training in the use of assistive products, assistive technology, and compensatory strategies for
	• Mobility, activities of daily living, and skin care		• Hearing aids and hearing loops[d]
	• Vision loss (such as white canes, braille displays, magnification, and other aids)		
	• Communication devices		

table continues next page

Table 15.1 Essential Package of Rehabilitation Interventions (continued)

Intervention area	Platform for delivery		
	Community[a]	Primary health center	Hospital[b]
Cross-cutting areas	Self-care training		Prescription[c] of self-care techniques customized to the condition and individual
	Early childhood development rehabilitation interventions (such as motor, sensory, and language stimulation)		
	Environmental modifications (such as a grab rail or ramp installation)		

Note: This table identifies a package of essential rehabilitation interventions that an effective rehabilitation system must be able to provide. The interventions selected are based on expert opinion from key stakeholders representing a broad range of rehabilitation disciplines.

- Interventions in red are considered acute and urgent.
- All interventions assigned to a given level also should be available at higher levels.
- Medications (such as pain medication to assist with pain management, and antispasmodic medication to assist with tone or spasticity) are not included here, but they may be essential adjuncts to these interventions.
- Interventions have been broadly categorized into intervention areas for the purposes of readability; however, substantial overlap exists in interventions between categories. For example, a person may require mobility training for musculoskeletal, cardiorespiratory, and neurological conditions; however, within the package it has been categorized under the musculoskeletal system intervention area.

A glossary of intervention terms is available in annex 15A.

a. The rehabilitation interventions in the community may need to be delivered by a specialized rehabilitation provider, whereas others may be delivered by generalist community-health workers or other care providers. The level of skill required of the provider depends on the complexity of a person's needs. Where warranted, interventions should be done under the prescription or supervision of a specialized rehabilitation provider based in the community or in the hospital setting.

b. Hospital-based rehabilitation interventions, in first-level and third-level hospitals, are highly variable across countries. Thus, first-level and third-level hospitals are considered as a single delivery setting for the purposes of this package.

c. A rehabilitation prescription is the provision of interventions customized for an individual's condition or specific needs, for ongoing self-management, or to be carried out by another provider. Education is provided to the individual and others involved in the individual's care to enable them to carry out the prescribed interventions safely and effectively. Such education may include instruction on correct technique, precautions, and specifications of the regime. Prescription and education usually require the input of a specialized rehabilitation provider.

d. This intervention also can occur in outpatient settings, although it usually takes place in hospitals.

e. This intervention requires access to immobilizing materials (such as thermoplastic, casting, or locally sourced materials) and knowledge of fabrication and application principles, techniques, and precautions.

f. This intervention can be done only if the providers are adequately trained in compression bandaging or garment fitting and provision and only if they are aware of precautions and contraindications. It is usually provided in a specialist outpatient service setting (such as a burn unit, plastic surgery facility, or vascular clinic).

of interventions. Specialized rehabilitation providers include but are not limited to physiatrists, physiotherapists, occupational therapists, and speech and language pathologists, who together have the capability to provide interventions across the full scope of needs existing in populations. However, the availability of such a workforce is rare in countries where rehabilitation is young and underdeveloped. In such cases, the skills required to conduct basic-level rehabilitation interventions (those that do not require complex clinical reasoning and are compatible with foundational health knowledge, skills, and competencies) may be distributed across the existing health workforce by using transdisciplinary approaches and by developing or strengthening a mid-level rehabilitation workforce. Where possible, models of service delivery in which supervision or oversight by a rehabilitation professional is provided to less qualified providers can expand access to services while reducing the risk of inappropriate interventions.

The package does not indicate specific rehabilitation disciplines that will be held responsible for providing the interventions, so as to be applicable to a range of settings and levels of rehabilitation workforce capability. However, an underlying assumption exists that providers at the primary health center level will be generalists with minimal rehabilitation training, whereas hospital-based providers will have specialized training. Unlike other areas, rehabilitation interventions in the community may need to be delivered by a specialized rehabilitation provider, whereas others may be delivered by generalist community-health workers or other providers. In the Essential Package of Interventions, a broad spectrum of skills is required to deliver many of the interventions, largely dependent on the complexity of the needs of the person (such as the presence of comorbidities, the severity of the health condition, and other personal and environmental factors). The effectiveness of the interventions depends heavily on a provider's skills, experience, and clinical reasoning. At a minimum, interventions need to be delivered on the basis of the person's underlying health condition; applying interventions irrespective of etiology can be both dangerous and ineffective.

Although interventions ideally should be customized to specific conditions and individual needs and goals (referred to as "prescriptions" in the package), the provision of rehabilitation should not be dependent on such an approach. Prescribing customized interventions requires a level of clinical reasoning that may be available by providers at the hospital level, but beyond the capabilities of a mid-level rehabilitation provider or generalist health worker in primary health centers or the community. In such instances, interventions can be delivered according to standardized protocols on the basis of presentation and condition. In the package, it is assumed that interventions delivered in the community may be delivered by providers capable of following preexisting standardized protocols for different presentations that, although not customized, can have great effect. Providers at the primary health center level, where a diagnosis may be more readily available, may be capable of delivering condition-specific interventions, but may not be able to customize them according to individual or complex needs.

Given the variability in training and level of specialization of the rehabilitation workforce in LMICs, for the sake of both quality and safety, countries and services must consider the competencies of their workforce (as well as other resource and contextual factors) when planning to implement the package. Annex 15A is a glossary that provides a brief description of the interventions that can be used to further guide decision making.

The interventions are organized across three service delivery platforms: community, primary health centers, and inpatient hospitals. Because of the substantial global variability in the rehabilitation capacity of first-level and referral hospitals, no differentiation is made between these settings. The service delivery platforms do not correspond with the providers' level of expertise; some community and primary health center–based interventions (such as recommendations for specific environmental modifications and cognitive interventions) should be delivered by specialist providers. The package reflects the necessity of providing rehabilitation in both the community and hospital settings. Delivery of the intervention is not restricted to the service delivery platform under which it is positioned; this positioning reflects only the intervention's typical point of delivery. In particular, the package has been targeted to low-resource health systems; systems with greater resource availability should aim to provide the most comprehensive package of services possible at the most accessible level of the delivery.

Substantial evidence supports the provision of rehabilitation at the earliest possible stages and across the continuum of care: acute, subacute, and long-term care (Choi and others 2008; Parker, Sricharoenchai, and Needham 2013; Scivoletto, Morganti, and Molinari 2005; Stucki and others 2005). Depending on the etiology of their condition, people may need to access rehabilitation at any level of the health system and likely will continue to require services as they move in and between levels. Community-based services are necessary to ensure that those people requiring rehabilitation who are not in hospital systems (such as children with sensory and developmental conditions) are identified and receive early intervention. Provision of rehabilitation in hospitals (including acute wards) is similarly imperative to prevent complications, to speed recovery, and to link people to follow-up care beyond discharge (Stucki and others 2005).

AVAILABLE TOOLS TO INFORM REHABILITATION SYSTEM PLANNING

The WHO has developed tools to assist countries in strengthening rehabilitation in their health systems, including the following:

- **The WHO Rehabilitation System Assessment Tool**[1]
  The Rehabilitation System Assessment Tool comprises (1) a survey-based tool on system-wide rehabilitation capacity and (2) a field component that assesses the rehabilitation system performance. A clear understanding of the various elements of the rehabilitation system that are available and how the system is working is essential to inform which interventions should be offered and how best to deliver them.
- *Rehabilitation in Health Systems*
  The publication *Rehabilitation in Health Systems* outlines nine fundamental recommendations for strengthening rehabilitation in health systems (WHO 2017). The recommendations highlight the strong need for rehabilitation to be integrated across all levels of the health system, as well as the need for financial allocation to ensure sustainable, quality service delivery.

Further information on both resources, as well as others under development (such as a toolkit for rehabilitation development), is available at the WHO rehabilitation website: http://www.who.int/disabilities /care/en/.

PRIORITIES FOR ACTION

The following actions are key for policy makers seeking to strengthen and extend quality rehabilitation services:

- Establish education and certification pathways for dedicated rehabilitation providers.
- Ensure the availability of appropriately skilled rehabilitation providers in specialized inpatient settings.
- Include rehabilitation in national health plans and financing schemes.
- Ensure that health insurance (where it exists or is to be implemented) covers rehabilitation interventions.
- Integrate rehabilitation into both community- and hospital-based health services.
- Implement financial and procurement policies to ensure that high-quality assistive products (as well as training in their proper use) are available to all who need them.

Research Priorities

Critical gaps exist in the evidence base for rehabilitation. A substantial increase in research is urgently needed to guide priority setting for system planning and to increase the availability and effectiveness of rehabilitation services. Several of the research priorities included in the WHO's *Rehabilitation in Health Systems* (WHO 2017) are particularly pertinent to rehabilitation policy:

- Research to ascertain the cost benefit of rehabilitation
- Research to identify facilitators and barriers to accessing rehabilitation
- Research to enable a standardized measure of rehabilitation effect.

CONCLUSIONS

Given the increasing demand for rehabilitation around the world, the need to extend the availability of essential rehabilitation interventions is urgent. Commendable efforts in several LMICs demonstrate the feasibility of improving rehabilitation capacity and performance in resource-poor settings. The *DCP3* package of essential rehabilitation interventions is designed to help scale up rehabilitation services to reach those who need them most. The package is informed by expert consensus and the limited evidence base available. As further evidence emerges, future iterations may reflect changes to the package of interventions.

To have the greatest effect on population health, careful attention needs to be given to the systems that deliver rehabilitation services, the training and skills of the rehabilitation workforce, and the financing and monitoring of rehabilitation delivery. Whereas rehabilitation plays a critical role in optimizing health outcomes, advances in the field have lagged those in other areas with comparable effects. Recognizing rehabilitation's contribution to improving functioning and the quality of life and its importance to the effectiveness of other health interventions is fundamental to correcting this disparity.

ANNEX

The annex to this chapter is as follows. It is available at http://www.dcp-3.org/DCP.

- Annex 15A. Glossary of Rehabilitation Intervention Terminology

ACKNOWLEDGMENTS

The following people contributed to the development of the Essential Package of Rehabilitation Interventions through research and peer review: Li-Rong Cheng (International Association of Logopedics and Phoniatrics), Christoph Gutenbunner and Boya Nugraha (International Society of Physical and Rehabilitation Medicine), Kaloyan Kamenov (WHO and Instituto de Salud Carlos III, Centro de Investigación Biomédica en Red, CIBERSAM), Pauline Kleinitz (Ludwig-Maximillians University), Ritchard Ledgerd (World Federation of Occupational Therapists), Chiara Retis (Handicap International), and Catherine Sykes (World Confederation of Physical Therapy).

NOTES

World Bank Income Classifications as of July 2014 are as follows, based on estimates of gross national income (GNI) per capita for 2013:

- Low-income countries (LICs) = US$1,045 or less
- Middle-income countries (MICs) are subdivided:
  (a) lower-middle-income = US$1,046 to US$4,125
  (b) upper-middle-income (UMICs) = US$4,126 to US$12,745
- High-income countries (HICs) = US$12,746 or more.

1. The WHO Rehabilitation System Assessment tool is not publicly available but is provided by the WHO on request when appropriate. Contact details are located on the home page: http://www.who.int/disabilities/care/en.

REFERENCES

Aisen, M. L., D. Kerkovich, J. Mast, S. Mulroy, T. A. Wren, and others. 2011. "Cerebral Palsy: Clinical Care and Neurological Rehabilitation." *The Lancet Neurology* 10 (9): 844–52.

Anchique Santos, C. V., F. Lopez-Jimenez, B. Benaim, G. Burdiat, R. Fernandez Coronado, and others. 2014. "Cardiac Rehabilitation in Latin America." *Progression in Cardiovascular Diseases* 57 (3): 268–78.

Atijosan, O., V. Simms, H. Kuper, D. Rischewski, and C. Lavy. 2009. "The Orthopaedic Needs of Children in Rwanda: Results from a National Survey and Orthopaedic Service Implications." *Journal of Pediatric Orthopedics* 29 (8): 948–51.

Bardos, M., H. Burak, and Y. Ben-Shalom. 2015. *Assessing the Cost and Benefits of Return-to-Work Programs.* Consultant report by Mathematica Policy Research for the U.S. Department of Labor, Washington, DC. https://www.dol .gov/odep/topics/pdf/RTW_Costs-Benefits_2015-03.pdf.

Beal, R. W. 2007. "Survey of Rehabilitation and Return-to-Work Practices among U.S. Disability Carriers." Report prepared by Milliman Consultants and Actuaries for Cornell University School of Industrial and Labor Relations, Ithaca, NY. http://digitalcommons.ilr.cornell.edu/cgi/viewcontent .cgi?article=1445&context=gladnetcollect.

Beswick, A. D., K. Rees, P. Dieppe, S. Ayis, R. Gooberman-Hill, and others. 2008. "Complex Interventions to Improve Physical Function and Maintain Independent Living in Elderly People: A Systematic Review and Meta-Analysis." *The Lancet* 371 (9614): 725–35.

Choi, J. H., M. Jakob, C. Stapf, R. S. Marshall, A. Hartmann, and H. Mast. 2008. "Multimodal Early Rehabilitation and Predictors of Outcome in Survivors of Severe Traumatic Brain Injury." *Journal of Trauma* 65 (5): 1028–35.

Dalal, H. M., P. Doherty, S. Rod, and R. S. Taylor. 2015. "Cardiac Rehabilitation." *BMJ* 351: h5000.

Dias, J. M., B. F. Mazuquin, F. Q. Mostagi, T. B. Lima, M. A. Silva, and others. 2013. "The Effectiveness of Postoperative Physical Therapy Treatment in Patients Who Have Undergone Arthroscopic Partial Meniscectomy: Systematic Review with Meta-Analysis." *Journal of Orthopaedic & Sports Physical Therapy* 43 (8): 560–76.

European Agency for Safety and Health at Work. 2016. *Research Review on Rehabilitation and Return to Work.* Luxembourg: European Union.

Fleury, A. M., S. A. Salih, and N. M. Peel. 2013. "Rehabilitation of the Older Vascular Amputee: A Review of the Literature." *Geriatrics & Gerontology International* 13 (2): 264–73.

Franche, R. L., K. Cullen, J. Clarke, E. Irvin, S. Sinclair, and others. 2005. "Workplace-Based Return-to-Work Interventions: A Systematic Review of the Quantitative Literature." *Journal of Occupational Rehabilitation* 15 (4): 607–31.

GBD 2015 Disease and Injury Incidence and Prevalence Collaborators. 2016. "Global, Regional, and National Incidence, Prevalence, and Years Lived with Disability for 310 Diseases and Injuries, 1990–2015: A Systematic Analysis for the Global Burden of Disease Study 2015." *The Lancet* 388: 1545–602.

Gillespie, L. D., M. C. Robertson, W. J. Gillespie, C. Sherrington, S. Gates, and others. 2012. "Interventions for Preventing Falls in Older People Living in the Community." *Cochrane Database of Systematic Reviews* (9): CD007146.

Godlwana, L., A. Stewart, and E. Musenge. 2015. "Mobility during the Intermediate Stage of Rehabilitation after Lower Limb Amputation from an Under Resourced Community: A Randomized Controlled Trial." *Physiotherapy* 101 (1): e458.

Gosselin, R., D. A. Spiel, R. Coughlin, and L. G. Zirkle. 2009. "Injuries: The Neglected Burden in Developing Countries." *Bulletin of the World Health Organization* 87: 246.

Grantham-McGregor, S., Y. B. Cheung, S. Cueto, P. Glewwe, L. Richter, and others. 2007. "Developmental Potential in the First 5 Years for Children in Developing Countries." *The Lancet* 369 (9555): 60–70.

Gupta, N., C. Castillo-Laborde, and M. D. Landry. 2011. "Health-Related Rehabilitation Services: Assessing the Global Supply of and Need for Human Resources." *BMC Health Services Research* 11 (1): 1.

Guzman, J. M., and E. G. Salazar. 2014. "Disability and Rehabilitation in Mexico." *American Journal of Physical Medicine & Rehabilitation* 29 (1 Suppl 1): 36–38.

Hyman, S., R. Parikh, P. Y. Collins, and V. Patel. 2015. "Adult Mental Disorders." In *Disease Control Priorities* (third edition): Volume 4, *Mental, Neurological, and Substance Use Disorders*, edited by V. Patel, D. Chisholm, T. Dua, R. Laxminarayan, and M. E. Medina-Mora. Washington, DC: World Bank.

Jolliffe, J. A., K. Rees, R. S. Taylor, D. Thompson, N. Oldridge, and others. 2000. "Exercise-Based Rehabilitation for Coronary Heart Disease." *Cochrane Database of Systematic Reviews* (4): Cd001800.

Kurichi, J. E., D. S. Small, B. E. Bates, J. A. Prvu-Bettger, P. L. Kwong, and others. 2009. "Possible Incremental Benefits of Specialized Rehabilitation Bed Units among Veterans after Lower Extremity Amputation." *Medical Care* 47 (4): 457–65.

Mock, C. N., S. Nguyen, R. Quansah, C. Arreola-Risa, R. Viradia, and M. Joshipura. 2006. "Evaluation of Trauma Care Capabilities in Four Countries Using the WHO-IATSIC Guidelines for Essential Trauma Care." *World Journal of Surgery* 30: 946-56. doi:10.1007/s00268-005-0768-4, PMID :16736320.

Na, W. 2016. "Cost-Benefit Analysis of Vocational Rehabilitation Program for Persons with Significant Disabilities in Korea." *Niepełnosprawność—Zagadnienia, Problemy, Rozwiązania* 2 (19): 7–15.

Nas, K., L. Yazmalar, V. Şah, A. Aydin, and K. Öneş. 2015. "Rehabilitation of Spinal Cord Injuries." *World Journal of Orthopedics* 6 (1): 8.

Nielsen, P. R., J. Andreasen, M. Asmussen, and H. Tonnesen. 2008. "Costs and Quality of Life for Prehabilitation and Early Rehabilitation after Surgery of the Lumbar Spine." *BMC Health Services Research* 8: 209.

Novak, I., S. Mcintyre, C. Morgan, L. Campbell, L. Dark, and others. 2013. "A Systematic Review of Interventions for Children with Cerebral Palsy: State of the Evidence." *Developmental Medicine & Child Neurology* 55 (10): 885–910.

Oldridge, N. B., M. T. Pakosh, and R. J. Thomas. 2016. "Cardiac Rehabilitation in Low- and Middle-Income Countries: A Review on Cost and Cost-Effectiveness." *International Health* 8 (2): 77–82.

Parker, A., T. Sricharoenchai, and D. M. Needham. 2013. "Early Rehabilitation in the Intensive Care Unit: Preventing Impairment of Physical and Mental Health." *Current Physical Medicine and Rehabilitation Reports* 14: 307–14.

Proctor, F. 2010. "Rehabilitation of the Burn Patient." *Indian Journal of Plastic Surgery* 43 (Suppl): S101–13.

Scivoletto, G., B. Morganti, and M. Molinari. 2005. "Early versus Delayed Inpatient Spinal Cord Injury Rehabilitation: An Italian Study." *Archives of Physical and Rehabilitation Medicine* 86 (3): 512–16.

Scott, J. G., C. Mihalopoulos, H. E. Erkskine, J. Roberts, and A. Rahman. 2015. "Childhood Mental and Developmental Disorders." In *Disease Control Priorities* (third edition): Volume 4, *Mental, Neurological, and Substance Use Disorders*, edited by V. Patel, D. Chisholm, T. Dua, R. Laxminarayan, and M. E. Medina-Mora. Washington, DC: World Bank.

Stroke Unit Trialists' Collaboration. 2013. "Organised Inpatient (Stroke Unit) Care for Stroke." *Cochrane Database of Systematic Reviews* 9: Cd000197.

Stucki, G., M. Stier-Jarmer, E. Grill, and J. Melvin. 2005. "Rationale and Principles of Early Rehabilitation Care after an Acute Injury or Illness." *Disability and Rehabilitation* 27 (7–8): 353–59.

Taylor, R. S., H. Dalal, K. Jolly, T. Moxham, and A. Zawada. 2010. "Home-Based versus Centre-Based Cardiac Rehabilitation." *Cochrane Database of Systematic Reviews* (1): Cd007130.

Turner-Stokes, L., H. Williams, A. Bill, P. Bassett, and K. Sephton. 2016. "Cost-Efficiency of Specialist Inpatient Rehabilitation for Working-Aged Adults with Complex Neurological Disabilities: A Multicentre Cohort Analysis of a National Clinical Dataset." *BMJ Open* 6 (2).

UN (United Nations). 2015. *World Population Ageing 2015.* New York: Department of Economic and Social Affairs, UN.

WHO (World Health Organization). 2001. *International Classification of Functioning, Disability and Health: ICF.* Geneva: WHO.

———. 2014. "Injuries and Violence: The Facts 2014." WHO, Geneva.

———. 2015. *World Report on Ageing and Health.* Geneva: WHO.

———. 2016a. *World Health Statistics 2016: Monitoring Health for the SDGs.* Geneva: WHO.

———. 2016b. "Global Health Observatory (GHO) Data." http://www.who.int/gho/child_health/mortality/mortality _under_five_text/en/.

———. 2016c. *International Classification of Health Interventions.* Geneva: WHO. http://www.who.int /classifications/ichi/en/.

———. 2017. *Rehabilitation in Health Systems.* Geneva: WHO.

WHO (World Health Organization) and World Bank. 2011. *World Report on Disability.* Geneva: WHO.

World Bank. 2016. "Population Ages 0–14 (% of Total)." http:// data.worldbank.org/indicator/SP.POP.0014.TO.ZS.

Part 5

Intersectoral and International Topics

Chapter 16

Development Assistance for Health

Eran Bendavid, Trygve Ottersen, Liu Peilong, Rachel Nugent,
Nancy Padian, John-Arne Rottingen, and Marco Schäferhoff

INTRODUCTION

Development assistance holds promise for alleviating the death and suffering of impoverished children, women, and men from readily preventable and treatable conditions and to support global economic development, demographic sustainability, and political stability. Although the desirability of these goals is widely shared, there is little agreement on who should shoulder the financial responsibility or how best to use development assistance to achieve these goals.

How much financing should be provided and in what form, who is eligible, and what health areas and interventions should be prioritized? How should institutions balance the financing for current interventions and for future priorities? Should funding for research and development (R&D) be a health aid priority? And what exactly counts as health aid? Does a favorable loan to build a hospital in rural China count? How about in rural Mali? How much health aid flows through recognized channels, and how much falls outside well-documented channels? What criteria should be used to allocate scarce health aid resources? Which countries and populations have the strongest claims to assistance or favorable financing? This chapter provides frameworks for addressing these questions and understanding the crossroads for foreign aid to the health sector. This chapter does not provide a systematic review of current patterns of health aid allocation. The descriptive epidemiology of health aid—the

patterns of sources, channels, flows, and targets of donor resources—is available from other sources, which we reference throughout this chapter. Instead, we address key questions that challenge our understanding of the present and planning for the future of international cooperation on health.

The first section addresses the measurement of health aid, including an overview of common definitions and measurements of how health aid flows, from whom, to whom, and to what intended ends. The section also summarizes recent efforts to reconsider the scope of health aid, including aid originating in non–Organisation for Economic Co-operation and Development (OECD) countries and support for R&D and other global public goods.

The second section addresses the normative landscape of health aid: What are the goals for the provision of health aid and the criteria guiding its allocation? We illustrate the role of the implicit and explicit goals of health aid, including the alleviation of death and suffering, human development, national relationships, global health equity, and international security. We also address how implicit and explicit goals guide the provision of health aid across regions and countries and across disease and intervention areas.

The third section provides two case studies that illustrate patterns of health aid sources and the breadth of health aid efforts. The fourth draws lessons learned from the experience with health aid and identifies guiding principles for organizing and implementing health aid resources. We end with a summary and recommendations for future health aid investments. Investing these resources wisely will play an important role in achieving a grand convergence in global health and a decent life for all (Jamison and others 2013).

TRACKING HEALTH AID

Health aid can be broadly defined as the transfer of resources from multilateral organizations, foundations, or governments to the health sector of a country or a population. Although much health aid is in the form of grants and in-kind gifts, some is in the form of concessionary agreements, loans, and preferable trade agreements. Beneath the broad definitions, however, lie several major challenges to the definitions and measurement of health aid.

Definitions

An important challenge to any discussion on prioritization of health aid is the lack of agreement on what exactly counts as health aid. This section describes two data sources that track health aid and highlights the differences between them.

The most detailed source of data on health aid comes from the OECD's Development Assistance Committee (DAC). The DAC is charged with tracking and measuring all forms of donor financing, including official development assistance (ODA).[1] ODA includes mostly grants and loans that are concessional in character and contain a grant element of at least 25 percent. The OECD maintains the Creditor Reporting System (CRS), a database of ODA coded into 36 broad sectors, including two sectors that are noted as "health" and "population and reproductive health." The database contains information on grants and loans starting as early as 1973, but health aid data are sparse before 2000. Thirty donor nations (mostly members of the DAC); several multilateral organizations, such as the World Health Organization (WHO) and the African Development Bank; as well as the Bill & Melinda Gates Foundation provide specific information about the purpose, amount, and intended recipients of grants and loans qualifying as development assistance.

Because the CRS database has become an important public source of health aid data, its limitations deserve further mention. First, information about the purpose of an aid item may be too general for many health purposes. For example, the CRS lacks a code for reproductive, maternal, newborn, and child health. As a result, recent initiatives that aim to monitor the international flow of resources for such priorities use different measurements, producing different results (IHME 2016a; PMNCH 2014; Victora and others 2015). In addition, information on the purpose of a grant or loan in the CRS can be vague or short, often no longer than a few words, making it difficult to link the resources with their intended priorities.

The second data source contains *development assistance for health*, a term introduced by the Institute for Health Metrics and Evaluation (IHME) in 2009 that quickly became commonly used in the global health community. In contrast to ODA, development assistance for health includes financing from private sources and financial transfers that target the private sector such as advance market commitments. Unlike the CRS, which contains project-level information on more than 3 million projects, IHME's data contain global health financing data aggregated by source, channel, recipient, and disease areas (IHME 2016a).

Largely lacking from both the CRS and IHME databases is information on investments in global public goods. Such goods include R&D for diseases that disproportionately affect people living in poor countries or for priorities with global benefits such as epidemic outbreak preparedness. The extent to which investments in global public goods should count as health aid is an area of active debate. The concept of *health ODA plus* attempts to provide a more complete picture of donor flows to global health by including flows to global functions (Schäferhoff and others 2015). Specifically, health ODA plus includes (1) health aid reported by donors to the OECD and (2) public funding for R&D for neglected diseases, including funding channeled by donors to organizations working on R&D without a specific focus on low- and middle-income countries (LMICs). For example, ODA plus includes financing by the Swedish government for research on antimicrobial resistance through the Karolinska Institute, as well as financing of research on a vaccine to prevent human immunodeficiency virus/acquired immunodeficiency syndrome (HIV/ AIDS) through federal institutions such as the National Institutes of Health or private pharmaceutical and biotechnology companies. Because these resources do not flow to LMICs and support research priorities with global importance, this funding is not included in the CRS and IHME databases. The concept of health ODA plus posits that funding for health priorities that affect lower-income countries is a valuable component of health aid even if it does not flow directly to LMICs (and adds to the complexity of health aid measurements).

What other types of assistance are not measured or tracked reliably? Aid to priority areas such as neglected tropical diseases may be substantially underrepresented in the CRS and other data sets. Aid for noncommunicable diseases (NCDs) is not officially represented at all.

Health aid from non-OECD countries such as Brazil, China, India, and South Africa is substantial, but these countries do not report to the DAC. Data on South-South cooperation are hard to track and may include items not considered aid by other definitions, even though it makes up an important supplement to more established forms of assistance (described in case study 2 in this chapter).

In addition, substantial amounts of aid, including health aid, flow between Arab nations and territories. Data on the magnitude or nature of this aid are very limited. Kuwait and the United Arab Emirates report to the CRS, and Qatar publishes aggregate information on aid provided mostly to other Arab nations (Kharas 2015). The United Arab Emirates has been increasing its ODA contributions since 2010, including a 608 percent increase in real terms in 2013 (mainly support to the Arab Republic of Egypt), of which a little less than 10 percent is designated for health. Support for health multilaterals is also growing. For example, Oman, Qatar, Saudi Arabia, and the United Arab Emirates all provide funding to Gavi, the Vaccine Alliance. Changing the CRS database to include reporting from non-DAC donor countries could add to our understanding of international cooperation and unmet needs. There is precedent for expanding the CRS database: several non-DAC donors already report ODA funding to the CRS, including Lithuania, Saudi Arabia, and Thailand. Expanding the global accounting of ODA—including health aid—would relieve areas of great uncertainty in deciding on resource allocations to countries and regions with limited information. For example, the resource flows to conflict regions such as Syria from non-OECD sources are largely unknown and likely substantial.

Sources and Flows of Health Aid

Growth in health aid slowed considerably between 2010 and 2015. During the "golden age of global health" (2000–10), health aid grew 11.4 percent a year on average. Since then, average growth has dropped to 1.2 percent. In 2015, health aid (as measured by the IHME) totaled US$36.4 billion, below the 2013 peak level of US$38.0 billion (see IHME 2016a). Much donor support for health originates in national budgets supported by taxes and other sources of national income in wealthier countries. Unlike domestic health spending that originates from governments that are, in many cases, accountable to the populations they serve, health aid is unstable. Because a donor government does not have the same fiduciary relationship to the population of another country as it does to its own population, health aid amounts and priorities may shift for reasons that have little to do with

needs in the recipient country. The dependence of health aid on nonhealth priorities and dynamics that may be entirely exogenous to events in the recipient country makes health aid particularly vulnerable to swings. The impact of volatility may be particularly detrimental to funding streams that finance health services with few substitutes and long-term commitments, such as antiretroviral therapy.

As shown in figure 16.1, substantial variation was experienced in the global increase in health aid. Between 2002 and 2014, some countries have given increasing amounts of health aid (for example, the United States), while others have given stable or declining amounts (Norway).

Global political and economic cycles also shape donor priorities, with recessions leading governments to rearrange their spending priorities, often in ways that do not favor foreign aid. Following the 2007–08 recession, the 2010 health aid budget of OECD countries became more volatile and that of the United States stagnated. In 2005, several OECD countries committed to tethering foreign aid—including health aid—to a portion (0.7 percent) of their gross domestic product. If the recommendation to peg foreign aid to gross domestic product is followed, health aid will grow during economic booms and shrink during economic downturns, making future levels of commitment highly uncertain. Following the 2016 elections in the United States, the new administration expressed decreasing commitment to foreign aid programs, including explicit large reductions in health aid.

Private sources and foundations have been playing an increasingly important role in the health aid landscape. Overall, private sources made up more than 25 percent of health aid between 2010 and 2015, a relatively small component of direct contributions. The Bill & Melinda Gates Foundation was the third-largest overall contributor of health aid between 2010 and 2015, above most European countries (IHME 2016a). However, the influence of private aid transcends its direct financial contribution. Unencumbered by public interests, organizations such as the Bill & Melinda Gates Foundation and the Hewlett Foundation are at relative liberty to take strategic risks and set new agendas. The Bill & Melinda Gates Foundation, for example, provided critical early financing to Gavi, the Vaccine Alliance, and its emphasis on financing novel technological solutions for global health problems has generated funding for more than 1,000 exploratory high-risk, high-reward projects such as farming grasshoppers as a source of protein or developing odorants to block the ability of malaria-causing *Anopheles* mosquitoes to detect humans. The Hewlett Foundation has been a leader in advancing rigorous program evaluations to

Figure 16.1 Health Aid as a Percentage of Total Aid for Major Country Donors, 2002–14

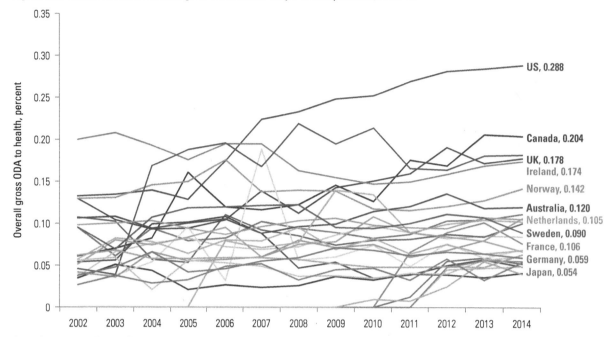

Source: Organisation for Economic Co-operation and Development Creditor Reporting System, gross disbursements in constant prices (sector codes 120 and 130) and imputed multilateral contributions to the health sector. Development Assistance Committee Secretariat estimates (as of January 2016).
Note: ODA = overseas development assistance.

understand what works, such as through its support for the International Initiative for Impact Evaluation and leadership of the Effective Philanthropy Group.

More than 300 foundations were registered with the U.S. Agency for International Development (USAID) in 2014, and most of them operate independently (USAID 2015). Their portfolios can be wide, including infectious diseases, reproductive health, and complementary areas such as education, health systems, and governance. One implication of the relatively small size of each foundation and their independent operation is that foundations commonly identify their own (often narrow) strategic focus rather than align their investments within a streamlined, global strategy.

Health financing is distributed unevenly across health areas. Since 2000, the launch year of the Millennium Development Goals (MDGs), the largest growth in health aid funding has been related to the control of infectious diseases, particularly HIV/AIDS and malaria. Child health and especially maternal and reproductive health have received more modest attention. (This trend has changed somewhat since 2010 following the launch

of several global initiatives, such as the Group of Eight's Muskoka Initiative on Maternal, Newborn and Child Health.) Health areas not targeted by the MDGs have received even less attention. These overlooked conditions include NCDs such as cardiovascular disease and cancers as well as neglected tropical diseases, even though the burden of these diseases is large in many aid-recipient countries.

Of the total amount of health aid in 2015, 30 percent and 28 percent were allocated to HIV/AIDS and to maternal, child, and newborn health, respectively, while 6 percent was targeted to malaria control, and only 1 percent to NCDs, even though NCDs are responsible for more deaths than any other major category in every region except Sub-Saharan Africa (Dieleman and others 2015). Box 16.1 discusses this issue in greater detail.

Financing has shifted slightly with the launch of global initiatives focusing on child health, maternal health, and nutrition (Darmstadt and others 2014; Kirton, Kulik, and Bracht 2014). Mirroring these shifts, health aid for HIV/AIDS and tuberculosis has declined from peak levels in 2013 (IHME 2016a).

Funding for Noncommunicable Diseases

Unlike in many other areas of health, households bear much of the burden of noncommunicable diseases (NCDs). Governments in low- and middle-income countries have allocated very little to NCD prevention and care. More than 50 percent of current spending for cardiovascular diseases in low-income countries is out of pocket from patients and their households, 33 percent is from domestic governments, and 13 percent is from donors; in high-income countries, out-of-pocket spending on NCDs is a far lower share of the total (WHO n.d.). Government financing for NCDs also varies substantially across countries.

Figure B16.1.1 provides estimates of development assistance for NCDs and all health aid from 2000 to 2014.

If health aid declines or stagnates in the coming years, domestic governments will have to provide the bulk of new funding. The following actions could help align NCD funding with needs:

* Aim for a closer alignment of funders' health aid with health burden in poor countries
* Link funders' priorities with NCD prevention and treatment programs—for example, integrate NCD prevention, such as blood pressure management, into primary care settings
* Link investments in health system strengthening with investments in NCD prevention.

Figure B16.1.1 Development Assistance for Noncommunicable Diseases and All Health, 2000–14, 2011 US$

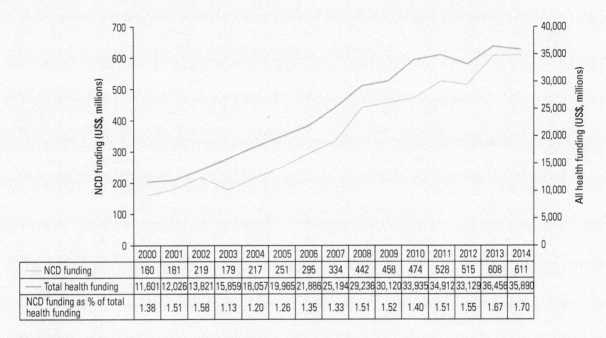

	2000	2001	2002	2003	2004	2005	2006	2007	2008	2009	2010	2011	2012	2013	2014
NCD funding	160	181	219	179	217	251	295	334	442	458	474	528	515	608	611
Total health funding	11,601	12,026	13,821	15,859	18,057	19,965	21,886	25,194	29,236	30,120	33,935	34,912	33,129	36,456	35,890
NCD funding as % of total health funding	1.38	1.51	1.58	1.13	1.20	1.26	1.35	1.33	1.51	1.52	1.40	1.51	1.55	1.67	1.70

Source: IHME 2016a.
Note: NCD = noncommunicable disease.

GOALS AND CRITERIA FOR ALLOCATING HEALTH AID

Donors' and recipients' normative views and goals inherently shape decisions about whether to provide aid, how much, in what form, to whom, toward what, and how (Centre on Global Health Security Working Group on Health Financing 2014). These views and goals underpin the variation in health aid across countries and partly explain, for example, why health aid per capita ranges from US$0.7 to US$32 in LMICs (IHME 2016a). This section examines stated and unstated goals underlying the allocation of health aid and discusses criteria for guiding the allocation of health aid resources across geographic and health areas.

Goals of Health Aid

Averting preventable deaths and suffering, especially in countries with limited domestic capacity to address health needs, is a shared goal of health aid providers and recipients. For example, the mission of the Global Fund is to invest the world's money to defeat HIV/AIDS, tuberculosis, and malaria, and the global health mission of USAID is to support partner countries in preventing and managing major health challenges of poor, underserved, and vulnerable people (Global Fund 2016a; USAID 2012). Between 2000 and 2015, many donors also explicitly sought to help countries reach the MDGs on child mortality (MDG 4); maternal health (MDG 5); and HIV/AIDS, tuberculosis, and other major diseases (MDG 6) (Ravishankar and others 2009). These priorities and funding streams remained dominant even after the deadline for the MDG 2 at the end of 2015. At the same time, many donors cite broader goals for health aid, including goals related to poverty alleviation, economic growth, educational outcomes, and security. Starting in 2016 with the Sustainable Development Goals, health-related aims could be further integrated with broader development objectives.

Donors may also have goals that have less to do with recipient need and more to do with donor interests. These goals can occasionally be gleaned from revealed donor preferences without being made explicit. For example, some donors provide health aid to protect their own populations, such as targeting rapidly spreading infectious diseases, like Ebola virus disease; or to promote their political and economic interests (Berthélemy 2006; Hoeffler and Outram 2011). Irrespective of whether explicit or implicit goals are pursued, the Paris Declaration on Aid Effectiveness calls for donors to align their support, whenever possible, with recipient-country government priorities.

Criteria for Allocation across Geographic Areas

Guiding the allocation of health aid across countries or geographic areas is often of importance to donors. Recent and ongoing economic transitions, however, have made decisions about country allocation more difficult for donors seeking to direct health aid toward individuals or communities with large needs relative to their capacity (rather than to countries that may have large relatively well-off populations). Economic growth rates have been impressive in many countries, including many formerly low-income countries (LICs), over the past two decades, and many countries have moved from low-income to middle-income status, including populous countries such as China, India, and Nigeria. At the same time, many of these countries have pronounced inequalities in income and health. One consequence is that most of the world's poor and the world's disease burden are no longer located in LICs, but in middle-income countries (MICs) (IHME 2016b; Sumner 2012).

Questions arise about the role of MICs with regard to health aid and, more generally, the central role currently given to mean national income, such as gross national income (GNI) per capita, in allocation decisions. Agreement is growing that GNI per capita is an inadequate basis for deciding which countries are eligible for health aid and how much each country should receive. Therefore, with respect to cross-country allocation of health aid, a central task for many donors in the coming years will be to consider resituating GNI per capita as one tool among several in the overall decision-making process.

The larger debate about how health aid can better target the communities and individuals in greatest need revolves around three broad approaches. One is determining whether GNI per capita thresholds should be used at all to determine eligibility for health aid. Many have called for donors to raise their thresholds, in effect reducing the role GNI per capita plays in determining eligibility. What other criteria should be used if GNI per capita does not provide an eligibility benchmark remains an open issue. Second, others argue for maintaining GNI per capita as a criterion, but supplementing it with criteria directly linked to health needs in the country. For example, the Global Fund hosted the Equitable Access Initiative in 2015, which concluded that countries' health needs and fiscal capacity are important factors for donors to consider when allocating funds (Global Fund 2016b). Again, the specific metrics to use and how to integrate them remain open issues. Finally, some suggest that donors ought to go beyond countries and average measures such as GNI per capita and focus more on the subnational allocation of health aid. Options for linking eligibility and other allocation criteria directly to subnational units need more study.

Criteria for Allocation across Health Areas

Allocation across disease and health priorities requires additional consideration. Health aid resources cannot fully subsidize the health sector of even the poorest countries, and decisions for prioritizing disease areas and programs are unavoidable. In 2014, US$10.8 billion and US$10.1 billion were allocated to HIV/AIDS and maternal and child health, respectively, while US$2.4 billion was allocated to malaria and only US$475 million to NCDs (IHME 2016a). What accounts for such variation? What principles appear to guide—and ought to guide—the distribution of health aid?

Although some donors clearly state their general priorities, few provide the explicit criteria used to allocate health aid across disease areas. Perhaps the most straightforward way to prioritize financing decisions would be to allocate resources in proportion to the burden of disease such that if the death and disability from disease A is twice that from disease B, then twice the resources should go toward controlling disease A (Sridhar and Batniji 2008). While the equitability of this resource-allocation heuristic is appealing, its principal shortcoming is that, without considering the cost of reducing disease burden, allocation proportional to burden may not reduce as much disease burden as prioritizing diseases for which the most cost-effective interventions exist. Disease burden estimates can be useful for identifying the conditions causing the most mortality and morbidity, but they do not show where health aid resources could yield the greatest benefits (Bendavid and others 2015). For example, stroke is a leading cause of death and disability in China, but financing stroke treatment in China may yield relatively few benefits in comparison with treating and preventing tuberculosis (Coyle and others 2013; Prabhakaran, Ruff, and Bernstein 2015). To identify the investment priorities that provide the greatest benefits with the available health aid resources, information is needed on the cost-effectiveness of potential interventions. One of the principal objectives of the third edition of *Disease Control Priorities* is to provide this information.

A third proposed criterion for choosing disease priorities for health aid (in addition to disease burden and cost-effectiveness of interventions) would be to provide resources to the diseases the afflict the most ill, globally or nationally (Ottersen and others 2014). For example, priority could be assigned to interventions benefiting persons with lower healthy life expectancy. Although this criterion might yield different allocation guidance than a cost-effectiveness criterion, many interventions will score high on both—for example, cheap and highly effective interventions targeting potentially life-threatening conditions, such as diarrhea, malaria, and pneumonia, in children living in poverty.

Epidemiological and other transitions are creating new challenges for allocating health aid across disease areas. NCDs now account for almost 60 percent of the global burden of disease (Murray and others 2015), and 80 percent of NCD deaths occur in LMICs. Donors need to carefully balance their responses to NCDs with their responses to maternal, neonatal, and child health problems and with the unfinished agenda of infectious diseases. Weighing these choices may involve further inquiry into how criteria related to cost-effectiveness, disease burden, and the worse off can be specified and traded off. At the same time, transnational health threats, including pandemics and antimicrobial resistance, are increasingly being viewed as within the purview of health aid. Chapter 18 of *Major Infectious Diseases* (volume 6 of this series) on antimicrobial infections provides additional arguments supporting the role of health aid in curbing antimicrobial resistance (Miller-Petrie, Pant, and Laxminarayan 2017). What share of health aid should be allocated to these kinds of threats will be a key question. The interpretation and generation of cost-effectiveness estimates for interventions in these areas will also be important because such estimates are currently lacking or are highly uncertain.

CASE STUDIES

This section presents two case studies illustrating the historical trajectory of health aid and the changing landscape of donor-recipient relationships. The first describes the role played by the U.S. President's Emergency Plan for AIDS Relief (PEPFAR) and illustrates the tensions in setting priorities and strategies with ambiguous goals and motivations. While the PEPFAR case study delves into the challenges of archetypal health aid institutions, the second case study—describing China's approach to development cooperation on health (South-South cooperation)—represents a complementary approach to health aid.

Case Study 1: PEPFAR

The spread of HIV/AIDS in Sub-Saharan Africa and the United States in the 1980s and 1990s preceded—and arguably caused—the expansion of health aid in the 1990s and 2000s. Health aid for HIV/AIDS increased from effectively zero in the mid-1990s to the largest single disease priority a decade later. The rapid global response was related to the spread of HIV/AIDS in Europe and the United States, where it became the leading cause of death among young men and created a groundswell of activism and growing recognition of the security and economic threats of infectious diseases in an increasingly globalized world. The United Nations General Assembly Declaration of Commitment on HIV/AIDS, endorsed in 2001, singled out HIV/AIDS as an exceptional priority.

That exceptionalism was backed by substantial increases in commitments and new disbursements toward global control of HIV/AIDS. The largest of those commitments, announced in early 2003, became PEPFAR. In this section, we draw on published materials and an interview with a former director of the Office of the U.S. Global AIDS Coordinator, the agency tasked with implementing PEPFAR, to understand historical and future trajectories of health aid and the challenges of identifying and standing by clear goals and criteria in aid allocation.

PEPFAR changed what was considered possible in health aid, directing billions of U.S. dollars annually toward a single issue in a small group of high-priority countries. The model adopted by PEPFAR involved rapid and concentrated deployment of resources as a response to a global public health emergency. The trade-offs of this approach included occasionally downplaying long-term considerations, such as international parity in resource allocation, that are more characteristic of multilateral organizations like the World Bank or United Nations agencies and that may lead to these thinly spread organizations' relatively slow operations.

The program funded implementers with established track records, including multilateral U.S.-based organizations such as Columbia University, the Elizabeth Glaser Pediatric AIDS Foundation, the Harvard School of Public Health, and Catholic Relief Services. Driven by expediency, the first phase of implementation included capacity building and service provision that largely circumvented the public sector in partner countries and created a tension that is still evident today: success from PEPFAR's perspective meant creating a parallel system of health care delivery. This allowed for short-term reduction in mortality, but created longer-term challenges. It took several years before PEPFAR prioritized capacity building in its partner countries and began moving U.S.-based partners to a technical assistance role. That model, in which in-country partners were supported to provide health services and the role of U.S.-based partners was more advisory, was viewed as more sustainable.

This tension between short-term goals and long-term vision is evident in many of PEPFAR's decisions. As recently as 2016, efforts to shift contracts to in-country organizations were met with resistance from the original U.S.-based implementers. Shifting to in-country organizations was thought to enable further scale-up of services (by eliminating the payment of overhead to U.S.-based organizations) and to foster local capacity, sustainability, and competence (Vermund and others 2012).

However, many of PEPFAR's U.S.-based partners resisted the withdrawal of support, resulting in a gradual and (as of 2016) still-incomplete transition of implementation to local organizations.

Another example of an effort to bridge short-term and long-term goals is PEPFAR's support for medical education in partner countries. Through a large grant program, PEPFAR supported the creation of a dozen medical training programs in Sub-Saharan African partner countries (Fogarty International Center 2015; Kim and Evans 2014). While this program reflects a commitment to creating long-term, in-country capacity, it also represents a rethinking of PEPFAR's original priorities.

PEPFAR receives little credit for its attempts to balance short-term targets and long-range vision. These tensions were an integral part of PEPFAR's implementation. In part because of the need for an epidemic control strategy that is responsive to a changing epidemic and in part because of changing leadership, PEPFAR has altered its strategy from responding to emergencies to increasing country ownership and integration, and, more recently, to achieving global public health goals that extend beyond HIV/AIDS control (Fauci and Folkers 2012).

The challenges facing PEPFAR's strategic decisions possibly reflect its attempts to balance short-term and long-term strategic goals. For example, the U.S. Global AIDS Coordinator at the end of the George W. Bush administration was replaced swiftly after President Obama took office, and the future of PEPFAR was, for a while, highly uncertain (McNeil 2010). By 2017, PEPFAR had matured into an established health aid program with wide-ranging support and a broad mandate. From this position, it could adopt a long-term, stable set of guiding principles that could help relieve some of the pressures to shift strategies in response to leadership and funding changes.

Many see an opportunity for PEPFAR to leverage the infrastructure it created to focus on multiple diseases, including NCDs, and, in the process, to integrate with other health sectors (Fogarty International Center 2016). Although this may be an intuitive direction for improving the care of HIV/AIDS patients treated in PEPFAR-supported programs, it also signals a broadening of PEPFAR's mandate at the same time that PEPFAR is poised to deepen its commitment to the highly ambitious goals of achieving both "90-90-90" (90 percent of persons with HIV/AIDS aware of their status, 90 percent in regular treatment, and 90 percent of those in treatment virally suppressed) and an "AIDS-free generation." If "90-90-90" is achieved, 55 million individuals are estimated to need treatment by 2030, more than 3.5 times the number of people on treatment at the end of 2016 (Hoos, El-Sadr, and Dehne 2016).

Successfully broadening and deepening its mandates, possibly with flat or declining resources, is likely to be among PEPFAR's principal challenges.

Case Study 2: China's Contributions to Global Health

Health aid is an integral part of China's foreign aid, which it has been providing for more than 60 years, mostly as South-South partnerships (Zhou, Zhang, and Zhang 2015). Beginning in 1950 with aid to socialist neighboring countries and extending in the mid-1950s to LMICs in other regions, notably Africa, China has provided a large quantity of goods and materials in support of development projects.[2] After the political and economic reform in 1978 and the subsequent rise in national income, China continued to expand the level of foreign aid and the diversity of aid forms. As of 2009, China's total foreign aid equaled US$37.6 billion after increasing nearly 30 percent annually from 2003 to 2009 (China State Council 2011; Zhou, Zhang, and Zhang 2015). From 2010 to 2012, China contributed an additional US$14.4 billion in foreign aid (China State Council 2014). During this period, China focused more on LICs; basic infrastructure projects such as roads, ports, and water supply; social projects linked to personal welfare; and technical training (Zhou, Zhang, and Zhang 2015).

China's health aid, although a small portion of overall Chinese foreign aid, increased over time, especially to Africa, with the launch of the Forum on China-Africa Cooperation. Unlike most OECD donors, China does not offer direct transfers to the health sector. It uses a project approach and provides health aid through grants. China's in-kind health aid focuses more on specific aspects of the health system, such as the delivery of health care services; provision of essential medical products, procedures, and traditional Chinese medicine technologies; improvement of health infrastructure; development of a health workforce; and, more recently, malaria control and emergency response to the Ebola epidemic. The main focus is Africa, where almost 90 percent of the dispatched medical teams and 80 percent of donated health facilities—the dominant forms of China's regular health aid—are targeted.

China's variable aid components emerged gradually. In 1963, China first dispatched medical teams with donated drugs and medical equipment. Since 1970, China has constructed health facilities, and in 2000, it launched the Human Resources Development Fund for Africa. Since 2006, China has been involved in malaria control, and in 2014, it provided four rounds of emergency aid, totaling US$120 million, to control the Ebola outbreak in West Africa. Recently, to support the 2030 Agenda for Sustainable Development, a series of new initiatives has helped establish an African Union Center for Disease Control and regional medical research centers, assisted African countries to improve disease surveillance systems, and funded 100 maternal and child health projects for LMICs. China also contributes to the Global Fund; Gavi, the Vaccine Alliance; the WHO; the African Union; the World Food Programme; and the United Nations' health programs. China's normative approaches to health aid have also evolved, with more emphasis on mutually beneficial goals and shared development, while emphasizing noninterference in internal affairs and avoiding political conditions for aid.

Official data on the financial flows of China's health aid are not available. According to Liu and others (2014), between 2007 and 2011, Chinese medical teams in Africa were equivalent to about US$60 million in aid annually, donated facilities were about the same, and total health aid to Africa averaged about US$150 million annually. However, these data include only central government health aid. They do not include basic salaries of medical team members, which are covered by their home hospitals; support provided by provincial governments to the medical teams they dispatch; scholarships for students from LMICs to study medicine in China, which are funded by the Ministry of Education; or R&D on neglected tropical diseases, which is funded by other sources.

China's role in health and development is not limited to the direct provision of health aid through bilateral channels. Since the outbreak of severe acute respiratory syndrome, China has participated in global action on health security. China has also engaged in global health policy debates and worked with global health institutions. Although not counted as health aid by most historical yardsticks, these activities support shared global functions with benefits to LMICs.

GUIDING PRINCIPLES FOR THE NEXT DECADE

Health Aid Effectiveness

A growing body of evidence suggests that the surge in health aid, especially since 2000, has helped reduce the morbidity and mortality from many infectious diseases and the burden of child and maternal mortality in many LMICs, occasionally to levels approaching those in wealthier regions (Bendavid 2014b; Bendavid and Bhattacharya 2014). The declines in child mortality during the past 30 years coincided with the increase in health aid targeting the causes of child mortality such as vaccine-preventable illnesses. While this supports the role of health aid in the decline of child mortality, direct attribution is difficult because child mortality has declined for many reasons. The proliferation of effective organizations committed to expanding the provision of highly efficacious, low-cost child health goods, such as insecticide-treated bednets and vaccinations, suggests that health aid has played an important role, in addition to factors such as economic growth, improved education and nutrition, and the diffusion of knowledge such as the benefits of breastfeeding (Levine 2004). Health aid is associated with the convergence of mortality rates not only among different countries, but also within countries. The geographic and wealth distribution of child mortality has been narrowing within most aid-recipient countries, most precipitously after 2000, coinciding with the largest rise in health aid (Bendavid 2014a).

Changing Aid Commitments

Economic development of aid recipients, changing distribution of disease burden, and growing recognition of the importance of global functions are creating new conditions and new opportunities that would intuitively lead to shifts in the allocation and emphasis of health aid. As countries are increasingly able to finance the delivery of health goods, and mortality from causes financed by health aid continue to decline (for example, vaccine-preventable illnesses or malaria), the allocation of health aid resources may be better used to address new priorities.

Outside of a spike in funding earmarked for Ebola response, health aid funding remained largely flat between 2010 and 2016. Unless new resources become available, any increases in financing of some priorities will require trade-offs and the deprioritization of existing high priorities. This is a challenging endeavor for some streams of health aid, where resources are tied up in long-term commitments. A striking example of this limited flexibility is the financing of antiretroviral therapy (ART) for millions of persons living with HIV/AIDS. ART is costly, life saving, and lifelong, and efforts to move ART programs from donor to domestic funding have been met with vociferous resistance (McNeil 2010).

Liberating aid committed from long-term programs would bring flexibility in responding to new challenges and opportunities, but the transition will be gradual and may not be feasible in the near term. In the meantime, resources could be diverted from low-value priorities lacking long-term commitments with relatively low opportunity cost. It could be expedient to start examining such priorities before tackling entitlements and long-term commitments.

Increasing the domestic ownership of health investments is one way to shift the allocation of health aid commitments. National governments in aid-recipient countries can finance some if not most health care delivery for their own populations. In the past 20 years, health aid grew, in part, because many countries did not adequately finance priorities that donors perceived as urgent (for example, HIV/AIDS) or exceptionally high value (for example, vaccinations). However, as countries continue to develop economically, including many in Latin America, South and South-East Asia, and Sub-Saharan Africa, the domestic resources dedicated to supporting health care could grow with, or even faster than, general economic growth (Moon and Omole 2013; Resch, Ryckman, and Hecht 2015). Additional domestic resources could finance goods and services, including child health, maternal health, reproductive health, and the prevention and treatment of some infectious diseases such as soil-transmitted helminths and malaria.

Which Health Aid Investments Work?

Health aid would have more impact if resources were guided by evidence of effectiveness and cost-effectiveness. A proliferation of randomized field trials during the past two decades has added a new layer of specificity to the evidence on what works for health improvements in LMICs. However, similar to the role of randomized clinical trials in clinical medicine, the interventions examined in each trial are specific, and the study populations may not be broadly representative. This limited generalizability notwithstanding, the widespread popularity of randomized controlled trials could point to other ways in which evidence could improve health aid.

Randomized evaluations could be incorporated into the design of major programs. Currently, most randomized evaluations are organized by academic institutions and result in attempts to infer generalizable insights about the process of successful development from high-quality evidence in specific instances. Despite the proliferation of randomized evaluations, however, concerns about generalizability of trial insights have only increased over time (Deaton 2009; Pritchett 2004). A shift in focus would greatly improve their utility: randomized evaluations could replace traditional monitoring and evaluation. Trials provide credible estimates of the effectiveness of specific interventions and the mechanisms of action. They are less biased than traditional monitoring and evaluation and could be streamlined so that routine field evaluations could be carried out. Using rigorous evidence to guide the allocation of health aid would lend credibility, improve resource allocation, and ultimately improve health.

Randomized trials are not the only approach to discovering "what works." They are part of a broader context of scientific understanding and discovery.

For many issues in global health, randomized trials may not be feasible for practical or ethical reasons. For example, studying the effect of good governance on health is not readily amenable to randomized assignment (Kudamatsu 2012). For such questions, observational analyses are the only way to discover meaningful insights. The accumulation of evidence is a gradual process, but lessons learned through cumulating evidence have been important in guiding interventions that save many lives (Glassman and Levine 2016).

Identifying Investment Opportunities

The burden (or projected burden) of disease is a predominant consideration in choosing new health aid investments, with high-burden conditions arguably deserving more attention than low-burden conditions. However, *efficient* distribution of resources is also needed. To allocate resources efficiently, the cost-effectiveness of available interventions must be taken into account. For example, coronary bypass surgery may be an efficacious option for a high-burden condition, but it is not cost-effective relative to preventing coronary artery disease (Basu, Bendavid, and Sood 2015).

Interventions that are similarly cost-effective may have different effectiveness (and different costs). Decision makers may have to choose among options that provide greater benefits to fewer people and similarly cost-effective options that provide fewer benefits to more people. A stylized example is a trade-off between two interventions with similar cost-effectiveness. Intervention A averts 1.0 disability-adjusted life year per person, while intervention B averts only 0.1 disability-adjusted life year per person; intervention A also costs 10 times more than intervention B to treat one person. With a fixed budget, choosing intervention A yields the same population-level benefits at the same cost as intervention B, and while only one-tenth of the people can be treated, people successfully treated with intervention A will realize greater gains (on average) than those treated with intervention B (Rose 2001). An efficiency (cost-effectiveness) framework cannot distinguish between the two interventions. The greater number of beneficiaries could advantage intervention B under an equity framework, but the greater effectiveness of intervention A may reduce the uncertainty about impact, which may be an important consideration in some circumstances.

Effectiveness and cost-efficiency are important criteria for health aid (Denny and Emanuel 2008), but aid displacement is also a consideration. Health aid flowing to disease areas from which domestic resources could easily be diverted is likely to lead to displacement, possibly outside the health sector. This is especially true if the

aid recipient believes that the sum total of health aid and domestic resources flowing to the same area exceeds the social optimum. The evidence for health aid displacement is consistent with this process (Lu and others 2010). To prevent or reduce the likelihood of displacement, donors might fund interventions for diseases that are relatively underfunded.

Using health aid to fund cost-effective interventions for underfunded high-burden diseases could yield high returns. Local context will determine the appeal of a particular intervention, given that the burden, cost (cost-effectiveness), domestic prioritization, and effectiveness of an intervention are locally determined. Future work comparing the appeal of interventions based on local conditions could have important implications for health aid decisions.

Investments in Global Functions

The *Lancet* Commission on Investing in Health made the case that, as LMICs undergo economic growth, the value of health aid investments in "global functions"—that is, the provision of global public goods and protection against global cross-border health threats (Jamison and others 2013)—might become more appealing in comparison with country-specific investments. This concept has been echoed in several high-impact policy analyses (Blanchet and others 2014; Centre on Global Health Security Working Group on Health Financing 2014; Frenk and Moon 2013; Ottersen and others 2014).

Based on work by the *Lancet* Commission on Investing in Health, one study estimated how much donors spend on global functions versus how much they spend on country-specific support (Schäferhoff and others 2015). Global functions were characterized by their ability to address transnational issues and were divided into those providing global public goods (conducting R&D of new health tools, generating and sharing knowledge), those managing cross-border externalities (preparing for outbreaks, tackling antimicrobial resistance), and those fostering leadership and stewardship (convening leaders to build consensus). Country-specific support, in contrast, tackles current health priorities that justify international collective action. The study found that about one-fifth of health ODA plus was for key global health functions, with the rest channeled to country-specific support. Strengthening donor support for global functions could have several benefits that are not immediately obvious.

First, every country benefits from investments in global health, and the costs of inaction are potentially very high—for example, a severe influenza pandemic could result in as much as US$3 trillion in global losses

(Gostin and Friedman 2015). The returns on investing in R&D are potentially among the largest of all investments in global health, but actual investments in R&D for neglected and poverty-related diseases are limited. For example, a 70 percent efficacious vaccine would reduce new HIV/AIDS infections by 44 percent (Harmon and others 2016), leading to large reductions in incidence and potential epidemic control. The WHO has therefore called for a doubling of current R&D expenditures for poverty-related and neglected diseases—from US$3 billion to US$6 billion a year, approximately 3 percent of total health R&D (Consultative Expert Working Group on Research and Development: Financing and Coordination 2012). Market-shaping activities such as advanced market commitments also have led to important gains, especially in the fields of immunization and diagnostics. However, only a small fraction of current health aid has market-shaping effects.

Second, enhanced capacity for global disease surveillance and detection and improved international coordination are important for responding to emerging health threats, such as the Ebola outbreak in West Africa. Donors invested less than US$1 billion in 2013 for management of cross-border externalities (including outbreak preparedness but also environmental challenges and other global threats). In the years leading up to the Ebola outbreak, the WHO's budget for outbreak and crisis response was cut from US$469 million in 2012–13 to US$241 million in 2014–15. A pandemic of larger proportions could be extraordinarily costly, estimated at about US$500 billion per year in losses (Fan, Jamison, and Summers 2016). On the other hand, implementing a framework to improve preparedness for such an event is estimated to cost about US$4.5 billion a year and could lead to large savings (Sands, Mundaca-Shah, and Dzau 2016).

Third, investments in global functions would help address the "middle-income country dilemma": although most of the poor now live in pockets of poverty in MICs and face high mortality rates, these countries are considered to be sufficiently wealthy to finance health care for their entire populations and are therefore commonly not eligible for health aid. Poor individuals in MICs would benefit from donor support for global functions, such as R&D, knowledge sharing, market shaping, and better systems for controlling and managing outbreaks. China and India, for example, would substantially benefit from collective purchasing of commodities, market shaping to reduce drug prices, and international efforts to control multidrug-resistant tuberculosis. These countries would also benefit from greater global leadership and dialogue on topics such as how to fight the double burden of infectious and noncommunicable diseases,

how to design and implement taxation polices to increase domestic financing, and how to engage in cross-sectoral work, including human rights and education.

CONCLUSIONS

Health aid is a relatively large component of all health expenditures in LICs and one of the key tools for reducing preventable death and suffering among the world's poorest. Several key challenges and opportunities exist for the future of health aid:

- *Health aid has an opportunity to continue driving health improvements among the poorest.* Although more deliberate and nuanced allocation is needed, especially across countries, populations, and disease areas, opportunities exist for high-impact investments in programs that address high-burden disease, finance cost-effective interventions, and address domestically underfunded priorities.
- *Donors should clarify and explicitly state their goals and their criteria for health aid allocation.* There are many legitimate goals for providing health aid, including reducing global inequalities, averting preventable human suffering, engaging in self-protection from border-crossing threats, and promoting peaceful national bonds. However, these goals are often only implicit. Clear standards are needed to align strategy with goals. In their absence, organizational priorities remain vague, and short-term pressures may move organizations away from their core priorities. Poor alignment with core priorities may jeopardize success, which in the case of health aid has important human costs because it reduces the potential benefits to the poorest.
- *As domestic resources rise in LMICs, a growing portion of health care should be financed by domestic resources, and a declining portion should be financed by health aid.* In other words, many LMICs should require less health aid as their own domestic resources grow. However, such transitions will need to occur carefully because abrupt shifts may disrupt aid-dependent health programs and jeopardize health gains (Isenman 2015; Katz, Bassett, and Wright 2013).
- *Health aid should gradually target global functions.* Enormous benefits could be gained from the discovery of new vaccines and therapeutics or the design of effective pandemic surveillance systems. As more countries make the transition from health aid, donor funding could be directed to global functions. This shift would help support poor populations in all countries. However, the value of

these investments is incompletely understood and should be a research priority.

- *As the composition of donors, channels, and forms of health aid changes, data systems need to capture a fuller breadth of health aid.* Newer donors like China engage in global health in ways that are poorly captured in the current data systems, and changing this situation would have large benefits.

NOTES

World Bank Income Classifications as of July 2014 are as follows, based on estimates of gross national income (GNI) per capita for 2013:

- Low-income countries (LICs) = US$1,045 or less
- Middle-income countries (MICs) are subdivided:
  (a) lower-middle-income = US$1,046 to US$4,125
  (b) upper-middle-income (UMICs) = US$4,126 to US$12,745
- High-income countries (HICs) = US$12,746 or more.

1. Two important exclusions from ODA are other official flows (broadly, financial transfers that are not clearly intended to promote development of the recipient country) and grants from private sources. More details on the exact definition of these concepts are available at http://www.oecd.org/dac/stats/dac-glossary.htm#ODA.
2. Complete projects refer to construction or civil projects completed in recipient countries supported by Chinese grants or interest-free loans. The Chinese side is responsible for all or part of the construction process. After a project is completed, China hands it over to the recipient country.

REFERENCES

Basu, S., E. Bendavid, and N. Sood. 2015. "Health and Economic Implications of National Treatment Coverage for Cardiovascular Disease in India: Cost-Effectiveness Analysis." *Circulation: Cardiovascular Quality and Outcomes* 8 (6): 541–51.

Bendavid, E. 2014a. "Changes in Child Mortality over Time across the Wealth Gradient in Less-Developed Countries." *Pediatrics* 134 (6): e1551–59.

———. 2014b. "Is Health Aid Reaching the Poor? Analysis of Household Data from Aid-Recipient Countries." *PLoS One* 9 (1): e84025.

Bendavid, E., and J. Bhattacharya. 2014. "The Relationship of Health Aid to Population Health Improvements." *JAMA Internal Medicine* 174 (6): 881–87.

Bendavid, E., A. Duong, C. Sagan, and G. Raikes. 2015. "Health Aid Is Allocated Efficiently, but Not Optimally: Insights from a Review of Cost-Effectiveness Studies." *Health Affairs* 34 (7): 1188–95.

Berthélemy, J. C. 2006. "Bilateral Donors' Interest vs. Recipients' Development Motives in Aid Allocation: Do All Donors Behave the Same?" *Review of Development Economics* 10 (2): 179–94.

Blanchet, N., M. Thomas, R. Atun, D. Jamison, F. Knaul, and others. 2014. "Global Collective Action in Health: The WDR+ 20 Landscape of Core and Supportive Functions." WIDER Working Paper, United Nations University World Institute for Development Economics Research, Helsinki.

Centre on Global Health Security Working Group on Health Financing. 2014. *Shared Responsibilities for Health: A Coherent Global Framework for Health Financing.* London: Chatham House.

China State Council. 2011. "China's Foreign Aid." Information Office of the State Council, Beijing. http://www.gov.cn /english/official/2011-04/21/content_1849913.htm.

———. 2014. "China's Foreign Aid." Information Office of the State Council, Beijing. http://news.xinhuanet.com/english /china/2014-07/10/c_133474011.htm.

Consultative Expert Working Group on Research and Development: Financing and Coordination. 2012. *Research and Development to Meet Health Needs in Developing Countries: Strengthening Global Financing and Coordination.* Geneva: WHO.

Coyle, D., K. Coyle, C. Cameron, K. Lee, S. Kelly, and others. 2013. "Cost-Effectiveness of New Oral Anticoagulants Compared with Warfarin in Preventing Stroke and Other Cardiovascular Events in Patients with Atrial Fibrillation." *Value in Health* 16 (4): 498–506.

Darmstadt, G. L., M. V. Kinney, M. Chopra, S. Cousens, L. Kak, and others. 2014. "Who Has Been Caring for the Baby?" *The Lancet* 384 (9938): 174–88.

Deaton, A. S. 2009. "Instruments of Development: Randomization in the Tropics, and the Search for the Elusive Keys to Economic Development." Working Paper 14690, National Bureau of Economic Research, Cambridge, MA.

Denny, C. C., and E. J. Emanuel. 2008. "U.S. Health Aid beyond PEPFAR." *Journal of the American Medical Association* 300 (17): 2048–51.

Dieleman, J. L., C. Graves, E. Johnson, T. Templin, M. Birger, and others. 2015. "Sources and Focus of Health Development Assistance, 1990–2014." *Journal of the American Medical Association* 313 (23): 2359–68.

Fan, V. Y., D. J. Jamison, and L. H. Summers. 2016. "The Inclusive Loss of Pandemic Influenza Risk." NBER Working Paper No. 22137, National Bureau of Economic Research, Cambridge, MA.

Fauci, A. S., and G. K. Folkers. 2012. "The World Must Build on Three Decades of Scientific Advances to Enable a New Generation to Live Free of HIV/AIDS." *Health Affairs* 31 (7): 1529–36.

Fogarty International Center. 2015. *Global Health Matters Newsletter* (September-October). https://www.fic.nih.gov /News/GlobalHealthMatters/september-october-2015 /Pages/default.aspx.

———. 2016. "Research to Guide Practice: Enhancing HIV/ AIDS Platforms to Address NCDs in Low-Resource Settings." Fogarty International Center, Washington, DC. https://www .fic.nih.gov/About/Staff/Policy-Planning-Evaluation/Pages /pepfar-ncd-project.aspx.

Frenk, J., and S. Moon. 2013. "Governance Challenges in Global Health." *New England Journal of Medicine* 368 (10): 936–42.

Glassman, A., and R. Levine. 2016. *Millions Saved: New Cases of Proven Success in Global Health*. Washington, DC: Brookings Institution Press.

Global Fund. 2016a. "History of the Global Fund." Global Fund, Geneva. http://www.theglobalfund.org/en/history/.

———. 2016b. "Overview: Equitable Access Initiative." Global Fund, Geneva. http://www.theglobalfund.org/en/equitableaccessinitiative/.

Gostin, L. O., and E. A. Friedman. 2015. "A Retrospective and Prospective Analysis of the West African Ebola Virus Disease Epidemic: Robust National Health Systems at the Foundation and an Empowered WHO at the Apex." *The Lancet* 385 (9980): 1902–9.

Harmon, T. M., K. A. Fisher, M. G. McGlynn, J. Stover, M. J. Warren, and others. 2016. "Exploring the Potential Health Impact and Cost-Effectiveness of AIDS Vaccine within a Comprehensive HIV/AIDS Response in Low- and Middle-Income Countries." *PLoS One* 11 (1): e0146387.

Hoeffler, A., and V. Outram. 2011. "Need, Merit, or Self-Interest—What Determines the Allocation of Aid?" *Review of Development Economics* 15 (2): 237–50.

Hoos, D., W. El-Sadr, and K. L. Dehne. 2016. "Getting the Balance Right: Scaling up Treatment and Prevention." *Global Public Health* (April): 1–15.

IHME (Institute for Health Metrics and Evaluation). 2016a. "Financing Global Health 2015: Development Assistance Steady on the Path to New Global Goals." IHME, Seattle, WA.

———. 2016b. "Global Burden of Disease Study 2013 (GBD 2013) Results by Location, Cause, and Risk Factor." IHME, Seattle, WA.

Isenman, P. 2015. "Defining Development Drastically Downward: Premature Graduation from IDA and ODA." Brookings Institution blog, Washington, DC, March 5. http://www.brookings.edu/blogs/future-development/posts/2015/03/05-ida-eligibility-isenman.

Jamison, D. T., L. H. Summers, G. Alleyne, K. J. Arrow, S. Berkley, and others. 2013. "Global Health 2035: A World Converging within a Generation." *The Lancet* 382 (9908): 1898–955.

Katz, I. T., I. V. Bassett, and A. A. Wright. 2013. "PEPFAR in Transition: Implications for HIV Care in South Africa." *New England Journal of Medicine* 369 (15): 1385–87.

Kharas, H. 2015. "Trends and Issues in Qatari Foreign Aid." Working Paper 15-11, Silatech, Doha.

Kim, J. Y., and T. G. Evans. 2014. "Redefining the Measure of Medical Education: Harnessing the Transformative Potential of MEPI." *Academic Medicine* 89 (8): S29–31.

Kirton, J., J. Kulik, and C. Bracht. 2014. "The Political Process in Global Health and Nutrition Governance: The G-8's 2010 Muskoka Initiative on Maternal, Child, and Newborn Health." *Annals of the New York Academy of Sciences* 1331 (1): 186–200.

Kudamatsu, M. 2012. "Has Democratization Reduced Infant Mortality in Sub-Saharan Africa? Evidence from Micro Data." *Journal of the European Economic Association* 10 (6): 1294–317.

Levine, R. 2004. *Millions Saved: Proven Successes in Global Health*. Washington, DC: Peterson Institute.

Liu, P., Y. Guo, X. Qian, S. Tang, Z. Li, and others. 2014. "China's Distinctive Engagement in Global Health." *The Lancet* 384 (9945): 793–804.

Lu, C., M. T. Schneider, P. Gubbins, K. Leach-Kemon, D. Jamison, and others. 2010. "Public Financing of Health in Developing Countries: A Cross-National Systematic Analysis." *The Lancet* 375 (9723): 1375–87.

McNeil, D., Jr. 2010. "At Front Lines, AIDS War Is Falling Apart." *New York Times,* May 9. http://www.nytimes.com/2009/01/31/health/31aids.html.

Miller-Petrie, M., S. Pant, and R. Laxminarayan. 2017. "Drug Resistant Infections." In *Disease Control Priorities* (third edition), Volume 6, *Major Infectious Diseases*. Edited by K. K. Holmes, S. Bertozzi, B. R. Bloom, and P. Jha. Washington, DC: World Bank.

Moon, S., and O. Omole. 2013. "Development Assistance for Health: Critiques and Proposals for Change." Chatham House, London.

Murray, C. J., R. M. Barber, K. J. Foreman, A. A. Ozgoren, F. Abd-Allah, and others. 2015. "Global, Regional, and National Disability-Adjusted Life Years (DALYs) for 306 Diseases and Injuries and Healthy Life Expectancy (HALE) for 188 Countries, 1990–2013: Quantifying the Epidemiological Transition." *The Lancet* 386 (10009): 2145–91.

Ottersen, T., A. Kamath, S. Moon, and J.-A. Røttingen. 2014. "Development Assistance for Health: Quantitative Allocation Criteria and Contribution Norms." Centre on Global Health Security Working Group Paper, Chatham House, London.

PMNCH (Partnership for Maternal, Newborn, and Child Health). 2014. *The PMNCH 2014 Accountability Report: Tracking Financial Commitments to the Global Strategy for Women's and Children's Health*. Geneva: World Health Organization, PMNCH.

Prabhakaran, S., I. Ruff, and R. A. Bernstein. 2015. "Acute Stroke Intervention: A Systematic Review." *Journal of the American Medical Association* 313 (14): 1451–62.

Pritchett, L. 2004. "An Homage to the Randomistas on the Occasion of the J-PAL 10th Anniversary: Development as a Faith-Based Activity." Center for Global Development blog, Washington, DC, March 10. http://www.cgdev.org/blog/homage-randomistas-occasion-j-pal-10th-anniversary-development-faith-based-activity.

Ravishankar, N., P. Gubbins, R. J. Cooley, K. Leach-Kemon, C. M. Michaud, and others. 2009. "Financing of Global Health: Tracking Development Assistance for Health from 1990 to 2007." *The Lancet* 373 (9681): 2113–24.

Resch, S., T. Ryckman, and R. Hecht. 2015. "Funding AIDS Programmes in the Era of Shared Responsibility: An Analysis of Domestic Spending in 12 Low-Income and Middle-Income Countries." *The Lancet Global Health* 3 (1): e52–61.

Rose, G. 2001. "Sick Individuals and Sick Populations." *International Journal of Epidemiology* 30 (3): 427–32.

Sands, P., C. Mundaca-Shah, and V. J. Dzau. 2016. "The Neglected Dimension of Global Security: A Framework for Countering Infectious-Disease Crises." *New England Journal of Medicine* 374 (13): 1281–87.

Schäferhoff, M., S. Fewer, J. Kraus, E. Richter, L. H. Summers, and others. 2015. "How Much Donor Financing for Health Is Channelled to Global versus Country-Specific Aid Functions?" *The Lancet* 386 (10011): 2436–41.

Sridhar, D., and R. Batniji. 2008. "Misfinancing Global Health: A Case for Transparency in Disbursements and Decision Making." *The Lancet* 372 (9644): 1185–91.

Sumner, A. 2012. "Where Do the Poor Live?" *World Development* 40 (5): 865–77.

USAID (U.S. Agency for International Development). 2012. *USAID's Global Health Strategic Framework: Better Health for Development.* Washington, DC: USAID.

———. 2015. *2015 VolAg Report: The Report of Voluntary Agencies Engaged in Overseas Relief and Development.* Washington, DC: USAID.

Vermund, S. H., M. Sidat, L. F. Weil, J. A. Tique, T. D. Moon, and others. 2012. "Transitioning HIV Care and Treatment Programs in Southern Africa to Full Local Management." *AIDS* 26 (10): 1303–10.

Victora, C. G., J. H. Requejo, A. J. Barros, P. Berman, Z. Bhutta, and others. 2015. "Countdown to 2015: A Decade of Tracking Progress for Maternal, Newborn, and Child Survival." *The Lancet* 387 (10032): 2049–59.

WHO (World Health Organization). n.d. "Health Accounts." WHO, Geneva. http://www.who.int/health-accounts/en.

Zhou, H., J. Zhang, and M. Zhang. 2015. *Foreign Aid in China.* Berlin: Springer Verlag and Social Sciences Academic Press (China).

Chapter 17

Pandemics: Risks, Impacts, and Mitigation

Nita Madhav, Ben Oppenheim, Mark Gallivan,
Prime Mulembakani, Edward Rubin, and Nathan Wolfe

INTRODUCTION

Pandemics are large-scale outbreaks of infectious disease that can greatly increase morbidity and mortality over a wide geographic area and cause significant economic, social, and political disruption. Evidence suggests that the likelihood of pandemics has increased over the past century because of increased global travel and integration, urbanization, changes in land use, and greater exploitation of the natural environment (Jones and others 2008; Morse 1995). These trends likely will continue and will intensify. Significant policy attention has focused on the need to identify and limit emerging outbreaks that might lead to pandemics and to expand and sustain investment to build preparedness and health capacity (Smolinsky, Hamburg, and Lederberg 2003).

The international community has made progress toward preparing for and mitigating the impacts of pandemics. The 2003 severe acute respiratory syndrome (SARS) pandemic and growing concerns about the threat posed by avian influenza led many countries to devise pandemic plans (U.S. Department of Health and Human Services 2005). Delayed reporting of early SARS cases also led the World Health Assembly to update the International Health Regulations (IHR) to compel all World Health Organization member states to meet specific standards for detecting, reporting on, and responding to outbreaks (WHO 2005). The framework put into place by the updated IHR contributed to a more coordinated global response during the 2009 influenza pandemic (Katz 2009). International donors also have begun to invest in improving preparedness through refined standards and funding for building health capacity (Wolicki and others 2016).

Despite these improvements, significant gaps and challenges exist in global pandemic preparedness. Progress toward meeting the IHR has been uneven, and many countries have been unable to meet basic requirements for compliance (Fischer and Katz 2013; WHO 2014). Multiple outbreaks, notably the 2014 West Africa Ebola epidemic, have exposed gaps related to the timely detection of disease, availability of basic care, tracing of contacts, quarantine and isolation procedures, and preparedness outside the health sector, including global coordination and response mobilization (Moon and others 2015; Pathmanathan and others 2014). These gaps are especially evident in resource-limited settings and have posed challenges during relatively localized epidemics, with dire implications for what may happen during a full-fledged global pandemic.

For the purposes of this chapter, an *epidemic* is defined as "the occurrence in a community or region of cases of an illness . . . clearly in excess of normal expectancy" (Porta 2014). A *pandemic* is defined as "an epidemic occurring over a very wide area, crossing international boundaries, and usually affecting a large number of people" (Porta 2014). Pandemics are, therefore, identified by their geographic scale rather than the severity of illness. For example, in contrast to annual seasonal influenza epidemics, *pandemic influenza* is

Corresponding Author: Nita Madhav, MSPH, Metabiota, San Francisco, California, United States; nmadhav@metabiota.com.

defined as "when a new influenza virus emerges and spreads around the world, and most people do not have immunity" (WHO 2010).

This chapter does not consider endemic diseases—those that are constantly present in particular localities or regions. Endemic diseases are far more common than pandemics and can have significant negative health and economic impacts, especially in low- and middle-income countries (LMICs) with weak health systems. Additionally, given the lack of historical data and extreme uncertainty regarding bioterrorism, this chapter does not specifically consider bioterrorism-related events, although bioterrorism could hypothetically lead to a pandemic.

This chapter covers the following findings concerning the risks, impacts, and mitigation of pandemics as well as knowledge gaps:

Risks

- Pandemics have occurred throughout history and appear to be increasing in frequency, particularly because of the increasing emergence of viral disease from animals.
- Pandemic risk is driven by the combined effects of spark risk (*where* a pandemic is likely to arise) and spread risk (*how likely* it is to diffuse broadly through human populations).
- Some geographic regions with high spark risk, including Central and West Africa, lag behind the rest of the globe in pandemic preparedness.
- Probabilistic modeling and analytical tools such as exceedance probability (EP) curves are valuable for assessing pandemic risk and estimating the potential burden of pandemics.
- Influenza is the most likely pathogen to cause a severe pandemic. EP analysis indicates that in any given year, a 1 percent probability exists of an influenza pandemic that causes nearly 6 million pneumonia and influenza deaths or more globally.

Impacts

- Pandemics can cause significant, widespread increases in morbidity and mortality and have disproportionately higher mortality impacts on LMICs.
- Pandemics can cause economic damage through multiple channels, including short-term fiscal shocks and longer-term negative shocks to economic growth.
- Individual behavioral changes, such as fear-induced aversion to workplaces and other public gathering places, are a primary cause of negative shocks to economic growth during pandemics.

- Some pandemic mitigation measures can cause significant social and economic disruption.
- In countries with weak institutions and legacies of political instability, pandemics can increase political stresses and tensions. In these contexts, outbreak response measures such as quarantines have sparked violence and tension between states and citizens.

Mitigation

- Pathogens with pandemic potential vary widely in the resources, capacities, and strategies required for mitigation. However, there are also common prerequisites for effective preparedness and response.
- The most cost-effective strategies for increasing pandemic preparedness, especially in resource-constrained settings, consist of investing to strengthen core public health infrastructure, including water and sanitation systems; increasing situational awareness; and rapidly extinguishing sparks that could lead to pandemics.
- Once a pandemic has started, a coordinated response should be implemented focusing on maintenance of situational awareness, public health messaging, reduction of transmission, and care for and treatment of the ill.
- Successful contingency planning and response require surge capacity—the ability to scale up the delivery of health interventions proportionately for the severity of the event, the pathogen, and the population at risk.
- For many poorly prepared countries, surge capacity likely will be delivered by foreign aid providers. This is a tenable strategy during localized outbreaks, but global surge capacity has limits that likely will be reached during a full-scale global pandemic as higher-capacity states focus on their own populations.
- Risk transfer mechanisms, such as risk pooling and sovereign-level catastrophe insurance, provide a viable option for managing pandemic risk.

Knowledge Gaps

- Spending and costs specifically associated with pandemic preparedness and response efforts are poorly tracked.
- There is no widely accepted, consistent methodology for estimating the economic impacts of pandemics.
- Most data regarding the impacts of pandemics and the benefits and costs of mitigation measures come from high-income countries (HICs), leading to biases and potential blind spots regarding the risks, consequences, and optimal interventions specific to LMICs.

PANDEMIC RISKS AND CONSEQUENCES

Importance of Pandemics

Pandemics can cause sudden, widespread morbidity and mortality as well as social, political, and economic disruption. The world has endured several notable pandemics, including the Black Death, Spanish flu, and human immunodeficiency virus/acquired immune deficiency syndrome (HIV/AIDS) (table 17.1).

Because the definition of pandemic primarily is geographic, it groups together multiple, distinct types of events and public health threats, all of which have their own severity, frequency, and other disease characteristics. Each type of event requires its own optimal preparedness and response strategy; however this chapter also discusses common prerequisites for effective response. The variety of pandemic threats is driven by the great diversity of pathogens and their interaction with humans. Pathogens vary across multiple dimensions, including the mechanism and dynamics of disease transmission, severity, and differentiability of associated morbidities. These and other factors determine whether cases will be identified and contained rapidly or whether an outbreak will spread (Fraser and others 2004). As a result, pathogens with pandemic potential also vary widely in the scale of their potential health, economic, and sociopolitical impacts as well as the resources, capacities, and strategies required for mitigation.

One must distinguish between several broad categories of pandemic threats. At one extreme are pathogens that have high potential to cause truly global, severe pandemics. This group includes pandemic influenza viruses. These pathogens transmit efficiently between humans, have sufficiently long asymptomatic infectious periods to facilitate the undetected movement of infected persons, and have symptomatic profiles that present challenges for differential diagnosis (particularly in the early periods of infection). A second group of pathogens presents a moderate global threat. These agents (for example, Nipah virus and H5N1 and H7N9 influenzas) have not demonstrated sustained human-to-human transmission but could become transmitted more efficiently as a result of mutations and adaptation. A third group of pathogens (for example, Ebola, Marburg, Lassa) has the potential to cause regional or interregional epidemics, but the risk of a truly global pandemic is limited because of the slow pace of transmission or high probability of detection and containment.

Among all known pandemic pathogens, influenza poses the principal threat because of its potential severity and semiregular occurrence since at least the 16th century (Morens and others 2010). The infamous 1918 influenza pandemic killed an estimated 20 million

Table 17.1 Notable Epidemics and Pandemics since the Middle Ages

Starting year	Event	Geographic extent	Estimated direct morbidity or mortality	Estimated economic, social, or political impact
1347	Bubonic plague (Black Death) pandemic	Eurasia	30–50 percent mortality of the European population (DeWitte 2014)	Likely hastened end of the feudal system in Europe (Platt 2014)
Early 1500s	Introduction of smallpox	Americas	More than 50 percent mortality in some communities (Jones 2006)	Destroyed native societies, facilitating the hegemony of European countries (Diamond 2009)
1881	Fifth cholera pandemic	Global	More than 1.5 million deaths (9.7 per 10,000 persons) (Chisholm 1911)	Sparked attacks on Russian tsarist government and medical officials (Frieden 1977)
1918	Spanish flu influenza pandemic	Global	20 million–100 million deaths (111–555 deaths per 10,000 persons) (Johnson and Mueller 2002)	GDP loss of 3 percent in Australia, 15 percent in Canada, 17 percent in the United Kingdom, 11 percent in the United States (McKibbin and Sidorenko 2006)
1957	Asian flu influenza pandemic	Global	0.7 million–1.5 million deaths (2.4–5.1 deaths per 10,000 persons) (Viboud and others 2016)	GDP loss of 3 percent in Canada, Japan, the United Kingdom, and the United States (McKibbin and Sidorenko 2006)
1968	Hong Kong flu influenza pandemic	Global	1 million deaths (2.8 deaths per 10,000 persons) (Mathews and others 2009)	US$23 billion–US$26 billion direct and indirect costs in the United States (Kavet 1977)

table continues next page

Table 17.1 Notable Epidemics and Pandemics since the Middle Ages (continued)

Starting year	Event	Geographic extent	Estimated direct morbidity or mortality	Estimated economic, social, or political impact
1981	HIV/AIDS pandemic	Global	More than 70 million infections, 36.7 million deaths (WHO Global Health Observatory data, http://www.who.int/gho/hiv/en/)	2–4 percent annual loss of GDP growth in Africa (Dixon, McDonald, and Roberts 2001)[a]
2003	SARS pandemic	4 continents, 37 countries	8,098 possible cases, 744 deaths (Wang and Jolly 2004)	GDP loss of US$4 billion in Hong Kong SAR, China; US$3 billion–US$6 billion in Canada; and US$5 billion in Singapore (Keogh-Brown and Smith 2008)
2009	Swine flu influenza pandemic	Global	151,700–575,500 deaths (0.2–0.8 per 10,000 persons) (Dawood and others 2012)	GDP loss of US$1 billion in the Republic of Korea (Kim, Yoon, and Oh 2013)
2012	MERS epidemic	22 countries	1,879 symptomatic cases, 659 deaths (Arabi and others 2017)	US$2 billion loss in the Republic of Korea, triggering US$14 billion in government stimulus spending (Jun 2015; Park and Kim 2015)
2013[b]	West Africa Ebola virus disease epidemic	10 countries	28,646 cases, 11,323 deaths (WHO 2016a)	US$2 billion loss in Guinea, Liberia, and Sierra Leone (World Bank 2014)
2015	Zika virus pandemic	76 countries	2,656 reported cases of microcephaly or central nervous system malformation (WHO 2017)	US$7 billion–US$18 billion loss in Latin America and the Caribbean (UNDP 2017)

Note: List of events is illustrative rather than exhaustive. All U.S. dollar amounts are rounded to nearest billion. GDP = gross domestic product; HIV/AIDS = human immunodeficiency virus/acquired immunodeficiency syndrome; MERS = Middle East respiratory syndrome; SARS = severe acute respiratory syndrome.

a. Studies of the effects of HIV/AIDS on per capita gross national product have found smaller effects.

b. The West Africa Ebola virus outbreak occurred from 2013 to 2016, but the peak and international response efforts began in 2014.

to 100 million persons globally, with few countries spared (Johnson and Mueller 2002). Its severity reflects in part the limited health technologies of the period, when no antibiotics, antivirals, or vaccines were available to reduce transmission or mortality (Murray and others 2006).

During the 1918 pandemic, populations experienced significantly higher mortality rates in LMICs than in HICs, likely as a result of higher levels of malnutrition and comorbid conditions, insufficient access to supportive medical care, and higher rates of disease transmission (Brundage and Shanks 2008; Murray and others 2006). The mortality disparity between HICs and LMICs likely would be even greater today for a similarly severe event, because LMICs have disproportionately lower medical capacity, less access to modern medical interventions, and higher interconnectivity between population centers.

Origin of Pandemics

Most new pandemics have originated through the "zoonotic" transmission of pathogens from animals to humans (Murphy 1998; Woolhouse and Gowtage-Sequeria 2005), and the next pandemic is likely to be a zoonosis as well. Zoonoses enter into human populations from both domesticated animals (such as farmed swine or poultry) and wildlife. Many historically significant zoonoses were introduced through increased human-animal interaction following domestication, and potentially high-risk zoonoses (including avian influenzas) continue to emerge from livestock production systems (Van Boeckel and others 2012; Wolfe, Dunavan, and Diamond 2007). Some pathogens (including Ebola) have emerged from wildlife reservoirs and entered into human populations through the hunting and consumption of wild species (such as bushmeat), the wild animal trade, and other contact with wildlife (Pike and others 2010; Wolfe, Dunavan, and Diamond 2007).

Zoonotic pathogens vary in the extent to which they can survive within and spread between human hosts. As shown in table 17.2, the degree of zoonotic adaptation spans a continuum from transmission only within animal populations (stage 1) to transmission only within human populations (stage 5). Most zoonotic pathogens are not well adapted to humans (stages 2–3), emerge sporadically through spillover events, and may lead to localized outbreaks, called stuttering chains (Pike and others 2010; Wolfe and others 2005). These episodes of "viral chatter" increase pandemic risk by providing opportunities for viruses to become better adapted to spreading within a human population. Pathogens that are past stage 3 are of the greatest concern, because they are sufficiently adapted to humans to cause long transmission chains between humans (directly or indirectly through vectors), and their geographic spread is not constrained by the habitat range of an animal reservoir.

Pandemic Risk Factors

Pandemic risk, as noted, is driven by the combined effects of spark risk and spread risk. The foci of both risk factors often overlap, especially in some LMICs (such as in Central and West Africa and Southeast Asia), making these areas particularly vulnerable to pandemics and their negative consequences.

Spark Risk

A zoonotic spark could arise from the introduction of a pathogen from either domesticated animals or wildlife. Zoonoses from domesticated animals are concentrated in areas with dense livestock production systems, including areas of China, India, Japan, the United States, and Western Europe. Key drivers for spark risk from domesticated animals include intensive and extensive farming and livestock production systems and live animal markets, as well as the potential for contact between livestock and wildlife reservoirs (Gilbert and others 2014; Jones and others 2008). Wildlife zoonosis risk is distributed far more broadly, with foci in China, India, West and Central Africa, and the Amazon Basin (Jones and others 2008). Risk drivers include behavioral factors (such as bushmeat hunting and use of animal-based traditional medicines), natural resource extraction (such as sylviculture and logging), the extension of roads into wildlife habitats, and environmental factors (including the degree and distribution of animal diversity) (Wolfe and others 2005).

Spread Risk

After a spark or importation, the risk that a pathogen will spread within a population is influenced by pathogen-specific factors (including genetic adaptation and mode of transmission) and human population-level factors (such as the density of the population and the susceptibility to infection; patterns of movement driven by travel, trade, and migration; and speed and effectiveness of public health surveillance and response measures) (Sands and others 2016).

Table 17.2 Pathogen Adaptation and Pandemic Risk

Stage	Transmission to humans[a]	Pathogen example	Simplified transmission diagram
Stage 1: animal reservoir transmission only	None	H3N8 equine influenza virus	
Stage 2: primary infection	Only from animals	Anthrax	
Stage 3: limited outbreaks	Few human-to-human transmission chains	Marburg virus	
Stage 4: sustained outbreaks	Many human-to-human transmission chains	Pandemic A (H1N1) 2009 influenza virus	
Stage 5: predominant human transmission	Human-to-human	Smallpox virus	

Source: Adapted from Wolfe, Dunavan, and Diamond 2007.
a. Direct or indirect transmission through vector.

Dense concentrations of population, especially in urban centers harboring overcrowded informal settlements, can act as foci for disease transmission and accelerate the spread of pathogens (Neiderud 2015). Moreover, social inequality, poverty, and their environmental correlates can increase individual susceptibility to infection significantly (Farmer 1996). Comorbidities, malnutrition, and caloric deficits weaken an individual's immune system, while environmental factors such as lack of clean water and adequate sanitation amplify transmission rates and increase morbidity and mortality (Toole and Waldman 1990). Collectively, all these factors suggest that marginalized populations, including refugees and people living in urban slums and informal settlements, likely face elevated risks of morbidity and mortality during a pandemic.

A country's expected ability to curtail pandemic spread can be expressed using a preparedness index developed by Oppenheim and others (2017). The index illustrates global variation in institutional readiness to detect and respond to a large-scale outbreak of infectious disease. It draws on the IHR core capacity metrics and other publicly accessible cross-national indicators. However, it diverges from the IHR metrics in its breadth and focus on measuring underlying and enabling institutional, infrastructural, and financial capacities such as the following (Oppenheim and others 2017):

- Public health infrastructure capable of identifying, tracing, managing, and treating cases
- Adequate physical and communications infrastructure to channel information and resources
- Fundamental bureaucratic and public management capacities
- Capacity to mobilize financial resources to pay for disease response and weather the economic shock of the outbreak
- Ability to undertake effective risk communications.

Well-prepared countries have effective public institutions, strong economies, and adequate investment in the health sector. They have built specific competencies critical to detecting and managing disease outbreaks, including surveillance, mass vaccination, and risk communications. Poorly prepared countries may suffer from political instability, weak public administration, inadequate resources for public health, and gaps in fundamental outbreak detection and response systems.

Map 17.1 presents the global distribution of epidemic preparedness, with countries grouped into quintiles. A geographic analysis of preparedness shows that some areas of high spark risk also are the least prepared. Geographic areas with high spark risk from domesticated animals (including China, North America, and Western Europe) have relatively higher levels of preparedness,

Map 17.1 Global Distribution of Epidemic Preparedness, 2017

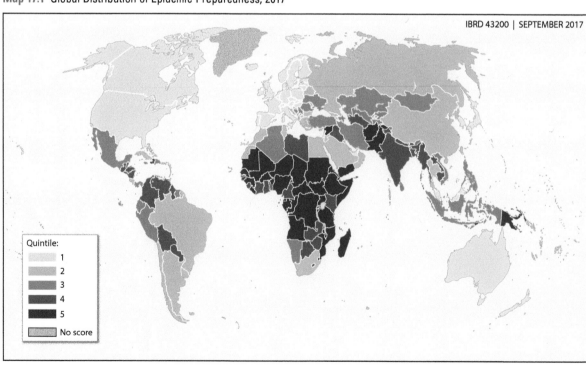

Note: Countries are grouped into quintiles of epidemic preparedness (1 = most prepared, 5 = least prepared).

although China lags behind its counterparts. However, geographic areas with high spark risk from wildlife species (including Central and West Africa) have some of the lowest preparedness scores globally, indicating a potentially dangerous overlap of spark risk and spread risk.

Table 17.3 presents the average epidemic preparedness quintile across each of the World Bank's country income groups. National income alone offers an incomplete and potentially misleading metric of preparedness. Although income is correlated with epidemic preparedness, many countries are substantially better or worse prepared than expected, given their gross national income per capita.

Burden of Pandemics

Quantifying the morbidity and mortality burden from pandemics poses a significant challenge. Although estimates are available from historical events (table 17.1), the historical record is sparse and incomplete. To overcome these gaps in estimating the frequency and severity of pandemics, probabilistic modeling techniques can augment the historical record with a large catalog of hypothetical, scientifically plausible, simulated pandemics that represent a wide range of possible scenarios. Modeling can also better account for changes that have occurred since historical times, such as medical advances, changing demographics, and shifting travel patterns.

Scenario modeling of epidemics and pandemics can be achieved through large-scale computer simulations of global spread, dynamics, and illness outcomes of disease (Colizza and others 2007; Tizzoni and others 2012). These models allow for specification of parameters that may drive the likelihood of a spark (for example, location and frequency) and determinants of severity (for example, transmissibility and virulence). The models then simulate at a daily time step the spread of disease

from person to person via disease transmission dynamics and from place to place via incorporation of long-range and short-range population movements. The models also can incorporate mitigation measures, seasonality, stochastic processes, and other factors that can vary during an epidemic. Millions of these simulations can be run with wide variation in the initial conditions and final outcomes.

These millions of simulations can be used to quantify the burden of pandemics through a class of probabilistic modeling called catastrophe modeling, which the insurance industry uses to understand risks posed by infrequent natural disasters such as hurricanes and earthquakes (Fullam and Madhav 2015; Kozlowski and Mathewson 1997). When applied to pandemics, this approach requires statistically fitting distributions of the parameters. These parameter distributions provide weightings of the likelihood of the different events. Through correlated statistical sampling based on the parameter weights, scenarios are selected for inclusion in an event catalog of simulated pandemic events. A schematic diagram shows how the catastrophe modeling process is used to develop the event catalog (figure 17.1).

Analysis of the event catalog yields annual EP curves (for example, as shown in figure 17.2), which provide a metric of the likelihood that an event of a given severity, or worse, begins in any given year. The EP curve is a visualization of the event catalog, in which the number of estimated deaths for each event is ranked in descending order. Because the event catalog includes scenarios incorporating spark probabilities and estimates of disease propagation, the EP curve includes the combined impacts of both spark risk and spread risk. Although a global curve is shown in figure 17.2, EP curves can be estimated for other geographic resolutions, such as a country or province.

Table 17.3 Epidemic Preparedness Score, by Country Income Group, 2017

Country income group[a]	Mean epidemic preparedness quintile[b]	Top-performing country in group	Bottom-performing country in group
High-income	1.3	Norway	Trinidad and Tobago
Upper-middle-income	2.9	Malaysia	Equatorial Guinea
Lower-middle-income	3.7	Armenia	Mauritania
Low-income	4.8	Nepal	Somalia

Source: The epidemic preparedness index draws on indicators from the World Health Organization, World Bank, United Nations agencies, and nongovernmental sources (see Oppenheim and others 2017).

a. Income groups follow World Bank income classifications for fiscal 2018, based on estimates of 2016 gross national income per capita and calculated using the World Bank Atlas method: high-income (US$12,236 or more), upper-middle-income (US$3,956–US$12,235), lower-middle-income (US$1,006–US$3,955), and low-income (US$1,005 or less). For further explanation, see https://datahelpdesk.worldbank.org/knowledgebase/articles/906519-world-bank-country-and-lending-groups.

b. Countries are grouped into quintiles of epidemic preparedness (1 = most prepared, 5 = least prepared).

Figure 17.1 Process for Generating the Event Catalog

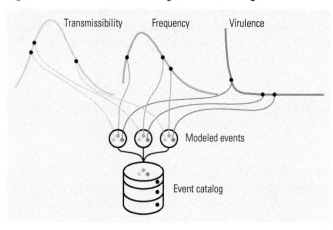

Figure 17.2 Estimated Annual Exceedance Probability Curve for Global Pneumonia and Influenza Deaths Caused by Influenza Pandemics, 2017

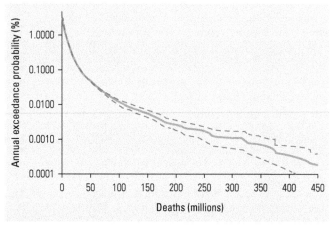

Source: Metabiota simulations.
Note: Annual exceedance probability is the likelihood that an event of a given severity, or worse, begins in any given year. Dashed lines indicate the 5th and 95th percentile bands.

The EP curve is a powerful tool that yields several key findings regarding the frequency and severity of potential pandemics. Applied to influenza pandemics, we find the following:

- An influenza pandemic having the global mortality rate observed during the 2009 Swine flu pandemic (0.2–0.8 deaths per 10,000 persons) or worse has about a 3 percent probability of occurring in any given year.
- In any given year, the probability of an influenza pandemic causing nearly 6 million pneumonia and influenza deaths (8 deaths per 10,000 persons) or more globally is 1 percent.
- The annual probability of an influenza pandemic's meeting or exceeding the global mortality rate of the 1918 Spanish flu pandemic (111–555 deaths per 10,000 persons) is less than 0.02 percent.
- As indicated by the heavy tail of the EP curve, most of the potential burden from influenza pandemics comes from the most severe pandemics.

Table 17.4 shows select EPs for influenza pandemics in low-, middle-, and high-income countries, based on further analysis of the event catalog. For example, in any given year, all LICs combined have a 3 percent probability of experiencing at least 140,000 deaths attributable to an influenza pandemic and a 0.1 percent chance of experiencing at least 8.3 million deaths. LICs bear a substantial burden of mortality risk from influenza pandemics. Strikingly, LICs contain only about 9 percent of the global population, yet they would contribute nearly 25 percent of deaths during an influenza pandemic.

Based on the event catalog, the average estimated global mortality from pneumonia and influenza during

Table 17.4 Select Annual Exceedance Probabilities for Pneumonia and Influenza Deaths Caused by Influenza Pandemics, by Country Income Level, 2017

Annual exceedance probability (%)	Deaths (millions)			
	Low income	Middle income	High income	Total
3.0	0.1	0.4	0.05	0.6
2.0	0.6	1.5	0.1	2.2
1.0	1.5	4.0	0.4	5.9
0.5	2.7	7.6	0.9	11.2
0.2	5.5	14.8	1.7	22.0
0.1	8.3	22.5	2.5	33.3

Source: Metabiota simulations.
Note: Annual exceedance probability is the likelihood that an event of a given severity, or worse, begins in any given year. Rows may not sum to total value due to rounding.

an influenza pandemic is more than 7.3 million deaths. However, because influenza pandemics occur on average once every 25–30 years, the average annual pneumonia and influenza mortality from influenza pandemics is a little more than 230,000 deaths. This is comparable to seasonal influenza, which worldwide causes at least 250,000 deaths annually (WHO 2016b). Although both numbers reflect an annual average, they differ in the combination of frequency and severity. Seasonal influenza deaths occur every year, but pandemic influenza deaths occur much less frequently, are concentrated in larger spikes, and affect a younger demographic.

When pandemics cause large morbidity and mortality spikes, they are much more likely to overwhelm health systems. Overwhelmed health systems and other indirect effects may contribute to a 2.3-fold increase in all-cause mortality during pandemics, although attribution of the causative agent is difficult (Simonsen and others 2013). If indirect deaths are taken into account, the average annual global deaths from influenza pandemics could be greater than 520,000, although there is a significant uncertainty in the estimate.

Pandemics caused by pathogens other than influenza also must be considered. Novel coronaviruses (such as SARS-CoV), filoviruses (such as Ebola virus), and flaviviruses (such as Zika virus) have caused large epidemics and pandemics. These viruses, like influenza, are ribonucleic acid viruses that have high mutation rates. Noninfluenza viruses typically cause more frequent, smaller epidemics but also an overall lower burden of morbidity and mortality than pandemic influenza. For diseases caused by coronaviruses and filoviruses, the lower burden stems from the mode of transmission, which often requires closer and more sustained contact than influenza does to spread.

Consequences of Pandemics

Health Impacts

The direct health impacts of pandemics can be catastrophic. During the Black Death, an estimated 30–50 percent of the European population perished (DeWitte 2014). More recently, the HIV/AIDS pandemic has killed more than 35 million persons since 1981 (WHO Global Health Observatory data, http://www.who.int/gho/hiv/en).

Pandemics can disproportionately affect younger, more economically active segments of the population (Charu and others 2011). During influenza pandemics (as opposed to seasonal outbreaks of influenza), the morbidity and mortality age distributions shift to younger populations, because younger people have lower immunity than older people, which significantly increases the years of life lost (Viboud and others 2010). Furthermore, many infectious diseases can have chronic effects, which can become more common or widespread in the case of a pandemic. For example, Zika-associated microcephaly has lifelong impacts on health and well-being.

The indirect health impacts of pandemics can increase morbidity and mortality further. Drivers of indirect health impacts include diversion or depletion of resources to provide routine care and decreased access to routine care resulting from an inability to travel, fear, or other factors. Additionally, fear can lead to an upsurge of the "worried well" seeking unnecessary care, further burdening the health care system (Falcone and Detty 2015).

During the 2014 West Africa Ebola epidemic, lack of routine care for malaria, HIV/AIDS, and tuberculosis led to an estimated 10,600 additional deaths in Guinea, Liberia, and Sierra Leone (Parpia and others 2016). This indirect death toll nearly equaled the 11,300 deaths directly caused by Ebola in those countries (WHO 2016a). Additionally, diversion of funds, medical resources, and personnel led to a 30 percent decrease in routine childhood immunization rates in affected countries (UNDP 2014). During the 2009 influenza pandemic, a greater surge in hospital admissions for influenza and pneumonia was associated with statistically significant increases in deaths attributable to acute myocardial infarction and stroke (Rubinson and others 2013). However, during a pandemic, distinguishing which deaths are attributable to the pandemic itself and which are merely coincidental may be impossible.

During the 2014 West Africa Ebola epidemic, facilities closures as a result of understaffing and fear of contracting the disease played a large role in lack of access to or avoidance of routine health care. One study of 45 public facilities in Guinea found that the Ebola outbreak led to a 31 percent decrease in outpatient visits for routine maternal and child health services (Barden-O'Fallon and others 2015). Among children under age five years, hospitals witnessed a 60 percent decrease in visits for diarrhea and a 58 percent decrease in visits for acute respiratory illness (ARI), while health centers saw a 25 percent decrease in visits for diarrhea and a 23 percent decrease in visits for ARI. In Sierra Leone, visits to public facilities for reproductive health care fell by as much as 40 percent during the outbreak (UNDP 2014).

The availability of health care workers also decreases during a pandemic because of illness, deaths, and fear-driven absenteeism. Viral hemorrhagic fevers such as Ebola take an especially severe toll on health care workers, who face significant exposure to infectious material:

- *During the first Ebola outbreak* in the Democratic Republic of Congo in 1976 (then called Zaire), the Yambuku Mission Hospital—at the epicenter of the outbreak—was closed because 11 out of the 17 staff members had died of the disease (WHO 1978).
- *During the Kikwit Ebola outbreak in 1995* in the same country, 24 percent of cases occurred among known or possible health care workers (Rosello and others 2015).
- *During the 2014 West Africa Ebola epidemic,* health care workers experienced high mortality rates: 8 percent of doctors, nurses, and midwives succumbed to Ebola in Liberia, 7 percent in Sierra Leone, and 1 percent in Guinea (Evans, Goldstein, and Popova 2015).

Even if health care workers do not die, their ability to provide care may be reduced. At the peak of a severe influenza pandemic, up to 40 percent of health care workers might be unable to report for duty because they are ill themselves, need to care for ill family members, need to care for children because of school closures, or are afraid (Falcone and Detty 2015; U.S. Homeland Security Council 2006).

Economic Impacts

Pandemics can cause acute, short-term fiscal shocks as well as longer-term damage to economic growth. Early-phase public health efforts to contain or limit outbreaks (such as tracing contacts, implementing quarantines, and isolating infectious cases) entail significant human resource and staffing costs (Achonu, Laporte, and Gardam 2005). As an outbreak grows, new facilities may need to be constructed to manage additional infectious cases; this, along with increasing demand for consumables (medical supplies, personal protective equipment, and drugs) can greatly increase health system expenditures (Herstein and others 2016).

Diminished tax revenues may exacerbate fiscal stresses caused by increased expenditures, especially in LMICs, where tax systems are weaker and government fiscal constraints are more severe. This dynamic was visible during the 2014 West Africa Ebola epidemic in Liberia: while response costs surged, economic activity slowed, and quarantines and curfews reduced government capacity to collect revenue (World Bank 2014).

During a mild or moderate pandemic, unaffected HICs can offset fiscal shocks by providing increased official development assistance (ODA) to affected countries, including direct budgetary support. However, during a severe pandemic where HICs confront the same fiscal stresses and may be unable or unwilling to provide assistance, LMICs could face larger budget shortfalls, potentially leading to weakened public health response or cuts in other government spending.

The direct fiscal impacts of pandemics generally are small, however, relative to the indirect damage to economic activity and growth. Negative economic growth shocks are driven directly by labor force reductions caused by sickness and mortality and indirectly by fear-induced behavioral changes. Fear manifests itself through multiple behavioral changes. As an analysis of the economic impacts of the 2014 West Africa Ebola epidemic noted, "Fear of association with others . . . reduces labor force participation, closes places of employment, disrupts transportation, motivates some governments to close land borders and restrict entry of citizens from affected countries, and motivates private decision makers to disrupt trade, travel, and commerce by canceling scheduled commercial flights and reducing shipping and cargo services" (World Bank 2014). These effects reduce labor force participation over and above the pandemic's direct morbidity and mortality effects and constrict local and regional trade.

The indirect economic impact of pandemics has been quantified primarily through computable general equilibrium simulations; the empirical literature is less developed. World Bank economic simulations indicate that a severe pandemic could reduce world gross domestic product (GDP) by roughly 5 percent (Burns, Van der Mensbrugghe, and Timmer 2006). The reduction in demand caused by aversive behavior (such as the avoidance of travel, restaurants, and public spaces, as well as prophylactic workplace absenteeism) exceeds the economic impact of direct morbidity- and mortality-associated absenteeism.

These results align with country-specific estimates: an analysis of pandemic influenza's impact on the United Kingdom found that a low-severity pandemic could reduce GDP by up to 1 percent, whereas a high-severity event could reduce GDP by 3–4 percent (Smith and others 2009). The World Bank's estimates from the 2014 West Africa Ebola epidemic suggest that economic disruption in low-income countries (LICs) could be even greater. For example, the 2015 economic growth estimate for Liberia was 3 percent (against a pre-Ebola estimate of 6.8 percent); for Sierra Leone, it was −2 percent (against a pre-Ebola estimate of nearly 9 percent) (Thomas and others 2015).

Finally, estimates of fiscal and growth shocks are significant but do not include the intrinsic value of lives lost. Fan, Jamison, and Summers (2016) consider this additional dimension of economic loss by estimating the value of excess deaths across varying levels of modeled pandemic severity, finding that the bulk of the expected annual loss from pandemics is driven by the direct cost of mortality, particularly in the case of low-probability, severe events.

During a severe pandemic, all sectors of the economy—agriculture, manufacturing, services—face disruption, potentially leading to shortages, rapid price increases for staple goods, and economic stresses for households, private firms, and governments. A sustained, severe pandemic on the scale of the 1918 influenza pandemic could cause significant and lasting economic damage.

Social and Political Impacts

Evidence suggests that epidemics and pandemics can have significant social and political consequences, creating clashes between states and citizens, eroding state capacity, driving population displacement, and heightening social tension and discrimination (Price-Smith 2009).

Severe premodern pandemics have been associated with significant social and political upheaval, driven by large mortality shocks and the resulting demographic shifts. Most notably, deaths arising from the introduction of smallpox and other diseases to the Americas led directly to the collapse of many indigenous societies and weakened the indigenous peoples' institutions and military capacity to the extent that they became vulnerable to European conquest (Diamond 2009; see table 17.1). Subsequent pandemics have not had such dramatic effects on political and social stability, primarily because the potential mortality shock has been attenuated by improvements in prevention and care.

Evidence does suggest that epidemics and pandemics can amplify existing political tensions and spark unrest, particularly in fragile states with legacies of violence and weak institutions. During the 2014 West Africa Ebola epidemic, steps taken to mitigate disease transmission, such as the imposition of quarantines and curfews by security forces, were viewed with suspicion by segments of the public and opposition political leaders. This led directly to riots and violent clashes with security forces (McCoy 2014). Latent political tensions from previously warring factions in Liberia also reemerged early in the epidemic and were linked with threats to health care workers as well as attacks on public health personnel and facilities.

The Ebola epidemic also greatly amplified political tensions in Guinea, Liberia, and Sierra Leone, with incumbent politicians accused of leveraging the crisis and disease control measures to cement political control and opposition figures accused of hampering disease response efforts (ICG 2015). Whereas growing tensions did not lead to large-scale political violence or instability, they did complicate public health response efforts. In Sierra Leone, quarantine in opposition-dominated regions was delayed because of concerns that it would be seen as politically motivated (ICG 2015). In countries with high levels of political polarization, recent civil war, or weak institutions, sustained outbreaks could lead to more sustained and challenging political tensions.

Pandemics also can have longer-term impacts on state capacity (Price-Smith 2001). The HIV/AIDS pandemic offers one notable example. The 1990s and early 2000s saw extremely high HIV/AIDS prevalence rates among African militaries, leading to increased absenteeism, decreased military capacity, and decreased readiness (Elbe 2002). Similar effects may occur during shorter, more acute pandemics, reducing state capacity to manage instability. The weakening of security forces can, in turn, amplify the risk of civil war and other forms of violent conflict (Fearon and Laitin 2003).

Large-scale outbreaks of infectious disease have direct and consequential social impacts. For example, widespread public panic during disease outbreaks can lead to rapid population migration. A 1994 outbreak of plague in Surat, India, caused only a small number of reported cases, but fear led some 500,000 people (roughly 20 percent of the city's population, including a disproportionately large number of clinicians) to flee their homes (Barrett and Brown 2008). Sudden population movements can have destabilizing effects, and migrants face elevated health risks arising from poor sanitation, poor nutrition, and other stressors (Toole and Waldman 1990). Migration also poses the risk of further spreading an outbreak.

Finally, outbreaks of infectious disease can cause already vulnerable social groups, such as ethnic minority populations, to be stigmatized and blamed for the disease and its consequences (Person and others 2004). During the Black Death, Jewish communities in Europe faced discrimination, including expulsion and communal violence, because of stigma and blame for disease outbreaks (Cohn 2007). Modern outbreaks have seen more subtle forms of discrimination, such as shunning and fear, directed at minority populations linked with disease foci. For example, Africans in Hong Kong SAR, China, reported experiencing social isolation, anxiety, and economic hardship resulting from fears of their association with Ebola (Siu 2015).

Trends Affecting Pandemic Risk

In recent decades, several trends have affected pandemic probability, preparedness, and mitigation capacity. Various factors—population growth, increasing urbanization, greater demand for animal protein, greater travel and connectivity between population centers, habitat loss, climate change, and increased interactions at the human-animal interface—affect the likelihood of pandemic events by increasing either the probability of a spark event or the potential spread of a pathogen (Tilman and Clark 2014; Tyler 2016; Zell 2004). With global population estimated to reach 9.7 billion by 2050 and with travel and trade steadily intensifying, public health systems will have less time to detect and contain a pandemic before it spreads (Tyler 2016).

As for poverty, the trends are mixed. On the positive side, enormous gains in poverty reduction have decreased the number of people living in extreme poverty. This may attenuate the mortality shock of a mild pandemic somewhat. On the negative side, extreme poverty is now concentrated in a small number of low-growth, high-poverty countries (Chandy, Kato, and Kharas 2015). In such countries, progress in building health system capacity also has been far slower.

Likewise, for a subset of countries with endemically weak institutions, building institutional capacity for complex tasks like pandemic mitigation and response is likely to be a slow process even under the most optimistic assumptions (Pritchett, Woolcock, and Andrews 2013). Many of these countries are in areas with high spark risk, particularly in Central and West Africa, and thus may remain vulnerable and require significant international assistance during a pandemic.

Other environmental and population trends that could increase the severity of pandemics include the persistence of slums, unresponsive health systems, higher prevalence of comorbidities, weaker sanitation, and aging populations (Arimah 2010; UNDESA 2015). The increasing threat posed by antibiotic resistance also could amplify mortality during pandemics of bacterial diseases such as tuberculosis and cholera and even viral diseases (especially for influenza, in which a significant proportion of deaths is often the result of bacterial pneumonia coinfections) (Brundage and Shanks 2008; Van Boeckel and others 2014).

PANDEMIC MITIGATION: PREPAREDNESS AND RESPONSE

Pandemic preparedness and response interventions can be classified by their timing with respect to pandemic occurrence: the prepandemic period, the spark period, and the spread period, as shown in box 17.1.

Whereas some interventions clearly fall under the purview of a single authority, responsibility for implementing and scaling up many critical aspects of preparedness and response is spread across multiple authorities, which

---

Box 17.1

Examples of Pandemic Preparedness and Response Activities, by Time Period

Prepandemic period (before a pandemic starts)
- Stockpile building
- Continuity planning
- Public health workforce training
- Simulation exercises
- Risk transfer mechanism set-up
- Situational awareness[a]

Spark period (as a pandemic starts)
- Initial outbreak detection
- Pathogen characterization or laboratory confirmation
- Risk communication and community engagement
- Animal disease control

- Contact tracing, quarantine, and isolation
- Situational awareness[a]

Spread period (after a pandemic starts)
- Global pandemic declaration
- Risk communications
- Contact tracing, quarantine, and isolation
- Social distancing
- Stockpile deployment
- Vaccine or antiviral administration
- Care and treatment
- Situational awareness[a]

a. Situational awareness includes passive and active animal and human disease surveillance and monitoring of public health facilities and resources.

play complementary, interlocking, and, in some cases, overlapping roles (Brattberg and Rhinard 2011). The governance of pandemic preparedness and response is complex, with authority fragmented across international, national, and subnational institutions, as well as among multiple organizations with functional responsibility for specific tasks (Hooghe and Marks 2003). Pandemic preparedness requires close coordination across public and private sector actors: vaccine development requires close coordination between government and vaccine producers; whereas critical response measures—such as managing quarantines—requires engagement between nonprofit organizations (hospitals, clinics, and nongovernmental organizations), public health authorities, affected communities and civil society groups, and the security sector.

Historical pandemics offer only a partial view to guide preparedness and response activities. Many countries and organizations have used the historical influenza pandemics in 1918, 1957, and 1968 to estimate the potential morbidity and mortality burden during a future pandemic (WHO 2016c). However, using these moderate-to-severe events to plan for a mild pandemic (for example, the 2009 influenza pandemic) can lead to an overzealous response—such as widespread mandatory school closures—that may create unintended negative economic consequences (Kelly and others 2011). And although the 1918 influenza pandemic is sometimes considered a "worst-case scenario" for planning purposes, possible scenarios today could be far more damaging—such as if a highly transmissible, highly virulent influenza virus were to emerge. Especially in LMICs, intensive care unit (ICU) beds and therapies for acute respiratory distress syndrome are in short supply, which could lead to many casualties (Osterholm 2005).

Situational Awareness

Situational awareness—in the context of pandemic preparedness—can be defined as having an accurate, up-to-date view of potential or ongoing infectious disease threats (including through traditional surveillance in humans and animals) and the resources (human, financial, informational, and institutional) available to manage those threats (ASPR 2014). Situational awareness is a crucial activity at all stages of a pandemic, including prepandemic, spark, and spread periods. It requires the support of health care resources (such as hospitals, doctors, and nurses), diagnostic infrastructure, and communications systems. It also requires the population to have access to and trust in the health care system.

Situational awareness supports policy decisions by tracking if and where disease transmission is occurring, detecting the most effective methods to reduce transmissibility, and deciding where to allocate resources. During a pandemic, situational awareness allows for monitoring to understand the course a pandemic is taking and whether intervention measures are effective.

The ability to detect the presence of a pandemic requires the health care workforce to recognize the illness and to have the technical and laboratory capacity to identify the pathogen (or rule out known pathogens) and respond to surges of clinical specimens in a timely manner. Rapid identification reduces risk by enabling infected persons to be isolated and given appropriate clinical care. During the 2003 SARS pandemic, a one-week delay in applying control measures may have nearly tripled the size of the outbreak and increased its duration by four weeks (Wallinga and Teunis 2004).

Endemic infectious diseases can affect pandemic detection by complicating the differential diagnosis and rapid identification of pandemic cases. Overlapping symptoms between endemic and emerging pathogens— for instance, between dengue and Zika or between malaria and Ebola—have hampered the early identification of cases (de Wit and others 2016; Waggoner and Pinsky 2016). This difficulty suggests a role for investment in the development and deployment of rapid diagnostic tests in regions with a high burden of endemic pathogens and high risk of disease emergence or importation (Yamey and others 2017). Additional constraints affecting epidemic and pandemic situational awareness in LMICs are described in box 17.2.

Preventing and Extinguishing Pandemic Sparks

Although most pandemic preparedness activities focus on reducing morbidity and mortality after a pandemic has spread widely, certain activities may prevent and contain pandemic sparks before they become a wider threat. At the core of pandemic prevention is the concept of One Health, an approach that considers human health, animal health, and the environment to be fundamentally interconnected (Zinsstag and others 2005).[1] Activities that focus on understanding and controlling zoonotic pathogens may prevent spillover events and subsequent pandemics (Morse and others 2012).

To understand the etiology of pandemics, important One Health activities include the surveillance of zoonotic pathogens of pandemic potential at the human-animal interface, the modeling of evolutionary dynamics, the risk assessments of zoonotic pathogens, and other methods of understanding the interplay between environmental changes and pathogen emergence (Paez-Espino and others 2016; Wolfe and

Situational Awareness Constraints in Low- and Middle-Income Countries

Perhaps the greatest challenge in epidemic and pandemic response is the timely identification and notification of the first pandemic case. However, low- and middle-income countries are substantially slower than high-income countries to identify and communicate infectious disease outbreaks (Chan and others 2010). In most outbreaks, the first (or index) case is found retrospectively. Reporting delays result from multiple factors, which are discussed here. Moreover, the epidemiological characteristics of the index case often are difficult to ascertain, particularly in settings with limited diagnostic and laboratory capacity.

Patients infected with potentially pandemic pathogens may present with nonspecific symptoms, making discriminating between endemic and novel or significant pathogens difficult unless differential diagnostic tools are available. Gaps in health system access and surveillance system coverage also hamper identification and reporting. In such cases, an incipient epidemic will be identified only after sufficient deaths have occurred to draw the attention of health authorities. Particularly in areas where health system gaps are significant, monitoring unofficial sources of information, including rumors, may be useful (Samaan and others 2005).

Even once a potentially unusual or significant case has been identified, delays can be caused by low statistical capacity, low data management capacity, and low communication capacity among local frontline health workers. Delays also can arise from how surveillance and reporting systems are designed—for example, if health workers routinely report potentially significant cases at the end of the month rather than when they are identified.

Another constraint arises from inconsistencies in real-time reporting of data. During an outbreak response, national and regional health authorities must have strong relationships with local health providers to understand how data are generated and reported at the clinical level. Robust monitoring and data validation procedures, such as the use of global positioning systems and case-based systems, along with positive incentives for correct reporting, may help to alleviate such problems (Mancini and others 2014).

others 2005). For example, the PREDICT project of the U.S. Agency for International Development (USAID) has invested a significant amount of resources in understanding and characterizing zoonotic risk (Anthony and others 2013).[2]

Countries can focus their spark mitigation efforts on policies designed to control animal reservoirs; monitor high-risk populations such as people working at the animal interface (for example, those involved in animal husbandry, animal slaughter, and so on); and maintain robust animal health infrastructure, biosecurity, and veterinary public health capacities (Jonas 2013; Pike and others 2010; Watts 2004; Yu and others 2014).

Risk Communications

Risk communications can play a significant role in the control of an emerging epidemic or pandemic by providing information that people can use to take protective and preventive action (WHO 2013c). The dissemination of basic information (such as how the pathogen is transmitted, guidance on managing patient care, high-risk practices, and protective behavioral measures) can rapidly and significantly reduce the transmission of disease.

The way in which risk communications are framed and transmitted matters a great deal; they must be clear, simple, timely, and delivered by credible messengers. Factors such as literacy rates, cultural sensitivities, familiarity with scientific principles (such as the germ theory of disease), and reliance on oral versus written traditions all have implications for how messages should be designed and delivered (Bedrosian and others 2016).

Public health officials also need to identify and address misinformation, rumors, and anxieties. This can be a significant challenge. During the 2014 West Africa Ebola epidemic, many communities reached for culturally familiar explanations of disease transmission and rejected disease control practices that clashed with their traditional healing and burial practices (Roca and others 2015). Still other individuals spread rumors about the source of the infection; for example, in Liberia some community leaders claimed that the disease was created by the government (Epstein 2014).

Rumors can impede disease control and can be amplified by mistrust of government officials, which is a significant challenge in LMICs with high levels of corruption or legacies of violent conflict and social division. Research has found that in unstable contexts, people tend to believe rumors that confirm their preexisting beliefs and anxieties (Greenhill and Oppenheim 2017). This finding suggests that countering rumors with facts alone will not be sufficient. Risk communications need to be both factual and empathetic, addressing unfolding events and underlying fears through the lens of community experiences, histories, and perceptions.

The effectiveness of risk communications is difficult to measure. However, previous risk communication efforts have brought forth overarching themes that may be beneficial during the next epidemic or pandemic. One notable model comes from a Nipah virus outbreak in Bangladesh in 2010. In that outbreak, investigators found that messages about the sources of infection and potential strategies to reduce risk were more effective when conveyed by trusted local leaders and in terms that were relevant and grounded in the shared experiences of the affected community (Parveen and others 2016).

Reducing Pandemic Spread

Once a pandemic has begun in earnest, public health efforts often focus on minimizing its spread. Limiting the spread of a pandemic can help to reduce the number of total people who are infected and thus also mitigate some of the indirect health and economic effects. Strategies to minimize pandemic spread include the following (Ferguson and others 2005):

- *Curtailing interactions* between infected and uninfected populations: for example, through patient isolation, quarantine, social distancing practices, and school closures
- *Reducing infectiousness* of symptomatic patients: for example, through antiviral and antibiotic treatment and infection control practices
- *Reducing susceptibility* of uninfected individuals: for example, through vaccines.

During the prepandemic period, plans for implementing those measures should be developed and tested through simulation exercises.

Curtailing Interactions between Infected and Uninfected Populations

The methods for curtailing interactions between infected and uninfected populations include patient isolation, quarantine, social distancing practices, school closures, use of personal protective equipment, and travel restrictions.

The practice of quarantine began in the fourteenth century in response to the Black Death and continues today (Mackowiak and Sehdev 2002). Quarantine and social distancing (such as the prohibition of mass gatherings) during the 1918 influenza pandemic reduced spread and mortality rates, particularly when implemented in the early stages of the pandemic (Bootsma and Ferguson 2007; Hollingsworth, Ferguson, and Anderson 2006). During SARS and Ebola outbreaks, health agencies and hospitals limited disease spread by isolating symptomatic patients, quarantining patient contacts, and improving hospital infection control practices (Cohen and others 2016; Twu and others 2003). During the 2003 SARS pandemic, none of the health care workers in hospitals in Hong Kong SAR, China, who reported appropriate and consistent use of masks, gloves, gowns, and hand washing (as recommended under droplet and contact precautions) were infected (Seto and others 2003).

Travel restrictions are sometimes implemented by governments to curtail disease spread. Fear and lack of scientific understanding may motivate the imposition of travel restrictions (Flahault and Valleron 1990). As such, these measures are sometimes implemented for inappropriate pathogens or too late to contain an outbreak and can cause substantial economic damage and public anxiety. Travel restrictions are more beneficial for pathogens that do not have a significant asymptomatic carrier state and have a relatively long incubation period (for example, SARS and Ebola). However, such restrictions may be of limited efficacy for influenza pandemics unless initiated when there are fewer than 50 cases at the spark site (Ferguson and others 2005).

Reducing Infectiousness and Susceptibility

Vaccines, antibiotics, and antiviral drugs can play a critical role in mitigating a pandemic by reducing the infectiousness of symptomatic patients and the susceptibility of uninfected individuals. Antivirals may reduce influenza transmission, although the extent of their effectiveness is unclear (Ferguson and others 2005; Jefferson and others 2014). A systematic review of clinical trial data among treated adults showed that oseltamivir reduced the duration of influenza symptoms by 17 hours, but prophylaxis trials found no significant reduction of transmission (Jefferson and others 2014).

If available, vaccines can reduce susceptibility. Significant efforts have focused on speeding up vaccine development and scaling up production. However, the availability of vaccines—particularly in LMICs—depends on the affected area's capacity for distribution (including the scale and integrity of the cold chain), its capacity for last-mile delivery to rural areas, and the population's willingness to adopt the vaccine. Vaccination strategies targeting younger populations may be especially beneficial, in part because influenza transmissibility is higher among younger populations during pandemics (Miller and others 2008).

The effectiveness of antivirals, antibiotics, and vaccines in reducing spread diminishes if the pandemic is already global, if LMICs cannot afford adequate vaccine stocks for their populations, or if specific populations (for example, the poor or the socially vulnerable) cannot access vaccines. Additionally, pandemics may be caused by a pathogen without an available vaccine or efficacious biomedical therapy. Efforts to improve the vaccine development pipeline are underway (box 17.3).

Care and Treatment to Reduce the Severity of Pandemic Illness

During a pandemic, health authorities work to reduce the severity of illness through patient care and treatment, which can help decrease the likelihood of severe outcomes such as hospitalizations and deaths. Treatments may range from nonspecific, supportive care to disease-specific drugs. During the prepandemic period, plans to implement these measures should be developed and tested through simulation exercises.

Maintaining supportive care during an epidemic or pandemic can improve mortality rates by alleviating the symptoms of disease. During the 2014 West Africa Ebola epidemic, for example, evidence suggests that earlier case identification, supportive care, and rehydration therapy modestly reduced mortality (Walker and Whitty 2015). Indeed, despite the unavailability of antivirals or vaccines, efforts to engage communities with added medical supplies and trained clinicians decreased the case-fatality ratio moderately as more patients trusted, sought, and received clinical care (Aylward and others 2014).

Box 17.3

Vaccine Research and Development to Meet Pandemic Threats

Current vaccine research, development, and production time lines are not conducive to quick responses to pandemic threats. For example, despite biomedical advances, most influenza vaccines are produced through vaccine platforms that rely on the availability of embryonated chicken eggs and can take several months to produce (Reperant, Rimmelzwaan, and Osterhaus 2014). Vaccines that are in development may take decades to become available for human use. For example, Ebola vaccines were in development for more than a decade, with the first vaccine approved for clinical use only in 2015 (Henao-Restrepo and others 2016; Richardson and others 2010).

Several areas of active research seek to hasten and strengthen vaccine development. Of note is the World Health Organization's Global Action Plan for Influenza Vaccines, whose mission, in part, is to increase the capacity to produce vaccines for global influenza pandemics, quicken the production of vaccines, and research a universal influenza vaccine (Nannei and others 2016). Egg-independent cell culture platforms also have become a reality: in 2013 the U.S. Food and Drug Administration approved an influenza vaccine produced in insect cell lines (Milián and Kamen 2015).

In preparation for a noninfluenza pandemic, the public-private Coalition for Epidemic Preparedness Innovations (CEPI) is building a bank of potential vaccines for viral diseases, such as SARS and MERS (Middle East respiratory syndrome), that are not currently of commercial interest. CEPI's goal is to focus on the development or licensure and manufacturing of high-potential viral vaccines through early-stage human trials and to purchase small stockpiles to mitigate the next pandemic (Mullard 2016).

Medical supplies that may be needed for supportive care during a pandemic include hospital beds, disinfectants, ICU supplies (such as ventilators), and personal protective equipment (WHO 2015b).

Medical interventions for pandemic influenza include antiviral drugs and antibiotics to treat bacterial coinfections. Antivirals especially may reduce mortality when given within 48 hours of symptom onset (Domínguez-Cherit and others 2009; Jain and others 2009). However, because of delays in case identification and antiviral deployment (as discussed in box 17.2), LMICs may experience only limited benefits from antiviral drugs.

Potential for Scaling Up

The term *scaling up* refers to the expansion of health intervention coverage (Mangham and Hanson 2010). In the context of pandemic preparedness, successfully scaling up requires health systems to expand services to accommodate rapid increases in the number of suspected cases. Scaling up is facilitated by *surge capacity* (the ability to draw on additional clinical personnel, logisticians, and financial and other resources) as well as preexisting operational relationships and plans linking government, nongovernmental organizations, and the private sector. Ultimately, scaling up consists of having both local surge capacity and the absorptive capacity to accept outside assistance.

Local capacity building is vital, and some capacities may have particularly important positive externalities during outbreaks. During the 2014 Ebola importation into Nigeria, surge capacity that existed because of polio eradication efforts contributed to a more successful outbreak response (Yehualashet and others 2016). Key elements included national experience running an emergency operations center and the use of global positioning systems to support contact tracing (Shuaib and others 2014; WHO 2015a).

Stockpiling of vaccines, medicines (including antibiotics and antivirals), and equipment (such as masks, gowns, and ventilators) also can be useful for building local surge capacity (Dimitrov and others 2011; Jennings and others 2008; Morens, Taubenberger, and Fauci 2008; Radonovich and others 2009). During a pandemic, health systems can tap into stockpiles more quickly than they can procure supplies from external sources or boost production. However, there are five important considerations for keeping stockpiles:

- Building a stockpile requires significant up-front costs, which can be especially prohibitive for LICs (Oshitani, Kamigaki, and Suzuki 2008).

- Prepandemic vaccines may not be closely matched to the pathogen causing the pandemic.
- The optimal size of a stockpile can be challenging to determine.
- Stockpiles need to be refreshed regularly, because pharmaceuticals and equipment can reach expiration dates.
- Robust health systems and channels for disseminating and using the stockpiles also must exist.

Boosting local production capacity for necessary supplies may be a viable strategy for pandemic preparedness and may circumvent some of the challenges associated with amassing stockpiles.

The 2009 influenza pandemic demonstrated how scaling up can affect the success rate of a mass vaccination campaign (table 17.5). Vaccination rates increased according to country income level, suggesting that vaccination campaigns were most successful in HICs, likely because of the size of their stockpiles, increased manufacturing capacity for vaccines, increased availability of vaccines, and more streamlined logistics in vaccine deployment.

Building local capacity to scale up is challenging, especially in LMICs. The biggest challenges include infrastructural gaps (such as weak road, transportation, and communications networks) and shortfalls in human resources (such as logisticians, epidemiologists, and clinical staff). Bilateral and multilateral aid organizations have channeled substantial funding into building and sustaining local technical capacities in LMICs. This type of investment is critically important. But, particularly in LMICs with weak health system capacity, progress in expanding local surge capacity likely will be slow.

Another key component of scaling up, especially in LMICs, is the ability to use external assistance effectively.

Table 17.5 Vaccination Rates during the 2009 Influenza Pandemic, by Country Income Level

Country income level[a]	Number of countries with data	Share of population vaccinated (%)
Low-income	13	5.7
Middle-income	42	8.5
High-income	31	16.8

Sources: Mihigo and others 2012; Tizzoni and others 2012; WHO 2013b.
a. Income groups follow World Bank income classifications for fiscal 2018, based on estimates of 2016 gross national income per capita and calculated using the World Bank Atlas method: low-income (US$1,005 or less), middle-income (US$1,006–US$12,235), and high-income (US$12,236 or more). For further explanation, see https://datahelpdesk.worldbank.org /knowledgebase/articles/906519-world-bank-country-and-lending-groups.

During the 2014 West Africa Ebola epidemic, a surge of foreign clinicians, mobile medical units, and epidemiologists and other public health personnel was required to bolster limited local resources. LMICs can improve systems to facilitate and coordinate surges of foreign support in the following ways:

- Streamline customs processes for critical medical supplies and drugs.
- Establish mechanisms to coordinate the deployment and operations of foreign medical teams.
- Build mechanisms to coordinate between military and humanitarian units involved in crisis response.

Even so, local absorptive capacity (that is, the ability to channel and use foreign assistance effectively) has its limits. Constraints in bureaucratic capacity, financial controls, logistics, and infrastructure all are likely to be most severe in the countries that most need foreign assistance to manage infectious disease crises.

Furthermore, although external assistance is a viable strategy during localized epidemics, it has limitations that are likely to arise during large-scale pandemics. First, supply constraints exist, including limits to the number of medical personnel (especially those with crisis response and infectious disease competencies) and the number of specialized resources (such as integrated mobile medical clinics available for deployment).

Second, during a severe pandemic, countries are likely to use such resources locally before providing medical assistance abroad. The global humanitarian system provides a critical reservoir of crisis response capacity and shock absorption. However, the humanitarian system currently is straining under the pressure of other crises, including upsurges in violent conflict (Stoddard and others 2015). A severe epidemic or pandemic can quickly outstrip international resources. Médecins Sans Frontières (Doctors Without Borders), an international health organization with deep experience providing Ebola treatment, found itself "pushed to the limits and beyond" during the 2014 West Africa Ebola epidemic (MSF 2015).

Risk Transfer Mechanisms

As with any other type of natural disaster, the risk from pandemics cannot be eliminated. Despite prevention efforts, pandemics will continue to occur and will at times overwhelm the systems that have been put in place to mitigate their health, societal, and economic effects. The residual risk may be significant, particularly for LMICs that lack the resilience or resources to absorb

shocks to public health and public finances. Risk transfer mechanisms (such as specialized insurance facilities) offer an additional tool to manage this risk.

Risk-based insurance products are increasingly deployed in LMICs to pay for remediation and reconstruction costs following natural catastrophes such as hurricanes, floods, and droughts (ARC 2016; IFRC 2016). Insurance products for epidemics and pandemics require specific characteristics. First, insurance policies should be designed to release discretionary funds early in the course of an outbreak. In situations where financing poses a constraint to mobilizing personnel, drugs, or other supplies, payouts can be used to mobilize a public health response and mitigate further spread of disease, reducing the potential health and economic impacts of the pandemic. Second, because pandemics do not stay contained in national borders, a strong case can be made for mobilizing bilateral and multilateral financing of LMICs' insurance premiums as a cost-effective way to improve global preparedness and support mitigation efforts. Third, risk transfer systems require the availability of rigorously and transparently compiled data to trigger a payout. In the context of pandemic insurance, the development of risk transfer systems requires countries to build the following capacities, among others:

- Robust surveillance data to identify when an outbreak has reached sufficient scale to require the release of funds
- Laboratory capacity to confirm the causative agent
- Predefined contingency and response plans to spend the funds effectively upon their release.

Insurance facilities can create positive incentives for LMICs to invest in planning and capacity building. Insurance mechanisms may have other positive externalities: most notably, the potential release of funds may provide a strong incentive for the timely reporting of surveillance data. However, insurance facilities also may introduce perverse incentives (including incentives to distort surveillance data) and potential moral hazards (such as permitting riskier activities). These incentive problems may be mitigated in the design of the risk transfer mechanism, such as by providing coverage only when minimum requirements for surveillance accuracy are met, by having preset phased triggers for payouts, and by including incentive payouts for successfully containing an outbreak.

Relative to investments in basic health provision, building capacity in infectious disease surveillance systems and other dimensions of pandemic preparedness has uncertain and potentially distant benefits. In LICs where near-term health needs are acute, this can complicate the political and economic logic for investing in pandemic preparedness (Buckley and Pittluck 2016). The use of catastrophe modeling tools (such as EP curves) can clarify the benefit-cost rationale and the relevant time horizon for investments in preparedness, and it can inform the design and financial structure of pandemic insurance policies.

Figure 17.3 shows a country's hypothetical pandemic preparedness budget allocation and the portion of risk transfer in estimated total costs of spread response. In this example, a country has a total budget of US$100 million to cover all aspects of pandemic preparedness during the prepandemic, spark, and spread periods. After allocating half of the funds for prepandemic and spark response activities, US$50 million is left for pandemic spread response. On the basis of its risk tolerance, the country makes a decision to manage its risk at the 3 percent annual probability point on its EP curve. Modeling estimates indicate that a successful response to a pandemic at this level would require at least US$125 million, which would fund spread response activities, shown in box 17.1. Because only US$50 million is left after allocation to prepandemic and spark response activities, this would leave a shortfall of US$75 million. Some or all of this shortfall could be offloaded to another entity, such as a catastrophe risk insurance pool, which would give the country access to a payout during a pandemic.

Innovations in pandemic financing have been developed in response to the significant burden that a pandemic can place on a country's financial resources. One such innovation is the World Bank's Pandemic Emergency Financing Facility (PEF) (Katz and Seifman 2016).[3] A type of disaster risk pool, the PEF provides poorly resourced countries with an infusion of funds to help with the costs of response in the early stages of an epidemic or pandemic. The maximum total coverage over a three-year period is US$500 million. Notably, the US$500 million coverage is much lower than the estimated US$3.8 billion cost of the multinational response to the 2014 West Africa Ebola epidemic (USAID and CDC 2016). Because the PEF is designed to trigger early in an outbreak, the anticipated funding is less than would be required for a full-fledged response once a widespread pandemic is under way.

Risk transfer mechanisms such as insurance offer an injection of financial resources to help insured parties rapidly scale up disease response activities. As such, the utility of risk transfer mechanisms depends, in large part, on the absorptive capacity of the insured party. A country must have the ability to use insurance payouts effectively to access additional human resources

Figure 17.3 Hypothetical Pandemic Preparedness Budget and Response Shortfall, Which Could Be Managed via Risk Transfer Mechanisms

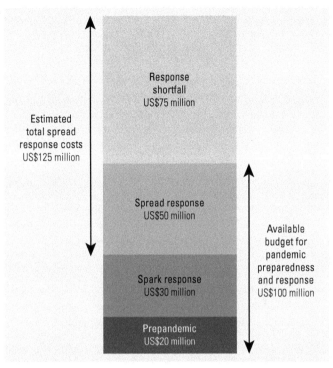

Source: Metabiota.
Note: Numbers are provided solely for illustrative purposes.

(clinicians, community health workers), personal protective equipment and other medical equipment consumables, and vaccines and therapeutics, from either domestic or international resources.

Adequacy of Evidence on Pandemics in LMICs

Much of the available data regarding pandemics (including the morbidity and mortality impacts of historical pandemics) and the effectiveness of different preparedness efforts and interventions come from HICs and upper-middle-income countries. Understanding of the prevalence of risk drivers, especially regarding spark risk, has improved markedly in both high- and low-income contexts. However, gaps in surveillance and reporting infrastructure in LMICs mean that, during a pandemic, many cases may never be detected or reported to the appropriate authorities (Katz and others 2012). Particularly in LICs, empirical data on outbreak occurrences may be biased downward systematically.

Additionally, the means to disseminate collected data rapidly may not exist. For example, data may be kept in paper archives, so resource-intensive digitization may be required to analyze and report data to a wider audience.

Data dissemination challenges are further compounded by a publication bias that results in overrepresentation of HICs in the scientific literature (Jones and others 2008).

SUMMARY OF PANDEMIC INTERVENTION COSTS AND COST-EFFECTIVENESS

Few data are available regarding costs and cost-effectiveness of pandemic preparedness and response measures, and they focus almost exclusively on HICs. The available data suggest that the greatest cost-related benefits in pandemic preparedness and response are realized from early recognition and mitigation of disease—that is, catching and stopping sparks before they spread. Costs can be reduced if action is taken before an outbreak becomes a pandemic. Similarly, once a pandemic has begun, preventing illness generally is more cost-effective than treating illness, especially because hospitalizations typically have the highest direct cost per person. High costs also may occur as a result of interventions (such as quarantines and school closures) that lead to economic disruption. These interventions may be more cost-effective during a severe pandemic.

Program and Health System Costs

No systematic time-series data exist on global spending on pandemic preparedness, and arriving at an exact figure is complicated by the fact that many investments in building basic health system capacity also support core dimensions of pandemic preparedness. An analysis of global health spending found that roughly 1 percent of global ODA spending on health in 2013 (approximately US$204 million) focused specifically on pandemic preparedness (Schäferhoff and others 2015). Other, non-ODA spending on pandemic preparedness is similarly difficult to measure but likely to be significant; in 2013, the U.S. Department of Defense spent roughly US$256 million on efforts to build global biosurveillance and response capacities (KFF 2014).

Globally, the current funding for pandemic preparedness and response falls short of what is needed. In 2016, the international Commission on a Global Health Risk Framework for the Future recommended an additional US$4.5 billion annual global investment for upgrading pandemic preparedness at the country level, for funding infectious disease research and development efforts, and for establishing or replenishing rapid-response financing mechanisms such as the World Bank's PEF (Sands, Mundaca-Shah, and Dzau 2016).

Costs for efforts associated with prepandemic preparedness activities also are not well quantified, although investment in One Health activities is likely to be cost-effective (World Bank 2012). The USAID PREDICT project has estimated that discovery and detection of the majority of zoonotic viruses would cost US$1.6 billion (Anthony and others 2013). The Global Virome Project, a more comprehensive study aiming to characterize more than 99 percent of the world's viruses, is estimated to cost US$3.4 billion over 10 years (Daszak and others 2016). Building on efforts to identify and describe the ecology of potential pandemic viruses, the Coalition for

Figure 17.4 Unit Costs for Selected Influenza Pandemic Response Activities

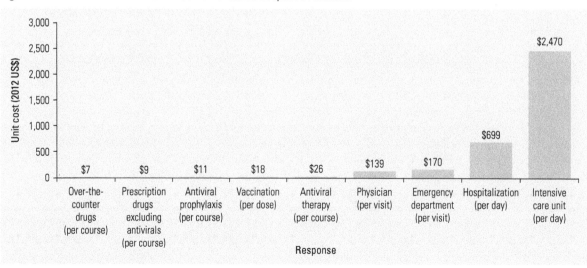

Source: Based on Lugnér and Postma 2009.
Note: Includes studies from France, Israel, the Netherlands, Singapore, the United Kingdom, and the United States.

Epidemic Preparedness Innovations (CEPI) estimated a cost of US$1 billion over five years to develop vaccine candidates against known emerging infectious diseases (for example, Ebola virus) and to build technology platforms and production facilities to accelerate vaccine response to outbreaks of known or unknown pathogens (Brende and others 2017).

Instituting response measures after a pandemic has begun can be expensive, with most of the direct cost borne by the health care sector, although response costs typically are not reported in a cohesive manner. As noted, the response to the 2014 West Africa Ebola epidemic cost more than US$3.8 billion, including donations from several countries (USAID and CDC 2016). Additionally, the World Bank Group mobilized US$1.6 billion from the International Development Association and the International Finance Corporation to stimulate economic recovery in the three worst-affected countries of Guinea, Liberia, and Sierra Leone (World Bank 2016). Taken together, at US$5.4 billion, these values amount to a cost of US$235 per capita for these three countries.

When total costs for response are not available, unit costs for response activities provide valuable insights. Figure 17.4 shows estimated unit costs for selected response measures, based on modeling studies for pandemic influenza in HICs. Vaccinations and medicines have the lowest unit costs; in LMICs, large-scale purchasing and subsidies could push drug costs down even more. Conversely, hospital care has the highest unit costs. Costs per day of hospitalization (especially those with ICU involvement) can add up quickly when aggregated at the national level. However, these medical care costs are potentially bounded by capacity limits (such as a finite number of hospital beds), especially during more severe pandemics.

Pandemic severity itself can play a role in the drivers of cost and the effects of mitigation efforts. One study based on modeling simulations in an Australian population found that, in low-severity pandemics, most costs borne by the larger economy (not just the health care system) come from productivity losses related to illness and social distancing. In higher-severity pandemics, the largest drivers of costs are hospitalization costs and productivity loss because of deaths (Milne, Halder, and Kelso 2013).

Costs per Death Prevented

Figure 17.5 depicts a compilation of data from 18 scientific publications that examined costs and benefits associated with response during the 2009 influenza pandemic. The lowest costs per deaths prevented were found for contact tracing, face masks, and surveillance. Pharmaceutical interventions such as vaccines and antiviral therapies were in the midrange.

Figure 17.5 Health Care System and Economic Costs per Death Prevented for Selected Interventions during the 2009 Influenza Pandemic

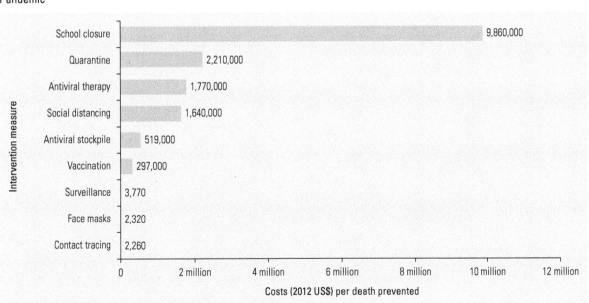

Source: Based on data from Pasquini-Descomps, Brender, and Maradan 2016.
Note: Includes studies from Australia, Brazil, Canada, China, Singapore, Sweden, the United Kingdom, and the United States.

Measures that decreased person-to-person contact, including social distancing, quarantine, and school closures, had the greatest cost per death prevented, most likely because of the amount of economic disruption caused by those measures. Social distancing includes avoidance of large gatherings and public places where economic activities occur. School closures often lead to lost productivity because they cause workplace absenteeism among caretakers of school-age children. Macroeconomic model simulations also have identified school closures as a potential source of GDP loss during a moderately severe pandemic (Smith and others 2009).

The information shown in figure 17.5 is subject to several caveats:

• The data come from only a few studies covering a handful of countries.
• Cost-utility analyses of pandemic preparedness and response for LMICs are rare. Because the underlying data for these studies were drawn primarily from HICs, the estimates may not accurately represent the relative benefit-cost of interventions in LMICs. For example, in countries with high unemployment and underemployment, school closures may not lead to increased workforce absenteeism and thus might have a lower cost per death prevented.
• The 2009 influenza pandemic is considered a relatively mild pandemic. In a more severe influenza pandemic,

the cost per death prevented could decrease for some interventions, such as school closures.
• Results are sensitive to assumptions about the value of a prevented death and estimated costs of different interventions.
• The data cover only pandemics caused by influenza. For pandemics caused by other types of pathogens, the cost-utility values may be different, and not all intervention measures may be available.

Data on antiviral stockpiles provide some insight into how the cost utility of pandemic preparedness efforts may vary by country income level. Figure 17.6 shows the cost utility of antiviral stockpiling by country income level, based on simulation studies.

A more recent study found that antiviral stockpiling in Cambodia (a lower-middle-income country) would cost between US$3,584 and US$115,168 per death prevented; however, this result is highly sensitive to assumptions about the timing between pandemics (Drake, Chalabi, and Coker 2015).

Although based only on a handful of countries, the results suggest that antiviral stockpiling in LICs has an extremely high cost per death prevented, whereas countries at other income levels are clustered within much lower ranges. Antiviral stockpiling is not cost-effective or feasible for LICs, primarily because of the high cost of antiviral agents. For stockpiling to be a cost-effective

Figure 17.6 Cost Utility of Antiviral Stockpiling for Pandemic Influenza Preparedness, by Share of Population Covered and Country Income Level, 2011

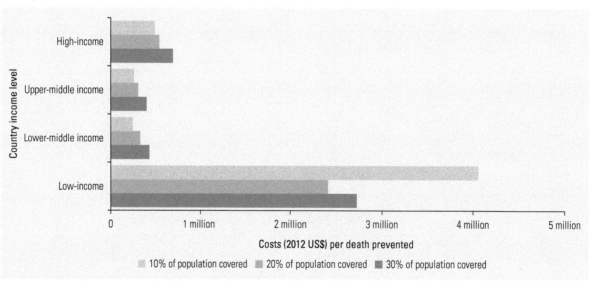

Source: Based on data from Carrasco and others 2011.
Note: Includes data from one low-income country (Zimbabwe), three lower-middle-income countries (Guatemala, India, and Indonesia), two upper-middle-income countries (Brazil and China), and four high-income countries (New Zealand, Singapore, the United Kingdom, and the United States).

strategy for LICs, almost all of the costs would have to be subsidized. The associated costs also may be reduced by the increased availability of generic antiviral drugs. Additionally, the efficacy of antivirals is not assured, particularly for LICs, which may not be able to identify cases early enough to administer antivirals efficaciously.

Cost-Effectiveness

Pérez Velasco and others (2012) synthesized information from 44 studies that contained economic evaluations of influenza pandemic preparedness and response strategies in HICs (figure 17.7). In their analysis, the following interventions among the general population had the potential to provide cost savings: vaccines, antiviral treatment, social distancing, antiviral prophylaxis plus antiviral treatment, and vaccines plus antiviral treatment. The cost savings from antiviral drugs found in this study are likely to be diminished in LMICs, as inability to deploy antivirals in a timely manner poses a serious challenge to their efficacious use.

Depending on the characteristics of a pandemic and how mitigation efforts are implemented, some mitigation strategies could become highly cost-*ineffective*. For example, a costly vaccination campaign that is carried out in an area well after a pandemic peaks is not nearly

as effective in reducing transmission as having vaccines available and distributed earlier in the pandemic.

Allocation of limited resources (by creating priority groups for vaccines and antivirals) is an important consideration during a pandemic. Modeling studies from the 2009 influenza pandemic investigated the most cost-effective strategies for allocating vaccines. Those studies found that vaccinating high-risk individuals was more cost-effective than prioritizing children. Favoring children decreased the overall infection rate, but high-risk individuals were the predominant drivers of direct costs during the pandemic, because they were more likely to be hospitalized (Lee and others 2010). However, these studies did not account for the indirect costs of school closures and absenteeism. Consideration of these factors could reveal increased cost savings from vaccinating children.

Another key question for benefit-cost analyses related to pandemics is the extent to which stockpiles of vaccines, antiviral drugs, and protective equipment should be assembled in advance of a pandemic. Vaccines for a novel influenza virus can take several months to develop, and vaccines for other pathogens (for example, Ebola and Zika) can take even longer to develop. Studies have examined the cost-effectiveness of stockpiling prepandemic vaccines that have lower efficacy than reactive vaccines but can be deployed

Figure 17.7 Cost-Effectiveness of Selected Interventions for Pandemic Influenza Preparedness and Response in High-Income Countries

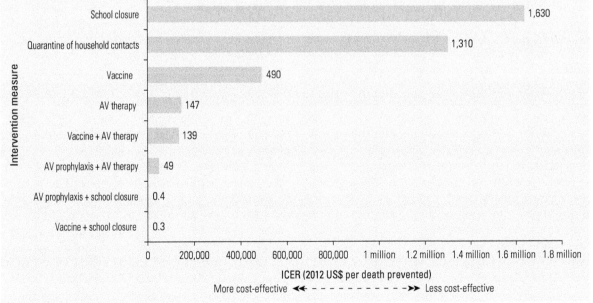

Source: Based on Pérez Velasco and others 2012.
Note: AV = antiviral; ICER = incremental cost-effectiveness ratio.

more quickly. One study found that cost savings can be obtained as long as prepandemic vaccines have at least 30 percent efficacy. However, cost-effectiveness differs by pandemic severity and the percentage of the population that receives the vaccine during the vaccination campaign (Halder, Kelso, and Milne 2014).

Antiviral drugs to fight pandemic influenza also can be stockpiled ahead of time. However, the optimal number of doses to stockpile depends on factors including the effectiveness of concurrent interventions and the likelihood of antiviral wastage on noninfluenza respiratory infections (Greer and Schanzer 2013).

Most pandemic-related benefit-cost studies focus on pharmaceutical interventions for high-income and upper-middle-income countries. The studies have largely neglected the question of how to allocate strained resources in low- and lower-middle-income countries. Furthermore, few evaluations have been conducted of the cost-effectiveness of general investment in health systems, infrastructure, and capacity building as a means to achieve pandemic preparedness (Drake, Chalabi, and Coker 2012).

CONCLUSIONS AND RECOMMENDATIONS FOR PRIORITIZING INVESTMENTS TO MITIGATE PANDEMIC RISK IN RESOURCE-LIMITED SETTINGS

Preparing for a pandemic is challenging because of a multitude of factors, many of which are unique among natural disasters. Pandemics are rare events, and the risk of occurrence is influenced by anthropogenic changes in the natural environment. In addition, accountability for preparedness is diffuse, and many of the countries at greatest risk have the most limited capacity to manage and mitigate pandemic risk.

Unlike most other natural disasters, pandemics do not remain geographically contained, and damages can be mitigated significantly through prompt intervention. As a result, there are strong ethical and global health imperatives for building capacity to detect and respond to pandemic threats, particularly in countries with weak preparedness and high spark and spread risk.

Investments to improve pandemic preparedness may have fewer immediate benefits, particularly relative to other pressing health needs in countries with heavy burdens of endemic disease. Therefore, characterizing pandemic risk and identifying gaps in pandemic preparedness are essential for prioritizing and targeting capacity-building efforts. Thinking about risks in terms of frequency and severity, notably using probabilistic modeling and EP curves, can quantify the potential pandemic risks facing each country and clarify the benefit-cost case for investing in pandemic preparedness.

No single, optimal response to a public health emergency exists; strategies must be tailored to the local context and to the severity and type of pandemic. However, overarching lessons emerge after multiple regional epidemics and global pandemics. For example, because of their high spark and spread risks, many LMICs would benefit most from building situational awareness and health care coordination capacity; public health response measures are far more cost-effective if they are initiated quickly and if scarce resources are targeted appropriately.

Building pandemic situational awareness is complex, requiring coordination across bureaucracies, across the public and private sectors, and across disciplines with different training and different norms (including epidemiology, clinical medicine, logistics, and disaster response). However, an appropriately sized and trained health workforce (encompassing doctors, nurses, epidemiologists, veterinarians, laboratorians, and others) that is supported by adequate coordination systems is a fundamental need—the World Health Organization has recommended a basic threshold of 23 skilled health professionals per 10,000 people (WHO 2013a).

Increasing the trained health workforce also will increase the capacity to detect whether any particular population (for example, human, farm animal, or wildlife) is suffering from a pathogen with high pandemic risk. Increasing the health workforce also will improve the overall resiliency of the health system, an improvement that can be applied to any emergency that results in morbidity and mortality shocks.

Additionally, building situational awareness will require sustained investment in infectious disease surveillance, crisis management, and risk communications systems. Investments in these capacities are likely to surge after pandemic or epidemic events and then abate as other priorities emerge. Hence, stable investment to build sustained capacity is critical.

Risk transfer mechanisms such as catastrophe risk pools offer a viable strategy for countries to manage pandemic risk. Further developing these mechanisms will allow countries to offload portions of pandemic risk and response that are beyond their immediate budgetary capacity. For this reason, risk transfer solutions should be designed with the needs and constraints of LMICs in mind. However, countries must have predefined contingency and response plans as well as the absorptive capacity to use the emergency financing offered by such solutions. Broad and effective use of pandemic insurance will require parallel investments in capacity building and emergency response planning.

Finally, researchers must address the significant knowledge gaps that exist regarding LMICs' pandemic preparedness and response. Improving the tracking of spending and aid flows specifically tied to pandemic prevention and preparedness is vital to tracking gaps and calibrating aid flows for maximum efficiency. Systematic data on response costs in low-income settings are scarce, including data regarding spending on clinical facilities, supplies, human resources, and response activities such as quarantines. Bridging these data gaps can improve pandemic preparedness planning and response through evidence-based decision making and support efforts to prevent and mitigate epidemics and pandemics.

ACKNOWLEDGMENTS

The authors would like to thank Ron Waldman, Dean Jamison, Steve Morse, Peter Sands, Mukesh Chawla and the Secretariat of the International Working Group on Financing Preparedness, Kimberly Dodd, Mary Guttieri, Patrick Ayscue, Damien Joly, Sarah Barthel, Joseph Krilanovich, Jonathan Koshi, Mike Gahan, Kierste Miller, Cathine Lam, Catherine Planey, Nicole Stephenson, Volodymyr Serhiyenko, Ming Yii Goh, Alessandro Vespignani, Qian Zhang, Matteo Chinazzi, Ana Pastore y Piontti, Marco Schäferhoff, and Jessica Kraus for their valuable technical and editorial contributions to the chapter.

NOTES

This chapter uses World Bank Income Classifications for 2018 as follows, based on estimates of gross national income (GNI) per capita for 2015:

- Low-income countries (LICs) = US$1,005 or less
- Middle-income countries (MICs) are subdivided:
  (a) lower-middle-income = US$1,006 to US$3,995
  (b) upper-middle-income countries (UMICs) = US$3,996 to US$12,235
- High-income countries (HICs) = US$12,236 or more.

1. One Health considers individual, community, and animal health as interconnected and requires the collaboration of human, animal, and environmental health professionals to recognize and alleviate the problems on one level to reduce the downstream health effects on another level (for example, rabies in animals and humans). For more information, see the U.S. Centers for Disease Control and Prevention's webpage, https://www.cdc.gov/onehealth/basics/index.html.

2. PREDICT, a project of USAID's Emerging Pandemic Threats Program, was initiated in 2009 to strengthen global capacity for detection and discovery of zoonotic viruses with pandemic potential. Working with partners in 31 countries, PREDICT is building platforms for conducting disease surveillance and for identifying and monitoring pathogens that can be shared between animals and people. Using the One Health approach, the project is investigating the behaviors, practices, and ecological and biological factors driving the emergence, transmission, and spread of disease. For more information, see the project website, http://www.vetmed.ucdavis.edu/ohi/predict/.

3. For more information about the PEF, see the brief on the World Bank website, "Pandemic Emergency Financing Facility: Frequently Asked Questions," http://www.worldbank.org/en/topic/pandemics/brief/pandemic-emergency-facility-frequently-asked-questions.

REFERENCES

Achonu, C., A. Laporte, and M. A. Gardam. 2005. "The Financial Impact of Controlling a Respiratory Virus Outbreak in a Teaching Hospital: Lessons Learned from SARS." *Canadian Journal of Public Health* 96 (1): 52–54.

Anthony, S. J., J. H. Epstein, K. A. Murray, I. Navarrete-Macias, C. M. Zambrana-Torrelio, and others. 2013. "A Strategy to Estimate Unknown Viral Diversity in Mammals." *MBio* 4 (5): e00598-13.

Arabi, Y. M., H. H. Balkhy, F. G. Hayden, A. Bouchama, T. Luke, and others. 2017. "Middle East Respiratory Syndrome." *New England Journal of Medicine* 376 (6): 584–94.

ARC (African Risk Capacity). 2016. "African Risk Capacity Strategic Framework 2016–2020." Strategy and policy document, ARC, Johannesburg, South Africa.

Arimah, B. C. 2010. "The Face of Urban Poverty: Explaining the Prevalence of Slums in Developing Countries." In *Urbanization and Development: Multidisciplinary Perspectives*, edited by Jo Beall, Basudeh Guha-Khasnobis, and Ravi Kanbur, 143–64. Oxford: Oxford University Press.

ASPR (Assistant Secretary for Preparedness and Response). 2014. "Public Health and Medical Situational Awareness Strategy." Strategy document for situational awareness implementation plan, U.S. Department of Health and Human Services, Washington, DC.

Aylward, B., P. Barboza, L. Bawo, E. Bertherat, P. Bilivogui, and others. 2014. "Ebola Virus Disease in West Africa—The First 9 Months of the Epidemic and Forward Projections." *New England Journal of Medicine* 371 (16): 1481–95.

Barden-O'Fallon, J., M. A. Barry, P. Brodish, and J. Hazerjian. 2015. "Rapid Assessment of Ebola-Related Implications for Reproductive, Maternal, Newborn, and Child Health Service Delivery and Utilization in Guinea." *PLoS Currents Outbreaks* (August): 7. doi:10.1371/currents.outbreaks.0b0ba06009dd091bc39ddb3c6d7b0826.

Barrett, R., and P. J. Brown. 2008. "Stigma in the Time of Influenza: Social and Institutional Responses to Pandemic

Emergencies." *Journal of Infectious Diseases* 197 (Suppl 1): S34–S37.

Bedrosian, S. R., C. E. Young, L. A. Smith, J. D. Cox, C. Manning, and others. 2016. "Lessons of Risk Communication and Health Promotion—West Africa and United States." *Morbidity and Mortality Weekly Report (MMWR) Supplements* 65 (3): 68–74.

Bootsma, M. C. J., and N. M. Ferguson. 2007. "The Effect of Public Health Measures on the 1918 Influenza Pandemic in U.S. Cities." *Proceedings of the National Academy of Sciences of the United States of America* 104 (18): 7588–93.

Brattberg, E., and M. Rhinard. 2011. "Multilevel Governance and Complex Threats: The Case of Pandemic Preparedness in the European Union and the United States." *Global Health Governance* 5 (1): 1–21.

Brende, B., J. Farrar, D. Gashumba, C. Moedas, T. Mundel, and others. 2017. "CEPI—A New Global R&D Organisation for Epidemic Preparedness and Response." *The Lancet* 389 (10066): 233–35.

Brundage, J. F., and G. D. Shanks. 2008. "Deaths from Bacterial Pneumonia during 1918–19 Influenza Pandemic." *Emerging Infectious Diseases* 14 (8): 1193–99.

Buckley, G. J., and R. E. Pittluck. 2016. *Global Health Risk Framework: Pandemic Financing: Workshop Summary.* Washington, DC: National Academies Press.

Burns, A., D. Van der Mensbrugghe, and H. Timmer. 2006. "Evaluating the Economic Consequences of Avian Influenza." Working Paper 47417, World Bank, Washington, DC.

Carrasco, L. R., V. J. Lee, M. I. Chen, D. B. Matchar, J. P. Thompson, and others. 2011. "Strategies for Antiviral Stockpiling for Future Influenza Pandemics: A Global Epidemic-Economic Perspective." *Journal of the Royal Society Interface* 8 (62): 1307–13.

Chan, E. H., T. F. Brewer, L. C. Madoff, M. P. Pollack, A. L. Sonricker, and others. 2010. "Global Capacity for Emerging Infectious Disease Detection." *Proceedings of the National Academy of Sciences of the United States of America* 107 (50): 21701–6.

Chandy, L., H. Kato, and H. Kharas, eds. 2015. *The Last Mile in Ending Extreme Poverty.* Washington, DC: Brookings Institution Press.

Charu, V., G. Chowell, L. S. Palacio Mejia, S. Echevarría-Zuno, V. H. Borja-Aburto, and others. 2011. "Mortality Burden of the A/H1N1 Pandemic in Mexico: A Comparison of Deaths and Years of Life Lost to Seasonal Influenza." *Clinical Infectious Diseases* 53 (10): 985–93.

Chisholm, H. 1911. "Cholera." *Encyclopedia Britannica* 11 (6): 265–66.

Cohen, N. J., C. M. Brown, F. Alvarado-Ramy, H. Bair-Drake, G. A. Benenson, and others. 2016. "Travel and Border Health Measures to Prevent the International Spread of Ebola." *Morbidity and Mortality Weekly Report (MMWR) Supplements* 65 (3): 57–67.

Cohn, S. K. 2007. "The Black Death and the Burning of Jews." *Past and Present* 196 (1): 3–36.

Colizza, V., A. Barrat, M. Barthelemy, A. J. Valleron, and A. Vespignani. 2007. "Modeling the Worldwide Spread of Pandemic Influenza: Baseline Case and Containment Interventions." *PLoS Medicine* 4 (1): 95–110.

Daszak, P., D. Carroll, N. Wolfe, and J. Mazet. 2016. "The Global Virome Project." *International Journal of Infectious Diseases* 53 (Suppl): 36.

Dawood, F. S., A. D. Iuliano, C. Reed, M. I. Meltzer, D. K. Shay, and others. 2012. "Estimated Global Mortality Associated with the First 12 Months of 2009 Pandemic Influenza A H1N1 Virus Circulation: A Modelling Study." *The Lancet Infectious Diseases* 12 (9): 687–95.

de Wit, E., D. Falzarano, C. Onyango, K. Rosenke, A. Marzi, and others. 2016. "The Merits of Malaria Diagnostics during an Ebola Virus Disease Outbreak." *Emerging Infectious Diseases* 22 (2): 323–26.

DeWitte, S. N. 2014. "Mortality Risk and Survival in the Aftermath of the Medieval Black Death." *PLoS One* 9 (5): e96513.

Diamond, J. 2009. *Guns, Germs, and Steel: The Fates of Human Societies.* New York: Norton.

Dimitrov, N., S. Goll, N. Hupert, B. Pourbohloul, and L. Meyers. 2011. "Optimizing Tactics for Use of the U.S. Antiviral Strategic National Stockpile for Pandemic Influenza." *PloS One* 6 (1): e16094.

Dixon, S., S. McDonald, and J. Roberts. 2001. "AIDS and Economic Growth in Africa: A Panel Data Analysis." *Journal of International Development* 13 (4): 411–26.

Domínguez-Cerit, G., S. E. Lapinsky, A. E. Macias, R. Pinto, L. Espinosa-Perez, and others. 2009. "Critically Ill Patients with 2009 Influenza A(H1N1) in Mexico." *Journal of the American Medical Association* 302 (17): 1880–87.

Drake, T. L., Z. Chalabi, and R. Coker. 2012. "Cost-Effectiveness Analysis of Pandemic Influenza Preparedness: What's Missing?" *Bulletin of the World Health Organization* 90 (12): 940–41.

———. 2015. "Buy Now, Saved Later? The Critical Impact of Time-to-Pandemic Uncertainty on Pandemic Cost-Effectiveness Analyses." *Health Policy and Planning* 30 (1): 100–10.

Elbe, S. 2002. "HIV/AIDS and the Changing Landscape of War in Africa." *International Security* 27 (2): 159–77.

Epstein, H. 2014. "Ebola in Liberia: An Epidemic of Rumors." *New York Review of Books* 61 (20): 91–95.

Evans, D. K., M. Goldstein, and A. Popova. 2015. "Health-Care Worker Mortality and the Legacy of the Ebola Epidemic." *The Lancet Global Health* 3 (8): e439–e440.

Falcone, R. E., and A. Detty. 2015. "The Next Pandemic: Hospital Response." *Emergency Medical Reports* 36 (26): 1–16.

Fan, V. Y., D. T. Jamison, and L. S. Summers. 2016. "The Inclusive Cost of Pandemic Influenza Risk." NBER Working Paper 22137, National Bureau of Economic Research, Cambridge, MA.

Farmer, P. 1996. "Social Inequalities and Emerging Infectious Diseases." *Emerging Infectious Diseases* 2 (4): 259–69.

Fearon, J. D., and D. D. Laitin. 2003. "Ethnicity, Insurgency, and Civil War." *American Political Science Review* 97 (1): 75–90.

Ferguson, N. M., D. A. T. Cummings, S. Cauchemez, C. Fraser, S. Riley, and others. 2005. "Strategies for Containing an Emerging Influenza Pandemic in Southeast Asia." *Nature* 437 (7056): 209–14.

Fischer, J. E., and R. Katz. 2013. "Moving Forward to 2014: Global IHR (2005) Implementation." *Biosecurity and Bioterrorism: Biodefense Strategy, Practice, and Science* 11 (2): 153–56.

Flahault, A., and A. J. Valleron. 1990. "HIV and Travel, No Rationale for Restrictions." *The Lancet* 336 (8724): 1197–98.

Fraser, C., S. Riley, R. M. Anderson, and N. M. Ferguson. 2004. "Factors That Make an Infectious Disease Outbreak Controllable." *Proceedings of the National Academy of Sciences of the United States of America* 101 (16): 6146–51.

Frieden, N. M. 1977. "The Russian Cholera Epidemic, 1892–93, and Medical Professionalization." *Journal of Social History* 10 (4): 538.

Fullam, J. D., and N. Madhav. 2015. "Quantifying Pandemic Risk." *The Actuary* 12 (1): 29–34.

Gilbert, M., N. Golding, H. Zhou, G. R. W. Wint, T. P. Robinson, and others. 2014. "Predicting the Risk of Avian Influenza A H7N9 Infection in Live-Poultry Markets across Asia." *Nature Communications* 5 (May): 1–7.

Greenhill, K., and B. Oppenheim. 2017. "Rumor Has It: The Adoption of Unverified Information in Conflict Zones." *International Studies Quarterly* 61 (3).

Greer, A. L., and D. Schanzer. 2013. "Using a Dynamic Model to Consider Optimal Antiviral Stockpile Size in the Face of Pandemic Influenza Uncertainty." *PLoS One* 8 (6): e67253.

Halder, N., J. K. Kelso, and G. J. Milne. 2014. "A Model-Based Economic Analysis of Pre-Pandemic Influenza Vaccination Cost-Effectiveness." *BMC Infectious Diseases* 14 (1): 266–85.

Henao-Restrepo, A. M., A. Camacho, I. M. Longini, C. H. Watson, W. J. Edmunds, and others. 2016. "Efficacy and Effectiveness of an rVSV-Vectored Vaccine in Preventing Ebola Virus Disease: Final Results from the Guinea Ring Vaccination, Open-Label, Cluster-Randomised Trial (Ebola Ça Suffit!)." *The Lancet* 389 (10068): 505–18.

Herstein, J. J., P. D. Biddinger, C. S. Kraft, L. Saiman, S. G. Gibbs, and others. 2016. "Initial Costs of Ebola Treatment Centers in the United States." *Emerging Infectious Diseases* 22 (2): 350.

Hollingsworth, T. D., N. M. Ferguson, and R. M. Anderson. 2006. "Will Travel Restrictions Control the International Spread of Pandemic Influenza?" *Nature Medicine* 12 (5): 497–99.

Hooghe, L., and G. Marks. 2003. "Unraveling the Central State, but How? Types of Multi-Level Governance." *American Political Science Review* 97 (2): 233–43.

ICG (International Crisis Group). 2015. *The Politics behind the Ebola Crisis*. Crisis Group Africa Report 232, International Crisis Group, Brussels, October 28.

IFRC (International Federation of Red Cross and Red Crescent Societies). 2016. *World Disasters Report, Resilience: Saving Lives Today, Investing for Tomorrow*. Geneva: IFRC.

Jain, S., L. Kamimoto, A. M. Bramley, A. M. Schmitz, S. R. Benoit, and others. 2009. "Hospitalized Patients with 2009 H1N1 Influenza in the United States, April–June 2009." *New England Journal of Medicine* 361 (20): 1935–44.

Jefferson, T., M. Jones, P. Doshi, E. A. Spencer, I. Onakpoya, and others. 2014. "Oseltamivir for Influenza in Adults and Children: Systematic Review of Clinical Study Reports and Summary of Regulatory Comments." *British Medical Journal* 348 (April): g2545.

Jennings, L. C., A. A. Monto, P. K. Chan, T. D. Szucs, and K. G. Nicholson. 2008. "Stockpiling Prepandemic Influenza Vaccines: A New Cornerstone of Pandemic Preparedness Plans." *The Lancet Infectious Diseases* 8 (10): 650–58.

Johnson, N. P. A. S., and J. Mueller. 2002. "Updating the Accounts: Global Mortality of the 1918–1920 'Spanish' Influenza Pandemic." *Bulletin of the History of Medicine* 76 (1): 105–15.

Jonas, O. B. 2013. "Pandemic Risk." Background paper for *World Development Report 2014: Risk and Opportunity; Managing Risk for Development*, World Bank, Washington, DC.

Jones, D. S. 2006. "The Persistence of American Indian Health Disparities." *American Journal of Public Health* 96 (12): 2122–34.

Jones, K. E., N. G. Patel, M. A. Levy, A. Storeygard, D. Balk, and others. 2008. "Global Trends in Emerging Infectious Diseases." *Nature* 451 (7181): 990–93.

Jun, K. 2015. "MERS Outbreak Prompts South Korean Stimulus Package." *Wall Street Journal*, June 25.

Katz, M. A., B. D. Schoub, J. M. Heraud, R. F. Breiman, M. K. Njenga, and others. 2012. "Influenza in Africa: Uncovering the Epidemiology of a Long-Overlooked Disease." *Journal of Infectious Diseases* 26 (Suppl 1): S1–S4.

Katz, R. 2009. "Use of Revised International Health Regulations during Influenza A (H1N1) Epidemic, 2009." *Emerging Infectious Diseases* 15 (8): 1165–70.

Katz, R., and R. Seifman. 2016. "Opportunities to Finance Pandemic Preparedness." *The Lancet Global Health* 4 (11): e782–e783.

Kavet, J. 1977. "A Perspective on the Significance of Pandemic Influenza." *American Journal of Public Health* 67 (11): 1063–70.

Kelly, H. A., P. C. Priest, G. N. Mercer, and G. K. Dowse. 2011. "We Should Not Be Complacent about Our Population-Based Public Health Response to the First Influenza Pandemic of the 21st Century." *BMC Public Health* 11 (1): 78.

Keogh-Brown, M. R., and R. D. Smith. 2008. "The Economic Impact of SARS: How Does the Reality Match the Predictions?" *Health Policy* 88 (1): 110–20.

KFF (Henry J. Kaiser Family Foundation). 2014. "The U.S. Government and Global Emerging Infectious Disease Preparedness and Response." Fact sheet, December 8, http://kff.org/global-health-policy/fact-sheet/the-u-s-government-global-emerging-infectious-disease-preparedness-and-response/.

Kim, Y.-W., S.-J. Yoon, and I.-H. Oh. 2013. "The Economic Burden of the 2009 Pandemic H1N1 Influenza in Korea." *Scandinavian Journal of Infectious Diseases* 45 (5): 390–96.

Kozlowski, R. T., and S. B. Mathewson. 1997. "A Primer on Catastrophe Modeling." *Journal of Insurance Regulation* 15 (3): 322.

Lee, B. Y., S. T. Brown, G. W. Korch, P. C. Cooley, R. K. Zimmerman, and others. 2010. "A Computer Simulation of Vaccine Prioritization, Allocation, and Rationing during the 2009 H1N1 Influenza Pandemic." *Vaccine* 28 (31): 4875–79.

Lugnér, A. K., and M. J. Postma. 2009. "Mitigation of Pandemic Influenza: Review of Cost-Effectiveness Studies." *Expert Review of Pharmacoeconomics and Outcomes Research* 9 (6): 547–58.

Mackowiak, P. A., and P. S. Sehdev. 2002. "The Origin of Quarantine." *Clinical Infectious Diseases* 35 (9): 1071–72.

Mancini, S., M. E. Coldiron, A. Ronsse, B. K. Ilunga, K. Porten, and others. 2014. "Description of a Large Measles Epidemic in Democratic Republic of Congo, 2010–2013." *Conflict and Health* 8 (1): 9.

Mangham, L. J., and K. Hanson. 2010. "Scaling Up in International Health: What Are the Key Issues?" *Health Policy and Planning* 25 (2): 85–96.

Mathews, J. D., J. M. Chesson, J. M. McCaw, and J. McVernon. 2009. "Understanding Influenza Transmission, Immunity, and Pandemic Threats." *Influenza and Other Respiratory Viruses* 3 (4): 143–49.

McCoy, T. 2014. "Why the Brutal Murder of Several Ebola Workers May Hint at More Violence to Come." *Washington Post*, September 19.

McKibbin, W. J., and A. A. Sidorenko. 2006. "Global Macroeconomic Consequences of Pandemic Influenza." Analysis, Lowy Institute for International Policy, Sydney, Australia.

Mihigo, R., C. V. Torrealba, K. Coninx, D. Nshimirimana, M. P. Kieny, and others. 2012. "2009 Pandemic Influenza A Virus Subtype H1N1 Vaccination in Africa—Successes and Challenges." *Journal of Infectious Diseases* 206 (Suppl 1): S22–S28.

Milián, E., and A. A. Kamen. 2015. "Current and Emerging Cell Culture Manufacturing Technologies for Influenza Vaccines." *BioMed Research International* 2015 (1): 1–11.

Miller, M. A., C. Viboud, D. R. Olson, R. F. Grais, M. A. Rabaa, and others. 2008. "Prioritization of Influenza Pandemic Vaccination to Minimize Years of Life Lost." *Journal of Infectious Diseases* 198 (3): 305–11.

Milne, G. J., N. Halder, and J. K. Kelso. 2013. "The Cost-Effectiveness of Pandemic Influenza Interventions: A Pandemic Severity Based Analysis." *PLoS One* 8 (4): e61504.

Moon, S., D. Sridhar, M. A. Pate, J. K. Jha, C. Clinton, and others. 2015. "Will Ebola Change the Game? Ten Essential Reforms before the Next Pandemic. The Report of the Harvard–LSHTM Independent Panel on the Global Response to Ebola." *The Lancet* 386 (10009): 2204–21.

Morens, D. M., J. K. Taubenberger, and A. S. Fauci. 2008. "Predominant Role of Bacterial Pneumonia as a Cause of Death in Pandemic Influenza: Implications for Pandemic Influenza Preparedness." *Journal of Infectious Diseases* 198 (7): 962–70.

Morens, D. M., J. K. Taubenberger, G. K. Folkers, and A. S. Fauci. 2010. "Pandemic Influenza's 500th Anniversary." *Clinical Infectious Diseases* 51 (12): 1442–44.

Morse, S. S. 1995. "Factors in the Emergence of Infectious Diseases." *Emerging Infectious Diseases* 1 (1): 7–15.

Morse, S. S., J. A. K. Mazet, M. Woolhouse, C. R. Parrish, D. Carroll, and others. 2012. "Prediction and Prevention of the Next Pandemic Zoonosis." *The Lancet* 380 (9857): 1956–65.

MSF (Médecins Sans Frontières). 2015. *Pushed to the Limit and Beyond: A Year into the Largest Ever Ebola Outbreak.* Report, MSF, London.

Mullard, A. 2016. "New Vaccine Coalition Targets Epidemics." *Nature Reviews Drug Discovery* 15 (10): 669.

Murphy, F. A. 1998. "Emerging Zoonoses." *Emerging Infectious Diseases* 4 (3): 429–35.

Murray, C. J., A. D. Lopez, B. Chin, D. Feehan, and K. H. Hill. 2006. "Estimation of Potential Global Pandemic Influenza Mortality on the Basis of Vital Registry Data from the 1918–20 Pandemic: A Quantitative Analysis." *The Lancet* 368 (9554): 2211–18.

Nannei, C., S. Goldin, G. Torelli, H. Fatima, K. Kumar, and others. 2016. "Stakeholders' Perceptions of 10 Years of the Global Action Plan for Influenza Vaccines (GAP)—Results from a Survey." *Vaccine* 34 (45): 5393–99.

Neiderud, C.-J. 2015. "How Urbanization Affects the Epidemiology of Emerging Infectious Diseases." *Infection Ecology and Epidemiology* 5: 27060. doi:/10.3402/iee .v5.27060.

Oppenheim, B., M. D. Gallivan, N. Madhav, N. Brown, V. Serhiyenko, and others. 2017. "Global Preparedness for the Next Pandemic." Unpublished manuscript.

Oshitani, H., T. Kamigaki, and A. Suzuki. 2008. "Major Issues and Challenges of Influenza Pandemic Preparedness in Developing Countries." *Emerging Infectious Diseases* 14 (6): 875–80.

Osterholm, M. T. 2005. "Preparing for the Next Pandemic." *New England Journal of Medicine* 352 (18): 1839–42.

Paez-Espino, D., E. A. Eloe-Fadrosh, G. A. Pavlopoulos, A. D. Thomas, M. Huntemann, and others. 2016. "Uncovering Earth's Virome." *Nature* 536 (7617): 425–30.

Park, J., and J. Kim. 2015. "Hong Kong Sets 'Serious' Response to South Korea's MERS Outbreak." Reuters, June 8.

Parpia, A. S., M. L. Ndeffo-Mbah, N. S. Wenzel, and A. P. Galvani. 2016. "Effects of Response to 2014–2015 Ebola Outbreak on Deaths from Malaria, HIV/AIDS, and Tuberculosis, West Africa." *Emerging Infectious Diseases* 22 (3): 433–41.

Parveen, S., M. S. Islam, M. Begum, M. Alam, H. M. S. Sazzad, and others. 2016. "It's Not Only What You Say, It's Also How You Say It: Communicating Nipah Virus Prevention Messages during an Outbreak in Bangladesh." *BMC Public Health* 16 (1): 726–37.

Pasquini-Descomps, H., N. Brender, and D. Maradan. 2016. "Value for Money in H1N1 Influenza: A Systematic Review of the Cost-Effectiveness of Pandemic Interventions." *Value in Health* 20 (6): 819–27.

Pathmanathan, I., K. A. O'Connor, M. L. Adams, C. Y. Rao, P. H. Kilmarx, and others. 2014. "Rapid Assessment of Ebola Infection Prevention and Control Needs—Six Districts, Sierra Leone, October 2014." *Morbidity and Mortality Weekly Report (MMWR)* 63 (49): 1172–74.

Pérez Velasco, R., N. Praditsitthikorn, K. Wichmann, A. Mohara, S. Kotirum, and others. 2012. "Systematic Review of Economic Evaluations of Preparedness Strategies and Interventions against Influenza Pandemics." *PloS One* 7 (2): e30333.

Person, B., F. Sy, K. Holton, B. Govert, A. Liang, and others. 2004. "Fear and Stigma: The Epidemic within the SARS Outbreak." *Emerging Infectious Diseases* 10 (2): 358–63.

Pike, B. L., K. E. Saylors, J. N. Fair, M. Lebreton, U. Tamoufe, and others. 2010. "The Origin and Prevention of Pandemics." *Clinical Infectious Diseases* 50 (12): 1636–40.

Platt, C. 2014. *King Death: The Black Death and Its Aftermath in Late-Medieval England.* Oxon, U.K.: Routledge.

Porta, M., ed. 2014. *A Dictionary of Epidemiology.* 6th ed. Oxford: Oxford University Press.

Price-Smith, A. T. 2001. *The Health of Nations: Infectious Disease, Environmental Change, and Their Effects on National Security and Development.* Cambridge, MA: MIT Press.

———. 2009. *Contagion and Chaos: Disease, Ecology, and National Security in the Era of Globalization.* Cambridge, MA: MIT Press.

Pritchett, L., M. Woolcock, and M. Andrews. 2013. "Looking Like a State: Techniques of Persistent Failure in State Capability for Implementation." *Journal of Development Studies* 49 (1): 1–18.

Radonovich, L. J., P. D. Magalian, M. K. Hollingsworth, and G. Baracco. 2009. "Stockpiling Supplies for the Next Influenza Pandemic." *Emerging Infectious Diseases* 15 (6): e1.

Reperant, L. A., G. F. Rimmelzwaan, and A. D. M. E. Osterhaus. 2014. "Advances in Influenza Vaccination." *F1000 Prime Reports* 6: 47.

Richardson, J. S., J. D. Dekker, M. A. Croyle, and G. P. Kobinger. 2010. "Recent Advances in Ebolavirus Vaccine Development." *Human Vaccines* 6 (6): 439–49.

Roca, A., M. O. Afolabi, Y. Saidu, and B. Kampmann. 2015. "Ebola: A Holistic Approach Is Required to Achieve Effective Management and Control." *Journal of Allergy and Clinical Immunology* 135 (4): 856–67.

Rosello, A., M. Mossoko, S. Flasche, A. J. Van Hoek, P. Mbala, and others. 2015. "Ebola Virus Disease in the Democratic Republic of the Congo, 1976–2014." *eLife* 2015 (4): e09015.

Rubinson, L., R. Mutter, C. Viboud, N. Hupert, T. Uyeki, and others. 2013. "Impact of the Fall 2009 Influenza A(H1N1) pdm09 Pandemic on US Hospitals." *Medical Care* 51 (3): 259–65.

Samaan, G., M. Patel, B. Olowokure, M. C. Roces, H. Oshitani, and others. 2005. "Rumor Surveillance and Avian Influenza H5N1." *Emerging Infectious Diseases* 11 (3): 463–66.

Sands, P., A. El Turabi, P. A. Saynisch, and V. J. Dzau. 2016. "Assessment of Economic Vulnerability to Infectious Disease Crises." *The Lancet* 388 (10058): 2443–48.

Sands, P., C. Mundaca-Shah, and V. J. Dzau. 2016. "The Neglected Dimension of Global Security—A Framework for Countering Infectious-Disease Crises." *New England Journal of Medicine* 374 (March): 1281–87.

Schäferhoff, M., S. Fewer, J. Kraus, E. Richter, L. H. Summers, and others. 2015. "How Much Donor Financing for Health Is Channelled to Global versus Country-Specific Aid Functions?" *The Lancet* 386 (10011): 2436–41.

Seto, W. H., D. Tsang, R. W. H. Hung, T. Y. Ching, T. K. Ng, and others. 2003. "Effectiveness of Precautions against Droplets and Contact in Prevention of Nosocomial Transmission of Severe Acute Respiratory Syndrome (SARS)." *The Lancet* 361 (9368): 1519–20.

Shuaib, F., R. Gunnala, E. O. Musa, F. J. Mahoney, O. Oguntimehin, and others. 2014. "Ebola Virus Disease Outbreak—Nigeria, July–September 2014." *Morbidity and Mortality Weekly Report (MMWR)* 63 (39): 867–72.

Simonsen, L., P. Spreeuwenberg, R. Lustig, R. J. Taylor, D. M. Fleming, and others. 2013. "Global Mortality Estimates for the 2009 Influenza Pandemic from the GLaMOR Project: A Modeling Study." *PLoS Medicine* 10 (11): e1001558.

Siu, J. Y. M. 2015. "Influence of Social Experiences in Shaping Perceptions of the Ebola Virus among African Residents of Hong Kong during the 2014 Outbreak: A Qualitative Study." *International Journal for Equity in Health* 14 (1): 88.

Smith, R. D., M. R. Keogh-Brown, T. Barnett, and J. Tait. 2009. "The Economy-Wide Impact of Pandemic Influenza on the UK: A Computable General Equilibrium Modelling Experiment." *British Medical Journal* 339 (November): b4571.

Smolinsky, M. S., M. A. Hamburg, and J. Lederberg, eds. 2003. *Microbial Threats to Health: Emergence, Detection, and Response.* Washington, DC: National Academies Press.

Stoddard, A., A. Harmer, K. Haver, G. Taylor, and P. Harvey. 2015. *The State of the Humanitarian System: 2015 Edition.* London: Active Learning Network for Accountability and Performance in Humanitarian Action/Overseas Development Institute.

Thomas, M. R., G. Smith, F. H. G. Ferreira, D. Evans, M. Maliszewska, and others. 2015. "The Economic Impact of Ebola on Sub-Saharan Africa: Updated Estimates for 2015." Working Paper 93721, World Bank, Washington, DC.

Tilman, D., and M. Clark. 2014. "Global Diets Link Environmental Sustainability and Human Health." *Nature* 515 (7528): 518–22.

Tizzoni, M., P. Bajardi, C. Poletto, J. J. Ramasco, D. Balcan, and others. 2012. "Real-Time Numerical Forecast of Global Epidemic Spreading: Case Study of 2009 A/H1N1pdm." *BMC Medicine* 10 (1): 165.

Toole, M. J., and R. J. Waldman. 1990. "Prevention of Excess Mortality in Refugee and Displaced Populations in Developing Countries." *Journal of the American Medical Association* 263 (24): 3296–302.

Twu, S-J., T-J. Chen, C-J. Chen, S. J. Olsen, L-T. Lee, and others. 2003. "Control Measures for Severe Acute Respiratory Syndrome (SARS) in Taiwan." *Emerging Infectious Diseases* 9 (6): 718–20.

Tyler, T. 2016. "IATA 2016 Annual Review." Annual review publication, International Air Transport Association (IATA), Montreal.

UNDESA (United Nations Department of Economic and Social Affairs). 2015. "World Population Prospects: The 2015 Revision, Key Findings and Advance Tables." Report ESA/P/WP.241, UNDESA, New York.

UNDP (United Nations Development Programme). 2014. "Assessing the Socio-Economic Impacts of Ebola Virus Disease in Guinea, Liberia, and Sierra Leone: The Road to Recovery." Synthesis report, UNDP, New York.

———. 2017. "A Socio-Economic Impact Assessment of the Zika Virus in Latin America and the Caribbean: With a Focus on Brazil, Colombia, and Suriname." Synthesis report, UNDP, New York.

USAID (U.S. Agency for International Development) and CDC (Centers for Disease Control and Prevention). 2016. "West Africa—Ebola Outbreak, Fact Sheet #11, Fiscal Year (FY) 2016." Fact sheet, USAID, CDC, June 24.

U.S. Department of Health and Human Services. 2005. "HHS Pandemic Influenza Plan." Strategic, guidance, and operational planning document, U.S. Department of Health and Human Services, Washington, DC.

U.S. Homeland Security Council. 2006. "Implementation Plan for the National Strategy for Pandemic Influenza." Plan document, U.S. Homeland Security Council, Executive Office of the President of the United States, Washington, DC.

Van Boeckel, T. P., S. Gandra, A. Ashok, Q. Caudron, B. T. Grenfell, and others. 2014. "Global Antibiotic Consumption 2000 to 2010: An Analysis of National Pharmaceutical Sales Data." *The Lancet Infectious Diseases* 14 (8): 742–50.

Van Boeckel, T. P., W. Thanapongtharm, T. Robinson, C. M. Biradar, X. Xiao, and others. 2012. "Improving Risk Models for Avian Influenza: The Role of Intensive Poultry Farming and Flooded Land during the 2004 Thailand Epidemic." *PLoS One* 7 (11): e49528.

Viboud, C., M. Miller, D. R. Olson, M. Osterholm, and L. Simonsen. 2010. "Preliminary Estimates of Mortality and Years of Life Lost Associated with the 2009 A/H1N1 Pandemic in the US and Comparison with Past Influenza Seasons." *PLoS Currents* 20 (March): RRN1153.

Viboud, C., L. Simonsen, R. Fuentes, J. Flores, M. A. Miller, and others. 2016. "Global Mortality Impact of the 1957–1959 Influenza Pandemic." *Journal of Infectious Diseases* 212 (11): 738–45.

Waggoner, J. J., and B. A. Pinsky. 2016. "Zika Virus: Diagnostics for an Emerging Pandemic Threat." *Journal of Clinical Microbiology* 54 (4): 860–67.

Walker, N. F., and C. J. Whitty. 2015. "Tackling Emerging Infections: Clinical and Public Health Lessons from the West African Ebola Virus Disease Outbreak." *Clinical Medicine* 15 (5): 457–60.

Wallinga, J., and P. Teunis. 2004. "Different Epidemic Curves for Severe Acute Respiratory Syndrome Reveal Similar Impacts of Control Measures." *American Journal of Epidemiology* 160 (6): 509–16.

Wang, M-D., and A. M. Jolly. 2004. "Changing Virulence of the SARS Virus: The Epidemiological Evidence." *Bulletin of the World Health Organization* 82 (7): 547–48.

Watts, J. 2004. "China Culls Wild Animals to Prevent New SARS Threat." *The Lancet* 363 (9403): 134.

WHO (World Health Organization). 1978. "Ebola Haemorrhagic Fever in Zaire, 1976. Report of an International Commission." *Bulletin of the World Health Organization* 56 (2): 271–93.

———. 2005. *International Health Regulations.* Geneva: WHO.

———. 2010. "What Is a Pandemic?" WHO, February 24. http://www.who.int/csr/disease/swineflu/frequently_asked _questions/pandemic/en/.

———. 2013a. "Global Health Workforce Shortage to Reach 12.9 Million in Coming Decades." News release, November 11.

———. 2013b. *Global Survey on National Vaccine Deployment and Vaccination Plans for Pandemic A(H1N1) 2009 Vaccine—2010.* Report of survey findings, WHO, Geneva.

———. 2013c. "IHR Core Capacity Monitoring Framework: Checklist and Indicators for Monitoring Progress in the Development of IHR Core Capacities in States Parties." International Health Regulations (2005) document, Reference WHO/HSE/GCR/2013.2, WHO, Geneva.

———. 2014. "Summary of States Parties 2013 Report on IHR Core Capacity Implementation: Regional Profiles." International Health Regulations (2005) document, Reference WHO/HSE/GCR/2014.10, WHO, Geneva.

———. 2015a. "Successful Ebola Responses in Nigeria, Senegal, and Mali." In *One Year into the Ebola Epidemic: A Deadly, Tenacious, and Unforgiving Year.* Paper Series, January 2015, WHO, Geneva.

———. 2015b. "WHO Model List of Essential Medicines, 19th ed." WHO, Geneva.

———. 2016a. *Ebola Situation Report.* Weekly data report, April 15.

———. 2016b. "Influenza (Seasonal)." Fact sheet, November. http://www.who.int/mediacentre/factsheets/fs211/en/.

———. 2016c. "Pandemic Influenza Preparedness Framework Partnership Contribution: Annual Report 2015." Document WHO/OHE/PED/2016.01, Pandemic Influenza Preparedness (PIP) Secretariat, WHO, Geneva.

———. 2017. *Situation Report: Zika Virus, Microcephaly, Guillain-Barré Syndrome.* Weekly data report, February 2.

Wolfe, N. D., P. Daszak, A. M. Kilpatrick, and D. S. Burke. 2005. "Bushmeat Hunting, Deforestation, and Prediction of Zoonotic Disease." *Emerging Infectious Diseases* 11 (12): 1822–27.

Wolfe, N. D., C. P. Dunavan, and J. Diamond. 2007. "Origins of Major Human Infectious Diseases." *Nature* 447 (7142): 279–83.

Wolicki, S. B., J. B. Nuzzo, D. L. Blazes, D. L. Pitts, J. K. Iskander, and others. 2016. "Public Health Surveillance: At the Core of the Global Health Security Agenda." *Health Security* 14 (3): 185–88.

Woolhouse, M. E. J., and S. Gowtage-Sequeria. 2005. "Host Range and Emerging and Reemerging Pathogens." *Emerging Infectious Diseases* 11 (12): 1842–47.

World Bank. 2012. *People, Pathogens, and Our Planet, Volume 2: The Economics of One Health.* Report 69145, World Bank, Washington, DC.

————. 2014. "The Economic Impact of the 2014 Ebola Epidemic: Short and Medium Term Estimates for Guinea, Liberia, and Sierra Leone." Working Paper 90748, World Bank, Washington, DC.

————. 2016. "World Bank Group Ebola Response Fact Sheet." Fact sheet, World Bank, April 6. http://www.worldbank.org/en/topic/health/brief/world-bank-group-ebola-fact-sheet.

Yamey, G., M. Schäferhoff, O. K. Aars, B. Bloom, D. Carroll, and others. 2017. "Financing of International Collective Action for Epidemic and Pandemic Preparedness." *The Lancet Global Health* 5 (8): e742–e744.

Yehualashet, Y. G., P. Mkanda, A. Gasasira, T. Erbeto, A. Onimisi, and others. 2016. "Strategic Engagement of Technical Surge Capacity for Intensified Polio Eradication Initiative in Nigeria, 2012–2015." *Journal of Infectious Diseases* 213 (Suppl 3): S116–S23.

Yu, H., J. T. Wu, B. J. Cowling, Q. Liao, V. J. Fang, and others. 2014. "Effect of Closure of Live Poultry Markets on Poultry-to-Person Transmission of Avian Influenza A H7N9 Virus: An Ecological Study." *The Lancet* 383 (9916): 541–48.

Zell, R. 2004. "Global Climate Change and the Emergence /Re-emergence of Infectious Diseases." *International Journal of Medical Microbiology Supplements* 293 (Suppl 37): 16–26.

Zinsstag, J., E. Schelling, K. Wyss, and M. B. Mahamat. 2005. "Potential of Cooperation between Human and Animal Health to Strengthen Health Systems." *The Lancet* 366 (9503): 2142–45.

Chapter 18

The Loss from Pandemic Influenza Risk

Victoria Y. Fan, Dean T. Jamison, and Lawrence H. Summers

INTRODUCTION

The 2014–16 Ebola virus outbreak in West Africa reminded the world that enormous economic and human losses result from the uncontrolled spread of a deadly infection. Less noticed was the likelihood that a pandemic with characteristics similar to the 1918 influenza pandemic would have killed about 10 times as many people in Liberia, Guinea, and Sierra Leone as did Ebola. The global death total from such a pandemic could be 2,500 times higher than the World Health Organization's (WHO) estimate of 11,300 deaths from Ebola through March 16, 2016 (WHO 2016a).

Economic Loss

In addition to the enormous loss in terms of human suffering, an important dimension of loss lies in a pandemic's effect on income. Premature deaths reduce the size of the labor force, illness leads to absenteeism and reduced productivity, resources flow to treatment and control measures, and individual and societal measures to reduce disease spread can seriously disrupt economic activity. The World Bank has generated estimates of these losses (Burns, Mensbrugghe, and Timmer 2008; Jonas 2013) and found that a pandemic of the severity of that in 1918 could reduce global gross domestic product (GDP) by about 5 percent and that the disruptive effects of avoiding infection would account for about 60 percent of that total. McKibbin and Sidorenko (2006) examined the consequences of a range of pandemic severities (mild, moderate, severe, and ultra) and estimated income losses exceeding 12 percent of gross national income (GNI) worldwide and exceeding 50 percent in some low- and middle-income countries (LMICs).

Value of Lives Lost and Illness Suffered

The second major dimension of loss from a pandemic lies in the intrinsic value of lives prematurely lost and of illness suffered. Efforts to measure the dollar value of losses associated with premature mortality and illness remain imperfect. Nevertheless, extensive empirical findings appear in the economics literature, particularly for losses from premature mortality (Hammitt and Robinson 2011; Lindhjem and others 2011; Viscusi 2014). Although the valuation of a change in mortality appears most frequently in the environmental economics literature, the report of the *Lancet* Commission on Investing in Health—"Global Health 2035: A World Converging within a Generation," or Global Health 2035—systematically applied these methods to global health (Jamison and others 2013; OECD 2014). This chapter estimates the magnitude of this dimension of loss from pandemic influenza using standard methods.

This chapter assesses the *expected* annual loss from a pandemic with risk r, expressed as a percentage of the annual probability of a pandemic, and severity s, expressed as the fraction of the world population that

Corresponding author: Victoria Y. Fan. Myron B. Thompson School of Social Work, University of Hawai'i at Mānoa, Honolulu, Hawai'i, U.S.A.; vfan@hawaii.edu.

dies from the pandemic. It uses the historical and modeling literatures to generate expected values of r and s, and it uses those values to generate estimates of mortality and its associated losses. The estimated loss is relative to the counterfactual of no risk ($r = 0$). Box 18.1 places the results of our research into context.

REVIEW OF HISTORICAL PANDEMIC RISK AND SEVERITY

The literature defines pandemic "severity" in different ways. We define it in terms of mortality only. Paules and Fauci (2017) point to long-term morbidity and disability consequences of a range of potential pandemic pathogens. Global Health 2035 appendix 4 introduced the term *standardized mortality unit* (SMU) in which 1 SMU is 10^{-4}. For example, the pandemic of 1957–58 had a global death rate of 3 SMU (or 0.03 percent of the population).

In the world's 2015 population of 7.35 billion, 1 SMU corresponds to 735,000 deaths. Seasonal influenza causes about 250,000 to 500,000 deaths per year (WHO 2016b). We define *severe* pandemics as having mortality rates of 10 SMU or greater, and *moderately severe* pandemics as having a severity less than 10 SMU.

The historical record suggests that the 1918 influenza pandemic was an outlier, with unusual circumstances, including the co-occurrence of World War I. No other influenza pandemic had such devastatingly high mortality rates. The 1918 influenza pandemic had an estimated 20 million to 50 million (or more) excess deaths from 1918 to 1920, most of which were concentrated in 1918. In 1918, 20 million deaths would constitute 1.1 percent of the world's population. In addition to the severe pandemic of 1918, the sparse record suggests that 12 to 17 other pandemics have occurred since 1700. Of these, we identify six as having substantial excess mortality, with mortality rates in the range of 3–8 SMU (table 18.1).

Box 18.1

Research in Context

Evidence before This Study
We searched PubMed and Google Scholar for all studies on influenza epidemics and pandemics. We also searched libraries at Harvard University and the University of Hawai'i for historical documents and life tables. Studies were restricted to those with abstracts in English.

Our review showed a wide range in the estimates of deaths caused by the 1918 influenza pandemic. We found three studies that examined loss in national income from influenza pandemics of varying severity. A substantial literature exists that estimates the monetary value of mortality risk—the value of a statistical life—but we found only one paper in that literature that estimates the loss from elevated mortality associated with pandemics. Integrative estimates of the magnitude of pandemic risk were found in only two sources, both partially proprietary.

Added Value of This Study
This study provides the first assessment of the expected value of losses from pandemic influenza and, specifically, the value of intrinsic losses from

increased mortality. It uses an expected value framework to estimate losses from an uncertain and rare event over time. Past work found that income losses (US$80 billion per year) are much lower than the losses from increased mortality (US$490 billion per year). We further analyzed economic losses of national income levels by world regions and conducted sensitivity analyses on the value of a statistical life.

Implications of All of the Available Evidence
Estimates of intrinsic loss substantially exceed previous estimates of income loss. As significant as the direct effect of a pandemic on income appears to be, we conclude that intrinsic losses far exceed the income losses. This finding points to the need for more attention to pandemic risk in public policy and to the value of enhanced understanding of both the magnitude and the consequences of pandemic risk. Low- and middle-income countries would suffer more than high-income countries in mortality losses. Further studies to investigate the potential losses from pandemics from other causes are ongoing.

Table 18.1 Worldwide Mortality from Selected Influenza Pandemics, 1700–2000[a]

Year	Estimated worldwide pandemic-related deaths (millions)	Estimated world population (millions)	Severity, s (fraction of world population killed, SMU)[b]
1729[c]	0.4	720	6
1781–82[c]	0.7	920	8
1830–33[c]	0.8	1,150	7
1898–1900[c]	1.2	1,630	7
1918–20[c,d]	20.0–50.0	1,830	110–270
1957–58[c]	1.0	2,860	3
1968–69[c]	1.0–2.0	3,540	3–6

Note: SMU = standardized mortality unit.

a. The table includes pandemics dating from 1700 to 2000 for which severity could be ascertained from the literature. Morens and Fauci (2004) and Morens and Taubenberger (2011) identify 12 to 17 pandemics in the period from 1700 to 2000, but many of those resulted in lower mortality than those in this table (or had mortality levels that could not be ascertained).

b. The SMU represents a 10^{-4} mortality risk and is used to represent small numbers as integers. For example, the 1729 pandemic led to an elevation in mortality of 0.06 percent of the world's population, which is more conveniently expressed as 6 SMU. In the world's 2015 population, 1 SMU corresponds to 735,000 deaths.

c. See Potter (2001).

d. See Beveridge (1991); Ghendon (1994); Johnson and Mueller (2002).

Although the world may be expected to experience moderately severe to severe pandemics several times each century, there is consensus among influenza experts that an event on the very severe scale of the 1918 pandemic may be plausible but remains historically and biologically unpredictable (Taubenberger, Morens, and Fauci 2007). A modeling exercise conducted for the insurance industry concluded that 100 to 200 years would pass before a 1918-type pandemic returned, but the exercise acknowledged major uncertainty (Madhav 2013). Although a biological replica of the 1918 influenza pandemic would result in lower mortality rates than those that occurred in 1918 (Madhav 2013), other studies point to the possibility that exceptionally transmissible and virulent viruses could lead to global death rates substantially higher than in 1918 (McKibbin and Sidorenko 2006; Osterholm 2005).

In general, lower-income areas of the world suffered disproportionately in 1918; in particular, India suffered a major share of global pandemic mortality (Davis 1968). Similarly, Madhav (2013) and Morens and Fauci (2007) argue that a modern epidemic would disproportionately affect poor countries. However, China's mortality rate in 1918 was low, probably because of lower case fatality rates rather than lower incidence rates (Cheng and Leung 2007). This finding points to the possibility of heterogeneity between countries of comparable national income levels in a modern pandemic.

This chapter does not seek to provide a new review of the literature on mortality in previous pandemics but rather to select plausible values from that literature to define reference cases. With Taubenberger and others (2007), we emphasize the uncertainty inherent both in the history and in projections drawn from it. In light of this literature and its attendant uncertainty, we develop and report results for two representative levels of severity. Table 18.2 defines the severity levels we use and indicates the levels of annual risk assigned to them. Box 18.2 provides the background to the calculation of expected severity that table 18.2 summarizes.

METHODS

The effort proceeds in two steps. First, information on pandemic severity is used to generate increases in age-specific death rates for the world and for each of the World Bank's four income groups of countries. Second, the literature on valuation of changes in mortality rates is used to generate estimates of the age-specific losses from mortality increase and, by extension, of total loss.

We begin by estimating the change in a population's age-specific mortality rate for the two severity reference cases. Estimates of the age-specific excess mortality rates of different populations from the 1918 pandemic are consistent in their form of a unique inverted U-shaped distribution, whereby adults ages 15 to 60 years experienced elevated rates compared to elderly persons (greater than age 60 years) (Luk, Gross, and Thompson 2001; Murray and others 2006). We use the specific U.S. data for age distribution of excess

Table 18.2 Worldwide Pandemic Risk: Two Representative Scenarios, 2015

Parameter	Moderately severe pandemic (< 10 SMU)[a]	Severe pandemic (≥ 10 SMU)[b]	Any pandemic
1. Annual probability, r[a] (%)	2.0	1.6	3.6
2. Return time, $1/r$ (years)	50	63	28
3. Average severity (SMU)[c]	2.5	58	27
4. Expected severity, s[d] (SMU)	0.05	0.93	0.98

Note: SMU = standardized mortality unit.

a. The SMU represents a 10^{-4} mortality risk and is used to represent small numbers as integers. For example, the 1729 pandemic led to an elevation in mortality of 0.06 percent of the world's population, which is more conveniently expressed as 6 SMU. In the world's 2015 population, 1 SMU corresponds to 735,000 deaths.

b. These severity states are mutually exclusive. Hence, the annual probability of any pandemic is $[1 - (1 - 0.2)(1 - 0.016)] = 3.6\%$

c. The average severity of a pandemic in a given severity range is the expected value of severity given that a pandemic did in fact occur in that range. For example, 2.5 SMU is the expected severity given that a pandemic of severity $s < 10$ SMU has occurred.

d. "Expected severity" is average severity multiplied by the probability of occurrence $[s = \text{row (3)} \times \text{row (1)}]$.

Box 18.2

Estimating Pandemic Severity and Risk

Following its usage in the insurance industry, we define risk, r(s), in terms of "exceedance probability," the annual probability of a pandemic having a severity *exceeding s*. Again following insurance industry usage, the "return time" for s is the expected number of years before a pandemic of at least severity s will occur. If t(s) is the return time, then $\text{t}(s) = \text{r}(s)^{-1}$. For example, if the annual probability of a pandemic of severity at least s is 1%, then its return time will be 100 years.

If we had access to a function r(s) showing exceedance probability as a function of severity, our analysis could proceed using the expected value of severity of all pandemics. Because r(s) is the complementary cumulative of the density for s, we would have

$$\text{Expected value of } s = \int_0^\infty \text{r}(s)\,ds. \quad \text{(B18.2.1)}$$

Modeled estimates of the function r(s) are not (publicly) available, so we approximated in two steps. We label pandemics with global $s \geq 10$ SMU as "severe." (As defined in the text, 1 SMU corresponds to a 10^{-4} mortality risk.) We label pandemics with global $s < 10$ as moderately severe. For the first step in our assessment of expected severity, we use recent history as a straightforward guide to frequency and severity

of moderately severe pandemics. In particular, we assume two such pandemics per century in this severity range with the average severity of 2.5 SMU globally. The *expected* annual severity of moderately severe pandemics is $0.02 \times 2.5 = 0.05$ SMU, corresponding to just over 35,000 expected annual deaths worldwide.

We turn next to equation B18.2.2 to estimate the contributions to expected severity from pandemic severity greater than 10 SMU worldwide (or 4 SMU in the United States). Let $\text{s}^*(x)$ be the contribution of pandemic severity greater than x to expected pandemic severity. Information available from AIR and its Pandemic Flu Model (AIR Worldwide 2014) allows calibration of r(s) for the United States with $s \geq 4$:

$$\text{s}^\star(4) = \int_4^\infty \text{r}(s)\,ds. \quad \text{(B18.2.2)}$$

(Available data allow us to calibrate only an exceedance probability function, r(s), for the United States. Hence, we start with that and translate to world values from severity ratios available in Madhav [2013].) The calibration points to a very fat-tailed distribution. The hyperbolic family of complementary cumulative distributions provides natural candidates for r(s), and we parameterize the hyperbolic in terms of its expectation and the fatness of its tail

box continues next page

Box 18.2 (continued)

(see Jamison and Jamison 2011, table 2, in the formally identical context of discounting). Thus,

$$r(s) = [1 + m(1 - f)s]^{-[1 + 1/(1-f)]} \quad \text{(B18.2.3)}$$

where $1/m$ is the expected value of s, and f indicates the fatness of the tail (smaller values imply a fatter tail). Our calibration yields a value of $m = 1.8$ and $f = -2$. Hence, $s^*(0) = 1/1.8 = 0.56$. $s^*(4)$ is given as

$$s^*(4) = 0.56 - \int_0^4 (1 + 3ms)^{-1.33} ds, \quad \text{(B18.2.4)}$$

and the integral is approximately 0.38. (For small values of s, equation B18.2.3 substantially overestimates r when the equation for $r(s)$ has been calibrated to fit larger values of s and thus the need for this two-step procedure.) Hence, $s^*(4) = 0.56 - 0.38 = 0.18$, which is the contribution to expected severity in the United States of severity levels ≥ 4 SMU. We infer global severity from the severity in the United States using the approach described in the main text.

Madhav (2013), using the AIR model, estimates that a 1918-type pandemic would kill 21 million to 33 million people in today's world. She reports a mid-range severity for the United States of such a pandemic of 8.8 SMU with a return time of 100 to 200 years. Equation B18.2.3 predicts that the return time for a pandemic of at least that severity is about 175 years.

Our calibrated value of -2 for f, the tail fatness parameter in equation 2.1.3, suggests that the distribution of exceedance probabilities is very fat tailed indeed. An exponential distribution for $r(s)$ could be considered to be neither fat nor thin tailed.

Calibrating an exponential as we did for the hyperbolic—so that the contribution to expected severity of severity ≥ 4 SMU is equal to 0.18—gives $r(s) = e^{0 - 0.57s}$, and a return time for a 1918-type pandemic of 150 years, quite close to the 175 years of equation B18.2.3. However, for $s = 4$ in the United States (over 7 million deaths worldwide), the exponential gives an unrealistic return time of only 10 years whereas equation B18.2.3 gives 63 years. AIR (AIR Worldwide 2014) estimates that an extreme pandemic with $s = 30$ in the United States (and perhaps 100 million deaths worldwide) has a return time of 1,000 years, and equation 2.1.3 gives 875 years. The exponential would give 27 million years.

Clearly, uncertainty surrounds the numbers we use to reflect the likelihood of pandemics of varying levels of severity. In particular, we point to recent estimates (Madhav and others 2018) of exceedance probability and pandemic risk that use methods similar to those of AIR but come to a substantially smaller number of expected annual deaths. However, our numbers represent conservative choices that are broadly consistent with historical experience and modeling parameters. Substantially greater severities and likelihoods have been discussed by Madhav (2013) and colleagues elsewhere in the literature (Bruine De Bruin and others 2006; McKibbin and Sidorenko 2006; Osterholm 2005). As Morens and Taubenberger (1977, 277) stated, "With human influenza the only certain thing seems to be uncertainty." We would slightly modify that statement to assert the virtual certainty that, "sooner or later, the world will again suffer a severe pandemic."

deaths to generate age distributions for the world, adjusting for greater absolute increases elsewhere (Luk, Gross, and Thompson 2001). The fatality rate among young adults, although high in the 1918 influenza pandemic, was relatively low in the 1957 and 1968 epidemics (Simonsen and others 1998). We also use an alternative and more typical distribution of excess mortality, where young children and elderly persons are disproportionally affected, as well as a combination of the two, assuming the same proportional increase in mortality for all age groups. Our final calculations are based on the assumption that moderately severe pandemics will have age distributions like those of the 1957 and 1968 pandemics, whereas severe pandemics will

have age distributions of death like those of the 1918 pandemic.

Using the age distributions of populations and the life tables from the *World Population Prospects* of the United Nations Population Division (2015), we calculate excess deaths and the estimated reduction in life expectancy based on these age-specific mortality rates (Preston, Heuveline, and Guillot 2000). Table 18.3 shows the results for our severity categories. Our *expected* annual pandemic death total across both severities is 720,000 (or 1.2 percent of the number of deaths in 2015), resulting in a decrease in life expectancy at birth by 0.3–0.4 years in low-income countries (LICs) and LMICs.

Table 18.3 Expected Annual Influenza Pandemic Deaths, by Country Income Group, 2015[a]

Parameter	Income level[b]				
	Low	Lower-middle	Upper-middle	High	World
1. Population (millions)	640	2,900	2,400	1,400	7,350
2. Moderately severe pandemics					
2.1. Relative pandemic severity[c]	4	3	2	1	n.a.
2.2. *Expected* annual pandemic-related mortality rate (SMU)	0.08	0.06	0.04	0.02	0.05
2.3. *Expected* excess deaths per year [x = (1) × (2.2)]	5,100	18,000	9,600	2,800	37,000
3. Severe pandemics (all severities combined)					
3.1. Relative pandemic severity[c]	10	7	4	1	n.a.
3.2. *Expected* annual pandemic-related mortality rate (SMU)	1.8	1.26	0.72	0.18	0.93
3.3. *Expected* excess deaths per year [x = (1) × (3.2)]	120,000	370,000	170,000	25,000	680,000
4. *Expected* totals					
4.1. *Expected* mortality rate (SMU)	1.9	1.3	0.76	0.2	0.98
4.2. *Expected* excess deaths per year [x = (2.3) + (3.3)]	125,000	390,000	180,000	28,000	720,000
					(430,000–1,000,000)[a]

Note: n.a. = not applicable. In the "World" column, the rows on pandemic severity are not applicable because this column incorporates all pandemic severities.

a. Very substantial uncertainty adheres to all data in panels 2–4 of this table. We judge that ± 40 percent reasonably reflects this uncertainty. AIR's (AIR Worldwide 2014) mortality estimates for a 1918-type pandemic occurring today are given ± 22 percent, and we have amplified that somewhat (Madhav 2013). Rather than report a ± 40 percent range, this table reports only our point estimates except for our estimate of total annual expected deaths where we state the range.

b. We use the World Bank's income level classification of countries (World Bank 2015).

c. Relative severity indicates severity in each income group relative to the high-income group. This ratio is assumed to be different for each level of severity. Our estimates for severe pandemics come from AIR (Madhav 2013). AIR estimates a narrow range of mortality rates across high-income countries (6–11 SMU) for its model of a 1918-type pandemic, and the relative severities we indicate are consistent with the HIC rates and AIR's estimate of 21 million to 33 million deaths globally in such a pandemic. Evidence for the moderate pandemics of 1957–58 and 1968–69 suggest a more compressed range for these less severe pandemics, and our relative severity numbers in row 2.1 reflect this. Alternative estimates of relative severity in lower-income countries are lower than those for AIR that we use, resulting in a lower estimated global death total.

Next, we place dollar values on the changes in mortality rates. Our specific calculations followed the methods used in Global Health 2035 (Jamison and others 2013). We defined levels of our valuation metric v of 0.7, 1.0, 1.3, and 1.6 percent of income per capita per SMU of mortality increase, that is, per 1/10,000 increase in mortality risk for one year for countries in each of the World Bank's four income groups of countries: 0.7 percent was used for LICs; 1.0 percent for lower-middle-income countries; 1.3 percent for upper-middle-income countries (UMICs); and 1.6 percent for HICs. In calculating the value of change in mortality at age, we used as a reference the literature's value as a fraction of GNI per capita for age 35 years. This amount was adjusted up or down for ages other than 35 years in proportion to the ratio of life expectancies at those ages to life expectancy at age 35 years. Hence, for a given level of overall mortality, the value of mortality loss will depend on which of the age distributions of excess pandemic mortality described is assumed.

RESULTS

Table 18.4 shows the results of our calculation of the value of intrinsic loss from pandemic risk, using values of v of 0.7–1.6 percent of GNI per SMU, depending on income category. We stress that these are expected annual values of loss associated with the indicated risks of pandemics in the severity ranges we have chosen. Expected losses from an actual severe pandemic would be about 60 times as large. The World Bank expresses income loss figures as expected annual values but uses different values for annual pandemic risk.

Table 18.4 shows our estimate of the expected annual loss for the world as a whole from the intrinsic loss from pandemic risk to be -0.6 percent of global income or about US$490 billion per year. Loss varies by income group, from a little over 0.3 percent in HICs to 1.6 percent in lower-middle-income countries.

Although the direct effect of a pandemic on income appears to be significant, we conclude that intrinsic losses

Table 18.4 Value of Mortality Losses from Pandemic Risk, by Country Income Group, 2015 *(age-dependent VSMU)*

Parameter	Income level[a]				
	Low	Lower-middle	Upper-middle	High	World
1. Economic parameters					
1.1 Income, Y (trillions of 2013 US$)	0.7	6.0	20.0	54.0	80.0
1.2 Per person income, y (2013 US$)	780	2,300	8,200	41,000	11,000
1.3 v (%)[b]	0.7	1.0	1.3	1.6	n.a.
2. Losses from pandemic[c]					
2.1 *Expected* annual value of mortality loss, C (billions of 2013 US$)[d]	−7	−100	−200	−180	−490 (−290 to −690)
2.2 Annual mortality loss, c [as % of income = (2.1) ÷ (1.1)]	−1.1	−1.6	−1.0	−0.34	−0.62 (−0.37 to −0.87)

Note: n.a. = not applicable; VSMU = value of a standardized mortality unit. In the "World" column, row 1.3 on pandemic severity is not applicable because this column incorporates all pandemic severities.

a. We use the World Bank's income data and income level classification of countries (World Bank 2015).

b. We use "v" to denote the value of a 1-in-10,000 risk of death, expressed as a percentage of per capita GNI. The dominant position in the literature is that lower-income countries should have lower values for v (Hammitt and Robinson 2011). The literature provides weak quantitative guidance on how v should vary with y, if at all, and the numbers we have chosen should be viewed as reasonable assumptions within the spirit of the literature.

c. Very substantial uncertainty adheres to these cost estimates (see note a, table 18.3). We judge that ± 40 percent reasonably reflects this uncertainty but report that range for our estimates of worldwide costs only.

d. For any given value of s, our calculation of the value of intrinsic loss from a pandemic depends on the age distribution of deaths from the pandemic, and the calculations reported here use different age distributions for pandemics of different severities. In particular, for moderately severe pandemics, we assume an older age distribution of deaths, typical of such pandemics. For severe pandemics, we assume the younger age distribution of deaths that characterized the 1918 pandemic.

far exceed the loss from lost income. We referred to estimates in the literature of the income loss from pandemics of differing levels of severity (Burns, Mensbrugghe, and Timmer 2008; Jonas 2013; McDonald and others 2008; McKibbin and Sidorenko 2006). Though our severity categories differ from theirs, the values of 1 percent of global income from a moderately severe pandemic and 4 percent from a severe pandemic are consistent with estimates in the literature. Using our estimates of the annual probabilities of such pandemics (table 18.2), we find expected annual income losses globally of US$16 billion for moderately severe pandemics and US$64 billion for severe pandemics, for a cost of approximately US$80 billion per year. Table 18.4 shows an expected annual value of mortality loss from pandemics of US$490 billion, of which 95 percent is from severe pandemics. (See annex 18A for further details on research methods.)

DISCUSSION

Expected annual pandemic losses appear substantial. Comparing the loss from pandemic risk with losses from climate change is instructive. As with pandemic risk, much uncertainty is attached both to the magnitude of future climate change and to the possible losses (Moore and Diaz 2015). In contrast to the modest number of studies on potential pandemic loss, there are hundreds of studies on the cost of climate change and the social cost of carbon (Pizer and others 2014; Tol 2013). Global carbon dioxide emissions were on the order of 36,000 million tons in 2013, containing 6,200 million tons of carbon (Global Carbon Project 2015). Estimates of the social cost of carbon vary widely, but if it were around US$120 per ton, then the cost of carbon dioxide emissions in 2013 would be about 1 percent of world income; US$120 per ton is within the range of available estimates (Nordhaus 2010; Tol 2013). One must add the losses from carbon in carbon dioxide to the losses from methane, which are likely to be substantial (Smith and others 2013). The synthesis of the 2014 report of the Intergovernmental Panel on Climate Change (IPCC) assessed the literature and estimated that global economic losses for warming of 2.5°C higher than pre-industrial levels range from 0.2 to 2.0 percent of income (Pachauri and others 2014). In comparison, our expected annual intrinsic loss from pandemic risk (at 0.7 percent of global income) lies 25 percent higher than the low end of the range of the IPCC's estimated range for global warming.

Although most studies of the cost of climate change fail to include the intrinsic loss of increased mortality risk, the effect of doing so may be modest. The IPCC report anticipates increased risks, with very high confidence, of ill health owing to heat waves and fires, undernutrition from diminished food production in poor regions, and increased foodborne and waterborne diseases and some vectorborne and infectious diseases (Pachauri and others 2014). Modest reductions in cold-related mortality and morbidity will be offset by the magnitude and severity of the increased risks. Although the IPCC presents scenarios of health risks, the aggregate effect of climate change on mortality was not summarized. However, the gradual nature of warming allows time for costly adaptations that could be expected to reduce the mortality consequences. A recent paper points to potentially important mortality reductions in the United States resulting from efforts to keep U.S. emissions consistent with global warming of 2°C (Shindell, Lee, and Faluvegi 2016). These benefits appear to flow almost entirely from reduced pollution rather than slower atmospheric warming. Most health losses from climate change are then likely to be included in the income losses from adaptation rather than included separately.

Another useful comparator for pandemic risk lies in deaths from selected alternative causes. The expected annual number of pandemic influenza deaths for 2015 in our reference cases is 720,000 (table 18.3). One might reasonably add 300,000 deaths per year from seasonal influenza to this number for a total of over 1 million deaths (WHO 2016b). In comparison, Mathers (2018) reports new WHO estimates for the diseases of comparable magnitude for 2015 (table 18.5).

Earlier studies have estimated losses from disease that included valuation of mortality consequences. Ozawa and others (2011), for example, estimated the losses from vaccine-preventable diseases, and Watkins and Daskalakis (2015) estimated burdens from rheumatic

Table 18.5 Causes of Death with Magnitude Comparable to Expected Deaths from Pandemic Influenza, 2015

Cause of death	Magnitude of deaths
Tuberculosis	1.4 million
HIV/AIDS	1.1 million
Maternal mortality	0.3 million
Cancers	8.8 million
Ischemic heart disease	7.9 million
Stroke	6.2 million

Source: Mathers 2018.
Note: HIV/AIDS = human immunodeficiency virus/acquired immune deficiency syndrome.

heart disease using methods closely related to ours. Far more studies assess the losses from specific environmental risk factors (OECD 2014).

SENSITIVITY TESTS AND LIMITATIONS

Sensitivity to Assumptions

The methods used to value mortality risk have limitations. The valuation of health risks—including fatalities, illness, and injuries—is inherently difficult because money is often an ineffective substitute for dimensions of human well-being. In practice, however, these estimates are obtained from ex post observations of the labor market and reflect the way people differentially value and trade off very small fatality risks for income. Substantial variation exists both in the estimated value of a small mortality risk at a given age in the United States and in the way the valuation (v) should vary across ages and countries (Hammitt and Robinson 2011; Lindhjem and others 2011). Our calculations to test the sensitivity of our results to this alternative assumption found a change of only about 5 percent in our headline number of US$490 billion.

Hammitt and Robinson (2011) have assembled the evidence that the value of mortality risk as a percentage of income in LICs may be less than for HICs. Global Health 2035 did not include this potential effect in its calculations (Jamison and others 2013). This chapter does include an adjustment for this effect, which leaves estimates of losses in HICs unchanged but reduces our estimated cost for the world as a whole. We assessed the sensitivity of our results to alternative assumptions on this point and others and concluded our main findings to be robust to the specific assumptions made.

Limitations

A key limitation of this study is its use of historical mortality estimates and modeled estimates from various sources to estimate pandemic risk. As we have noted throughout, the estimates we use for pandemic risk, r, and severity, s, remain subject to substantial inherent uncertainty. Although the AIR modeling efforts (Madhav 2013) on which we rely explicitly account for potentially increased risks associated with increased air travel and mobility of persons and goods, as well as increased urbanization, we lacked access to the full results of that study. Similarly, whereas AIR attempted to account for decreased risks associated with increased incomes, schooling, and access to health care services—including vaccination, antiviral medications, improved infection control, increased surveillance, and real-time communications— we could use that information only indirectly.

A modeling effort separate from that by AIR uses similar methods but different assumptions, resulting in a smaller expected annual mortality, although in the same broad range (Madhav and others 2018). In contrast to the robustness of our conclusions with respect to how to value mortality risk, our findings respond sensitively to how we model r and s. Increased global temperature may reduce the case fatality rates of influenza, but it may also increase the transmissibility of the virus. Population-level immunity against a particular influenza strain likely varies by region and by age distribution, although the extent of that variation is not known. In 1918, a few countries did not experience the typical inverted U-shaped distribution of excess age-specific mortality from influenza. In Mexico, elderly persons were not spared from excess mortality in contrast to those in the United States, although its working-age population suffered as significantly as those in other regions. (Chowell and others 2010). In China, mortality rates were low at all ages. The characteristics of new pandemic viral strains depend on poorly understood patterns of immunity and the complex and poorly understood process of viral evolution and genetic re-assortment in dynamic ecosystems (Morens, Folkers, and Fauci 2004).

An additional limitation of this study is its omission of an estimated value of the intrinsic undesirability of non-fatal illness or of pandemic fear—significant characteristics of population response to SARS (severe acute respiratory syndrome) in Taiwan, China (Liu and others 2005). The high media salience and associated fear may also lead populations to overreact to mild pandemics, increasing the effect beyond what might be considered optimal (Brahmbhatt and Dutta 2008). The economics literature currently provides value estimates almost entirely for mortality risk. However, when appropriate valuations of illness and fear become available, our results may be shown to be underestimates for this reason.

A final limitation of this study is its estimation of losses from only pandemic influenza risk. Further work should extend this analysis to at least 11 additional pathogens that the WHO regards as known potential causes of pandemics or epidemics (Brende and others 2017). Including most other known pathogens may increase the risk to about 50 percent over that from influenza alone (personal communication, J. Douglas Fullam).

CONCLUSIONS

World Bank studies estimate approximately 5 percent of global income as the probable income loss from a pandemic as severe as that of 1918. This chapter estimates the value of intrinsic loss from the excess deaths from potential pandemics. Our estimate of the expected number of pandemic deaths per year is 720,000. The expected annual intrinsic cost that results for the world is US$490 billion, or 0.6 percent of global income. In comparison, the IPCC estimates that the likely cost of global warming falls in the range 0.2 to 2.0 percent of global income annually.

Posner (2004) has argued that economics and the social sciences generally fail to pay adequate attention to potentially catastrophic events, although literature is emerging (Barro and Jin 2011; Pike and others 2014; Pindyck and Wang 2013). Concluding that the academic and policy attention provided to pandemic risk falls well short of a sensibly estimated comparison of that risk with its consequences is reasonable. However, recent trends are encouraging. As he prepared to host the G-7 (Group of Seven) in 2016, Japanese Prime Minister Shinzo Abe placed high priority on dealing with health crises (Abe 2015). German Prime Minister Angela Merkel, as host for the meeting of the G-20 (Group of Twenty) in Hamburg in June 2017, maintained this high-level interest by including specific attention to pandemic preparedness. Hosted for the WHO and the World Bank by the U.S. National Academy of Medicine, a recent Commission on a Global Health Risk Framework for the Future pointed to practical and significant financial and organizational steps to improve pandemic preparedness and response (GHRF Commission 2016; Sands and others 2016). Despite these encouraging indicators, Moon and others (2017) have concluded that inadequate action followed the warning from the Ebola virus in West Africa.

In chapter 17 of this volume, Madhav and others (2018) assess the costs and probable effects of investments to reduce the likelihood or potential severity of a pandemic. These investments could range from research and development to a universal influenza vaccine to much-enhanced surveillance to pre-investment in manufacturing capacity for drugs and vaccines (Varney and others 2017). Important investments along these lines are indeed being made. Given this chapter's estimate of the intrinsic expected loss from pandemic risk, the economic benefits of further investments are likely to substantially exceed their cost.

ANNEX

The annex in this chapter is as follows. It is available at http://www.dcp-3.org/DCP.

• Annex 18.A. Materials and Methods

ACKNOWLEDGMENTS

The authors thank Branden Nakamura (University of Hawai'i) and Jennifer Nguyen (Susan G. Komen Foundation) for valuable research assistance. Kristie Ebi (University of Washington) provided guidance to the literature on carbon emission levels and their costs. Julian Jamison and Olga Jonas of the World Bank provided helpful suggestions. The Bill & Melinda Gates Foundation provided partial financial support for this research through grants to the University of California, San Francisco, for the Commission on Investing in Health, Phase 3 and to the University of Washington for the Disease Control Priorities Network.

NOTE

World Bank Income Classifications as of July 2014 are as follows, based on estimates of gross national income (GNI) per capita for 2013:

- Low-income countries (LICs) = US$1,045 or less
- Middle-income countries (MICs) are subdivided:
  (a) lower-middle-income = US$1,046 to US$4,125
  (b) upper-middle-income (UMICs) = US$4,126 to US$12,745
- High-income countries (HICs) = US$12,746 or more.

REFERENCES

Abe, S. 2015. "Japan's Vision for a Peaceful and Healthier World." *The Lancet* 386 (10011): 2367–69.

AIR Worldwide. 2014. "The AIR Pandemic Flu Model." AIR Worldwide, September 3. http://www.air-worldwide.com /Publications/AIR-Currents/2014/The-AIR-Pandemic -Flu-Model/.

Barro, R. J., and T. Jin. 2011. "On the Size Distribution of Macroeconomic Disasters." *Econometrica* 79 (5): 1567–89. doi:10.3982/ECTA8827.

Beveridge, W. I. 1991. "The Chronicle of Influenza Epidemics." *History and Philosophy of the Life Sciences* 13 (2): 223–34.

Brahmbhatt, M., and A. Dutta. 2008. "On SARS Type Economic Effects during Infectious Disease Outbreaks." Policy Research Working Paper 4466, World Bank, Washington, DC. http://dx.doi.org/10.1596/1813-9450-4466.

Brende, B., J. Farrar, D. Gashumba, C. Moedas, T. Mundel, and others. 2017. "CEPI-A New Global R&D Organisation for Epidemic Preparedness and Response." *The Lancet* 389 (10066): 233–35. doi:10.1016/S0140-6736(17)30131-9.

Bruine De Bruin, W., B. Fischhoff, L. Brilliant, and D. Caruso. 2006. "Expert Judgments of Pandemic Influenza Risks." *Global Public Health* 1 (2): 179–94. doi:10.1080/17441690600673940.

Burns, A., D. Mensbrugghe, and H. Timmer. 2008. "Evaluating the Economic Consequences of Avian Influenza." Working Paper 47417, World Bank, Washington, DC. http:// documents.worldbank.org/curated/en/2006/06/10247442 /evaluating-economic-consequences-avian-influenza.

Cheng, K. F., and P. C. Leung. 2007. "What Happened in China during the 1918 Influenza Pandemic?" *International Journal of Infectious Diseases* 11 (4): 360–64. doi:10.1016/j .ijid.2006.07.009.

Chowell, G., C. Viboud, L. Simonsen, M. A. Miller, and R. Acuna-Soto. 2010. "Mortality Patterns Associated with the 1918 Influenza Pandemic in Mexico: Evidence for a Spring Herald Wave and Lack of Preexisting Immunity in Older Populations." *Journal of Infectious Diseases* 202 (4): 567–75. doi:10.1086/654897.

Davis, K. 1968. *The Population of India and Pakistan.* New York: Russell and Russell.

Ghendon, Y. 1994. "Introduction to Pandemic Influenza through History." *European Journal of Epidemiology* 10 (4): 451–53.

GHRF Commission (Commission on a Global Health Risk Framework for the Future). 2016. *The Neglected Dimension of Global Security: A Framework to Counter Infectious Disease Crises.* Washington, DC: National Academies Press. http:// www.nap.edu/catalog/21891/the-neglected-dimension-of -global-security-a-framework-to-counter.

Global Carbon Project. 2015. "Global Carbon Atlas: CO_2 Emissions." http://www.globalcarbonatlas.org/?q=en /emissions.

Hammitt, J. K., and L. A. Robinson. 2011. "The Income Elasticity of the Value per Statistical Life: Transferring Estimates between High and Low Income Populations." *Journal of Benefit-Cost Analysis* 2 (01): 1–29. doi:10.2202 /2152-2812.1009.

Jamison, D. T., and J. Jamison. 2011. "Characterizing the Amount and Speed of Discounting Procedures." *Journal of Benefit-Cost Analysis* 2 (2). doi:10.2202/2152-2812.1031.

Jamison, D. T., L. H. Summers, G. Alleyne, K. J. Arrow, S. Berkley, and others. 2013. "Global Health 2035: A World Converging within a Generation." *The Lancet* 382 (9908): 1898–955. doi:10.1016/S0140-6736(13)62105-4.

Johnson, N. P. A. S., and J. Mueller. 2002. "Updating the Accounts: Global Mortality of the 1918–1920 'Spanish' Influenza Pandemic." *Bulletin of the History of Medicine* 76 (1): 105–15. doi:10.1353/bhm.2002.0022.

Jonas, O. B. 2013. "Pandemic Risk." World Development Report Background Paper, World Bank, Washington, DC. https://openknowledge.worldbank.org/bitstream /handle/10986/16343/WDR14_bp_Pandemic_Risk_Jonas .pdf?sequence=1&isAllowed=y.

Lindhjem, H., S. Navrud, N. A. Braathen, and V. Biausque. 2011. "Valuing Mortality Risk Reductions from Environmental, Transport, and Health Policies: A Global Meta-Analysis of Stated Preference Studies." *Risk Analysis* 31 (9): 1381–407. doi:10.1111/j.1539-6924.2011.01694.x.

Liu, J.-T., J. K. Hammitt, J.-D. Wang, and M.-W. Tsou. 2005. "Valuation of the Risk of SARS in Taiwan." *Health Economics* 14 (1): 83–91. doi:10.1002/hec.911.

Luk, J., P. Gross, and W. W. Thompson. 2001. "Observations on Mortality during the 1918 Influenza Pandemic." *Clinical Infectious Diseases* 33 (8): 1375–78. doi:10.1086/322662.

Madhav, N. 2013. "Modelling a Modern-Day Spanish Flu Pandemic." *AIR Worldwide.* February 21. http://www .air-worldwide.com/publications/air-currents/2013/modeli ng-a-modern-day-spanish-flu-pandemic/.

Madhav, N., B. Oppenheim, M. Gallivan, P. Mulembakani, E. Rubin, and others. 2018. "Pandemics: Risks, Impacts, and Mitigation." In *Disease Control Priorities* (third edition): Volume 9, *Disease Control Priorities: Improving Health and Reducing Poverty,* edited by D. T. Jamison, H. Gelband, S. Horton, P. Jha, R. Laxminarayan, C. N. Mock, and R. Nugent. Washington, DC: World Bank.

Mathers, C., G. Stevens, D. Hogan, A. Mahanani, and J. Ho. 2018. "Global and Regional Causes of Death: Patterns and Trends, 2000–15." In *Disease Control Priorities* (third edition): Volume 9, *Disease Control Priorities: Improving Health and Reducing Poverty,* edited by D. T. Jamison, H. Gelband, S. Horton, P. Jha, R. Laxminarayan, C. N. Mock, and R. Nugent. Washington, DC: World Bank.

McDonald, M., K.-B. Scott, W. J. Edmunds, P. Beutels, and R. D. Smith. 2008. "The Macroeconomic Costs of a Global Influenza Pandemic." Paper presented at the Global Trade Analysis Project 11th Annual Conference on Global Economic Analysis, "Future of Global Economy," Helsinki, June. http://www.gtap.agecon.purdue.edu/resources/download/3828.pdf.

McKibbin, W. J., and A. Sidorenko. 2006. "Global Macroeconomic Consequences of Pandemic Influenza." Lowy Institute for International Policy, Sydney, Australia.

Moon, S., J. Leigh, L. Woskie, F. Checchi, V. Dzau, and others. 2017. "Post-Ebola Reforms: Ample Analysis, Inadequate Action." *British Medical Journal* 356 (January): j280. doi:10.1136/bmj.j280.

Moore, F. C., and D. B. Diaz. 2015. "Temperature Impacts on Economic Growth Warrant Stringent Mitigation Policy." *Nature Climate Change* 5 (2): 127–31. doi:10.1038/nclimate2481.

Morens, D. M., and A. S. Fauci. 2007. "The 1918 Influenza Pandemic: Insights for the 21st Century." *Journal of Infectious Diseases* 195 (7): 1018–28. doi:10.1086/511989.

Morens, D. M., G. K. Folkers, and A. S. Fauci. 2004. "The Challenge of Emerging and Re-Emerging Infectious Diseases." *Nature* 430 (6996): 242–49. doi:10.1038/nature02759.

Morens, D. M., and J. K. Taubenberger. 2011. "Pandemic Influenza: Certain Uncertainties." *Reviews in Medical Virology* 21 (5): 262–84. doi:10.1002/rmv.689.

Murray, C. J. L., A. D. Lopez, B. Chin, D. Feehan, and K. H. Hill. 2006. "Estimation of Potential Global Pandemic Influenza Mortality on the Basis of Vital Registry Data from the 1918–20 Pandemic: A Quantitative Analysis." *The Lancet* 368 (9554): 2211–18. doi:10.1016/S0140-6736(06)69895-4.

Nordhaus, W. D. 2010. "Economic Aspects of Global Warming in a Post-Copenhagen Environment." *Proceedings of the National Academy of Sciences* 107 (26): 11721–26. doi:10.1073/pnas.1005985107.

OECD (Organisation for Economic Co-operation and Development). 2014. *The Cost of Air Pollution: Health Impacts of Raod Pollution.* Paris: OECD. http://www.oecd-ilibrary.org/content/book/9789264210448-en.

Osterholm, M. T. 2005. "Preparing for the Next Pandemic." *New England Journal of Medicine* 352 (18): 1839–42.

Ozawa, S., M. L. Stack, D. M. Bishai, A. Mirelman, I. K. Friberg, and others. 2011. "During the 'Decade Of Vaccines', the Lives of 6.4 Million Children Valued at $231 Billion Could Be Saved." *Health Affairs* 30 (6): 1010–20. doi:10.1377/hlthaff.2011.0381.

Pachauri, R., M. Allen, V. Barros, J. Broome, W. Cramer, and others, eds. 2014. "Climate Change 2014: Synthesis Report. Contribution of Working Groups I, II and II to the Fifth Assessment Report of the Intergovernmental Panel on Climate Change." Intergovernmental Panel on Climate Change, Geneva. http://ar5-syr.ipcc.ch/.

Paules, C. I., and A. S. Fauci. 2017. "Emerging and Reemerging Infectious Diseases: The Dichotomy between Acute Outbreaks and Chronic Endemicity." *Journal of the American Medical Association* 317 (7): 691–92. doi:10.1001/jama.2016.21079.

Pike, J., T. Bogich, S. Elwood, D. C. Finnoff, and P. Daszak. 2014. "Economic Optimization of a Global Strategy to Address the Pandemic Threat." *Proceedings of the National Academy of Sciences of the United States of America* 111 (52): 18519–23. doi:10.1073/pnas.1412661112.

Pindyck, R. S, and N. Wang. 2013. "The Economic and Policy Consequences of Catastrophes." *American Economic Journal: Economic Policy* 5 (4): 306–39. doi:10.1257/pol.5.4.306.

Pizer, W., M. Adler, J. Aldy, D. Anthoff, M. Cropper, and others. 2014. "Using and Improving the Social Cost of Carbon." *Science* 346 (6214): 1189–90.

Posner, R. A. 2004. *Catastrophe: Risk and Response.* Oxford, U.K.: Oxford University Press.

Potter, C. W. 2001. "A History of Influenza." *Journal of Applied Microbiology* 91 (4): 572–79.

Preston, S., P. Heuveline, and M. Guillot. 2000. *Demography: Measuring and Modeling Population Processes.* Malden, MA: Wiley-Blackwell.

Sands, P., A. El Turabi, P. A. Saynisch, and V. J. Dzau. 2016. "Assessment of Economic Vulnerability to Infectious Disease Crises." *The Lancet* 388 (10058): 2443–48. doi:10.1016/S0140-6736(16)30594-3.

Shindell, D. T., Y. Lee, and G. Faluvegi. 2016. "Climate and Health Impacts of US Emissions Reductions Consistent with 2°C." *Nature Climate Change* 6: 503–507. doi:10.1038/nclimate2935.

Simonsen, L., M. J. Clarke, L. B. Schonberger, N. H. Arden, N. J. Cox, and others. 1998. "Pandemic versus Epidemic Influenza Mortality: A Pattern of Changing Age Distribution." *Journal of Infectious Diseases* 178 (1): 53–60.

Smith, K. R., Manish A. Desai, J. V. Rogers, and R. A. Houghton. 2013. "Joint CO_2 and CH_4 Accountability for Global Warming." *Proceedings of the National Academy of Sciences* 110 (31): E2865–74.

Taubenberger, J. K., D. M. Morens, and A. S. Fauci. 2007. "The Next Influenza Pandemic: Can It Be Predicted?" *Journal of the American Medical Association* 297 (18): 2025–27. doi:10.1001/jama.297.18.2025.

Tol, R. S. J. 2013. "Climate Change. CO_2 Abatement." In *Global Problems, Smart Solutions: Costs and Benefits,* edited by B. Lomborg, 186–91. Cambridge, U.K.: Cambridge University Press.

UNPD (United Nations Population Division). 2015. *World Population Prospects, the 2015 Revision—Key Findings and Advance Tables*. New York: United Nations Department of Economic and Social Affairs. http://esa.un.org/unpd/wpp/.

Viscusi, W. K. 2014. "The Value of Individual and Societal Risks to Life and Health." In *Handbooks in Economics:* Vol. 1, *Economics of Risk and Uncertainty,* edited by M. Machina and W. K. Viscusi, 385–452. Amsterdam: North-Holland. http://www.sciencedirect.com/science/article/pii/B9780444536853000076.

Watkins, D. A., and A. Daskalakis. 2015. "The Economic Impact of Rheumatic Heart Disease in Developing Countries." *The Lancet Global Health* 3: S37.

World Bank. 2015. World Development Indicators database. http://data.worldbank.org/products/wdi.

WHO (World Health Organization). 2016a. "Ebola Situation Report—16 March 2016." http://apps.who.int/ebola/current-situation/ebola-situation-report-16-march-2016.

———. 2016b. "Influenza (Seasonal)." Fact Sheet, November, WHO, Geneva. http://www.who.int/mediacentre/factsheets/fs211/en/.

Yamey, G., M. Schäferhoff, O. K. Aars, B. Bloom, D. Carroll, and others. 2017. "Financing of International Collective Action for Epidemic and Pandemic Preparedness." *The Lancet Global Health.* doi:10.1016/S2214-109X(17)30203-6.

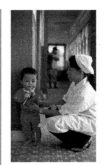

Chapter **19**

Fiscal Instruments for Health in India

Amit Summan, Nicholas Stacey, Karen Hofman, and
Ramanan Laxminarayan

INTRODUCTION

It has been recognized for some time that the primary determinants of population health and health inequalities, particularly in low- and middle-income countries (LMICs), lie outside of the health care system (CSDH 2008). These determinants include individual-level factors—such as access to clean water and sanitation, nutrition, and antenatal care—as well as environmental-level factors—such as pollution, walkability of neighborhoods, rates of open defecation, and tariffs on food imports and exports.

Exposure to these hazardous risk factors is the primary contributor to adverse health outcomes, which increase resource demands on health care systems and increase private and public health expenditures. The impetus for universal health coverage (UHC) in countries as diverse as Brazil, India, and South Africa has run up against the barrier of these broader determinants that hinder efforts to improve health. There are three additional challenges to UHC:

- The economic slowdown has significantly reduced growth rates and government revenues in LMICs. Annual growth rates in Brazil, the Russian Federation, India, China, and South Africa (BRICS) were a population weighted average of nearly two percentage points lower during 2011–15 than during the previous decade (World Bank and IHME 2016). As a result, government expenditures and the ability to increase spending on health care have tightened.

- The narrow fiscal space for health care, even in countries with relatively high growth rates, is a consequence of a low tax base and constrains health care spending by national and state governments. In India, although government health expenditures as a proportion of total government expenditures are comparable to similar countries, they lag when measured as a proportion of gross domestic product (GDP).

- Countries seeking to transition to UHC have weak health care systems that are challenged in delivering quality health care coverage even when additional resources are available. India and South Africa are examples of countries where the health care system serves a fairly small proportion of the population; large segments are excluded from even basic health coverage.

Despite the recognition that social determinants exercise a significant influence on population health in LMICs as direct interventions in the health sector, there remains a limited understanding of how existing fiscal policy instruments available to governments in LMICs can be leveraged to improve health.

This chapter presents the analytic framework for assessing the potential of fiscal instruments to improve population health. We describe the application of this method to specific interventions in India and discuss the implications of these policy changes. The goal is to inform policies at ministries of finance that have an effect on health, either through new

Corresponding author: Ramanan Laxminarayan, Center for Disease Dynamics, Economics and Policy, Washington, DC; ramanan@cddep.org.

policies or by examining existing policies that affect important health risk factors.

ROLE OF FISCAL POLICY INTERVENTIONS

Fiscal measures, including tax and subsidy reforms, offer an appealing complementary opportunity to improve health without reliance on additional budgetary allocations to ministries of health. In India (table 19.1), subsidies for food, fertilizer, and petroleum—three commodities that can have large direct and indirect health impacts—total US$42 billion and together account for twice the direct health expenditures of the roughly US$18 billion spent by the state and central governments on health. Tax and tariff policies are also important and can potentially modify health when applied to commodities that potentially affect health adversely, including alcohol, tobacco, salt, sugar, and trans fats. Current levels of taxes and subsidies for key influencers of health are described in table 19.2.

Fiscal policies can also implicitly influence health and increase public usage of health systems by modifying incentives for treatment of illness, prevention of illness, and promotion of healthy lifestyles. Additionally, fiscal policies can be used to influence the large portion of

Table 19.1 Current National Accounts for India: Combined Revenue and Capital Expenditures and Receipts for Central and State Governments

Item	US$ (Rs 65 = US$1)	GDP (percent)
GDP at current market prices (BE)	2.17 trillion	100.00
Revenue receipts (BE)	437 billion	20.15
Revenue expenditures (BE), including	488 billion	22.51
• Interest payments	67 billion	4.75
• Food subsidy	20 billion	0.92
• Fertilizer subsidy	11 billion	0.52
• Petroleum subsidy	5 billion	0.21
• Health expenditures (includes medical and public health, water supply, sanitation, and family welfare)	21 billion	0.96
• Defense	23 billion	1.07
Total capital expenditures, including loans and advances	95 billion	4.42
Total expenditures (revenue + capital)	583 billion	26.89

Source: Ministry of Finance 2016.
Note: BE = budget estimate; GDP = gross domestic product; Rs = Indian rupees.

Table 19.2 Current Levels of Taxes/Subsidies and Health Risk Factors and Outcomes in India

Commodity	Outcome	Risk factor	Instrument	Level of tax/subsidy in India
Cigarettes[a]	Cancers, heart disease	Smoking, chewing tobacco	Tax	33% plus Rs 2076 per thousand cigarettes (Central Board of Excise and Customs 2017)
Alcohol	Road traffic accidents, cancers, liver disease, STIs	Drunk driving, unsafe sex	Tax	Rates vary by state and product, including prohibition in five states
Condoms	STIs	Unsafe sex	Subsidy	Free condoms for high-risk groups (Ministry of Health and Family Welfare 2016a)
Vaccines	Infectious diseases	Measles, pneumococcal disease, other VPDs	Subsidy	Under Universal Immunization Programme, 10 free vaccines provided against VPDs (Ministry of Health and Family Welfare 2016b)

table continues next page

Table 19.2 Current Levels of Taxes/Subsidies and Health Risk Factors and Outcomes in India **(continued)**

Commodity	Outcome	Risk factor	Instrument	Level of tax/subsidy in India
Essential drugs for infectious disease	HIV, TB, malaria, bacterial infections	Lack of treatment	Subsidy	100% for ARTs (Ministry of Health and Family Welfare 2016c); 100% for TB DOTS (Ministry of Health and Family Welfare 2016d)
TB rapid diagnostics	TB	Lack of TB diagnosis	Subsidy	GeneXpert ceiling price of Rs 2,000 for private clinics receiving reduced pricing (Initiative for Promoting Affordable Quality TB Tests 2013)
Salt	Stroke	Hypertension	Tax	None (Central Board of Excise and Customs 2017)
Sugar-sweetened beverages	Cancer, heart disease, diabetes	Obesity	Tax	40% (Central Board of Excise and Customs 2017)
Trans fats	Heart disease, diabetes	Obesity	Tax	None
Diesel	COPD	Air pollution	Tax	18.6–27% (varies by state)
LPG to substitute for solid cooking fuels	TB, COPD	Air pollution (reduced)	Subsidy	Rs 568 per 14.2 kg cylinder (or Rs 40/kg)

Note: ARTs = antiretroviral therapies; COPD = chronic obstructive pulmonary disease; DOTs = directly observed treatment, short course; HIV = human immunodeficiency virus; kg = kilogram; LPG = liquefied petroleum gas; Rs = Indian rupees; STIs = sexually transmitted diseases; TB = tuberculosis; VPDs = vaccine preventable diseases.
a. Cigarettes not exceeding 65 mm in length.

health prevention expenditures still occurring in the private sector that are not directly paid for or monitored by the government. The government's role can be to encourage uptake of preventive health services using direct subsidy policies that are similar to the production level subsidy for antimalarial artemisinin-combination therapies initiated under the Affordable Medicines Facility-malaria (AMFm) financing mechanism. Fiscal policies are practical alternatives to regulation, particularly in areas where regulation is challenged by the number of actors. For example, subsidies for micronutrient fortification of food commodities may be more effective than compulsory fortification when there are many producers and it is difficult to enforce compliance (Chow, Klein, and Laxminarayan 2010). Fiscal policies can also be more effective than regulation in modifying incentives. For example, a package of regulatory interventions to reduce carbon emissions—efficiency standards for buildings, fuel efficiency standards for vehicles, and a carbon ceiling for energy production—could encourage the substitution of alternative energy sources and reductions in emissions intensity through greater efficiency; however, these regulations would still fail to reduce fuel demand (Parry and others 2014).

ANALYTIC FRAMEWORK

The consumption of commodities such as alcohol, cigarettes, condoms, and vaccines involves external effects that are not taken into consideration by those who consume them. In the case of alcohol and cigarettes, the externalities are negative—consumption of these goods causes secondhand smoke or fires (cigarettes) and drunk driving accidents (alcohol). In the case of condoms and vaccines, the externalities are positive because of reductions in the transmission of infections. Taxes can be levied to facilitate a socially optimal level of consumption of commodities with negative externalities; subsidies can be used for commodities with positive externalities. Paternalistic preferences—where the state's desire to improve societal welfare supersedes the individual's preferences—over health outcomes for other households are a common, although contentious, justification for government intervention. Paternalistic preferences recognize that the social marginal benefit from better health exceeds the private marginal benefit in the case of a positive consumption externality, thereby offsetting the distortion created by the subsidy instrument (Browning 1999.)

However, the optimal tax on a commodity may exceed any amount that might be justified on externality grounds alone if the commodity is a weaker substitute for leisure than the average consumption good; the optimal tax rises further the more inelastic the demand for the taxed commodity (Sandmo 1976).[1] Taxing leisure items—such as tobacco or alcohol—would discourage their use during leisure activities and consequently increase the labor supply. If these taxes offset labor taxes, which distort labor and leisure decisions, they would increase welfare. Therefore, a tax on individual products can increase welfare, but this will further depend on whether tax-neutrality is specified in legislation. Because extra tax revenues could end up funding more public spending rather than other tax reductions, the fiscal rationale for higher taxes may be undermined and would have to be evaluated under alternative possibilities for recycling of the revenues. In previous work, we estimated that the optimal tax on alcohol exceeds the level warranted on externality grounds by between 59 and 126 percent, because of the revenue-raising component of the optimal tax (Parry, Laxminarayan, and West 2009).

To assess the health and economic effects of tax and subsidy interventions in India, we use simple macrosimulation spreadsheet-based simulation models. Taxes reduce consumption of the taxed good (or increase it in the case of a subsidy—a negative tax), which changes exposure to risk factors within the affected populations. We employ statistical parameters called elasticities to estimate the change in consumption caused by changes in prices. We assume full pass-through of the tax to the consumer and zero tax evasion, except for the alcohol tax intervention. We employ a lagged population impact factor, which estimates the proportional reduction in risk from changing risk factor exposure, in conjunction with life tables to

calculate premature deaths averted and years of life gained (YLG). A lag factor is used to incorporate the delay in change in exposure to change in risk and to account for the irreversibility of the effects of some exposures. Incorporating fertility rates and trends in future mortality rates, we project the difference in the number of deaths and YLG over 15 years. We estimate changes in health expenditures (both private and public, except for tuberculosis diagnostic tools subsidies where only private expenditures are estimated) and government receipts. To capture uncertainty, we conduct Monte Carlo simulations with 1,000 iterations at the 95 percent confidence interval on relative risk and elasticity parameters.

The outcomes of taxation will significantly depend on the elasticity of demand. If demand is inelastic, a higher tax will cause only a small fall in demand. Most of the tax will be passed on to consumers. When demand is inelastic, governments will see a significant increase in tax revenue. However, if demand is elastic, the tax will be effective in reducing demand for the commodity, which is helpful in reducing its adverse health impact but may be less effective in raising revenue. Table 19.3 summarizes the evidence on price elasticity of demand for various categories of health-impacting commodities. The next section presents the results of our fiscal policy simulations and complementary policy recommendations.

Table 19.3 Price Elasticity of Demand for Various Commodities That Influence Health

Commodity	Elasticity	Country	Year	Source	Link
Tobacco (bidis)	−0.89	India	1999–2000	John (2008)	http://heapol.oxfordjournals.org/content/23/3/200/T5.expansion.html
Alcohol	−0.9495	India	1999–2000	John (2005)	http://oii.igidr.ac.in:8080/jspui/bitstream/2275/24/1/WP-2005-003.pdf
Condoms	−0.5 to −0.1	Pakistan	1998	Matheny (2004)	http://www.guttmacher.org/pubs/journals/3013404.html
	−0.29 to -2.68	Bangladesh, Haiti, Pakistan	1995	Matheny (2004)	http://www.guttmacher.org/pubs/journals/3013404.html
Vaccines	0 to −1.07 (influenza)	Japan	2001–02 and 2004–05	Kondo, Hoshi, and Okubo (2009)	http://www-ncbi-nlm-nih-gov.ezproxy.bu.edu/pubmed/?term=Does+subsidy+work%3F+Price+elasticity+of+demand+for+influenza+vaccination+among+the+elderly+in+Japan
Essential drugs for treating infectious diseases	−1.9 (Indinavir for HIV)	Morocco	2003	Srivastava and McGuire (2014)	http://www.biomedcentral.com/1471-2458/14/767
	−1.2 (Nevirapine for HIV)	Lebanon, Morocco	2003	Srivastava and McGuire (2014)	http://www.biomedcentral.com/1471-2458/14/768

table continues next page

Table 19.3 Price Elasticity of Demand for Various Commodities That Influence Health **(continued)**

Commodity	Elasticity	Country	Year	Source	Link
	−1.4 (Streptomycin for TB)	Morocco	2003	Srivastava and McGuire (2014)	http://www.biomedcentral.com/1471-2458/14/769
	−1.4 (Benzathine benzylpenicillin)	Morocco	2003	Srivastava and McGuire (2014)	http://www.biomedcentral.com/1471-2458/14/770
	−1.1 to −1.9 (Zidovudine for HIV)	Lebanon, Malaysia	2003	Srivastava and McGuire (2014)	http://www.biomedcentral.com/1471-2458/14/771
	−1.0 to −1.7 (Ceftriaxone)	various countries	2003	Srivastava and McGuire (2014)	http://www.biomedcentral.com/1471-2458/14/772
	−1.0 to −1.6 (Ciprofloxacin)	various countries	2003	Srivastava and McGuire (2014)	http://www.biomedcentral.com/1471-2458/14/773
	−1.5 to −1.2 (Co-trimoxazole)	Syria, Tunisia	2003	Srivastava and McGuire (2014)	http://www.biomedcentral.com/1471-2458/14/774
Sugar-sweetened beverages	−0.94	India	2009/10	Basu and others (2014)	http://www.plosmedicine.org/article/info%3Adoi%2F10.1371%2Fjournal.pmed.1001582
	−1.09	Mexico	1998–99	Barquera and others (2008)	http://jn.nutrition.org/content/138/12/2454.long
	−0.85	Brazil	2005–06	Claro and others (2012)	https://www.ncbi.nlm.nih.gov/pmc/articles/PMC3490548/
Grains (rice)	−0.247	India	1983–2004	Kumar and others (2011)	http://ageconsearch.umn.edu/bitstream/109408/2/1-P-Kumar.pdf
Grains (wheat)	−0.34	India	1983–2004	Kumar and others (2011)	http://ageconsearch.umn.edu/bitstream/109408/2/1-P-Kumar.pdf
Trans fats	−0.48	USA	1938–2007	Andreyeva, Long, and Brownell (2010)	http://www.ncbi.nlm.nih.gov/pmc/articles/PMC2804646/
Palm oil	−1.24	USA	1991/92–2010/11	Kojima, Parcell, and Cain (2014)	http://ageconsearch.umn.edu/bitstream/162472/2/A%20Demand%20Model%20of%20the%20Wholesale%20Vegetable%20Oils%20Market%20in%20the%20U.S.A%20(Revised%20in%20March%202014)%20(1).pdf
Diesel *(long-run value)*	−0.55	Korea. Rep.	1986–2011	Lim and others (2012)	http://www.mdpi.com/1996-1073/5/12/5055
LPG to substitute for solid cooking fuels	−0.92 to −1.05	India	1998–99	Gundimeda and Köhlin (2006)	http://www.eaber.org/node/22501

Note: A price elasticity of demand greater than −1 is considered elastic and less than −1 is considered inelastic. A price elasticity of demand equal to −1 would mean a 1 percent change in price results in a 1 percent change in demand. Inelastic goods tend to have fewer substitutes (gasoline), constitute a small percentage of expenditures (salt), or may be necessary for survival (for example, food). Bidi = a small, thin, hand-rolled cigarette made in Southeast Asian countries. HIV = human immunodeficiency virus; LPG = liquefied petroleum gas; TB = tuberculosis.

FISCAL POLICY ANALYSIS AND RECOMMENDATIONS

We explore both fiscal policies that have been adopted widely and those that have been introduced only recently. These include taxes on alcohol, tobacco, coal, transportation fuels, and sugar-sweetened beverages (SSBs) and subsidies for sugar, cooking fuels, and tuberculosis diagnostic tools. This section discusses the main results of our fiscal policy interventions and presents complementary policy recommendations. In many cases, the success of the tax and subsidy policy can be strengthened by implementing these complementary policies. Results from the models are highlighted in table 19.4.

Table 19.4 Results Summary—Health and Economic Effects of India's Main Fiscal Policies, 2017–2032

Intervention area	Product	Intervention	YLG (thousands)	Discounted YLG (thousands)	Deaths averted (thousands)	Tax revenue gains (US$,ᵃ millions)	Decreased health expenditures (US$, thousands)
Tobacco	Bidi	20% price increase (200% tax increase)	23,082 (13,742–33,131)	17,038 (10,203–24,427)	3,561 (2,020–5,231)	3,998 (3,345–4,521)	87,322 (63,692–114,307)
	Cigarette	50% price increase (90% tax increase)	7,108 (3,695–11,577)	5,410 (2,803–8,846)	851 (449–1,359)	16,200 (11,597–21,081)	40,743 (27,230–53,846)
Alcohol	Country Liquor	20% price increase (170% tax increase)	300 (114–482)	206 (74–339)	35 (13–56)	12,977 (12,303–13,554)	81,002 (60,307–114,769)
	Foreign Liquor	20% price increase (95% tax increase)	76 (−4–170)	58 (−3–130)	9 (−1–20)	24,828 (24,286–25,292)	63,127 (49,538–77,230)
Cooking fuel	LPG	25% of WQ 1 and 2 households receive LPG subsidy	25,839 (2,515–170,956)	67,633 (1,888–127,989)	12,197 (331–23,552)	0	399,548 (149,692–564,000)
Fossil fuels	Diesel	Rs 2.38/liter annual tax increase	86 (46–135)	64 (34–100)	13 (7–21)	268,508 (223,824–308,654)	544 (77–1,430)
	Gasoline	Rs 1.54/liter annual tax increase	26 (12–41)	20 (9–30)	5 (2–7)	146,170 (123,655–166,502)	30 (4–69)
	Coal	Rs 100 annual levy increase over 15 years	419 (216–607)	307 (158–444)	82 (42–118)	164,223 (157,008–171,320)	51,754 (8,153–113,692)
Food	Sugar	Removal of public distribution of sugar subsidy	5,570 (2,380–8,790)	4,331 (1,850–6,835)	437 (174–704)	10,385	27,278 (17,538–40,153)
	SSB Tax	20% price increase (114% tax increase)	267 (109–434)	200 (82–325)	41 (17–68)	74,277 (73,061–75,704)	2,559 (1,692–3,846)
Tuberculosis diagnostic tools	GeneXpert	Replace 1 million sputum smear tests with GeneXpert annually	5,463 (3,610–7,463)	4,131 (2,730–5,642)	704 (464–962)	0	105,287 (−83,384–284,769)

Note: LPG = liquified petroleum gas; Rs = Indian rupees; SSB = sugar-sweetened beverage; WQ = wealth quintile; YLG = years of life gained.
a. US$1 = Rs 65.

Taxation

Taxation of tobacco (cigarettes and bidis [small, thin, hand-rolled cigarettes made in Southeast Asian countries]), alcohol (country liquor and foreign liquor), fossil fuels (diesel, petrol, and coal), and SSBs are discussed in this section.

Tobacco

Tobacco taxation is one of India's most familiar and widely used health-directed fiscal policies. In 2016, roughly 29 percent of Indian adults used tobacco in some form (smoked or smokeless) (Ministry of Health and Family Welfare 2017). Over 900,000 lives are lost prematurely each year from tobacco-related diseases (IHME 2015). The Indian federal government and the states taxed tobacco products, with significant lack of

harmonization in taxes across states until July 2017, when the goods and services tax (GST) harmonized tobacco tax. In recent years, including the increase in tax due to GST implemenation, the real tax increase on cigarettes has been small, and bidi taxes remain significantly lower than levels recommended by the World Health Organization (WHO).

Our simulations focus on increased taxation of smoked tobacco products. Our modeling suggests that increasing the bidi tax by 200 percent could lead to 23.0 (95% confidence interval [CI]: 13.8–33.1) million YLG over 15 years and an increase in government tax revenues by US$3.9 (CI: $3.3–$4.5) billion. Health expenditures can decrease by US$87 (CI: $63–$114) million from the bidi tax increase. Increasing the cigarette tax by 90 percent can lead to 7.1 (CI: 3.6–11.6) million YLG over 15 years and an increase in government tax revenues of $16.2 (CI: $11.6–$21.0) billion. Health expenditures can decrease by US$40.7 (CI: $27.2–$53.8) million. Our estimates of health effects ignore the harms of secondhand smoke, resulting in an underestimation of possible health gains. Additional recommendations presented are directed at creating a more consistent tax structure throughout the country and stepping up the implementation of complementary interventions.

The following additional interventions could further improve health and ensure success of taxation:

- Increase state and union territory National Tobacco Control Programme (NTCP) fund transfers to be used for improved awareness and education campaigns, more effective smoking cessation centers, and greater enforcement of existing laws.
- Link current tobacco taxes to inflation.
- Allocate funds to retrain bidi workers and tobacco farmers.
- Remove tax exemptions for small bidi producers.
- Remove price controls on tendu leaves (a plant native to Asia that is used for making bidis).

Traditional economic theories suggest that as taxes increase, the incentives for smuggling and black market activity increase (Cnossen 2006). Black market activity, by its very nature, is difficult to gauge; for this reason, it is also difficult to measure black market activities that involve tobacco products that are smoked (Blecher and others 2015). However, it is well documented that many countries have successfully implemented high levels of tobacco taxation without drastic increases in black market activity (WHO 2015). In our analysis, we only simulate tax levels consistent with WHO recommendations for tobacco products that are smoked and additionally recommend greater resources for India's NTCP, which follows best practices for curtailing black market activity.

Alcohol

Alcohol taxation is another widely used health-directed fiscal policy. In 2015, alcohol consumption in India was implicated in nearly 360,000 premature deaths (IHME 2015). Alcohol taxes are levied at the state and central government levels and provide as much as 20 percent of state government income except in the states of Bihar, Gujarat, Manipur, Mizoram, and Nagaland, where alcohol is prohibited. Like tobacco, alcohol taxes are complex and inconsistent. Alcohol regulation is further complicated by the presence of a large illicit liquor market; some estimates suggest that up to 50 percent of alcohol

is illicitly produced. Increasing Indian liquor taxation and foreign liquor taxation by 170 percent and 95 percent, respectively, could result in 300,000 (CI: 114,000–482,000) YLG and 76,000 (CI: –4,000–170,000) YLG, respectively, over 15 years. Tax revenues can increase by US$13.0 (CI: $12.3–$13.5) billion from country liquor taxation and by US$24.8 (CI: $24.3–$25.3) billion from foreign liquor taxation, over 15 years.[2] Health expenditures can decrease by US$81 (CI: $60–$114) million from country liquor taxation and by US$63 (CI: $49–$77) million over 15 years from foreign liquor taxation. In our analysis of health effects, we exclude externalities, which would include individuals killed by drunk drivers or alcohol-induced violence against others, resulting in an underestimate of the health effects. These health gains and any excess gains are contingent on strong tax administration and control of illicit liquor production. We make four complementary recommendations:

- Formulate a national strategy on alcohol policy to guide state-level alcohol policy.
- Use alcohol tax revenue for research on alcohol consumption patterns and unrecorded alcohol production.
- Restrict the marketing of alcohol products to youth.
- Earmark alcohol tax revenues for strengthening enforcement to reduce the consumption of illicitly produced liquor.
- Increase funding for alcohol addiction centers.

In the case of alcohol taxation, the presence of a very large illicit market for Indian-made liquor may challenge the success of future tax increases and possibly exacerbate the current illicit liquor problem. Therefore, it is necessary to first ensure that future tax increases do not result in increased illicit liquor production by providing greater monitoring of the alcohol market and increased resources for tax administration.

Fossil Fuels

Fossil fuel taxes—on coal, diesel, and gasoline—are designed to reduce air pollution and its massive deleterious health consequences in India. Ambient particulate matter pollution costs the Indian economy an estimated Rs 3.1 trillion per year, or 0.89 percent of GDP (World Bank 2016). The two major sources of air pollution are emissions from coal-fired power plants and vehicles. An annual increase of Rs 2.38 and Rs 1.54 per liter in the diesel and gasoline taxes over 15 years could result in 86,000 (CI: 46,000–135,000) and 26,000 (CI: 12,000–41,000) YLG respectively, and an increase in aggregate tax revenues of US$414 (CI: $436–$474) billion.

Aggregate health expenditures could decrease by US$574,000 (CI: $81,000–$1,494,000). Complementary recommendations include the following:

- Allocate tax revenues for public transportation investments.
- Implement toll roads or congestion charges.
- Establish new parking fines and enforce current fines.
- Facilitate the adoption of improved emission standards for vehicles.
- Reduce and control fuel adulteration.

Annually increasing the coal levy, which is now largely a means of raising revenue for the National Clean Energy Fund (NCEF), by Rs 100 over 15 years could prevent 82,000 (CI: 42,000–118,000) premature deaths and result in 419,000 (CI: 216,000–607,000) YLG while increasing tax revenues by US$164 (CI: $157–$171) billion over 15 years. Health expenditures could decrease by US$51 (CI: $8–$113) million. We only consider the health effects from changes in coal used for power generation and exclude the 30 percent of coal used for other purposes, resulting in a conservative estimate of the possible health effects. Complementary recommendations for coal taxation are as follows:

- Increase the coal levy revenue allocation to the NCEF.
- Increase transparency in the use of NCEF funds and use them for the intended purposes.
- Prioritize NCEF allocations for improving the grid infrastructure.
- Allocate revenues to increase the efficiency of coal-fired power plants to reduce emissions.
- Allocate coal levy revenues to expand continuous emissions monitoring systems in power plants.

Sugar-Sweetened Beverages

An increase in the tax on SSBs could help to curb the nascent obesity epidemic in India. An SSB tax was first imposed in 2014 and was increased to 21 percent in 2017. This tax had not dampened demand sufficiently, and following India's Committee on Goods and Services Tax's recommendation, the tax was increased to 40 percent under the GST. We found that a tax increase of 114 percent, corresponding to a tax rate of 40 percent, could result in 267,000 (CI: 109,000–434,000) YLG over 15 years and increase tax revenues by US$74 (CI: $73–$76) billion. Health expenditures can decrease by $2.5 (CI: $1.7–$3.8) million. Complementary policies include the following:

- Conduct education and awareness campaigns on healthy diets.
- Label the sugar content of drinks clearly to make nutritional information accessible to consumers.

- Restrict advertisements for sugary beverages.
- Subsidize healthier food options.

Subsidies

The analysis of the remaining health-directed fiscal policies involve subsidies related to sugar, cooking fuels, and tuberculosis diagnostic tools.

Public Distribution Sugar Subsidy

The first policy examined the reduction or elimination of the existing public distribution sugar subsidy. The past sugar subsidy under the public distribution system (PDS) (US$692 million annually) provided sugar subsidies to poor households. This year, the Indian government announced it would not be funding the subsidy and left this option to the states. Recently, however, the government has decided to provide sugar subsidies to only the 25 million poorest families in the country. Historically, inclusion error has resulted in richer households also benefiting from the subsidy. Removal of the subsidy could result in 5.5 (CI: 2.3–8.8) million YLGs over 15 years. Our estimates suggest health expenditures could decrease by US$27.3 (CI: $17.5–$40.1) million. For our analysis, we have considered the effects of the intervention on body mass index (BMI) and added sugar consumption. Although individuals in the the lowest wealth quintile benefited from reduced added sugar consumption, including potential reductions in BMIs, there are concens about the negative health consequences of reduced BMIs. Therefore, we recommend that poorer households receive a replacement subsidy for healthy food products, such as fruits, vegetables, or grains, rather than a sugar subsidy, as the current policy has suggested. Although past PDS subsidies have sometimes failed to target their intended beneficiaries, some states have successfully implemented reforms in recent years that encourage us to suggest greater subsidies that target the poor in lieu of the sugar subsidy. For example, Bihar has been able to decrease leaks (diversion of subsidized food commodities to nonbeneficiaries) from 91 percent in 2004 to 24 percent in 2011, with further improvements in the past few years, by tracking coupon use and better targeting households who would benefit most from a reduced sugar subsidy (Dreze and Khera 2015). Complementary measures to promote healthy diets are similar to those discussed in the SSB tax section.

Cooking Fuel Subsidies

Improved targeting of the cooking fuel subsidy is modeled to estimate the effect of accelerated progress of the current liquefied petroleum gas (LPG) subsidy. The rationale for this government subsidy is to reduce the number of households relying on biomass fuel for indoor cooking, which takes a large toll on cardiovascular and respiratory health. Unfortunately, as implemented, the subsidy has not greatly benefited the target population—households in the lowest income quintile, particularly in rural areas—because of distribution challenges and preferences for biomass cooking. If 25 percent of households currently using biomass switched to LPG next year, the result would be 25.8 (CI: 2.5–170.9) million YLGs over 15 years. Health expenditures would decrease by US$399 (CI: $149–$565) million. To ensure the success of the intervention, it will be critical to invest in education and other behavioral change interventions to increase uptake of the LPG subsidy. Uptake of the LPG subsidy can even be considered a greater challenge than ensuring supply and accessibility, as has been demonstrated in previous studies (Grossman 2012; Hanna, Duflo, and Greenstone 2012). Employing innovative behavior change interventions will help increase demand for LPG cooking.

Tuberculosis Diagnostic Tools

The final intervention is a subsidy for tuberculosis diagnostic tools. India has the highest tuberculosis burden in the world. Progress in controlling tuberculosis has been hindered by poor diagnostic practices, related to long-standing problems in the Indian health care system—mainly in the predominant private sector. A large proportion of the population chooses to use private sector providers, who deliver almost half of India's tuberculosis services, many of which are of poor quality. Decreasing the price of accurate diagnostic technologies (including removing existing import tariffs), particularly for the private sector, and giving private practitioners incentives either to refer tuberculosis cases to the public sector for treatment or to improve their own treatment practices, would raise the overall quality of tuberculosis control. For example, provision of negotiated public sector pricing for more accurate diagnostic tools, such as GeneXpert MTB/RIF (mycobacterium tuberculosis/rifampicin) for India's large private sector can increase demand for these tools. Our modeling suggests that replacing one million sputum smear tests annually with the accurate GeneXpert MTB/RIF test would decrease tuberculosis incidence by 26 (CI: 19–34) per 100,000 people over 15 years and result in 5.4 (CI: 3.6–7.4) million YLGs. Private health expenditures would decrease by US$105 (CI: -$84 –$284) million.[3]

Complementary measures are as follows:

- Enable reduced pricing for all accurate and approved diagnostic tools in the private sector.
- Remove import duties on GeneXpert MTB/RIF.

- Conduct public awareness campaigns on Revised National Tuberculosis Control Program (RNTCP), and publicize tuberculosis prevention and treatment options.
- Engage private health care providers to improve their diagnostic and treatment practices.
- Promote public-private alliances (PPAs), including innovative schemes to incentivize notification and referral of patients to the RNTCP.
- Conduct periodic national surveys of tuberculosis prevalence and treatment practices.

Increased taxes will necessitate increases in tax administration resources. Our modeling results will be realized only if new taxes are actually collected. This may be more of a challenge for some items, such as alcohol, where additional resources must be employed to control illicit liquor production. Our complementary policies suggest some of the ways in which the unintended negative consequences can be mitigated and overall welfare gains maximized. These additional policies include assistance for affected workers and producers as they transition to alternative industries, investments in superior substitutes (in the case of fuels, for example), and strengthening monitoring and enforcement of regulations. Deploying a portion of the tax revenues could fund these policies.

Our analysis provides the lower bounds for the possible effects in three ways:

- We focus only on mortality, excluding morbidity.
- We do not consider externalities, except in the case of fossil fuel.
- We limit our analysis to health effects for older age groups for many of our interventions because of the lack of health risk data for all age groups.

DISCUSSION

Health outcomes are determined by the complex interplay of social, economic, biological, and environmental factors, which can be influenced through fiscal policies. Our report demonstrates that in times of fiscal exigency, taxation and subsidy reform for certain goods may deliver tremendous health gains while actually increasing government receipts. Even though challenged by large fiscal deficits and insufficient outlays for health care, India has great scope to use complementary fiscal policies to improve both population health and fiscal health. The results of the fiscal policy interventions modeled suggest that there are large potential health gains to be made from correcting market failures through tax and subsidy policies.

The gains in health are proportional to the changes in taxes or subsidies modeled, and the tax and subsidy levels we chose to model were determined by a number of factors, including the feasibility of uptake of the policy and the ability to administer and successfully enforce a tax or subsidy level. For tobacco, alcohol, and fossil fuels, theoretically, greater taxation could reduce health burdens by reducing exposure to the taxed product. However, tax officials may not have the resources to ensure the enforcement of a higher level of tax. For example, half of alcohol consumption is currently illicit; very large tax increases can further exacerbate this situation, if greater resources are not devoted to ensure successful implementation of the tax and elimination of potential black market activity.

Other welfare effects need to be considered as well. In the short run, these may include reduced employment; the medium- and long-term effects may be on economic growth through a more productive labor force or through effects on pension systems and health care costs. In the case of fossil fuel taxation, the long-term effects may be on economic growth or the costs of goods. Given the potential unintended consequences of our policies, it is critical that the complementary measures and the complete set of policy recommendations that accompany our tax and subsidy policy recommendations be given as much importance as the tax or subsidy recommendation itself.

Tax and subsidy policies cannot be undertaken in isolation: they require complementary policies to realize the potential health and revenue gains that our modeling results suggest. Two themes that recur in the complementary recommendations across the interventions are (a) education and awareness and (b) monitoring and enforcement of taxes and regulations. Other complementary policies are more specific and focus on minimizing any potential adverse consequences of policies—for example, by using the revenues or savings to invest in counseling and addiction services, alternative energy sources, and public transportation systems. These complementary measures involve revenue recycling into initiatives that may not be the purview of ministries of finance or excise departments. For example, the complementary policy recommendations for tobacco may involve the Ministry of Labour and Employment in retraining bidi workers or the Ministry of Education in conducting tobacco awareness campaigns in schools.

A holistic view of health and its importance needs to be adopted by all sectors of government. Subsidies by one department should not incentivize the use of coal, for example, while another department pushes for a coal levy. Coordination and communication will ensure that polices are consistent across departments. Given the complex and sometimes unanticipated

outcomes of government policies, stakeholder engagement with relevant government departments and affected populations will be crucial in the policy development process.

Limitations

It is important to recognize the limitations of our models. First, the results rely heavily on a few central parameters, such as relative risk and elasticity. We have attempted to employ estimates that would be suitable for the Indian population; however, these estimates, particularly with respect to elasticity, are calculated for certain populations in the past and may not be applicable to the populations in our study. Second, we only consider partial equilibrium effects of fiscal interventions and not the general equilibrium effects arising from the effect of these interventions on deficits, employment, growth, and debt. Third, limitations in data do not allow us to calculate health effects for all age groups, and we exclude calculation of externality costs potentially leading to lower-bound estimates of health outcomes. Finally, our consumption data for many interventions are based on household and individual surveys, which may not capture true consumption patterns, given the effects of recall bias and underreporting.

CONCLUSIONS

Although direct public health expenditures undoubtedly play an integral role in determining population health, health outcomes are determined by the complex interactions of social, economic, biological, and environmental factors. A wide range of viable fiscal policy interventions could modify these proximate factors. These are particularly useful when governments find themselves unable to expand direct health care expenditures. This chapter highlights that in times of fiscal exigency, reforming taxes and subsidies for certain commodities may yield tremendous health gains while increasing government receipts.

NOTES

World Bank Income Classifications as of July 2014 are as follows, based on estimates of gross national income (GNI) per capita for 2013:

- Low-income countries (LICs) = US$1,045 or less
- Middle-income countries (MICs) are subdivided:
  (a) lower-middle-income = US$1,046 to US$4,125
  (b) upper-middle-income (UMICs) = US$4,126 to US$12,745
- High-income countries (HICs) = US$12,746 or more.

1. Recent literature on green tax swaps provides more insight on this finding by decomposing two different links between taxes on products or inputs and the broader fiscal system (for example, Bovenberg and Goulder [2002]; Parry and Oates [2000]). First is the efficiency gain from using new revenue sources to reduce preexisting, distortionary taxes elsewhere in the economy. Second is a counteracting effect, because of the impact of commodity taxes on driving up the general price level, thereby reducing real household wages and slightly reducing the overall level of labor supply. For the average good, the second effect dominates the former, so fiscal considerations warrant setting commodity taxes below (rather than above) marginal external costs. However, the second effect is weaker, and possibly reverses sign, when the commodity in question is a relatively weak substitute (or complement) for leisure. Sgontz (1993) discusses the efficiency gains from recycling alcohol tax revenues in labor tax reductions. However, his partial equilibrium framework excludes impacts on labor supply from the increase in price of alcohol relative to the price of leisure.

2. This assumes 50 percent of country liquor is shifted from licit to illicit consumption, which has the same mortality risks as licit country liquor and does not get taxed.

3. This intervention assumes reduced public sector pricing for GeneXpert for private firms, which the private sectors can operate profitably. Health expenditure estimates assume access to reduced price GeneXpert for diagnosis and a shift from private to public treatment.

REFERENCES

Andreyeva, T., M. W. Long, and K. D. Brownell. 2010. "The Impact of Food Prices on Consumption: A Systematic Review of Research on the Price Elasticity of Demand for Food." *American Journal of Public Health* 100 (2): 216–222. http://doi.org/10.2105/AJPH.2008.151415.

Barquera, S., L. Hernandez-Barrera, M. L. Tolentino, J. Espinosa, S. W. Ng, J. A. Rivera, and B. M. Popkin. 2008. "Energy Intake from Beverages Is Increasing among Mexican Adolescents and Adults." *The Journal of Nutrition* 138 (12): 2454–61. http://doi.org/10.3945/jn.108.092163.

Basu, S., S. Vellakkal, S. Agrawal, D. Stuckler, B. Popkin, and S. Ebrahim. 2014. "Averting Obesity and Type 2 Diabetes in India through Sugar-Sweetened Beverage Taxation: An Economic-Epidemiologic Modeling Study." *PLoS Medicine* 11 (1): e1001582. http://doi.org/10.1371/journal.pmed.1001582.

Blecher, E., A. Liber, H. Ross, and J. Birckmayer. 2015. "Euromonitor Data on the Illicit Trade in Cigarettes." *Tobacco Control* 24 (1): 100–101. http://doi.org/10.1136/tobaccocontrol-2013-051034.

Bovenberg, A. L., and L. H. Goulder. 2002. "Environmental Taxation and Regulation." In *Handbook of Public Economics* (first edition): Volume 3, edited by A. J. Auerbach and M. Feldstein, 1471–1545. Amsterdam: Elsevier.

Browning, E. K. 1999. "The Myth of Fiscal Externalities." *Public Finance Review* 27: 3–18.

Central Board of Excise and Customs. 2017. "GST—Goods and Services Tax." http://www.cbec.gov.in/htdocs-cbec/gst/central-tax-notfns-2017.

Chow, J., E. Y. Klein, E. Y., and R. Laxminarayan. 2010. "Cost-Effectiveness of 'Golden Mustard' for Treating Vitamin A Deficiency in India." *PLoS ONE* 5 (8): e12046. http://doi.org/10.1371/journal.pone.0012046.

Claro, R. M., R. B. Levy, B. M. Popkin, and C. A. Monteiro. 2012. "Sugar-sweetened Beverage Taxes in Brazil." *American Journal of Public Health* 102 (1): 178–83. http://doi.org/10.2105/AJPH.2011.300313.

Cnossen, S. 2006. "Tobacco Taxation in the European Union." *FinanzArchiv/Public Finance Analysis* 62 (2): 305–22.

CSDH (Commission on Social Determinants in Health). 2008. *Closing the Gap in a Generation: Health Equity through Action on the Social Determinants of Health*. Geneva: CSDH.

Dreze, J., and R. Khera. 2015. "Understanding Leakages in the Public Distribution System." *Economic & Political Weekly* 1 (7): 39–42.

Grossman, D. 2012. *J-PAL Policy Briefcase: Up in Smoke*. Cambridge, MA: Abdul Latif Jameel Poverty Action Lab.

Gundimeda, H., and G. Köhlin. 2006. "Fuel Demand Elasticities for Energy and Environmental Policies: Indian Sample Survey Evidence." EABER working paper 9/2006. East Asian Bureau of Economic Research, Canberra. http://www.eaber.org/node/22501.

Hanna, R., E. Duflo, and M. Greenstone. 2012. "Up in Smoke: The Influence of Household Behavior on the Long-Run Impact of Improved Cooking Stoves." Faculty Research Working Paper Series 12–10, Department of Economics, Massachusetts Institute of Technology, Cambridge, MA.

Initiative for Promoting Affordable Quality TB Tests (IPAQT). 2013. "Initiative for Promoting Affordable Quality TB Tests," Slide presentation, IPAQT, New Delhi. http://www.who.int/tb/careproviders/ppm/IPAQT.pdf.

IHME (Institute for Health Metrics and Evaluation). 2015. *GBD Compare*. IHME. http://vizhub.healthdata.org/gbd-compare/patterns.

John, R. M. 2005. "Price Elasticity Estimates for Tobacco and Other Addictive Goods in India." Working Paper 117, eSocial Sciences. http://www.esocialsciences.org/Download/repecDownload.aspx?fname=Document90782282005530.3319818.pdf&fcategory=Articles&AId=117&fref=repec.

———. 2008. "Price Elasticity Estimates for Tobacco Products in India." *Health Policy and Planning* 23 (3): 200–9. http://doi.org/10.1093/heapol/czn007.

Kojima, Y., J. L. Parcell, and J. S. Cain. 2014. "A Demand Model of the Wholesale Vegetable Oils Market in the U.S.A." Paper no. 162472 presented at the Southern Agricultural Economics Association annual meeting, Dallas, TX, February 1–4. http://econpapers.repec.org/paper/agssaea14/162472.htm.

Kondo, M., S. Hoshi, and I. Okubo. 2009. "Does Subsidy Work? Price Elasticity of Demand for Influenza Vaccination among the Elderly in Japan." *Health Policy* 91 (3): 269–76.

Kumar, P., A. Kumar, S. Parappurathu, and S. S. Raju. 2011. "Estimation of Demand Elasticity for Food Commodities in India." *Agricultural Economics Research Review* 24 (June): 1–14. http://www.indianjournals.com/ijor.aspx?target=ijor:aerr&volume=24&issue=1&article=001.

Lim, K.-M., M. Kim, C. Kim, and S.-H. Yoo. 2012. "Short-Run and Long-Run Elasticities of Diesel Demand in Korea." *Energies* 5 (12): 5055–64. http://doi.org/10.3390/en5125055.

Matheny, G. 2004. "Family Planning Programs: Getting the Most for the Money." *International Family Planning Perspectives* 30 (3): 134.

Ministry of Finance, Government of India. 2016a. "Condom Promotion Programme." National Aids Control Organisation, Ministry of Health and Family Welfare, New Dehli. http://naco.gov.in/condom-promotion-programme.

———. 2016b. "Universal Immunization Programme." News release, Press Information Bureau, Ministry of Health and Family Welfare, New Dehli, December. http://pib.nic.in/newsite/PrintRelease.aspx?relid=154779.

———. 2016c. "ART Treatment." National Aids Control Organisation, Ministry of Health and Family Welfare, New Dehli. http://naco.gov.in/treatment.

———. 2016d. TB India 2016: Revised National TB Control Programme Annual Status Report. Ministry of Health and Family Welfare, New Dehli. http://www.tbcindia.nic.in/showfile.php?lid=3180.

———. 2017. *"Global Adult Tobacco Survey: GATS-2 India 2016–17 Highlights."* New Delhi: World Health Organization. http://www.searo.who.int/india/mediacentre/events/2017/gats2_india.pdf?ua=1.

Parry, I. W. H., D. Heine, E. Lis, and S. Li. 2014. *Getting Energy Prices Right: From Principles to Practice.* Washington, DC: International Monetary Fund.

Parry, I. W. H., R. Laxminarayan, and S. E. West. (2006) 2009. "Fiscal and Externality Rationales for Alcohol Taxes." Discussion paper, Resources for the Future, Washington, DC. http://www.rff.org/files/sharepoint/WorkImages/Download/RFF-DP-06-51-REV.pdf.

Parry, I. W. H., and W. E. Oates. 2000. "Policy Analysis in the Presence of Distorting Taxes." *Journal of Policy Analysis and Management* 19 (4): 603–13. http://doi.org/10.1002/1520-6688(200023)19:4<603::AID-PAM5>3.0.CO;2-3.

Sandmo, A. 1976. "Optimal Taxation." *Journal of Public Economics* 6: 37–54.

Sgontz, L. 1993. "Optimal Taxation: The Mix of Alcohol and Other Taxes." *Public Finance Review* 21 (3): 260–75.

Srivastava, D., and A. McGuire. 2014. "Analysis of Prices Paid by Low-Income Countries: How Price Sensitive Is Government Demand for Medicines?" *BMC Public Health* 14 (1): 767. http://doi.org/10.1186/1471-2458-14-767.

WHO (World Health Organization). 2015. *WHO Report on the Global Tobacco Epidemic, 2015: Raising Taxes on Tobacco*, 103. Geneva: WHO.

World Bank and IHME (Institute for Health Metrics and Evaluation). 2016. *The Cost of Air Pollution: Strengthening the Economic Case for Action.* Washington, DC: World Bank. http://documents.worldbank.org/curated/en/781521473177013155/pdf/108141-REVISED-Cost-of-PollutionWebCORRECTEDfile.pdf.

World Bank. 2016. *World Bank Development Indicators.* Washington, DC: World Bank. http://data.worldbank.org/products/wdi.

DCP3 Series Acknowledgments

Disease Control Priorities, third edition *(DCP3)* draws on the global health knowledge of institutions and experts from around the world, a task that required the efforts of over 500 individuals, including volume editors, chapter authors, peer reviewers, and research and staff assistants. The finalization of this series would not have been possible without the intellectual vision, enduring support, and invaluable contributions of these individuals.

We owe gratitude to the financial sponsor of this effort: the Bill & Melinda Gates Foundation. The Foundation provided sole financial support of the Disease Control Priorities Network (DCPN), of which *DCP3* is a main product. Many thanks to Program Officers Kathy Cahill, Philip Setel, Carol Medlin, Damian Walker, and (currently) David Wilson for their thoughtful interactions, guidance, and encouragement over the life of the project. We also thank program assistants Karolyne Carloss and Christine VanderWerf at the Foundation for working tirelessly to organize and execute several critical review meetings.

We are grateful to the University of Washington's Department of Global Health—and to successive chairs King Holmes and Judy Wasserheit—for creating a home base for the *DCP3* Secretariat, a base that provided intellectual collaboration, logistical coordination, and administrative support. We thank those who worked behind the scenes within the department to ensure this grant ran smoothly, including Athena Galdonez, Meghan Herman, Aimy Pham, and Ann Van Haney.

We are tremendously appreciative of the wisdom and guidance provided by the 36 members of the *DCP3* Advisory Committee to the Editors (ACE). Steered by Chair Anne Mills, the committee provided keen oversight and guidance on the scope and development of *DCP3* through chapter and document review, collaborative discussion, and yearly in-person meetings. They have ensured quality and intellectual rigor at the highest order and have helped maximize the impact and usefulness of *DCP3*. The ACE members are listed separately in this volume.

The U.S. National Academy of Medicine, in collaboration with the InterAcademy Medical Panel, coordinated the peer review process for *DCP3* chapters. Patrick Kelley, Gillian Buckley, Megan Ginivan, Rachel Pittluck, and Tara Mainero managed this effort and provided critical and substantive input.

The World Bank provided exceptional guidance and support throughout the demanding production and design process. Within the World Bank, Carlos Rossel and Mary Fisk oversaw the editing and publication of the series and served as champions of *DCP3*. We also thank Nancy Lammers, Rumit Pancholi, Deborah Naylor, Elizabeth Forsyth, and Sherrie Brown for their diligence and expertise. Additionally, we thank Jose de Buerba, Mario Trubiano, Yulia Ivanova, and Chiamaka Osuagwu of the World Bank for providing professional counsel on communications and marketing strategies.

We thank the many contractors and consultants who provided support to specific volumes in the form of economic analytical work, volume coordination, and chapter drafting: the Center for Disease Dynamics, Economics & Policy; Centre for Global Health Research; Emory University; Evidence to Policy Initiative; Harvard T. H. Chan School of Public Health; Public Health Foundation of India; QURE Healthcare; University of California, San Francisco; University of Waterloo; University of Queensland; and the World Health Organization.

We are grateful for the efforts of several institutions that contributed to the organization and execution of key consultation meetings and conferences that were convened as part of the preparation of this series. These institutions include the International Health Economics Association; National Cancer Institute; Pan American Health Organization; University of California, Berkeley School of Public Health; and the World Health Organization's Eastern Mediterranean Regional Office.

Formulation of the main messages of this volume benefited from a Policy Forum convened in London, September 16, 2016, jointly by DCP and EMRO under the leadership of Regional Director Emeritus Dr. Ala Alwan. We are grateful to the participants in that Forum, whose names are listed elsewhere in this volume.

Finally, we thank the individuals who served as members of the *DCP3* Secretariat over the life of the project. In particular, we thank Carol Levin, who provided indispensable inputs into our cost and cost-effectiveness analyses. Stéphane Verguet added valuable guidance in applying and improving the extended cost-effectiveness analysis method. Elizabeth Brouwer, Nazila Dabestani, Shane Murphy, Zachary Olson, Jinyuan Qi, David A. Watkins, and Daphne Wu provided exceptional research and analytic assistance, and often served as chapter authors. Kristen Danforth provided crucial guidance on strategic organization and implementation. Brianne Adderley served ably as Project Manager since the beginning. We owe her a very particular thanks. Jennifer Nguyen, Shamelle Richards, Jennifer Grasso, Sheri Sepanlou, and Tiffany Wilk contributed exceptional project coordination support. The efforts of these individuals were absolutely critical to producing this series, and we are thankful for their commitment.

Volume Editors

Dean T. Jamison

Dean T. Jamison is Emeritus Professor in Global Health Sciences at the University of California, San Francisco, and the University of Washington. He previously held academic appointments at Harvard University and the University of California, Los Angeles. Prior to his academic career, he was an economist on the staff of the World Bank, where he was lead author of the World Bank's *World Development Report 1993: Investing in Health*. He serves as lead editor for *DCP3* and was lead editor for the previous two editions. He holds a PhD in economics from Harvard University and is an elected member of the Institute of Medicine of the U.S. National Academy of Sciences. He recently served as Co-Chair and Study Director of *The Lancet's* Commission on Investing in Health.

Hellen Gelband

Hellen Gelband is an independent global health policy expert. Her work spans infectious disease, particularly malaria and antibiotic resistance, and noncommunicable disease policy, mainly in low- and middle-income countries. She has conducted policy studies at Resources for the Future, the Center for Disease Dynamics, Economics & Policy, the (former) Congressional Office of Technology Assessment, the Institute of Medicine of the U.S. National Academies, and a number of international organizations.

Susan Horton

Susan Horton is Professor at the University of Waterloo and holds the Centre for International Governance Innovation (CIGI) Chair in Global Health Economics in the Balsillie School of International Affairs there. She has consulted for the World Bank, the Asian Development Bank, several United Nations agencies, and the International Development Research Centre, among others, in work conducted in over 20 low- and middle-income countries. She led the work on nutrition for the Copenhagen Consensus in 2008, when micronutrients were ranked as the top development priority. She has served as associate provost of graduate studies at the University of Waterloo, vice-president academic at Wilfrid Laurier University in Waterloo, and interim dean at the University of Toronto at Scarborough.

Prabhat Jha

Prabhat Jha is the founding director of the Centre for Global Health Research at St. Michael's Hospital. He holds Endowed and Canada Research Chairs in Global Health in the Dalla Lana School of Public Health at the University of Toronto. He is lead investigator of the Million Death Study in India, which quantifies the cause of death and key risk factors in over two million homes over a 14-year period. He is also Scientific Director of the Statistical Alliance for Vital Events, which aims to expand reliable measurement of causes of death worldwide. His research includes the epidemiology and economics of tobacco control worldwide.

Ramanan Laxminarayan

Ramanan Laxminarayan is Director of the Center for Disease Dynamics, Economics & Policy in Washington, DC. His research deals with the integration of epidemiological models of infectious diseases and drug resistance into the economic analysis of public health problems.

He was one of the key architects of the Affordable Medicines Facility–malaria, a novel financing mechanism to improve access and delay resistance to antimalarial drugs. In 2012, he created the Immunization Technical Support Unit in India, which has been credited with improving immunization coverage in the country. He teaches at Princeton University.

Charles N. Mock

Charles N. Mock, MD, PhD, FACS, has training as both a trauma surgeon and an epidemiologist. He worked as a surgeon in Ghana for four years, including at a rural hospital (Berekum) and at the Kwame Nkrumah University of Science and Technology (Kumasi). In 2005–07, he served as Director of the University of Washington's Harborview Injury Prevention and Research Center. He worked at the WHO headquarters in Geneva from 2007 to 2010, where he was responsible for developing the WHO's trauma care activities. In 2010, he returned to his position as Professor of Surgery (with joint appointments as Professor of Epidemiology and Professor of Global Health) at the University of Washington.

His main interests include the spectrum of injury control, especially as it pertains to low- and middle-income countries: surveillance, injury prevention, prehospital care, and hospital-based trauma care. He was President of the International Association for Trauma Surgery and Intensive Care from 2013–15.

Rachel Nugent

Rachel Nugent is Vice President for Global Noncommunicable Diseases at RTI International. She was formerly a Research Associate Professor and Principal Investigator of DCPN in the Department of Global Health at the University of Washington. Previously, she served as Deputy Director of Global Health at the Center for Global Development, Director of Health and Economics at the Population Reference Bureau, Program Director of Health and Economics Programs at the Fogarty International Center of the National Institutes of Health, and senior economist at the Food and Agriculture Organization of the United Nations. From 1991–97, she was associate professor and department chair in economics at Pacific Lutheran University.

Contributors

Olusoji Adeyi
World Bank, Washington, DC

Zipporah Ali
Kenya Hospices and Palliative Care Association,
Nairobi, Kenya

Silvia Allende
Instituto Nacional de Cancerologia,
Mexico City, Mexico

Ala Alwan
Department of Global Health, University of Washington,
Seattle, Washington, United States

Shuchi Anand
Department of Medicine, Stanford University,
Palo Alto, California, United States

Hector Arreola-Ornelas
Fundación Mexicana para la Salud, Mexico City,
Mexico

Rifat Atun
Harvard T. H. Chan School of Public Health, Boston,
Massachusetts, United States

Eran Bendavid
Stanford University School of Medicine, Palo Alto,
California, United States

Stefano Bertozzi
University of California, Berkeley, School of Public
Health, Berkeley, California, United States

Melanie Y. Bertram
World Health Organization, Geneva,
Switzerland

Afsan Bhadelia
Harvard T. H. Chan School of Public Health, Boston,
Massachusetts, United States

Zulfiqar Bhutta
Aga Khan University Hospital, Division of Women and
Child Health, Karachi, Pakistan

Agnes Binagwaho
Former Minister of Health, Kigali, Rwanda

David Bishai
Johns Hopkins University Bloomberg School of Public
Health, Baltimore, Maryland, United States

Robert E. Black
Johns Hopkins University Bloomberg School of Public
Health, Baltimore, Maryland, United States

Mark Blecher
South Africa Treasury Department, Cape Town,
South Africa

Barry R. Bloom
Harvard T. H. Chan School of Public Health, Boston,
Massachusetts, United States

Edward Broughton
USAID, Washington DC, United States

Elizabeth Brouwer
University of Washington, Seattle, Washignton,
United States

Donald A. P. Bundy
Bill & Melinda Gates Foundation, London,
United Kingdom

Angela Y. Chang
Harvard T. H. Chan School of Public Health, Boston, Massachusetts, United States

Dan Chisholm
Department of Health System Financing, World Health Organization, Geneva, Switzerland

Annie Chu
Regional Office for the Western Pacific, World Health Organization, Manila, Philippines

Alarcos Cieza
World Health Organization, Geneva, Switzerland

Stephen Connor
National Palliative Care Research Center, Washington, DC, United States

Mark Cullen
Stanford University School of Medicine, Palo Alto, California, United States

Kristen Danforth
Department of Global Health, University of Washington, Seattle, Washington, United States

Liliana De Lima
International Association for Hospice and Palliative Care, Houston, Texas, United States

Nilanthi de Silva
University of Kelaniya, Colombo, Sri Lanka

Haile T. Debas
Global Health Institute, University of California, San Francisco, San Francisco, California, United States

Peter Donkor
Kwame Nkrumah University of Science and Technology, Kumasi, Ghana

Tarun Dua
Department of Mental Health and Substance Abuse, World Health Organization, Geneva, Switzerland

Beverley Essue
University of Sydney Medical School, Sydney, Australia

Victoria Y. Fan
Myron B. Thompson School of Social Work, University of Hawai'i at Mānoa, Honolulu, Hawaii, United States

Xiagming Fang
Department of Applied Economics, China Agricultural University, Beijing, China

John Flanigan
African Strategies for Advancing Pathology, Baltimore, Maryland, United States

Kenneth A. Fleming
Center for Global Health, National Cancer Institute, Bethesda, Maryland, United States

Mark Gallivan
Metabiota, San Francisco, California, United States

Patricia Garcia
Minister of Health, Lima, Peru

Atul Gawande
Brigham and Women's Hospital, Boston, Massachusetts, United States

Thomas Gaziano
Harvard Medical School, Boston, Massachusetts, United States

Abdul Ghaffar
The Alliance for Health Policy and Systems Research, Geneva, Switzerland

Roger Glass
Forgarty International Center, National Institutes of Health, Bethesda, Maryland, United States

Amanda Glassman
Center for Global Development, Washington, DC, United States

Eduardo González-Pier
Center for Global Development, Washington, DC, Untied States

Glenda Gray
Chris Hani Baragwanath Hospital, Johannesburg, South Africa

Brian Greenwood
London School of Hygiene & Tropical Medicine, London, United Kingdom

Liz Gwyther
University of Cape Town School of Public Health and Family Medicine, Cape Town, South Africa

Demissie Habte
International Clinical Epidemiological Network, Addis Ababa, Ethiopia

Ednin Hamzah
Chief Executive, Hospice Malaysia, Kuala Lampur, Malaysia

Jessica Ho
Department of Information, Evidence, and Research, World Health Organization, Geneva, Switzerland

Karen Hofman
University of Witwatersrand School of Public Health, Johannesburg, South Africa

Dan Hogan
Department of Health Statistics and Information Systems, World Health Organization, Geneva, Switzerland

King K. Holmes
Department of Global Health, University of Washington, Seattle, Washington, United States

Guy Hutton
WASH Section, United Nations Children's Fund, New York, New York, United States

Stephen Jan
The George Institute for Global Health, Sydney, Australia

Quach Thanh Khanh
The Institute for Palliative Medicine, San Diego, California, United States

Felicia Knaul
University of Miami, Institute for Advanced Study of the Americas, Miami, Florida, United States

Olive Kobusingye
Makerere University Medical School, Kampala, Uganda

Eric L. Krakauer
Massachusetts General Hospital, Boston, Massachusetts, United States

Margaret E. Kruk
Harvard T. H. Chan School of Public Health, Boston, Massachusetts, United States

Suresh Kumar
Institute of Palliative Medicine, Kerala, India

Modupe Kuti
University of Ibadan, College of Medicine, Ibadan, Nigeria

Xiaoxiao Kwete
Harvard T. H. Chan School of Public Health, Boston, Massachusetts, United States

Tracey Laba
University of Sydney Medical School, Sydney, Australia

Peter Lachmann
University of Cambridge, Cambridge, United Kingdom

Nestor Lago
University of Buenos Aires, Department of Pathology, Buenos Aires, Argentina

Carol Levin
University of Washington, Department of Global Health, Seattle, Washington, United States

Lai Meng Looi
University of Malaya, Kuala Lumpur, Malaysia

Emmanuel Luyirika
African Palliative Care Association, Kampala, Uganda

Nita Madhav
Metabiota, San Francisco, California, United States

Annet Mahanani
Department of Information, Evidence, and Research, World Health Organization, Geneva, Switzerland

Adel Mahmoud
Woodrow Wilson School of Public and International Affairs, Princeton University, Princeton, New Jersey, United States

Elaine Marks
Blindness and Deafness Prevention, Disability and Rehabilitation Unit, World Health Organization, Geneva, Switzerland

Colin Mathers
Department of Information, Evidence, and Research, World Health Organization, Geneva, Switzerland

Jean-Claude Mbanya
Faculty of Medicine, University of Yaoundé I, Yaoundé, Cameroon

Anthony R. Measham
World Bank (retired)

Maria Elena Medina-Mora
National Institute of Psychiatry Ramón de la Fuente Muñiz, Mexico City, Mexico

Carol Medlin
Independent Consultant

Oscar Mendez
Fundación Mexicana para la Salud, Mexico City, Mexico

Anne Merriman
Hospice Africa, Kampala, Uganda

Anne Mills
London School of Hygiene & Tropical Medicine, London, United Kingdom

Jody-Anne Mills
World Health Organization, Geneva, Switzerland

Hoang Van Minh
Hanoi University of Public Health, Center for Population Health Sciences, Hanoi, Vietnam

Jaime Montoya
Philippine Council for Health Research and Development, Taguig City, the Philippines

Egide Mpanumusingo
Butaro Hospital, Burera, Rwanda

Prime Mulembakani
Metabiota, Democratic Republic of the Congo

Mahendra Naidoo
National Cancer Institute Center for Global Health, Bethesda, Maryland, United States

Diana Nevzrova
Russian Health Ministry, Moscow, Russia

Liu Peilong
Global Health Department, Peking University, Beijing, China

Thi Kim Phoung Nguyen
World Health Organization, Hanoi, Vietnam

Ole Frithjof Norheim
University of Bergen Department of Global Public Health and Primary Care, Bergen, Norway

Christian Ntizimira
Kibagabaga Hospital, Kigali, Rwanda

Osondu Ogbuoji
Harvard T. H. Chan School of Public Health, Boston, Massachusetts, United States

Zachary Olson
University of California, Berkeley, School of Public Health, Berkeley, California, United States

Folashade Omokhodion
University College Hospital, Ibadan, Nigeria

Ben Oppenheim
Metabiota, San Francisco, California, United States

Toby Ord
University of Oxford, Oxford, United Kingdom

Hibah Osman
Lebanese Center for Palliative Care, Beirut, Lebanon

Trygve Ottersen
University of Oslo, Department of Community Medicine and Global Health, Oslo, Norway

Nancy Padian
University of California, Berkeley School of Public Health, Berkeley, California, United States

Vikram Patel
London School of Hygiene & Tropical Medicine, London, United Kingdom

George C. Patton
Murdoch Children's Research Institute, Melbourne, Australia

John Peabody
QURE Healthcare, San Francisco, California, United States

Pedro Perez-Cruz
Departamento de Medicina Interna, Facultad de Medicina, Pontificia Universidad Católica de Chile, Santiago, Chile

Dorairaj Prabhakaran
Public Health Foundation of India, New Delhi, India

Christopher Price
Tallahassee Memorial HealthCare, Tallahassee, Florida, United States

Jinyuan Qi
Office of Population Research, Princeton University, Princeton, New Jersey, United States

Lukas Radbruch
Malteser International, Cologne, Germany

M. R. Rajagopal
International Association for Hospice and Palliative Care, New Delhi, India

Teri A. Reynolds
World Health Organization, Geneva, Switzerland

Natalia Rodriguez
Research Support for Global Health, University of Miami, Miami, Florida, United States

John-Arne Rottingen
The Research Council of Norway, Oslo, Norway

Kun Ru
Allegheny General Hospital, Pittsburgh, Pennsylvania, United States

Sevket Ruacan
Koc University School of Medicine, Istanbul, Turkey

Andres Rubiano
Ashoka Colombia, Neiva, Colombia

Edward Rubin
Metabiota, San Francisco, California, United States

Rengaswamy Sankaranarayanan
International Agency for Research on Cancer, Lyon, France

Hendry Sawe
Muhimbili University of Health and Allied Sciences, Emergency Medicine Department, Dar es Salaam, Tanzania

Helen Saxenian
World Bank (retired), Washington, DC, United States

Marco Schäferhoff
SEEK Development, Berlin, Germany

Jaime Sepulveda
Global Health Sciences, University of California, San Francisco, San Francisco, California, United States

Melissa Sherry
Johns Hopkins Bloomberg School of Public Health, Baltimore, Maryland, United States

Riti Shimkhada
Center for Health Policy Research, University of California Los Angeles, Los Angeles, California, United States

Sang Do Shin
Seoul National University College of Medicine, Department of Emergency Medicine, Seoul, Republic of Korea

Richard Skolnik
Retired, Albuquerque, New Mexico, United States

Kirk R. Smith
University of California, Berkeley, School of Public Health, Berkeley, California, United States

Agnes Soucat
World Health Organization, Geneva, Switzerland

Dingle Spence
Hope Institute Hospital, Kingston, Jamaica

Nicholas Stacey
University of the Witwatersrand, Johannesburg, South Africa

Gretchen Stevens
Department of Health Statistics and Information Services, World Health Organization, Geneva, Switzerland

Mark Stoltenberg
Division of Palliative Care and Geriatric Medicine, Massachusetts General Hospital, Massachusetts, United States

Amit Summan
Center for Disease Dynamics, Economics, & Policy, New Delhi, India

Lawrence H. Summers
Harvard Kennedy School, Cambridge, Massachusetts, United States

Neo Tapela
Brigham and Women's Hospital, Boston, Massachusetts, United States

Marleen Temmerman
Aga Khan University East Africa, Nairobi, Kenya

Stephen Tollman
University of Witwatersrand, Johannesburg, South Africa

Stéphane Verguet
Harvard T. H. Chan School of Public Health, Boston, Massachusetts, United States

Damian Walker
Bill & Melinda Gates Foundation, Seattle, Washington, United States

Neff Walker
Bloomberg School of Public Health, Johns Hopkins University, Baltimore, Maryland, United States

Huihui Wang
Senior Economist, World Bank Group, Washington DC, United States

Jianxiang Wang
Institute for Hematology, Chinese Academy of Medical Sciences, Beijing, China

Lee Wallis
University of Cape Town, Cape Town, South Africa

David A. Watkins
University of Washington School of Medicine, Seattle, Washington, United States

David Wilson
Bill & Melinda Gates Foundation, Seattle, Washington, United States

Michael Wilson
University of Colorado, Department of Pathology, Aurora, Colorado, United States

Nathan Wolfe
Metabiota, San Francisco, California,
United States

Yangfeng Wu
The George Institute, Beijing,
China

Gavin Yamey
Duke Global Health Institute, Durham, North Carolina,
United States

Kun Zhao
China National Health Development Research Center,
Beijing, China

Advisory Committee to the Editors

Reviewers

Jishnu Das
Development Research Group, World Bank,
New Delhi, India

Joseph L. Dieleman
Institute for Health Metrics and Evaluation, Seattle,
Washington, United States

Bernard Franck
World Education, Inc., Vientiane, Lao People's
Democratic Republic

Heike Geduld
African Federation for Emergency Medicine,
Cape Town, South Africa

Peter Heller
International Monetary Fund, Washington, DC,
United States

Peter Neumann
Center for the Evaluation of Value and Risk in Health
at the Institute for Clinical Research and Health
Policy Studies, Tufts Medical Center, Boston,
Massachusetts, United States

Zachary Olson
Berkeley School of Public Health, University of
California, Berkeley, Berkeley, California,
United States

Gayatri Palat
MNJ Institute of Oncology and Regional Cancer
Center, Hyderbad, India

Anna Vassall
London School of Hygiene and Tropical Medicine,
London, United Kingdom

Ron Waldman
Milken Institute School of Public Health, George
Washington University, Washington, DC,
United States

Policy Forum Participants

The following individuals provided valuable insights to improve this volume's key findings through participation in the Disease Control Priorities–World Health Organization, Regional Office for the Eastern Mediterranean policy forum on developing a universal health coverage package of high priority interventions. The forum was held in London, United Kingdom, on September 16, 2016, and was organized by Dr. Ala Alwan, Regional Director and member of the DCP3 Advisory Committee to the Editors.

Shaikh Dr Mohamed Bin Abdulla Al Khalifa
Chairman, Supreme Council of Health,
Manama, Bahrain

Ahmed Mohamed Al-Saidi
Minister of Health, Muscat, Oman

Mohammed Al-Thani
Director, Department of Public Health, Ministry of Public Health, Doha, Qatar

Fawzi Amin
Secretary General, Bahrain Red Crescent Society;
Formerly Director General of Primary Health Care,
Ministry of Health, Manama, Bahrain

Walid Ammar
Director General, Ministry of Public Health,
Beirut, Lebanon

Aysha Mubarak Buaneq
Undersecretary, Ministry of Health, Manama, Bahrain

Rassoul Dinarvand
Deputy Minister of Health and President, Iran Food and Drug Administration, Ministry of Health, Tehran, Islamic Republic of Iran

Ferozuddin Feroz
Minister of Public Health, Ministry of Public Health,
Kabul, Afghanistan

Assad Hafeez
Director General of Health,
Ministry of National Health Services,
Regulations and Coordination,
Islamabad, Pakistan

Ziad Memish
Professor, College of Medicine, Alfaisal University,
Riyadh, Saudi Arabia

Keshav Desiraju
Former Secretary of Health, Government of India,
New Delhi, India

Raj Shankar Ghosh
Deputy Director, Vaccine Delivery and Infectious
Disease, Bill & Melinda Gates Foundation,
New Delhi, India

Soonman Kwon
Chief, Health Sector Group, Asian Development Bank,
Manila, the Philippines

Index

Boxes, figures, maps, notes, and tables are indicated by b, f, m, n, and t following the page number.

B

Bangladesh
    burden of disease in, 133–34
    fiscal policy in, 362
    pandemics in, 329
    pathology services in, 228
BCA. *See* benefit-cost analysis
Bell, D., 204
Beltran-Sanchez, H., 98
Bendavid, Eran, 299
benefit-cost analysis (BCA), 10, 167–81, 169–73*t*
    cancer interventions, 179
    child health and mortality interventions,
        167, 179, 181
    communicable disease interventions, 168, 172–73
    drugs, 171, 173
    essential packages of care, 179–80
    extended cost-effectiveness analysis and, 157
    life expectancy and, 169, 171–75, 177, 181
    malaria interventions, 169, 172, 179
    morbidity and, 168–69, 174, 178
    neglected tropical disease interventions, 169, 171
    pandemic interventions, 168, 171
    policy interventions, 168, 178, 181
    role of, 167–68
    tuberculosis interventions, 172–73
    universal health coverage, 47
    vaccines and vaccinations, 173
    value per statistical life (VSL) in,
        174–77, 175–78*f*, 176*t*
Bertozzi, Stefano, 3
Bhadelia, Afsan, 235
Bhutta, Zulfiqar, 3
Bill & Melinda Gates Foundation, 178–79, 300–301
Binagwaho, Agnes, 3
birth control. *See* family planning
Bishai, David, 267
Black, Robert, 3
Blecher, Mark, 3
Bloom, Barry R., 3
body mass index (BMI)
    fiscal policy and, 366
    intersectoral policies on, 24
Brazil
    development assistance in, 301
    fiscal policy in, 359, 363
    pandemics in, 335–36
    pathology services in, 227
    rehabilitation services in, 287–88
breast cancer
    cost-effectiveness analysis for
        interventions, 150–51
    mortality rates, 96

    pathology services and, 221
    quality of care, 202
Broughton, Edward, 185
Brouwer, Elizabeth, 3
Bundy, Donald A. P., 3
burden of disease, 121–43
    cancer, 122, 126–28, 130, 132–33, 135
    cardiovascular disease, 122, 126–27, 130–35
    catastrophic and impoverishing health
        expenditures, 122–24, 126, 129–30
        defined, 122–23, 122*f*
        future research needs, 138
        indicators, 123, 123–24*t*
        measures of, 130–33, 131–35*f*
        policy recommendations, 137–38
        population-level estimates, 122–26
        prevalence, 126–28*t*, 126–30, 127*m*,
            129–30*f*, 130*t*
        relationship between, 123*b*
        universal health coverage and, 124–25*b*
    chronic diseases and chronic ill health,
        121–33, 135, 136–39
    chronic obstructive pulmonary
        disease (COPD), 126, 128
    communicable diseases, 126
    consequences of illness or injury, 32
    cost-effectiveness of interventions and, 3
    development assistance and, 305, 308
    distressed financing and, 133, 135*f*
    families and, 133–35
    financial risk protection (FRP) and, 121, 136–37
    heart disease, 126, 128
    HIV/AIDS, 122, 125–26, 128, 134–35
    influenza pandemic, 322–23, 325, 326, 347–48,
        352–53, 353*t*
    kidney diseases, 126, 128
    malaria, 126, 128, 134
    mental illnesses, 126, 128–29
    pandemics, 321–23, 322*f*, 322*t*, 325, 326, 347–48,
        352–53, 353*t*
    productivity changes, 132–33, 134*f*
    treatment discontinuation and, 133
    tuberculosis, 126, 134
    universal health coverage and, 46, 49, 121–25, 137
Burkina Faso, mortality rates in, 101, 114
Burundi, quality of care in, 194

C

Cambodia
    emergency care in, 250
    mortality rates in, 109, 115
    pandemics in, 336
    pathology services in, 218

Canada
    community health platforms in, 267
    development assistance from, 302, 302*f*
    pandemics in, 317–18, 335
    pathology services in, 227
cancer. *See also specific types*
    benefit-cost analysis for interventions, 179
    burden of disease in, 122, 126–28, 130,
        132–33, 135
    cost-effectiveness analysis for interventions,
        147, 150–51
    development assistance and, 302
    fiscal policy and, 360–61
    intersectoral policies on, 25
    mortality rates, 70–72, 74, 96, 98, 100
    palliative care and pain control, 240
    pathology services and, 215–16, 221, 225
    quality of care, 196–97, 202
    universal health coverage and, 51, 53
Canudas-Romo, V., 98
capacity
    burden of disease and, 121, 123, 126, 129
    community health platforms and, 279–80
    development assistance and, 304
    emergency care and, 252, 254–56, 261
    extended cost-effectiveness analysis and, 159
    pandemics and, 316–17, 320, 330–31, 338
    pathology services and, 217, 219–20
    rehabilitation services and, 286–87
    universal health coverage, 12, 14, 46, 58, 60, 62
cardiovascular disease
    burden of disease, 122, 126–27, 130–35
    cost-effectiveness analysis for
        interventions, 149–52
    development assistance and, 302–3
    extended cost-effectiveness analysis for
        interventions, 162
    mortality rates, 74, 98
    palliative care and pain control, 236–37
    pathology services and, 215
    quality of care, 193
catastrophic and impoverishing health expenditures
    burden of disease, 122–24, 126, 129–30
    defined, 122–23, 122*f*
    future research needs, 138
    indicators, 123, 123–24*t*
    measures of, 130–33, 131–35*f*
    policy recommendations, 137–38
    population-level estimates, 122–26
    prevalence, 126–28*t*, 126–30, 127*m*, 129–30*f*, 130*t*
    relationship between, 123*b*
    universal health coverage and, 124–25*b*
CCTs. *See* conditional cash transfer

CEA. *See* cost-effectiveness analysis
CEPI (Coalition for Epidemic Preparedness
        Innovations), 330, 335
Chang, Angela Y., 167
child health and mortality
    benefit-cost analysis for interventions,
        167, 179, 181
    community health platforms and, 273, 275
    cost-effectiveness analysis for
        interventions, 149, 153
    development assistance and, 300, 302,
        304, 305, 307–8
    intersectoral policies on, 27
    trends, 69–70, 72, 99–101, 106–7, 109–10, 110*t*,
        114–17, 117*f*
    universal health coverage and, 47, 48, 49,
        51, 53, 55, 56
Chile
    life expectancy in, 6
    mortality rates in, 106
China
    benefit-cost analysis in, 169, 179–80
    burden of disease in, 125, 127, 132–35
    development assistance from, 301, 304–5, 307
    emergency care in, 251
    extended cost-effectiveness analysis in, 162
    fiscal policy in, 359
    household coal use in, 29*b*
    influenza pandemic in, 355
    mortality rates in, 72, 116–17
    noncommunicable diseases in, 3
    pandemics in, 318–21, 325, 329, 335–36, 355
    pathology services in, 218, 226–28
    quality of care in, 190
    tobacco taxation in, 9–10
Chisholm, Dan, 3
Chongsuvivatwong, V., 132
chronic diseases and chronic ill health. *See also*
        specific diseases
    benefit-cost analysis for interventions, 180
    burden of disease, 121–33, 135, 136–39
    quality of care, 190, 204
chronic obstructive pulmonary disease (COPD)
    burden of disease, 126, 128
    emergency care, 261
    fiscal policy and, 361
    intersectoral policies on, 25
    mortality rates, 96–98
    palliative care and pain control, 236
Chu, Annie, 121
Cieza, Alarcos, 3, 285
cigarettes. *See* tobacco use
Cleary, James F., 235

immunizations. *See* vaccines and vaccinations
impoverishing health expenditures. *See* catastrophic
     and impoverishing health expenditures
incremental cost-effectiveness ratio (ICER),
     47, 159, 161, 337
incremental costs
    emergency care, 262
    quality of care, 205
    universal health coverage, 12–14, 50, 55
India
    benefit-cost analysis in, 169–70, 179–81
    burden of disease in, 127–28, 132–35
    development assistance in, 301, 304
    extended cost-effectiveness analysis in,
       158, 160–62
    fiscal policy in
       analytic framework, 361–62, 362–63*t*
       role of, 360–61, 360–61*t*
       subsidies, 364*t*, 366–67
       taxation, 364–66, 364*t*
    intersectoral policies in, 26
    Million Death Study, 61*b*
    mortality rates in, 71–72, 116–17
    pandemics in, 319, 325, 336, 349
    pathology services in, 218, 226–28, 230–31
    quality of care in, 186, 190–91, 202
    subsidies in, 364*t*, 366–67
    taxation in, 364–66, 364*t*
    tobacco use in, 26
    universal health coverage in, 61
Indonesia
    community health platforms in, 268, 273–75, 275*f*
    pandemics in, 336
    pathology services in, 227
infectious diseases. *See* communicable diseases
influenza pandemic, 347–58
    burden of disease, 322–23, 325, 326, 347–48,
       352–53, 353*t*
    cost-effectiveness of interventions, 335–37
    economic burden, 347
    mitigation of, 327, 329, 331, 335
    mortality rates, 316, 322, 323, 349*t*, 354
    risk of, 315–17, 348–49, 350–51*b*
    severity of, 348–49, 350–51*b*
    study methodology, 349–52, 352*t*
injuries
    catastrophic health expenditures and, 126, 128
    head injuries, 34–35*b*
    mortality rates, 69–70, 73, 98, 101
    rehabilitation services, 286
    road traffic, 12
Institute of Health Metrics and Evaluation (IHME), 70,
    72, 101, 106, 116, 300–305, 359, 364–65

Institute of Medicine, 200
insurance. *See also* universal health coverage
    access to health care and, 8
    extended cost-effectiveness analysis and, 159–62
    pandemics and, 333
    pathology services and, 228
intensive care unit (ICU), 190, 249–50, 327, 334
Intergovernmental Panel on Climate Change (IPCC),
    353–54
International Association for Trauma Surgery and
    Intensive Care, 199
International Classification of Diseases (ICD),
    70–71, 235
International Decision Support Initiative, 61–62
International Monetary Fund, 12
International Standards for Tuberculosis Care, 186
intersectoral policies and interventions, 11–12
    accountability and, 37
    cancer and, 25
    consequences of illness or injury addressed by,
       31–32, 34
    distal determinants of health and, 26–27, 26*t*
    essential packages and, 27–31, 28–29*t*, 29–30*b*, 37
    financial risk protection (FRP) and, 37
    health conditions and risk factors amenable to,
       24–27, 25*f*
    implementation of, 34–37
    life expectancy and, 26, 31
    priorities for, 23–42
    subsidy-related strategies, 37
    Sustainable Development Goals and, 37
    taxation-based strategies, 36–37
    universal health coverage and, 46
interventions. *See also* intersectoral policies and
    interventions; *specific interventions*
    barriers to uptake, 58
    benefit-cost analysis and, 167–68, 178. *See also*
       benefit-cost analysis
    cost, 16–17*t*, 16–18
    cost-effectiveness analysis, 147–48. *See also* cost-
       effectiveness analysis
    extended cost-effectiveness analysis, 158. *See also*
       extended cost-effectiveness analysis
    nutrition interventions, 152, 170
    pandemics and, 316
    rehabilitation services, 288
    universal health coverage and, 44, 49
IPCC (Intergovernmental Panel on Climate Change),
    353–54
Iran
    burden of disease in, 128
    intersectoral policies in, 34
    mortality rates in, 115

Ntizimira, Christian, 235
Nugent, Rachel, 3, 11, 23, 105, 299
nutrition interventions, 152, 170

O

obstetric care, 149, 151, 153, 251, 262
OECD countries
    benefit-cost analysis in, 175
    development assistance from, 301
official development assistance. *See* development
    assistance
Ogbuoji, Osondu, 105
Olson, Zachary, 3, 105
Omokhodion, Folashade, 3
Oppenheim, Ben, 3, 315
Ord, Toby, 3
Osman, Hibah, 235
Ottersen, Trygve, 299

P

packages. *See* essential packages of care
Padian, Nancy, 299
PAHO (Pan American Health Organization),
    269, 280
palliative care and pain control, 235–46
    access to, 238
    cancer, 240
    cardiovascular disease, 236–37
    chronic obstructive pulmonary disease
        (COPD), 236
    cost, 241–43, 242*t*
    cost-effectiveness analysis, 10–11
    equipment, 240
    essential package for, 235–36, 238–43, 239*t*
    extended cost-effectiveness analysis, 162
    families and, 236, 238, 240–43
    financial risk protection (FRP) and, 236, 243
    heart disease, 236–37
    heart failure, 236
    HIV/AIDS, 236–38
    hospitals and, 239–41
    human resources, 241
    intersectoral policies and, 31–32
    medicines, 239–40, 242–43
    need for, 236–38, 237*t*
    platforms for delivery, 235, 240, 242
    psychological and spiritual counseling, 240
    social supports, 240–41
    tuberculosis, 237
    universal health coverage and, 47–48, 54, 59
Pan American Health Organization
    (PAHO), 269, 280
Pandemic Influenza Preparedness (PIP), 336–37

pandemics, 315–46. *See also specific diseases*
    access to health care and, 354
    accountability and, 338
    benefit-cost analysis for interventions, 168, 171
    burden of, 321–23, 322*f*, 322*t*
    consequences of, 323–25
    cost-effectiveness analysis for interventions, 149
    development assistance and, 305, 310
    economic impacts of, 324–25
    health impacts of, 323–24
    intervention costs and cost-effectiveness,
        334–37*f*, 334–38
    investment priorities, 338–39
    knowledge gaps, 316
    mitigation, 316, 326–34, 326*b*
    pathology services and, 218
    patient care and treatment protocols, 330–31
    preparedness for, 7, 11, 316, 320*m*, 321*t*, 326–27,
        331–34, 336, 338, 340, 345, 355
    reducing spread of, 329–30
    risk communications and, 328–29
    risks, 316, 317–19*t*, 317–23, 320*m*, 338, 341,
        348, 351–55
    risk transfer mechanisms, 332–33, 333*f*
    situational awareness and, 327, 328*b*
    social and political impacts of, 325
    universal health coverage and, 51, 53, 61
    vaccines and, 330*b*, 331, 331*t*
Patel, Vikram, 3
pathology services, 8, 11, 215–34
    accountability and, 226–27
    accreditation, 225–27, 227*b*
    breast cancer and, 221
    cancer and, 215–16, 221, 225
    cardiovascular disease and, 215
    challenges in LMICs, 217–18
    communicable diseases and, 215, 218, 221
    continuing education, 222–24
    costs, 228–29
    data handling, 225
    economics of, 228–31*t*, 228–32
    education, 222–24
    emerging diseases and, 216, 219, 221, 225
    emerging technologies, 224–25, 224*b*
    essential package for, 215, 217, 219–32,
        220–21*t*, 220*b*
    financial risk protection (FRP) and, 219
    HIV/AIDS and, 215, 218–19, 225
    leadership and, 222–23
    maternal mortality and, 218
    misdiagnosis issues, 202, 202*b*
    neglected tropical diseases (NTDs) and, 218
    platforms for delivery, 224–25

point-of-care testing, 225
quality management, 202, 202b, 225–27, 226b
reimbursement policies, 227–28
services, 216–17, 217b, 217t, 221–22, 227–28
staffing inadequacies, 218
Sustainable Development Goals and, 218, 218–19t
training, 222–24
universal health coverage and, 52, 54
Patton, George C., 3
pay for performance (P4P), 193–94, 193b
Peabody, John, 3, 185
Peilong, Liu, 299
PEPFAR (President's Emergency Plan for
AIDS Relief), 305–7
Perez-Cruz, Pedro, 235
Peru
community health platforms in, 272, 276–77
mortality rates in, 109
pesticides, 30b
pharmaceutical drugs. See drugs
Philippines
benefit-cost analysis in, 169
burden of disease in, 124–25
mortality rates in, 114
quality of care in, 191–93, 202
physical inactivity, 24–26
PIP (Pandemic Influenza Preparedness), 336–37
platforms
community health platforms, 267–84. See also
community health platforms
defined, 7
development assistance and, 306, 308
intersectoral policies and, 4–5
palliative care and pain control, 235, 240, 242
pathology services, 224–25
quality of care, 189, 194, 199, 203
rehabilitation services, 289–91
universal health coverage and, 13–14, 45–46, 62
pneumonia
development assistance and, 305
emergency care, 249–50, 252, 254, 261–62
mortality rates, 98
pandemics and, 316, 322–23
quality of care, 196
policy interventions
benefit-cost analysis, 168, 178, 181
catastrophic and impoverishing health
expenditures, 137–38
development assistance and, 307
extended cost-effectiveness analysis, 157–61
fiscal policy, 359–68. See also fiscal policy
intersectoral policies, 24, 27–28. See also
intersectoral policies and interventions

pathology services and, 216
quality of care and, 186, 187–88, 194,
195–98t, 199, 205
population aging. See aging population
Prabhakaran, Dorairaj, 3
pregnancy. See maternal mortality; obstetric care
President's Emergency Plan for AIDS Relief
(PEPFAR), 305–7
Preston, S. H., 98
Price, Christopher P., 215
primary care
community health platforms and, 267,
273, 276–77
cost-effectiveness analysis, 150–51
quality of care and, 191
Progresa/Oportunidades (Mexico), 192b

Q
QALYs (quality-adjusted life years), 10
benefit-cost analysis and, 167
cost-effectiveness analysis and, 148, 150–52, 154
emergency care and, 262
rehabilitation services and, 288
universal health coverage and, 47–48
value of, 6
Qi, Jinyuan, 3, 43, 50, 105
Quality Improvement Demonstration Study (QIDS),
192–93, 193b
quality of care, 185–214
access to health care and, 199
accountability and, 187, 191, 194–95, 201, 203–4
affordability, 201
assessment challenges, 201–3
breast cancer, 202
cancer, 196–97, 202
cardiovascular disease, 193
chronic diseases and chronic ill health, 190, 204
conditional cash transfers (CCTs) and, 192–93
costs of improving, 204–5
effectiveness of interventions, 201
equity, 201–2
essential package for, 58–59
family planning and, 195, 199
financial risk protection (FRP) and, 204
framework for, 199–201, 199f, 200t
health care facilities and, 185, 191, 201
heart failure, 197
HIV/AIDS, 196, 198
hospitals and, 185, 190–92, 194–202, 204
incentives, 192–93
infrastructure requirements, 187–94, 195–98t
malaria, 198
measurement of, 187–90, 188t

misdiagnosis and, 202, 202*b*

morbidity and, 199–200, 202

patient focus, 201

perceptions of quality, 202–3

performance-based financing, 193–94, 193*b*, 194*f*

platforms for delivery, 189, 194, 199, 203

pneumonia, 196

policy interventions and, 186, 187–88, 194, 195–98*t*, 199, 205

primary care and, 191

safety and efficacy, 200–201

severe acute respiratory syndrome (SARS), 196, 198

standards, 190–91

supervision, 192

syphilis, 195

timeliness, 201

training, 191–92

tuberculosis, 196

universal health coverage and, 58–59, 201, 203

vaccinations and, 192, 196–98

variations in, 186–87

R

Radbruch, Lukas, 235

Rajagopal, M. R., 235

RBF (results-based financing), 59, 193–94

rehabilitation services, 285–95

    access to, 286–87

    cost-effectiveness, 287–88

    demand for, 286–87

    essential package, 288–92, 289–91*t*

    heart failure, 288

    hospitals and, 285–88, 290–92

    planning tools, 292

    platforms for delivery, 289–91

    policy priorities, 293

    universal health coverage and, 43

renal diseases

    burden of disease, 122, 126, 128–32, 134, 136–37

    pathology services and, 221

Republic of Korea

    burden of disease in, 127–28

    fiscal policy in, 363

    pandemics in, 318

respiratory diseases, 122, 126–30

results-based financing (RBF), 59, 193–94

Reynolds, Teri, 3, 247, 285

risk factors

    burden of disease and, 137

    community health platforms and, 269

    conceptual model for interactions among, 24–25, 25*f*

financial risk, 8–11, 121, 124

fiscal policy and, 360–62

influenza pandemic, 315–17, 348–49, 350–51*b*

intersectoral policies and, 24–27

mortality rates and, 115

pandemics, 315–17, 317–19*t*, 317–23, 320*m*, 338, 341, 348–49, 350–51*b*, 351–55

quality of care and, 191

risk reduction

    benefit-cost analysis and, 175, 177

    emergency care and, 252

    pathology services and, 219

risk transfer mechanisms, 332–33, 333*f*

Rodriguez, Natalia M., 235

rotavirus

    burden of disease, 128

    cost-effectiveness analysis for interventions, 151–52

Rottingen, John-Arne, 299

Ru, Kun, 215

Ruacan, Sevket, 3

Rubiano, Andrés M., 247

Rubin, Edward, 315

Russian Federation, fiscal policy in, 359

Rwanda

    emergency care in, 251

    mortality rates in, 109, 114–15

    palliative care and pain control in, 236, 242, 242*t*

    quality of care in, 194

S

Sample Registration System (SRS), 61, 71

Sanderson, W. C., 175

Sankaranarayanan, Rengaswamy, 3

SARA (Service Availability and Readiness Assessment), 194

SARS. *See* severe acute respiratory syndrome

Saudi Arabia, development assistance in, 301

Sawe, Hendry, 247

Saxenian, Helen, 23

Schäferhoff, Marco, 299

Scherbov, S., 175

SDGs. *See* Sustainable Development Goals

Sen, A., 8

Sepúlveda, Jaime, 3

Service Availability and Readiness Assessment (SARA), 194

severe acute respiratory syndrome (SARS)

    development assistance and, 307

    impact of, 315

    mitigation of, 329–30, 355

    quality of care, 196, 198

    risks of, 318

Sherry, Melissa, 267

Temmerman, Marleen, 3
Thailand
    benefit-cost analysis in, 181
    burden of disease in, 129
    development assistance in, 301
    intersectoral policies in, 35
    pathology services in, 226–27, 230–31
Timor-Leste, rehabilitation services in, 286
tobacco use
    benefit-cost analysis for interventions, 173
    community health platforms and, 269
    cost-effectiveness analysis for interventions, 150
    extended cost-effectiveness analysis for
        interventions, 162
    fiscal policy and, 360–65
    intersectoral policies and, 11–12, 23–24, 28, 31, 36
    taxation of, 9–10, 27, 173, 364–65, 364t
    universal health coverage and, 56
Tobago, pandemics in, 321
Tollman, Stephen, 3
Trans-Pacific Partnership Agreement, 227
tuberculosis
    benefit-cost analysis for interventions, 172–73
    burden of disease, 126, 134
    cost-effectiveness analysis for interventions,
        149–51, 153
    development assistance and, 302, 304
    diagnostic tool subsidies, 367
    emergency care, 252
    extended cost-effectiveness analysis for
        interventions, 158, 160–62
    fiscal policy and, 361–64, 366–67
    mortality rates, 56, 70–72, 105–9, 111,
        112t, 113–18
    palliative care and pain control, 237
    pandemics and, 323, 326, 354
    pathology services and, 215, 218, 220, 225
    quality of care, 196
    universal health coverage and, 48–49, 51,
        53, 56–57, 59
Tunisia, fiscal policy in, 363
Turkmenistan, mortality rates in, 114

U
Uganda
    community health platforms in, 277–78
    palliative care and pain control in, 238
    pathology services in, 218
UHC. *See* universal health coverage
UMICs. *See* upper-middle-income countries
UNAIDS, 70, 72, 100, 115
under-five mortality rates. *See* child health and
    mortality

United Arab Emirates, development
        assistance from, 301
United Kingdom
    household coal use in, 29b
    intersectoral policies in, 26
    pandemics in, 317, 324, 334–36
    pathology services in, 215, 218, 226–27, 229, 231
    rehabilitation services in, 288
    tobacco use in, 26
United Nations Children's Fund, 106, 267
United Nations Population Division, 14, 181, 351
United States
    benefit-cost analysis in, 167, 171, 173–76
    burden of disease in, 127–28
    community health platforms in, 267
    development assistance from, 301, 302, 302f, 305
    extended cost-effectiveness analysis in, 157
    influenza pandemic in, 350–51, 354–55
    intersectoral policies in, 23, 26, 31
    mortality rates in, 105, 116
    palliative care and pain control in, 235–36
    pandemics in, 315, 317, 319, 334–36, 350–51, 354–55
    pathology services in, 215–16, 218, 226–27, 229–31
    quality of care in, 185–86, 193, 201
    tobacco use in, 26
    universal health coverage in, 43
universal health coverage (UHC), 43–65
    access to health care and, 43–44, 59
    barriers to intervention uptake, 58
    burden of disease and, 46, 49, 121–25, 137
    cancer and, 51, 53
    catastrophic health expenditures and, 124–25b
    child health and mortality and, 47, 48, 49,
        51, 53, 55, 56
    communicable diseases and, 48, 51, 53, 56
    conditional cash transfers (CCTs) and, 59
    cost-effectiveness analysis, 44–45, 47–48, 58, 60, 147
    costs and, 12–14, 13–14t, 49–55, 51–55t
    development of, 45
    emergency care and, 247, 252, 261
    essential, 12–16, 12f
    extended cost-effectiveness analysis and, 44, 158
    family planning and, 46–47
    financial risk protection (FRP) and, 43–44, 47–48
    financing, 60
    fiscal policy and, 359
    governance and, 59–60
    health outcomes and, 56, 57t
    health workforce and, 60
    HIV/AIDS and, 48–51, 53–54, 56–60, 62
    hospitals and, 13–14, 45–46, 55
    identification of highest-priority package, 45–49
    implementation, 56–62, 59t, 61b

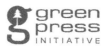